现代内科学学习指南

Current Medical Diagnosis and Treatment Study Guide, 2nd Edition

第2版·英文版

Gene R. Quinn, MD, MS
Division of Cardiovascular Disease
Department of Medicine
Beth Israel Deaconess Medical Center
Boston
Nathaniel W. Gleason, MD
Maxine A. Papadakis, MD
Stephen J. McPhee, MD
Department of Medicine
University of California
San Francisco

北京联合出版公司
Beijing United Publishing Co.,Ltd.

图书在版编目（CIP）数据

现代内科学学习指南：第2版：英文 /（美）奎恩,（美）格利森,（美）帕帕扎基斯著. — 北京：北京联合出版公司,2017.1
ISBN 978-7-5502-9363-2

Ⅰ.①现… Ⅱ.①奎… ②格… ③帕… Ⅲ.①内科学 —英文 Ⅳ.①R5

中国版本图书馆CIP数据核字(2016)第287730号

Gene R. Quinn,Nathaniel W. Gleason,Maxine A. Papadakis,Stephen J. McPhee
Current Medical Diagnosis and Treatment Study Guide,Second Edition
ISBN 978-0-07-184805-3

北京市版权局著作权合同登记号：01-2016-8869

现代内科学学习指南（第 2 版）

著　　者：Gene R. Quinn 等
选题策划：后浪出版公司
出版统筹：吴兴元
特约编辑：张忠丽
责任编辑：李　伟
营销推广：ONEBOOK
装帧制造：墨白空间·李　渔

北京联合出版公司出版
（北京市西城区德外大街 83 号楼 9 层　100088）
北京盛通印刷股份有限公司印刷　新华书店经销
字数1030千字　889毫米×1194毫米　1/16　36印张
2017 年 3 月第 1 版　2017 年 3 月第 1 次印刷
ISBN 978-7-5502-9363-2
定价：238.00 元

Contents

Preface

Purpose

Current Medical Diagnosis and Treatment (CMDT) is the leading internal medicine textbook known for its comprehensive coverage of current inpatient and outpatient care with diagnostic tools relevant to day-to-day practice. Facilitating its usefulness, this *CMDT Study Guide*, second edition, directs readers through a case analysis of 80 of the most common topics in internal medicine. The *CMDT Study Guide* provides a comprehensive and clearly organized synopsis of each medical topic that helps the reader review and study for a variety of examinations, such as the medicine clerkship shelf exam, USMLE Step 2 examinations, ABIM internal medicine boards, and recertification examinations. As such it will be very useful to medical, nursing (Adult and Family Nurse Practitioner Certification Exam), pharmacy, and other health professional students, Physician Assistant National Certifying Exam (PANCE), to house officers, and to practicing physicians. The *CMDT Study Guide* is engaging and patient-centered since each of the 80 topics begins with presentation of a typical patient to help the reader think in a step-wise fashion through the various clinical problem-solving aspects of the case. For each topic, the *CMDT Study Guide* provides PubMed's references to the most current and pertinent MEDLINE articles for that topic. Each reference provides PMID numbers to facilitate retrieval of the relevant articles.

Outstanding Features

- Eighty common internal medicine topics useful to learners and practitioners for patient care and to prepare for examinations
- Material drawn from the expert source, *Current Medical Diagnosis and Treatment 2016*, including tables about laboratory tests and treatments
- In-depth, consistent, and readable format organized in a way that allows for quick study and easy access to information
- Emphasis on a standard approach to clinical problem-solving with Learning Objectives, Salient Features, Symptoms and Signs, Treatment, Outcomes, When to Refer and When to Admit, and References

- Medical and nursing students, physician's assistants, nurse practitioners, house officers, and practicing physicians will find the clear organization and current literature references useful in devising proper management for patients with these conditions

Organization

The *CMDT Study Guide* provides comprehensive yet succinct information. Each *CMDT Study Guide* topic begins with a patient presentation, followed by Learning Objectives and 9 Questions to help the learner work through the topic in the context of the patient presented. Answers to the 9 questions are organized as Salient Features, How to Think Through the Problem, Key Features (which contain Essentials of Diagnosis, General Considerations, and Demographics), Symptoms and Signs, Differential Diagnosis, Laboratory, Imaging, and Procedural Findings, Treatments, Outcomes, and When to Refer and When to Admit. References are then provided that contain current literature citations complete with PubMed (PMID) numbers. The *CMDT Study Guide* is a complete source of patient care information for these 80 most common clinical problems! The 80 topics in the *CMDT Study Guide* were selected as the core topics for the learner because of their importance to the field of internal medicine.

The *CMDT Study Guide* follows the organization of *Quick Medical Diagnosis and Treatment (QMDT)* (or *Quick Dx & Rx* at www.accessmedicinemhmedical. com) and the *QMDT* App, and is divided into 11 sections:
- Skin Disorders
- Pulmonary/Ear, Nose, & Throat Disorders
- Heart/Hypertension/Lipid Disorders
- Hematologic Disorders
- Gastrointestinal/Liver/Pancreas Disorders
- Gynecologic/Urologic Disorders
- Musculoskeletal Disorders
- Kidney/Electrolyte Disorders
- Nervous System/Psychiatric Disorders
- Endocrine/Metabolic Disorders
- Infectious Disorders

Intended Audience

Medical students on their internal medicine clerkship will find this *Study Guide* a useful aid as they care for patients with these common medical problems. The *Study Guide* will assist medical students, PA students, and NP students taking their internal medicine rotation and house officers to review the core topics as they prepare for standardized examinations. Practicing physicians, physician assistants and nurse practitioners will similarly find the *CMDT Study Guide* useful in order to stay current in clinical problem-solving, while providing a concise summary of relevant diagnostic laboratory, microbiologic, and imaging studies and treatments, and recent relevant publications.

Acknowledgments

We thank our *Current Medical Diagnosis and Treatment* authors for their contributions to it and we are grateful to the many students, residents, and practitioners who have made useful suggestions to this book. We hope that you will share with us your comments about the *CMDT Study Guide*.

Gene R. Quinn, MD, MS
Nathaniel W. Gleason, MD
Maxine A. Papadakis, MD
Stephen J. McPhee, MD

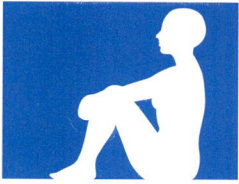

Skin Disorders

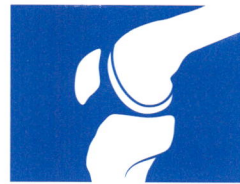

Musculoskeletal Disorders

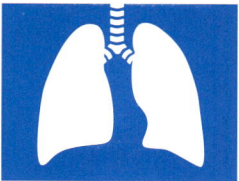

Pulmonary/Ear, Nose and Throat Disorders

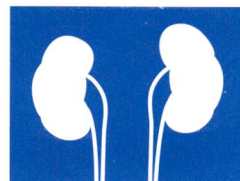

Kidney/Electrolyte Disorders

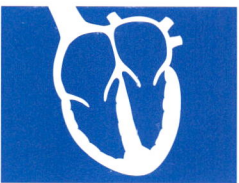

Heart/ Hypertension/ Lipid Disorders

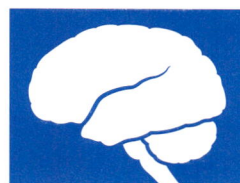

Nervous System/ Psychiatric Disorders

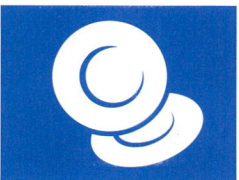

Hematologic Disorders

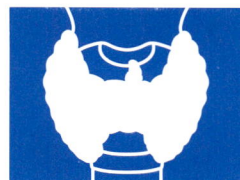

Endocrine/ Metabolic Disorders

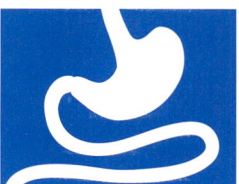

Gastrointestinal/ Liver/Pancreas Disorders

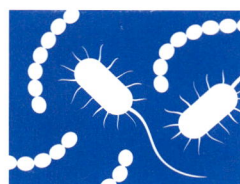

Infectious Disorders

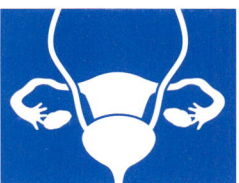

Gynecologic/ Urologic Disorders

Skin Disorders

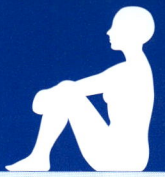

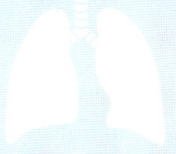

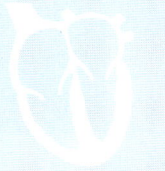

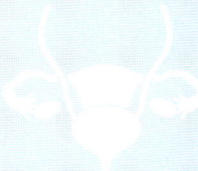

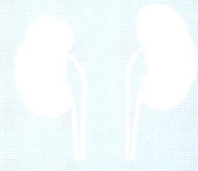

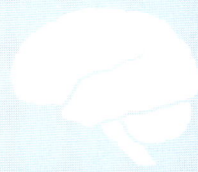

1

Atopic Dermatitis

A 30-year-old woman presents to her primary care clinician with an itchy rash on her hands, wrists, and arms. She states she has had similar rashes before, which had gone away with over-the-counter hydrocortisone cream, the first episode occurring when she was very young. Her past medical history includes asthma. She takes loratadine occasionally for allergic rhinitis. Physical examination reveals plaques on the hands, wrists, and antecubital folds, which are mildly exudative and without scale. Laboratory testing shows eosinophilia on a complete blood count with differential and an elevated serum immunoglobulin E (IgE) level.

LEARNING OBJECTIVES

▶ Learn the clinical manifestations and objective findings of atopic dermatitis, and the findings that distinguish it from other skin conditions
▶ Understand the associated diseases that predispose to atopic dermatitis
▶ Know the differential diagnosis of atopic dermatitis
▶ Learn the treatments for each clinical pattern of atopic dermatitis
▶ Know which patients are likely to have recurrent atopic dermatitis and how to prevent flares

QUESTIONS

1. What are the salient features of this patient's problem?
2. How do you think through her problem?
3. What are the key features, including essentials of diagnosis and general considerations, of atopic dermatitis?
4. What are the symptoms and signs of atopic dermatitis?
5. What is the differential diagnosis of atopic dermatitis?
6. What are the laboratory findings in atopic dermatitis?
7. What are the treatments for atopic dermatitis?
8. What are the outcomes, including complications, prognosis, and prevention, of atopic dermatitis?
9. When should patients with atopic dermatitis be referred to a specialist?

ANSWERS

1. Salient Features

Pruritic rash in distribution of hands, wrists, antecubital folds; similar symptoms starting in childhood; personal history of atopic conditions (asthma, allergic rhinitis); plaques with exudates and without scale; eosinophilia; and elevated serum IgE levels

2. How to Think Through

It is important to think broadly about possible causes of rash in this patient, despite her strong atopic history. Might this be seborrheic dermatitis? (Seborrheic dermatitis typically looks like greasy, scaly lesions on the central face and scalp.) A fungal infection? (Prior similar manifestations have resolved with topical corticosteroid treatment, making this unlikely.) Psoriasis? (The distribution and absence of silvery scale makes this unlikely.) Contact dermatitis? (This is a reasonable consideration. Contact dermatitis can be indistinguishable from atopic dermatitis, and in this case, the rash is similarly confined to exposed areas of the body.) What would raise your suspicion for contact dermatitis? (A history of new potential allergen or irritant exposure.)

After considering the above, a diagnosis of atopic dermatitis is most likely, given the prior atopy (asthma and allergic rhinitis), the recurrence of similar symptoms since childhood, the eosinophilia, and elevated IgE. How should she be treated? (Mid-potency topical corticosteroids twice daily with subsequent tapering to low-potency corticosteroids, and with emollient applied frequently. This patient's presentation is unlikely to require oral corticosteroid treatment. An oral antihistamine for itching may be helpful.) How would you counsel this patient to prevent future flares? (Avoid excessive bathing and hand washing. Use mild soaps. Apply emollient after washing. Trim fingernails and wrap affected areas at night to prevent scratching.)

3. Key Features

Essentials of Diagnosis

- Pruritic, exudative, or lichenified eruption on face, neck, upper trunk, wrists, hands, and antecubital and popliteal folds
- Personal or family history of allergies or asthma
- Tendency to recur
- Onset in childhood in most patients; onset after age 30 is very uncommon

General Considerations

- Also known as eczema
- Looks different at different ages and in people of different races
- Diagnostic criteria include
  — Pruritus
  — Typical morphology and distribution (flexural lichenification, hand eczema, nipple eczema, and eyelid eczema in adults)
  — Onset in childhood
  — Chronicity
- Also diagnostically helpful are
  — Personal history of asthma or allergic rhinitis
  — Family history of atopic disease (asthma, allergic rhinitis, atopic dermatitis)
  — Xerosis ichthyosis
  — Facial pallor with infraorbital darkening
  — Elevated serum IgE
  — Repeated skin infections

4. Symptoms and Signs

- Itching may be severe and prolonged
- Rough, red plaques usually without the thick scale and discrete demarcation of psoriasis affect the face, neck, and upper trunk; may be pruritic or exudative
- Flexural surfaces of elbows and knees are often involved
- In chronic cases, the skin is dry, leathery, and lichenified
- In black patients with severe disease, pigmentation may be lost in lichenified areas
- During acute flares, widespread redness with weeping, either diffusely or in discrete plaques

5. Differential Diagnosis

- Seborrheic dermatitis
- Impetigo
- Secondary staphylococcal infections
- Psoriasis
- Lichen simplex chronicus (circumscribed neurodermatitis)

6. Laboratory Findings

Laboratory Tests

- Eosinophilia and increased serum IgE levels may be present

7. Treatments

Medications

Local Treatments

- Corticosteroids
  — For treatment of lesions on the body (excluding genitalia, axillary or crural folds), begin with triamcinolone 0.1% ointment or a stronger corticosteroid, then taper to hydrocortisone 1% ointment or another slightly stronger mild corticosteroid (alclometasone 0.05% or desonide 0.05% ointment)
  — Apply sparingly once or twice daily
  — Taper off corticosteroids and substitute emollients as the dermatitis clears to avoid the side effects of corticosteroids and rebound
- Tacrolimus and pimecrolimus
  — Do not appear to cause corticosteroid side effects
  — Safe on the face and eyelids
  — Use sparingly and for as brief a time as possible
  — Avoid in patients at high risk for lymphoma (ie, those with HIV, iatrogenic immuno-suppression, prior lymphoma)
  — Tacrolimus 0.03% and 0.1% ointment applied twice daily
    ○ Effective as a first-line steroid-sparing agent
    ○ Burning on application occurs in about half but may resolve with continued treatment
  — Pimecrolimus 1% cream applied twice daily is similar but burns less

Systemic and Adjuvant Therapies

- Prednisone
  — Start at 40 to 60 mg orally daily
  — Taper to nil over 2 to 4 weeks
  — Use as long-term maintenance therapy is not recommended
- Bedtime doses of hydroxyzine, diphenhydramine, or doxepin may be helpful via their sedative properties in reducing perceived pruritus

- Antistaphylococcal antibiotics
  — Should only be used if indicated by bacterial culture
  — First-generation cephalosporins may be helpful
  — Doxycycline, if methicillin-resistant *Staphylococcus aureus* is suspected
- Phototherapy
- Oral cyclosporine, mycophenolate mofetil, methotrexate, interferon gamma, dupilumab, or azathioprine may be used for the most severe and recalcitrant cases

Treatment by Pattern and Stage of Dermatitis
- Acute weeping lesions
  — Staphylococcal or herpetic superinfection should be excluded
  — Use saline or aluminum subacetate solution (Domeboro tablets) or colloidal oatmeal (Aveeno) as soothing or wet dressings or astringent soaks for 10 to 30 minutes two to four times a day
- Lesions on the extremities may be bandaged for protection at night
  — Use high-potency corticosteroids after soaking but spare the face and body folds
  — Tacrolimus may not be tolerated; systemic corticosteroids are last resort
- Subacute or scaly lesions (lesions are dry but still red and pruritic)
  — Mid- to high-potency corticosteroids
    › In ointment form if tolerated—creams, if not
    › Should be continued until scaling and elevated skin lesions are cleared and itching is decreased
    › Then, begin a 2- to 4-week taper with topical corticosteroids
- Chronic, dry lichenified lesions (thickened and usually well demarcated)
  — High-potency to ultrahigh-potency corticosteroid ointments
  — Nightly occlusion for 2 to 6 weeks may enhance the initial response
  — Occasionally, adding tar preparations such as liquor carbonis detergens 10% in Aquaphor or 2% crude coal tar may be beneficial
- Maintenance treatment
  — Constant application of effective moisturizers is recommended to prevent flares
  — In patients with moderate disease, topical anti-inflammatory agents can be used on weekends only or three times weekly to prevent flares

8. Outcomes

Complications
- Treatment complications
  — Monitor for skin atrophy
  — Eczema herpeticum, a generalized herpes simplex infection manifested by monomorphic vesicles, crusts, or scalloped erosions superimposed on atopic dermatitis or other extensive eczematous processes
- Smallpox vaccination is absolutely contraindicated in patients with atopic dermatitis or a history thereof because of the risk of eczema vaccinatum

Prognosis
- Runs a chronic or intermittent course
- Affected adults may have only hand dermatitis
- Poor prognostic factors for persistence into adulthood: onset early in childhood, early generalized disease, and asthma; only 40% to 60% of these patients have lasting remissions

Prevention
- Avoid things that dry or irritate the skin: low humidity and dry air
- Other triggers: sweating, overbathing, animal danders, scratchy fabrics
- Do not bathe more than once daily and use soap only on armpits, groin, and feet
- After rinsing, pat the skin dry (not rub) and then, before it dries completely, cover with a thin film of emollient such as Aquaphor, Eucerin, petrolatum, Vanicream

9. When to Refer

- If there is a question about the diagnosis, recommended therapy is ineffective, or specialized treatment is necessary

SUGGESTED REFERENCES

Beck LA et al. Dupilumab treatment in adults with moderate-to-severe atopic dermatitis. *N Engl J Med.* 2014 Jul 10;371(2):130–139. [PMID: 25006719]

Coenraads PJ. Eczema. *N Engl J Med.* 2012 Nov;367(19):1829–1837. [PMID: 23134383]

Eichenfield LF et al. Guidelines of care for the management of atopic dermatitis: section 1. Diagnosis and assessment of atopic dermatitis. *J Am Acad Dermatol.* 2014 Feb;70(2):338–351. [PMID: 24290431]

Eichenfield LF et al. Guidelines of care for the management of atopic dermatitis: section 2. Guidelines of care for the management and treatment of atopic dermatitis with topical therapies. *J Am Acad Dermatol.* 2014 Jul;71(1):116–132. [PMID: 24813302]

Kwatra SG et al. The infra-auricular fissure: a bedside marker of disease severity in patients with atopic dermatitis. *J Am Acad Dermatol.* 2012 Jun;66(6):1009–1010. [PMID: 2258371]

Roekevisch E et al. Efficacy and safety of systemic treatments for moderate-to-severe atopic dermatitis: a systematic review. *J Allergy Clin Immunol.* 2014 Feb;133(2):429–438. [PMID: 24269258]

Sidbury R et al. Guidelines of care for the management of atopic dermatitis: section 3. Management and treatment with phototherapy and systemic agents. *J Am Acad Dermatol.* 2014 Aug;71(2):327–349. [PMID: 24813298]

Sidbury R et al. Guidelines of care for the management of atopic dermatitis: Section 4. Prevention of disease flares and use of adjunctive therapies and approaches. *J Am Acad Dermatol.* 2014 Dec; 71(6):1218–1233. [PMID: 25264237]

Sugerman DT. JAMA patient page. Atopic eczema. *JAMA.* 2014 Feb;311(6):636. [PMID: 24519314]

Contact Dermatitis

2

A 30-year-old woman presents to the clinic complaining that she has "an itchy rash all over the place." She noticed that her legs became red, itchy, and blistered about 2 days after she had been hiking in a heavily wooded area. She says that scratching broke the blisters and afterward the rash became much worse and spread all over. She is convinced that the rash could not be poison ivy because once before she was exposed to that plant and did not develop a rash. On examination, there are erythematous vesicles and bullae in linear streaks on both of her legs. Some areas are weepy, with a yellowish crust. There are ill-defined erythematous plaques studded with papulovesicles on the trunk and arms.

LEARNING OBJECTIVES

▶ Learn the clinical manifestations and morphologic type of eruption in contact dermatitis
▶ Understand the factors that predispose to contact dermatitis
▶ Know the differential diagnosis of contact dermatitis
▶ Learn the treatments for contact dermatitis by its severity
▶ Understand how to prevent contact dermatitis from recurring

QUESTIONS

1. What are the salient features of this patient's problem?
2. How do you think through her problem?
3. What are the key features, including essentials of diagnosis and general considerations, of contact dermatitis?
4. What are the symptoms and signs of contact dermatitis?
5. What is the differential diagnosis of contact dermatitis?
6. What are the laboratory and procedural findings in contact dermatitis?
7. What are the treatments for contact dermatitis?
8. What are the outcomes, including prognosis and prevention, of contact dermatitis?
9. When should patients with contact dermatitis be referred to a specialist?

ANSWERS

1. Salient Features

Itchy erythematous rash; history of pre-eruption exposure to the outdoors; previous initial exposure to same antigen; weeping, vesicles, and bullae in allergic type

2. How to Think Through

This patient's rash is severe, so it is important to think broadly about other causes besides those linked to the outdoor exposure. No symptoms or signs of systemic illness are mentioned, but a complete review of systems and physical examination (with vital signs) are essential. Could this be atopic dermatitis? (Unlikely—there is no history of atopy or prior similar symptoms.) Might this be seborrheic dermatitis? (No, since it typically involves the face and scalp.) A fungal infection? (The pace is too rapid and the rash is more consistent with dermatitis). Scabies? (No, due to the rapid pace and lack of focus in intertriginous areas.) Could this be impetigo? (Yes, careful examination is warranted to exclude impetigo.) What features of this case provide the strongest evidence for contact dermatitis? (Streaked appearance, a pattern confined to exposed areas of the body, recent possible exposure to poison ivy with prior contact with this antigen.) What are the two classes of causative agents in contact dermatitis? (Irritants and antigens.) What are common irritants or antigens?

How should she be treated—topically or systemically? (The weeping and bullae suggest that she may need systemic corticosteroids.) What complications may develop? (Superinfection, especially with *Streptococcus* spp and *Staphylococcus aureus*.)

3. Key Features

Essentials of Diagnosis

- Erythema and edema, with pruritus, often followed by vesicles and bullae in an area of contact with a suspected agent
- Later, weeping, crusting, or secondary infection
- A history of previous reaction to suspected contactant
- Patch test with agent positive

General Considerations

- An acute or chronic dermatitis that results from direct skin contact with chemicals or allergens
- Irritant contact dermatitis
  - Eighty percent of cases are due to excessive exposure to or additive effects of universal irritants such as soaps, detergents, or organic solvents
  - Appears red and scaly but not vesicular
- Allergic contact dermatitis
  - Most common causes are poison ivy, oak, or sumac; topically applied antimicrobials (especially bacitracin and neomycin), anesthetics (benzocaine); haircare products; preservatives; jewelry (nickel); rubber; essential oils; propolis (from bees); vitamin E; and adhesive tape
  - Occupational exposure is an important cause
- Weeping and crusting are typically due to allergic and not irritant dermatitis

4. Symptoms and Signs

- The acute phase is characterized by tiny vesicles and weepy and crusted lesions
- Resolving or chronic contact dermatitis presents with scaling, erythema, and possibly thickened skin; itching, burning, and stinging may be severe
- The lesions, distributed on exposed parts or in bizarre asymmetric patterns, consist of erythematous macules, papules, and vesicles
- The affected area is often hot and swollen, with exudation and crusting, simulating and, at times, complicated by infection

- The pattern of the eruption may be diagnostic (eg, typical linear streaked vesicles on the extremities in poison oak or ivy dermatitis)
- The location will often suggest the cause
  — Scalp involvement suggests hair dyes or shampoos
  — Face involvement, creams, cosmetics, soaps, shaving materials, nail polish; neck involvement, jewelry, hair dyes

5. Differential Diagnosis

- Impetigo
- Cellulitis
- Scabies
- Dermatophytid reaction (allergy or sensitivity to fungi)
- Atopic dermatitis
- Pompholyx
- Asymmetric distribution, blotchy erythema around the face, linear lesions, and a history of exposure help distinguish contact dermatitis from other skin lesions
- The most commonly confused diagnosis is impetigo, in which case Gram stain and culture will rule out impetigo or secondary infection (impetiginization)

6. Laboratory and Procedural Findings

Laboratory Tests

- Gram stain and culture will rule out impetigo or secondary infection (impetiginization)
- After the episode of allergic contact dermatitis has cleared, patch testing may be useful if triggering allergen is not known

Diagnostic Procedures

- If itching is generalized, then consider scabies

7. Treatments

- Table 2-1
- Vesicular and weepy lesions often require systemic corticosteroid therapy
- Localized involvement (except on the face) can often be managed with topical agents
- Irritant contact dermatitis is treated by protection from the irritant and use of topical corticosteroids as for atopic dermatitis

Local Measures

- Acute weeping dermatitis
  — Compresses are most often used
  — Lesions on the extremities may be bandaged with wet dressings for 30 to 60 minutes several times a day
  — Calamine or zinc oxide paste can be used between wet dressings, especially for intertriginous areas or when oozing is not marked
  — High-potency topical corticosteroids in gel or cream form (fluocinonide, clobetasol, or halobetasol) may help suppress acute contact dermatitis and relieve itching
  — Then, taper the number of high-potency topical steroid applications per day or use a mid-potency corticosteroid, such as triamcinolone 0.1% cream to prevent rebound of the dermatitis
  — A soothing formulation is 2 oz 0.1% triamcinolone acetonide cream in 7.5 oz Sarna lotion (0.5% camphor, 0.5% menthol, 0.5% phenol)
- Subacute dermatitis (subsiding)
  — Mid-potency (triamcinolone 0.1%) to high-potency corticosteroids (clobetasol 0.05%, fluocinonide 0.05%, desoximetasone 0.05%–0.25%) are the mainstays of the therapy
- Chronic dermatitis (dry and lichenified)
  — High- to super-potency corticosteroids are used in ointment form

Table 2-1. Useful topical dermatologic therapeutic agents for contact dermatitis.

Agent	Formulations, Strengths, and Prices[a]	Apply	Potency Class	Comments
Corticosteroids				
Hydrocortisone acetate	Cream 1% Ointment 1% Lotion 1%	Twice daily	Low	Not the same as hydrocortisone butyrate or valerate Not for poison oak OTC lotion (Aquanil HC) OTC solution (Scalpicin, T Scalp)
	Cream 2.5%	Twice daily	Low	Perhaps better for pruritus ani Not clearly better than 1% More expensive Not OTC
Alclometasone dipropionate (Aclovate)	Cream 0.05% Ointment 0.05%	Twice daily	Low	More efficacious than hydrocortisone Perhaps causes less atrophy
Desonide	Cream 0.05% Ointment 0.05% Lotion 0.05%	Twice daily	Low	More efficacious than hydrocortisone Can cause rosacea or atrophy Not fluorinated
Clocortolone (Cloderm)	Cream 0.1%	Three times daily	Medium	Does not cross-react with other corticosteroids chemically and can be used in patients allergic to other corticosteroids
Prednicarbate (Dermatop)	Emollient cream 0.1% Ointment 0.1%	Twice daily	Medium	May cause less atrophy No generic formulations Preservative-free
Triamcinolone acetonide	Cream 0.1% Ointment 0.1% Lotion 0.1%	Twice daily	Medium	Caution in body folds, face Economical in 0.5-lb and 1-lb sizes for treatment of large body surfaces Economical as solution for scalp
	Cream 0.025% Ointment 0.025%	Twice daily	Medium	Possibly less efficacy and few advantages over 0.1% formulation
Fluocinolone acetonide	Cream 0.025% Ointment 0.025% Solution 0.01%	Twice daily	Medium	
Mometasone furoate (Elocon)	Cream 0.1% Ointment 0.1% Lotion 0.1%	Once daily	Medium	Often used inappropriately on the face or on children Not fluorinated
Diflorasone diacetate	Cream 0.05% Ointment 0.05%	Twice daily	High	
Amcinonide (Cyclocort)	Cream 0.1% Ointment 0.1%	Twice daily	High	
Fluocinonide (Lidex)	Cream 0.05% Gel 0.05 Ointment 0.05% Solution 0.05%	Twice daily	High	Economical generics Lidex cream can cause stinging on eczema Lidex emollient cream preferred
Betamethasone dipropionate (Diprolene)	Cream 0.05% Ointment 0.05% Lotion 0.05%	Twice daily	Ultra-high	Economical generics available
Clobetasol propionate (Temovate)	Cream 0.05% Ointment 0.05% Lotion 0.05%	Twice daily	Ultra-high	Somewhat more potent than diflorasone Limited to 50 g or less per week Limited to 2 continuous weeks of use Cream may cause stinging; use "emollient cream" formulation Generic available
Halobetasol propionate (Ultravate)	Cream 0.05% Ointment 0.05%	Twice daily	Ultra-high	Same restrictions as clobetasol Cream does not cause stinging Compatible with calcipotriene (Dovonex)
Flurandrenolide (Cordran)	Tape: 3" roll Lotion 0.05%	Every 12 h	Ultra-high	Protects the skin and prevents scratching
Nonsteroidal Anti-Inflammatory Agents				
Tacrolimus[a] (Protopic)	Ointment 0.1% Ointment 0.03%	Twice daily	N/A	Steroid substitute not causing atrophy or striae Burns in ≥ 40% of patients with eczema
Pimecrolimus[a] (Elidel)	Cream 1%	Twice daily	N/A	Steroid substitute not causing atrophy or striae

N/A, not applicable; OTC, over-the-counter.

[a]Topical tacrolimus and pimecrolimus should only be used when other topical treatments are ineffective. Treatment should be limited to an area and duration to be as brief as possible. Treatment with these agents should be avoided in persons with known immunosuppression, HIV infection, bone marrow and organ transplantation, lymphoma, at high risk for lymphoma, and those with a prior history of lymphoma.

Systemic Therapy

- For acute severe cases, give oral prednisone for 12 to 21 days
- Prednisone, 60 mg for 4 to 7 days, 40 mg for 4 to 7 days, and 20 mg for 4 to 7 days without a further taper is one useful regimen or dispense 78 prednisone 5-mg pills to be taken 12 the first day, 11 the second day, and so on
- The key is to use enough corticosteroid (and as early as possible) to achieve a clinical effect and to taper slowly enough to avoid rebound
- A Medrol Dosepak (methylprednisolone) with 5 days of medication is inappropriate on both counts

8. Outcomes

Prognosis

- Self-limited if reexposure is prevented but often takes 2 to 3 weeks for full resolution

Prevention

- Prompt and thorough removal of the causative oil by washing with liquid dishwashing soap (eg, Dial Ultra) may be effective if done within 30 minutes after exposure to poison oak or ivy
- Goop and Tecnu oil-removing skin cleansers are also effective but much more costly without increased efficacy
- The most effective over-the-counter barrier creams that are applied prior to exposure and prevent or reduce the severity of the dermatitis are
  — Stokogard
  — Hollister Moisture Barrier
  — Hydropel
- The mainstay of prevention is identification of the agent causing the dermatitis and avoidance of exposure or use of protective clothing and gloves

9. When to Refer

- Occupational allergic contact dermatitis should be referred to a dermatologist

SUGGESTED REFERENCES

Fonacier LS et al. Allergic contact dermatitis. *Ann Allergy Asthma Immunol*. 2014 Jul;113(1):9–12. [PMID: 24950843]

Holness DL. Occupational skin allergies: testing and treatment (the case of occupational allergic contact dermatitis). *Curr Allergy Asthma Rep*. 2014 Feb;14(2):410. [PMID: 24408535]

Tan CH et al. Contact dermatitis: allergic and irritant. *Clin Dermatol*. 2014 Jan–Feb;32(1):116–124. [PMID: 24314385]

Wolf R et al. Contact dermatitis: facts and controversies. *Clin Dermatol*. 2013 Jul–Aug;31(4):467–478. [PMID: 23806164]

Wolf R et al. Patch testing: facts and controversies. *Clin Dermatol*. 2013 Jul–Aug;31(4):479–486. [PMID: 23806165]

3

Psoriasis

A 25-year-old woman presents with a complaint of rash that has developed over the last several weeks and seems to be progressing. She describes the involved areas as mildly itchy. On examination, she is noted to have several plaque-like lesions over the extensor surfaces of both upper and lower extremities as well as similar lesions on her scalp. The plaques are erythematous, with silvery scales, and are sharply marginated.

LEARNING OBJECTIVES

▶ Learn the clinical manifestations and morphologic type of eruption in psoriasis
▶ Understand the factors that predispose to psoriasis
▶ Know the differential diagnosis of psoriasis
▶ Learn the treatments for psoriasis by its severity
▶ Understand the complications and prognosis of psoriasis

QUESTIONS

1. What are the salient features of this patient's problem?
2. How do you think through her problem?
3. What are the key features, including essentials of diagnosis and general considerations, of psoriasis?
4. What are the symptoms and signs of psoriasis?
5. What is the differential diagnosis of psoriasis?
6. What are the procedural findings in psoriasis?
7. What are the treatments for psoriasis?
8. What are the outcomes, including complications and prognosis, of psoriasis?
9. When should patients with psoriasis be referred to a specialist?

ANSWERS

1. Salient Features

Progressive rash; mild itching; plaque-like lesions; extensor surfaces of extremities and scalp distribution; sharp margins with silvery scales

2. How to Think Through

What are the common skin diseases in the differential diagnosis of this woman's eruption and what features about her presentation make psoriasis the most likely diagnosis? (Candidiasis, tinea, and atopic dermatitis are characterized by poorly demarcated lesions and typically present on the extensor surfaces. *Candida*, in particular, is found in the moist body folds and flexural surfaces. This patient's lesions are described as mildly pruritic, which is more typical of psoriasis than these alternative diagnoses. The scaly scalp plaques are particularly characteristic of psoriasis.) How does her presentation differ from that of seborrheic dermatitis?

What other manifestations should you explore? (Nail pitting is common in psoriasis and will help confirm your diagnosis. Joint pain and inflammation would raise the possibility psoriatic arthritis.)

3. Key Features

Essentials of Diagnosis
- Silvery scales on bright red, well-demarcated plaques, usually on the knees, elbows, and scalp
- Nail findings include pitting and onycholysis (separation of the nail plate from the bed)
- Mild itching (usually)
- May be associated with psoriatic arthritis
- Patients with psoriasis are at increased risk for metabolic syndrome and lymphoma
- Histopathology is not often useful and can be confusing

General Considerations
- A common benign, chronic inflammatory skin disease with both a genetic basis and known environmental triggers
- Injury or irritation of normal skin tends to induce lesions of psoriasis at the site (Koebner phenomenon)
- Obesity worsens psoriasis, and significant weight loss in persons with high body mass index may lead to substantial improvement
- Psoriasis has several variants—the most common is the plaque type

4. Symptoms and Signs

There are often no symptoms, but itching may occur
- Although psoriasis may occur anywhere, examine the scalp, elbows, knees, palms and soles, umbilicus, intergluteal fold, and nails
- The lesions are red, sharply defined plaques covered with silvery scales; the glans penis and vulva may be affected; occasionally, only the flexures (axillae, inguinal areas including genitalia) are involved ("inverse psoriasis")
- Fine stippling ("pitting") in the nails is highly suggestive; onycholysis (separation of the nail plate from its bed) may occur
- Patients with psoriasis often have a pink or red intergluteal fold
- There may be associated seronegative arthritis, often involving the distal interphalangeal joints
- Eruptive (guttate) psoriasis, consisting of myriad lesions 3 to 10 mm in diameter, occurs occasionally after streptococcal pharyngitis
- Plaque-type or extensive erythrodermic psoriasis with abrupt onset may accompany HIV infection

5. Differential Diagnosis

- Atopic dermatitis (eczema)
- Contact dermatitis
- Nummular eczema (discoid eczema, nummular dermatitis)
- Tinea
- Candidiasis
- Intertrigo

- Seborrheic dermatitis
- Pityriasis rosea
- Secondary syphilis
- Pityriasis rubra pilaris
- Onychomycosis (nail findings)
- Cutaneous features of reactive arthritis
- Cutaneous features of reactive lupus
- Cutaneous T-cell lymphoma (mycosis fungoides)

6. Procedural Findings

Diagnostic Procedures
- The combination of red plaques with silvery scales on elbows and knees, with scaliness in the scalp or nail pitting or onycholysis, is diagnostic
- Psoriasis lesions are well demarcated and affect extensor surfaces—in contrast to atopic dermatitis, with poorly demarcated plaques in flexural distribution
- In body folds and groin, scraping and culture for *Candida* and examination of scalp and nails will distinguish inverse psoriasis from intertrigo and candidiasis

7. Treatments

- Certain drugs, such as β-blockers, antimalarial agents, statins, and lithium, may flare or worsen psoriasis
- Even tiny doses of systemic corticosteroids given to psoriasis patients may lead to severe rebound flares of their disease
- Never use systemic corticosteroids to treat flares of psoriasis

Medications
- Topical corticosteroid cream or ointment (Table 3-1)
- Limited disease (< 10% of the body surface)
  — Restrict the highest potency corticosteroids to 2 to 3 weeks of twice daily use; then three or four times on weekends or switch to a mid-potency corticosteroid
  — Rarely induce a lasting remission
- Calcipotriene ointment 0.005% or calcitriol ointment 0.003%, both vitamin D analogs, is used twice daily
  — Initial treatment regimen: corticosteroids twice daily plus a vitamin D analog twice daily
  — Once lesions are cleared, vitamin D analog is used alone, once daily, and with corticosteroids, once daily, for several weeks
  — Then, once- or twice-daily application of the vitamin D analog is continued long term and topical corticosteroids are stopped
  — Calcipotriene usually cannot be applied to the groin or the face because of irritation
  — Calcipotriene is incompatible with many topical corticosteroids; it must be applied at a different time
  — Maximum dose for calcipotriene is 100 g/week and for calcitriol is 200 g/week
- Occlusion alone clears isolated plaques in 30% to 40% of patients
  — Thin, occlusive hydrocolloid dressings are placed on the lesions and left undisturbed for 5 to 7 days and then replaced
  — Responses may be seen within several weeks
- For the scalp
  — Start with a tar shampoo once daily
  — Thick scales: 6% salicylic acid gel (eg, Keralyt), P & S solution (phenol, mineral oil, and glycerin), or oil-based fluocinolone acetonide 0.01% (Derma-Smoothe/FS) under a shower cap at night, followed by a shampoo in the morning
  — In order of increasing potency, triamcinolone 0.1%, or fluocinolone, betamethasone dipropionate, fluocinonide or amcinonide, and clobetasol are available in solution form for use on the scalp twice daily

Table 3-1. Useful topical dermatologic therapeutic agents for psoriasis.

Agent	Formulations, Strengths	Application	Potency Class	Comments
Diflorasone diacetate	Cream 0.05% Ointment 0.05%	Twice daily	High	
Amcinonide (Cyclocort)	Cream 0.1% Ointment 0.1%	Twice daily	High	
Fluocinonide (Lidex)	Cream 0.05% Gel 0.05% Ointment 0.05% Solution 0.05%	Twice daily	High	Economical generics Lidex cream can cause stinging on eczema Lidex emollient cream preferred
Betamethasone dipropionate (Diprolene)	Cream 0.05% Ointment 0.05% Lotion 0.05%	Twice daily	Ultra-high	Economical generics available
Clobetasol propionate (Temovate)	Cream 0.05% Ointment 0.05% Lotion 0.05%	Twice daily	Ultra-high	Somewhat more potent than diflorasone Limited to two continuous weeks of use Limited to 50 g or less per week Cream may cause stinging; use "emollient cream" formulation Generic available
Halobetasol propionate (Ultravate)	Cream 0.05% Ointment 0.05%	Twice daily	Ultra-high	Same restrictions as clobetasol Cream does not cause stinging Compatible with calcipotriene (Dovonex)
Flurandrenolide (Cordran)	Tape: 80" × 3" roll Lotion 0.05%: 60 mL	Every 12 hours	Ultra-high	Protects the skin and prevents scratching

- Psoriasis in the body folds
  - Potent corticosteroids cannot be used
  - Tacrolimus ointment 0.1% or 0.03% or pimecrolimus cream 1% may be effective in penile, groin, and facial psoriasis
- Moderate disease (10%–30% of the body surface) to severe disease (> 30% of the body surface)
  - Methotrexate is very effective in doses up to 25 mg once weekly orally
  - Acitretin, a synthetic retinoid, is most effective for pustular psoriasis at 0.5 to 0.75 mg/ kg/day orally
    - Liver enzymes and serum lipids must be checked periodically
    - Acitretin is a teratogen and persists for 2 to 3 years in fat tissue. Women must wait at least 3 years after completing treatment before considering pregnancy
  - Cyclosporine dramatically improves severe cases of psoriasis
  - Tumor necrosis factor (TNF) inhibitors (etanercept, 50 mg twice weekly subcutaneously ×12, then once weekly; infliximab, 5 mg/kg once weekly intravenously at weeks 0, 2, and 6; and adalimumab, 40 mg every 2 weeks subcutaneously) can be effective; all three can also induce or worsen psoriasis
  - IL-12/23 monoclonal antibodies (ustekinumab [Stelara]) and IL-17 monoclonal antibodies (brodalumab, secukinumab, and ixekizumab)
    - Are effective in psoriasis
    - May be considered instead of using a TNF inhibitor

Therapeutic Procedures
- Limited to moderate disease: UV phototherapy
- Moderate-to-severe disease
  - The treatment of choice is narrow-band UVB light exposure three times weekly; clearing usually occurs in ~7 weeks; maintenance may be needed since relapses are frequent

— Severe disease unresponsive to UV light may be treated in a psoriasis day care center with the Goeckerman regimen, using crude coal tar for many hours and exposure to UVB light; this offers the best chance for prolonged remissions

— PUVA (psoralen plus ultraviolet A) may be effective even if standard UVB treatment has failed; may be used with other therapy, eg, acitretin

8. Outcomes

Complications

- Treatment with calcipotriene may result in hypercalcemia
- Long-term use of PUVA (> 250 doses) is associated with an increased risk of skin cancer (especially squamous cell carcinoma and perhaps melanoma)

Prognosis

- The course tends to be chronic and unpredictable, and the disease may be refractory to treatment
- Patients (especially those > 40 years of age) should be monitored for metabolic syndrome, which correlates with the severity of skin disease

9. When to Refer

- If there is a question about the diagnosis, if recommended therapy is ineffective, or if specialized treatment is necessary

SUGGESTED REFERENCES

Armstrong AW et al. Combining biologic therapies with other systemic treatments in psoriasis: evidence-based, best-practice recommendations from the Medical Board of the National Psoriasis Foundation. *JAMA Dermatol.* 2015 Apr;151(4):432–438 [PMID: 25517130]

Armstrong AW et al. Psoriasis and the risk of diabetes mellitus: a systematic review and meta-analysis. *JAMA Dermatol.* 2013 Jan;149(1):84–91. [PMID: 23407990]

Coumbe AG et al. Cardiovascular risk and psoriasis: beyond the traditional risk factors. *Am J Med.* 2014 Jan;127(1):12–18. [PMID: 24161194]

Debbaneh M et al. Diet and psoriasis, part I: impact of weight loss interventions. *J Am Acad Dermatol.* 2014 Jul;71(1):133–140. [PMID: 24709272]

Gelfand JM et al. Comparative effectiveness of commonly used systemic treatments of phototherapy for moderate to severe plaque psoriasis in the clinical practice setting. *Arch Dermatol.* 2012 Apr;148(4):487–494. [PMID: 22508874]

Hendriks AG et al. Combinations of classical time-honoured topicals in plaque psoriasis: a systematic review. *J Eur Acad Dermatol Venereol.* 2013 Apr;27(4):399–410. [PMID: 22779910]

Hsu S et al. Consensus guidelines for the management of plaque psoriasis. *Arch Dermatol.* 2012 Jan;148(1):95–102. [PMID: 22250239]

Kim IH et al. Comparative efficacy of biologics in psoriasis: a review. *Am J Clin Dermatol.* 2012 Dec 1;13(6):365–374. [PMID: 22967166]

Kupetsky EA et al. Psoriasis vulgaris: an evidence-based guide for primary care. *J Am Board Fam Med.* 2013 Nov–Dec;26(6):787–801. [PMID: 24204077]

Lynch M et al. Treating moderate to severe psoriasis—best use of biologics. *Expert Rev Clin Immunol.* 2014 Feb;10(2):269–279. [PMID: 24372444]

Mason A et al. Topical treatments for chronic plaque psoriasis: an abridged Cochrane Systematic Review. *J Am Acad Dermatol.* 2013 Nov;69(5):799–807. [PMID: 24124809]

Reich K et al. Efficacy of biologics in the treatment of moderate to severe psoriasis: a network meta-analysis of randomized controlled trials. *Br J Dermatol.* 2012 Jan;166(1):179–188. [PMID: 21910698]

Richard MA et al. Evidence-based recommendations on the role of dermatologists in the diagnosis and management of psoriatic arthritis: systematic review and expert opinion. *J Eur Acad Dermatol Venereol.* 2014 Aug;28(suppl 5):3–12. [PMID: 24985557]

Samarasekere EJ et al. Topical therapies for the treatment of plaque psoriasis: systematic review and network meta-analyses. *Br J Dermatol.* 2013 May;168(5):954–967. [PMID: 23413913]

Weigle N et al. Psoriasis. *Am Fam Physician.* 2013 May;87(9):626–633. [PMID: 23668525]

Pulmonary/Ear, Nose, and Throat Disorders

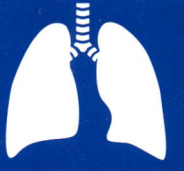

4

Asthma

A 25-year-old previously well woman presents to your office with complaints of episodic shortness of breath and chest tightness. She has had these symptoms on and off for about 2 years but states that they have worsened lately, occurring two or three times a month. She notes that the symptoms are worse during the spring months, and since her new roommate and his cat moved in. She has no exercise-induced or nocturnal symptoms. The patient smokes occasionally when out with friends, drinks socially, and has no history of recreational drug use. Examination is notable for mild end-expiratory wheezing.

LEARNING OBJECTIVES

▶ Learn the clinical manifestations and objective findings of asthma
▶ Understand the factors that predispose to asthma
▶ Know the differential diagnosis of asthma
▶ Learn the treatments for asthma
▶ Learn how to prevent asthma exacerbations

QUESTIONS

1. What are the salient features of this patient's problem?
2. How do you think through her problem?
3. What are the key features, including essentials of diagnosis, general considerations, and demographics, of asthma?
4. What are the symptoms and signs of asthma?
5. What is the differential diagnosis of asthma?
6. What are laboratory, imaging, and procedural findings in asthma?
7. What are the treatments for asthma?
8. What are the outcomes, including follow-up, complications, prognosis, and prevention, of asthma?
9. When should patients with asthma be referred to a specialist or admitted to the hospital?

ANSWERS

1. Salient Features

Intermittent shortness of breath and chest tightness; environmental triggers; family history; wheezing on physical examination

2. How to Think Through

What are other causes of shortness of breath, and what makes asthma the most likely cause in this patient? What are common environmental triggers to explore? What associated atopic diseases would you ask about? What are non-allergy-mediated exacerbating factors to explore? How can you best establish the severity of her asthma symptoms and the potential for life-threatening exacerbations? (History of emergency department visits, hospital admissions, and intubations.) If she did not have audible wheezing on examination, what more subtle signs could you look for? (Increased expiratory time, cough induced by rapid expiration.) What would her pulmonary function tests (PFTs) likely show? Once you begin treatment of her asthma, what should serve as your barometer for the degree of control? (Number of episodes per week, peak expiratory flow rate [PEFR].) At what point would you add a daily controller medication, and what would be your first choice? Beyond medication, what are other important interventions? (Allergen reduction, smoking cessation.)

3. Key Features

Essentials of Diagnosis

- Episodic or chronic symptoms of airflow obstruction
- Reversibility of airflow obstruction, either spontaneously or after bronchodilator therapy
- Symptoms frequently worse at night or in the early morning
- Prolonged expiration and diffuse wheezes on physical examination
- Limitation of airflow on pulmonary function testing or positive bronchoprovocation challenge

General Considerations

- Affects 8% to 10% of the population
- Accounts for 1.75 million emergency department visits, 480,000 hospital admissions, and > 3000 death annually in the United States
- Prevalence, hospitalizations, and fatal asthma have all increased in the United States over the past 20 years

Demographics

- Slightly more common in boys (< 14 years old) and in women
- Hospitalization rates have been highest among blacks and children
- Death rates for asthma are consistently highest among blacks aged 15 to 24 years

4. Symptoms and Signs

- Episodic wheezing and difficulty breathing, chest tightness, and cough
- Wheezing with normal breathing or a prolonged forced expiratory phase
- Excess sputum production
- Symptoms are frequently worse at night
- See Table 4-1 to estimate attack severity
- Common aeroallergens
  — Dust mites
  — Cockroaches
  — Cats
  — Pollen

Table 4-1. Evaluation and classification of severity of asthma exacerbations.

	Mild	Moderate	Severe	Respiratory Arrest Imminent
Symptoms				
Breathlessness	While walking	At rest, limits activity	At rest, interferes with conversation	While at rest, mute
Talks in	Sentences	Phrases	Words	Silent
Alertness	May be agitated	Usually agitated	Usually agitated	Drowsy or confused
Signs				
Respiratory rate	Increased	Increased	Often greater than 30/minute	Greater than 30/minute
Body position	Can lie down	Prefers sitting	Sits upright	Unable to recline
Use of accessory muscles; suprasternal retractions	Usually not	Commonly	Usually	Paradoxical thoracoabdominal movement
Wheeze	Moderate, often only end expiratory	Loud; throughout exhalation	Usually loud; throughout inhalation and exhalation	Absent
Pulse/minute	< 100	100–120	> 120	Bradycardia
Pulsus paradoxus	Absent, < 10 mm Hg	May be present 10–25 mm Hg	Often present, >25 mm Hg	Absence suggests respiratory muscle fatigue
Functional Assessment				
PEF or FEV$_1$ % predicted or % personal best	≥ 70%	40%–69%	< 40%	> 25%
Pao$_2$ (on air, mm Hg)	Normal[a]	≥ 60[a]	< 60: possible cyanosis	< 60: possible cyanosis
Pco$_2$ (mm Hg)	< 42 mm Hg[a]	< 42 mm Hg[a]	≥ to 42[a]	≥ to 42[a]
Sao$_2$ (on air, %)	> 95%[a]	90%–95%[a]	< 90%[a]	< 90%[a]

[a]Test not usually necessary

PEF, peak expiratory flow; Sao$_2$, oxygen saturation.

Adapted from National Asthma Education and Prevention Program. Expert Panel Report 3: Guidelines for the Diagnosis and Management of Asthma. National Institutes of Health Pub. No. 08-4051. Bethesda, MD, 2007. http://www.nhlbi.nih.gov/health-pro/guidelines/current/asthma-guidelines/.

- Nonspecific precipitants
  - Exercise
  - Respiratory tract infections, especially viral
  - Rhinitis, sinusitis
  - Postnasal drip
  - Aspiration
  - Gastroesophageal reflux
  - Changes in weather
  - Stress
- Tobacco smoke increases symptoms and decreases lung function
- Nasal findings consistent with allergy and evidence of allergic skin disorders
- Certain medications (including aspirin and nonsteroidal anti-inflammatory drugs) may be triggers (Table 4-2)

5. Differential Diagnosis

Upper Airway Disorders
- Vocal cord paralysis
- Vocal cord dysfunction syndrome
- Foreign body aspiration
- Laryngotracheal mass

Table 4-2. Medications that may precipitate asthma.

β-blockers
Aspirin
Nonsteroidal anti-inflammatory drugs
Histamine
Methacholine
Acetylcysteine
Aerosolized pentamidine
Any nebulized medication

- Tracheal stenosis
- Tracheobronchomalacia
- Airway edema (eg, angioedema or inhalation injury)

Lower Airway Disorders
- Chronic obstructive pulmonary disease
- Bronchiectasis
- Allergic bronchopulmonary aspergillosis
- Cystic fibrosis
- Eosinophilic pneumonia
- Bronchiolitis obliterans

Systemic Vasculitides
- Eosinophilic granulomatosis with polyangiitis (formerly known as Churg–Strauss syndrome)

Psychiatric
- Conversion disorder

6. Laboratory, Imaging, and Procedural Findings

Laboratory Tests
- PFTs: spirometry (FEV_1, FVC, FEV_1/FVC) before and after the administration of a short-acting bronchodilator
- Significant reversibility of obstruction is demonstrated by an increase of ≥ 12% and 200 mL in FEV_1 or ≥ 15% and 200 mL in FVC after inhaling a short-acting bronchodilator
- PEFR monitoring can
  — Establish peak flow variability
  — Quantify asthma severity
  — Provide objective measurements on which treatment decisions can be based
- PEFR should be measured in the morning before using a bronchodilator and in the afternoon after taking a bronchodilator
  — 20% change in PEFR values from morning to afternoon or from day to day suggests inadequately controlled asthma
  — Values < 200 L/min indicate severe airflow obstruction
- Arterial blood gases may show a respiratory alkalosis and an increase in the alveolar–arterial oxygen difference; in severe exacerbations, hypoxemia develops and the $Paco_2$ normalizes
- An increased $Paco_2$ and respiratory acidosis may portend respiratory failure

Imaging Studies
- Chest radiographs usually show only hyperinflation but may include bronchial wall thickening and diminished peripheral lung vascular shadows
- Chest imaging is indicated when pneumonia, another disorder mimicking asthma, or a complication of asthma (such as pneumothorax) is suspected

Diagnostic Procedures
- Bronchial provocation testing with inhaled histamine or methacholine
  — May be useful when asthma is suspected but spirometry is nondiagnostic
  — It is not recommended if the FEV_1 is < 65% of predicted

— A positive methacholine test is defined as a $\geq 20\%$ fall in the FEV_1 at exposure to a concentration of 16 mg/mL or less

— A negative test has a negative predictive value for asthma of 95%

• Exercise challenge testing may be useful in patients with symptoms of exercise-induced bronchospasm

• Skin testing for sensitivity to environmental allergens may be useful in persistent asthma

7. Treatments

Medications

• Long-term control therapy (see Tables 4-3 and 4-4)
  — Inhaled corticosteroids
  — Systemic corticosteroids
  — Inhaled long-acting β_2-agonists
  — Anticholinergics
  — Combination medications (inhaled corticosteroid and long-acting β_2-agonist)
  — Leukotriene modifiers
  — Mediator inhibitors
  — Phosphodiesterase inhibitors

Quick-Relief Therapy

• Short-acting inhaled β_2-agonists (Table 4-5)
• Inhaled anticholinergics
• Systemic corticosteroids
• Antimicrobials
  — No role in routine asthma exacerbations
  — May be beneficial when asthma is accompanied by fever and purulent sputum or evidence of pneumonia or bacterial sinusitis

Acute Exacerbations

• Repetitive or continuous use of inhaled short-acting β_2-agonist
• Early administration of systemic corticosteroids
• Treatment or removal of any identified trigger to the exacerbation
• Mild exacerbations (PEFR $\geq 70\%$ predicted or personal best)
  — Many patients respond quickly and fully to an inhaled short-acting β_2-agonist alone
  — However, an inhaled short-acting β_2-agonist may need to be continued at increased doses, eg, every 3 to 4 hours for 24 to 48 hours
  — In patients not taking an inhaled corticosteroid, consider starting this agent
  — In patients already taking an inhaled corticosteroid, a 7-day course of oral corticosteroids (0.5–1.0 mg/kg/d) may be necessary
  — Doubling the dose of inhaled corticosteroid is not effective and is not recommended in the National Asthma Education and Prevention Program 3 guidelines
• Moderate exacerbations (PEFR 40%–69% predicted or personal best)
  — Continuous administration of an inhaled short-acting β_2-agonist
  — Early administration of systemic corticosteroids
• Severe exacerbations (PEFR < 40% predicted or personal best)
  — Immediate treatment with oxygen, to maintain an $SaO_2 > 90\%$ or a $PaO_2 > 60$ mm Hg
  — High doses of an inhaled short-acting β_2-agonist (at least three metered-dose inhaler [MDI] or nebulizer treatments in the first hour; thereafter, treatment frequency depends on improvement in airflow)
  — Systemic corticosteroids
  — Ipratropium bromide reduces the rate of hospital admissions when added to inhaled short-acting β_2-agonists
  — If $FEV_1 < 25\%$ of predicted on presentation, or failure to respond to initial treatment, intravenous magnesium sulfate (2 g intravenously over 20 minutes) produces a detectable improvement in airflow and may reduce hospitalization rates

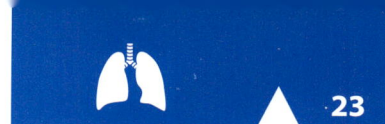

Table 4-3. Long-term control medications for asthma.

Medication	Dosage Form	Adult Dose	Comments
Inhaled Corticosteroids			**(See Table 4-4)**
Systemic Corticosteroids			**(Applies to all three corticosteroids)**
Methylprednisolone	2, 4, 6, 8, 16, 32 mg tablets	7.5–60 mg daily in a single dose in AM or every other day as needed for control	• Administer single AM dose either daily or on alternate days (alternate-day therapy may produce less adrenal suppression). Short courses or "bursts" are effective for establishing control when initiating therapy or during a period of gradual deterioration.
Prednisolone	5 mg tablets, 5 mg/5 mL, 15 mg/5 mL	Short-course "burst": to achieve control, 40–60 mg/d as single or two divided doses for 3–10 d	• There is no evidence that tapering the dose following improvement in symptom control and pulmonary function prevents relapse.
Prednisone	1, 2.5, 5, 10, 20, 50 mg tablets; 5 mg/mL, 5 mg/mL		
Inhaled Long-Acting β₂-Agonists			**Should not be used for symptom relief or exacerbations. Use with inhaled corticosteroids.**
Salmeterol	DPI 50 µg/blister	1 blister every 12 h	• Decreased duration of protection against EIB may occur with regular use.
Formoterol	DPI 12 µg /single-use capsule	1 capsule every 12 h	• Decreased duration of protection against EIB may occur with regular use. • Each capsule is for single use only; additional doses should not be administered for at least 12 hr. • Capsules should be used only with the Aerolizer™ inhaler and should not be taken orally.
Combined Medication			
Fluticasone/ Salmeterol	DPI 100 µg/50 µg, 250 µg/50 µg, or 500 µg/50 µg	One inhalation twice daily; dose depends on severity of asthma	• 100/50 DPI or 45/21 HFA for patient not controlled on low- to medium-dose inhaled corticosteroids.
			• 250/50 DPI or 115/21 HFA for patients not controlled on medium- to high-dose inhaled corticosteroids.
	HFA 45 µg/21 µg 115 µg/21 µg 230 µg/21 µg		
Budesonide/ Formoterol	HFA MDI 80 µg/4.5 µg 160 µg/4.5 µg	2 inhalations twice daily; dose depends on severity of asthma	• 80/4.5 for asthma not controlled on low- to medium-dose inhaled corticosteroids.
			• 160/4.5 for asthma not controlled on medium- to high-dose inhaled corticosteroids.
Cromolyn and Nedocromil			
Cromolyn	MDI 0.8 mg/puff	2 puffs four times daily	• 4–6 wk trial may be needed to determine maximum benefit.
	Nebulizer 20 mg/ampule	1 ampule four times daily	• Dose by MDI may be inadequate to affect hyperresponsiveness.
Nedocromil	MDI 1.75 mg/puff	2 puffs four times daily	• One dose before exercise or allergen exposure provides effective prophylaxis for 1–2 h. Not as effective for EIB as SABA. • Once control is achieved, the frequency of dosing may be reduced.
Inhaled Long-Acting Anti-Cholinergic			**Should not be used for symptom relief or exacerbations. Use with inhaled corticosteroids.**
Tiotropium	DPI 18 µg /blister	1 blister daily	
Leukotriene Modifiers			
Leukotriene Receptor Antagonists			
Montelukast	4 or 5 mg chewable tablet 10 mg tablet	10 mg each night at bedtime	• Exhibits a flat dose-response curve. Doses > 10 mg will not produce a greater response in adults.
Zafirlukast	10 or 20 mg tablet	40 mg daily (20 mg tablet twice daily)	• Administration with meals decreases bioavailability; take at least 1 h before or 2 h after meals. • Monitor for symptoms and signs of hepatic dysfunction.

(continued)

Table 4-3. Long-term control medications for asthma. (continued)

Medication	Dosage Form	Adult Dose	Comments
5-Lipoxygenase Inhibitor			
Zileuton	600 mg tablet	2400 mg daily (600 mg four times daily)	• Monitor hepatic enzymes (ALT).
Methylxanthines			
Theophylline	Liquids, sustained release tablets, and capsules	Starting dose 10 mg/kg/d up to 300 mg maximum; usual maximum dose 800 mg/d	• Adjust dosage to achieve serum concentration of 5–15 μg /mL at steady state (at least 48 h on same dosage). • Due to wide interpatient variability in theophylline metabolic clearance, routine serum theophylline level monitoring is important.
Immunomodulator			
Omalizumab	Subcutaneous injection, 150 mg/1.2 mL following reconstitution with 1.4 mL sterile water for injection	150–375 mg SC every 2–4 wk, depending on body weight and pretreatment serum IgE level	• Do not administer > 150 mg per injection site.
			• Monitor for anaphylaxis for 2 h following at least the first three injections.

DPI, dry power inhaler; EIB, exercise-induced bronchospasm; HFA, hydrofluoroalkaline; MDI, metered-dose inhaler; SABA, short-acting β_2-agonist.

Table 4-4. Estimated comparative daily dosages for inhaled corticosteroids for asthma.

Drug	Low Daily Dose Adult	Medium Daily Dose Adult	High Daily Dose Adult
Beclomethasone HFA 40 or 80 μg/puff	80–240 μg	> 240–480 μg	> 480 μg
Budesonide DPI 90, 180, or 200 μg/inhalation	180–600 μg	> 600–1200 μg	> 1200 μg
Flunisolide 250 μg/puff	500–1000 μg	> 1000–2000 μg	> 2000 μg
Flunisolide HFA 80 μg/puff	320 μg	> 320–640 μg	> 640 μg
Fluticasone HFA/MDI: 44, 110, or 220 μg/puff	88–264 μg	> 264–440 μg	> 440 μg
DPI: 50, 100, or 250 μg/inhalation	100–300 μg	> 300–500 μg	> 500 μg
Mometasone DPI 200 μg/puff	200 μg	400 μg	> 400 μg
Triamcinolone acetonide 75 μg/puff	300–750 μg	> 750–1500 μg	> 1500 μg

DPI, dry power inhaler; HFA, hydrofluoroalkaline; MDI, metered-dose inhaler.

Notes:
• The most important determinant of appropriate dosing is the clinician's judgment of the patient's response to therapy.
• Potential drug interactions:

A number of the inhaled corticosteroids, including fluticasone, budesonide, and mometasone, are metabolized in the gastrointestinal tract and liver by CYP 3A4 isoenzymes. Potent inhibitors of CYP 3A4, such as ritonavir and ketoconazole, have the potential for increasing systemic concentrations of these inhaled corticosteroids by increasing oral availability and decreasing systemic clearance. Some cases of clinically significant Cushing syndrome and secondary adrenal insufficiency have been reported.

Adapted from National Asthma Education and Prevention Program. Expert Panel Report 3: Guidelines for the Diagnosis and Management of Asthma. National Institutes of Health Pub. No. 08-4051. Bethesda, MD, 2007. http://www.nhlbi.nih.gov/health-pro/guidelines/current/asthma-guidelines/

Table 4-5. Quick-relief medications for asthma.

Medication	Dosage Form	Adult Dose	Comments
Inhaled Short-Acting β_2-Agonists			
	MDI		
Albuterol CFC	90 µg /puff, 200 puffs/canister	2 puffs 5 min before exercise	• An increasing use or lack of expected effect indicates diminished control of asthma.
Albuterol HFA	90 µg /puff, 200 puffs/canister	2 puffs every 4–6 h as needed	• Not recommended for long-term daily treatment. Regular use exceeding 2 d/wk for symptom control (not prevention of EIB) indicates the need to step up therapy.
Pirbuterol CFC	200 µg /puff, 400 puffs/canister		• Differences in potency exist, but all products are essentially comparable on a per puff basis. • May double usual dose for mild exacerbations. • Should prime the inhaler by releasing four actuations prior to use.
Levalbuterol HFA	45 µg /puff, 200 puffs/canister		• Periodically clean HFA activator, as drug may block/plug orifice. • Nonselective agents (ie, epinephrine, isoproterenol, metaproterenol) are not recommended due to their potential for excessive cardiac stimulation, especially in high doses.
	Nebulizer solution		
Albuterol	0.63 mg/3 mL 1.25 mg/3 mL 2.5 mg/3 mL 5 mg/mL (0.5%)	1.25–5 mg in 3 mL of saline every 4–8 h as needed	• May mix with budesonide inhalant suspension, cromolyn or ipratropium nebulizer solutions. May double dose for severe exacerbations.
Levalbuterol (R-albuterol)	0.31 mg/3 mL 0.63 mg/3 mL 1.25 mg/0.5 mL 1.25 mg/3 mL	0.63 mg–1.25 mg every 8 h as needed	• Compatible with budesonide inhalant suspension. The product is a sterile-filled, preservative-free, unit dose vial.
Anticholinergics			
	MDI		
Ipratropium HFA	17 µg /puff, 200 puffs/canister	2–3 puffs every 6 h	• Evidence is lacking for anticholinergics producing added benefit to β_2-agonists in long-term control asthma therapy.
	Nebulizer solution		
	0.25 mg/mL (0.025%)	0.25 mg every 6 h	
	MDI		
Ipratropium with albuterol	18 µg /puff of ipratropium bromide and 90 µg /puff of albuterol 200 puffs/canister	2–3 puffs every 6 h	
	Nebulizer solution		
	0.5 mg/3 mL ipratropium bromide and 2.5 mg/3 mL albuterol	3 mL every 4–6 h	• Contains EDTA to prevent discolorations of the solution. This additive does not induce bronchospasm.
Systemic Corticosteroids			
Methylprednisolone	2, 4, 6, 8, 16, 32 mg tablets	Short course "burst": 40–60 mg/d as single or 2 divided doses for 3–10 d	• Short courses or "bursts" are effective for establishing control when initiating therapy or during a period of gradual deterioration. • The burst should be continued until symptoms resolve and the PEF is at least 80% of personal best. This usually requires 3–10 d but may require longer. There is no evidence that tapering the dose following improvements prevents relapse.
Prednisolone	5 mg tablets, 5 mg/5 mL, 15 mg/5 mL		
Prednisone	1, 2.5, 5, 10, 20, 50 mg tablets; 5 mg/mL, 5 mg/5 mL		
	Repository injection		
(Methylprednisolone acetate)	40 mg/mL 80 mg/mL	240 mg IM once	• May be used in place of a short burst of oral corticosteroids in patients who are vomiting or if adherence is a problem.

CFC, chlorofluorocarbon; EIB, exercise-induced bronchospasm; HFA, hydrofluoroalkane; IM, intramuscular; MDI, metered-dose inhaler; PEF, peak expiratory flow.

Adapted from National Asthma Education and Prevention Program. Expert Panel Report 3: Guidelines for the Diagnosis and Management of Asthma. National Institutes of Health Pub. No. 08-4051. Bethesda, MD, 2007. http://www.nhlbi.nih.gov/health-pro/guidelines/current/asthma-guidelines/

Table 4-6. Assessing asthma control.

	Components of Control	Classification of Asthma Control (> 12 y of age)		
		Well Controlled	**Not Well Controlled**	**Very Poorly Controlled**
Impairment	Symptoms	≤ 2 d/wk	> 2 d/wk	Throughout the day
	Nighttime awakenings	≤ 2×/mo	1–3×/wk	≥ 4×/wk
	Interference with normal activity	None	Some limitation	Extremely limited
	Short-acting β_2-agonist use for symptom control (not prevention of EIB)	≤ 2 d/wk	> 2 d/wk	Several times/d
	FEV_1 or peak flow	> 80% predicted/personal best	60%–80% predicted/personal best	< 60% predicted/personal best
	Validated questionnaires			
	ATAQ	0	1–2	3–4
	ACQ	≤ 0.75[a]	≥ 1.5	N/A
	ACT	≥ 20	16–19	≤ 15
Risk	Exacerbations requiring oral system corticosteroids	0–1/y	≥ 2/y (see Note)	
		Consider severity and interval since last exacerbation		
	Progressive loss of lung function	Evaluation requires long-term follow-up care		
	Treatment-related adverse effects	Medication side effects can vary in intensity from none to very troublesome and worrisome. The level of intensity does not correlate to specific levels of control but should be considered in the overall assessment of risk		
Recommended Action for Treatment		• Maintain current step • Regular follow-ups every 1–6 mo to maintain control. • Consider step down if well controlled for at least 3 mo	• Step up 1 step and • Reevaluate in 2–6 wk • For side effects, consider alternative treatment options	• Consider short course of oral systemic corticosteroids, • Step up 1–2 steps, and • Reevaluate in 2 wk • For side effects, consider alternative treatment options

EIB, exercise-induced bronchospasm; ICU, intensive care unit.

[a]ACQ values of 0.76–1.4 are indeterminate regarding well-controlled asthma.

Notes:
- The stepwise approach is meant to assist, not replace, the clinical decision making required to meet individual patient needs.
- The level of control is based on the most severe impairment or risk category. Assess impairment domain by patient's recall of previous 2–4 weeks and by spirometry or peak flow measures. Symptom assessment for longer periods should reflect a global assessment, such as inquiring whether the patient's asthma is better or worse since the last visit.
- At present, there are inadequate data to correspond frequencies of exacerbations with different levels of asthma control. In general, more frequent and intense exacerbations (eg, requiring urgent, unscheduled care, hospitalization, or ICU admission) indicate poorer disease control. For treatment purposes, patients who had ≥ 2 exacerbations requiring oral systemic corticosteroids in the past year may be considered the same as patients who have not-well-controlled asthma, even in the absence of impairment levels consistent with not-well-controlled asthma.
- Validated questionnaires for the impairment domain (the questionnaire did not assess lung function or the risk domain).
- ATAQ = Asthma Therapy Assessment Questionnaire©
- ACQ = Asthma Control Questionnaire© (user package may be obtained at www.qoltech.co.uk or juniper@qoltech.co.uk)
- ACT = Asthma Control Test™
- Minimal Importance Difference: 1.0 for the ATAQ; 0.5 for the ACQ; not determined for the ACT.
- Before step up in therapy:
  — Review adherence to medication, inhaler
  — If an alternative treatment option was used in a step, discontinue and use the preferred treatment for that step.

Adapted from National Asthma Education and Prevention Program. Expert Panel Report 3: Guidelines for the Diagnosis and Management of Asthma. National Institutes of Health Pub. No. 08-4051. Bethesda, MD, 2007. http://www.nhlbi.nih.gov/health-pro/guidelines/current/asthma-guidelines/.

Chronic Asthma
- Treatment is guided by an assessment of asthma severity (Table 4-6)
- Mild intermittent asthma treatment
  — Short-acting β_2-agonists
  — Control therapy added if > 2 uses/wk
- Mild persistent asthma treatment
  — Daily use of either low-dose inhaled corticosteroid **or** cromolyn or nedocromil
  — Sustained-release theophylline or a leukotriene modifier is less desirable
  — Short-acting β_2-agonists

- Moderate persistent asthma treatment
  — Daily use of medium-dose **or** low-to-medium-dose inhaled corticosteroid with long-acting inhaled β_2-agonist
  — Daily use of long-acting inhaled β_2-agonist **or** sustained-release theophylline or long-acting β_2-agonist tablets
  — Short-acting β_2-agonists
- Severe persistent asthma treatment
  — Daily use of high-dose inhaled corticosteroid **and** long-acting bronchodilator or sustained-release theophylline or long-acting β_2-agonist tablets
  — Daily use of systemic corticosteroids
  — Short-acting β_2-agonists

Therapeutic Procedures
- Desensitization to specific allergens
- Intubation and mechanical ventilation for patients with impending respiratory failure; permissive hypercapnia to limit airway pressures

8. Outcomes

Follow-Up
- Patient self-assessment is a primary method of monitoring
- PEFR monitoring can provide objective measurement to guide treatment
  — A 20% change in PEFR from day to day or from morning to night suggests inadequate control
  — PEFR < 200 L/min indicates severe obstruction
- Follow-up visits should be at least biannual to maintain control and evaluate medication adjustments
- Repeat spirometry at least every 1 to 2 years after symptoms have stabilized

Complications
- Exhaustion, dehydration, and tussive syncope
- Airway infection
- Acute hypercapnic and hypoxic respiratory failure in severe disease
- Pneumothorax (rare)

Prognosis
- Good with regular follow-up and care

Prevention
- Patients should be taught to recognize early symptoms of an exacerbation and initiate a predetermined action plan
- Pneumococcal and annual influenza vaccinations
- Environmental measures to reduce exposure to allergens

9. When to Refer and When to Admit

When to Refer
- Atypical presentation or uncertain diagnosis of asthma, particularly if additional diagnostic testing is required (bronchoprovocation challenge, allergic skin testing, rhinoscopy, consideration of occupational exposure)
- Complicating comorbid problems, such as rhinosinusitis, tobacco use, multiple environmental allergies, suspected allergic bronchopulmonary mycosis
- Suboptimal response to therapy
- Patient not meeting goals of asthma therapy after 3 to 6 months of treatment
- Requires high-dose inhaled corticosteroids for control
- More than two courses of oral prednisone therapy in the past 12 months

- Any life-threatening asthma exacerbation or exacerbation requiring hospitalization in the past 12 months
- Presence of social or psychological issues interfering with asthma management

When to Admit
- Patients with acute exacerbations who have an inadequate response to initial therapy
- The duration and severity of symptoms, as well as severity of prior exacerbations and psychosocial issues, should be taken into account

SUGGESTED REFERENCES

Gibson PG et al. Asthma in older adults. *Lancet.* 2010 Sep 4;376(9743):803–813. [PMID: 20816547]

Hopkin JM. The diagnosis of asthma, a clinical syndrome. *Thorax.* 2012 Jul;67(7):660–662. [PMID: 22561527]

Lazarus SC. Clinical practice. Emergency treatment of asthma. *N Engl J Med.* 2010 Aug19;363(8): 755–764. [PMID: 20818877]

Mannam P et al. Analytic review: management of life-threatening asthma in adults. *J Intensive Care Med.* 2010 Jan–Feb;25(1):3–15. [PMID: 20085924]

National Asthma Education and Prevention Program: Expert panel report III: Guidelines for the diagnosis and management of asthma. Bethesda, MD: National Heart, Lung, and Blood Institute, 2007. (NIH publication No. 08-4051). http://www.nhlbi.nih.gov/guidelines/asthma/asthgdln.htm

Chronic Obstructive Pulmonary Disease

5

A 72-year-old man with chronic obstructive pulmonary disease (COPD) presents to the emergency department with progressively worsening shortness of breath. He usually uses 2 L/min of oxygen at home and is able to walk around the house without limitation, but over the past 4 days he has had increasing dyspnea on exertion. He has also noticed an increase in his chronic cough, which is once again productive of thick green sputum. He has not noted any chest pain or worsening of his chronic, mild ankle edema. He has smoked two packs of cigarettes daily for the past 50 years. Previous pulmonary function tests demonstrated a decreased FEV_1 and FEV_1/FVC ratio. On physical examination, he is tachycardic, has a respiratory rate of 28 breaths/min, and has bilaterally decreased breath sounds with diffuse wheezing. His arterial blood gas (ABG) measurement shows acidemia from a partially compensated respiratory acidosis. He is placed on noninvasive positive pressure ventilation with marked improvement of his acidemia.

LEARNING OBJECTIVES

▶ Learn the clinical manifestations and objective findings of chronic obstructive pulmonary disease, and what distinguishes chronic bronchitis from emphysema

▶ Understand the factors that predispose to chronic obstructive pulmonary disease

▶ Know the differential diagnosis of chronic obstructive pulmonary disease

▶ Recognize the spirometric and ABG findings suggestive of chronic obstructive pulmonary disease

▶ Learn the treatments that decrease mortality and control the symptoms of chronic obstructive pulmonary disease

QUESTIONS

1. What are the salient features of this patient's problem?

2. How do you think through his problem?

3. What are the key features, including essentials of diagnosis and general considerations, of chronic obstructive pulmonary disease?

4. What are the symptoms and signs of chronic obstructive pulmonary disease?

5. What is the differential diagnosis of chronic obstructive pulmonary disease?

6. What are laboratory and imaging findings in chronic obstructive pulmonary disease?

7. What are the treatments for chronic obstructive pulmonary disease?

8. What are the outcomes, including complications, prevention, and prognosis, of chronic obstructive pulmonary disease?

9. When should patients with chronic obstructive pulmonary disease be referred to a specialist or admitted to the hospital?

ANSWERS

1. Salient Features

Increasing dyspnea on exertion; change in cough and sputum; home oxygen requirement; 100-pack-year smoking history; obstructive pattern on spirometry; wheezing and respiratory distress; stable, not worsened lower extremity edema; acidemia with partially compensated respiratory acidosis; improvement on noninvasive positive pressure ventilation

2. How to Think Through

This patient with COPD presents in distress with a respiratory rate of 28 breaths/min. With a home oxygen requirement at baseline, he has little pulmonary reserve, and prompt management is needed. What test will be most instructive in assessing the severity of his pulmonary problem? (ABGs.) He has a component of acute respiratory acidosis on his ABGs and noninvasive positive pressure ventilation is appropriately initiated. What other diagnoses can exacerbate COPD or mimic a COPD exacerbation? (Community-acquired pneumonia, pulmonary embolism, heart failure, pneumothorax, and acute coronary syndrome.)

In addition to ventilatory support, what are the treatment priorities? (Corticosteroid, inhaled β-agonist, inhaled anticholinergic agents.) Are intravenous corticosteroids more effective? What clinical developments would necessitate transition to endotrachial intubation? (Altered mental status, failure to decrease $Paco_2$.)

Once the patient has recovered to baseline, what therapies are known to decrease COPD exacerbations? (Smoking cessation is the most important intervention. Inhaled corticosteroids, vaccinations for influenza, and pneumococcal pneumonia.) Are there medical therapies known to decrease mortality? (Home oxygen therapy.)

3. Key Features

Essentials of Diagnosis
• History of cigarette smoking
• Chronic cough, dyspnea, and sputum production
• Rhonchi, decreased intensity of breath sounds, and prolonged expiration on physical examination
• Airflow limitation on pulmonary function testing

General Considerations
• Airflow obstruction due to chronic bronchitis or emphysema; most patients have features of both
• Obstruction
  — Is progressive
  — May be accompanied by airway hyperreactivity
  — May be partially reversible
• Chronic bronchitis is characterized by excessive mucous secretions with productive cough for 3 months or more in at least 2 consecutive years
• Emphysema is abnormal enlargement of air spaces distal to terminal bronchiole, with destruction of bronchial walls without fibrosis

- Cigarette smoking is the most important cause
  — About 80% of patients have had a significant exposure to tobacco smoke
- Air pollution, airway infection, familial factors, and allergy have been implicated in chronic bronchitis
- α_1-Antiprotease deficiency has been implicated in emphysema

4. Symptoms and Signs

- Presentation
  — Usually at 40 to 50 years of age
  — Cough
  — Sputum production
  — Shortness of breath
- Dyspnea initially occurs only with heavy exertion, progressing to symptoms at rest in severe disease
- Exacerbation of symptoms beyond normal day-to-day variation, often including increased dyspnea, an increased frequency or severity of cough, increased sputum volume, or change in sputum character
- Infections (viral more commonly than bacterial) precede exacerbations in most patients
- Late-stage COPD characterized by
  — Hypoxemia
  — Pneumonia
  — Pulmonary hypertension
  — Cor pulmonale
  — Respiratory failure
- Clinical findings may be absent early
- Patients are often dichotomized as "pink puffers" or "blue bloaters" depending on whether emphysema or chronic bronchitis predominates (Table 5-1)

5. Differential Diagnosis

- Asthma
- Bronchiectasis, which features recurrent pneumonia and hemoptysis, with distinct radiographic findings
- Bronchopulmonary mycosis
- Central airflow obstruction
- Severe α_1-antiprotease deficiency
- Cystic fibrosis, which is usually first seen in children and young adults

6. Laboratory and Imaging Findings

Laboratory Tests

- Sputum examination may reveal
  — *Streptococcus pneumoniae*
  — *Haemophilus influenzae*
  — *Moraxella catarrhalis*
  — Cultures correlate poorly with exacerbations
- ECG shows sinus tachycardia, abnormalities consistent with cor pulmonale in severe disease, and/or supraventricular tachycardias and ventricular irritability
- ABGs
  — Unnecessary unless: hypoxemia or hypercapnia is suspected
  — An increased A–a D_{O_2} in early disease
  — Compensated respiratory acidosis with worsening acidemia during exacerbations
  — Hypoxemia in advanced disease
- Spirometry
  — Objectively measures pulmonary function and assesses severity
  — Early changes are reductions in midexpiratory flow and abnormal closing volumes

Table 5-1. Patterns of disease in advanced COPD.

	Type A: Pink Puffer (Emphysema Predominant)	Type B: Blue Bloater (Bronchitis Predominant)
History and physical examination	Major complaint is dyspnea, often severe, usually presenting after age 50. Cough is rare, with scant clear, mucoid sputum. Patients are thin, with recent weight loss common. They appear uncomfortable, with evident use of accessory muscles of respiration. Chest is very quiet without adventitious sounds. No peripheral edema.	Major complaint is chronic cough, productive of mucopurulent sputum, with frequent exacerbations due to chest infections. Often presents in late 30s and 40s. Dyspnea usually mild, though patients may note limitations to exercise. Patients frequently overweight and cyanotic but seem comfortable at rest. Peripheral edema is common. Chest is noisy, with rhonchi invariably present; wheezes are common.
Laboratory studies	Hemoglobin usually normal (12–15 g/dL). Pao_2 normal to slightly reduced (65–75 mm Hg) but Sao_2 normal at rest. $Paco_2$ normal to slightly reduced (35–40 mm Hg). Chest radiograph shows hyperinflation with flattened diaphragms. Vascular markings are diminished, particularly at the apices.	Hemoglobin usually elevated (15–18 g/dL). Pao_2 reduced (45–60 mm Hg) and $Paco_2$ slightly to markedly elevated (50–60 mm Hg). Chest radiograph shows increased interstitial markings ("dirty lungs"), especially at bases. Diaphragms are not flattened.
Pulmonary function tests	Airflow obstruction ubiquitous. Total lung capacity increased, sometimes markedly so. D_{LCO} reduced. Static lung compliance increased.	Airflow obstruction ubiquitous. Total lung capacity generally normal but may be slightly increased. D_{LCO} normal. Static lung compliance normal.
Special Evaluations		
$\dot{V}/\dot{Q}$ matching	Increased ventilation to high $\dot{V}/\dot{Q}$ areas, ie, high dead space ventilation.	Increased perfusion to low $\dot{V}/\dot{Q}$ areas.
Hemodynamics	Cardiac output normal to slightly low. Pulmonary artery pressures mildly elevated and increase with exercise.	Cardiac output normal. Pulmonary artery pressures elevated, sometimes markedly so, and worsen with exercise.
Nocturnal ventilation	Mild-to-moderate degree of oxygen desaturation not usually associated with obstructive sleep apnea.	Severe oxygen desaturation, frequently associated with obstructive sleep apnea.
Exercise ventilation	Increased minute ventilation for level of oxygen consumption. Pao_2 tends to fall; $Paco_2$ rises slightly.	Decreased minute ventilation for level of oxygen consumption. Pao_2 may rise; $Paco_2$ may rise significantly.

D_{LCO}, single-breath diffusing capacity for carbon monoxide; $\dot{V}/\dot{Q}$, ventilation-perfusion.

— FEV_1 and FEV_1/FVC are reduced later in the disease
— FVC is reduced in severe disease
— Lung volume measurements show an increase in total lung capacity (TLC), residual volume (RV), and an elevation of RV/TLC indicating air trapping
• Obtaining an α_1-antiprotease level may reveal a deficiency in a young patient with emphysema

Imaging Studies
• Radiographs of patients with chronic bronchitis typically show only nonspecific peribronchial and perivascular markings
• Plain radiographs are insensitive for the diagnosis of emphysema; they show hyperinflation with flattening of the diaphragm or peripheral arterial deficiency in about half of cases
• In advanced disease, radiographs that show enlarged central pulmonary arteries may indicate pulmonary hypertension
• Computed tomography (CT) of the chest is more sensitive and specific than plain radiographs for the diagnosis of emphysema
• Doppler echocardiography provides a noninvasive estimate pulmonary artery pressure

7. Treatments
Medications
• Supplemental oxygen
— Hypoxemic patients with pulmonary hypertension, chronic cor pulmonale, erythrocytosis, impaired cognitive function, exercise intolerance, nocturnal restlessness, or morning headache are likely to benefit from home oxygen therapy
— Benefits of home oxygen therapy in patients with hypoxemia include longer survival, reduced hospitalizations, and better quality of life
— Unless therapy is intended only for nighttime or exercise use, 15 hours of nasal oxygen per day is required

Table 5-2. Home oxygen therapy: requirements for Medicare coverage.[a]

Group I (Any of the Following):

1. $Pao_2 \leq 55$ mm Hg or $Sao_2 \leq 88\%$ taken while awake, at rest, breathing room air

2. During sleep (prescription for nocturnal oxygen use only):

    a. $Pao_2 \leq 55$ mm Hg or $Sao_2 \leq 88\%$ for a patient whose awake, resting, room air Pao_2 is ≥ 56 mm Hg or $Sao_2 \geq 89\%$

    or

    b. Decrease in $Pao_2 > 10$ mm Hg or decrease in $Sao_2 > 5\%$ associated with symptoms or signs reasonably attributed to hypoxemia (eg, impaired cognitive processes, nocturnal restlessness, insomnia)

3. During exercise (prescription for oxygen use only during exercise):

    a. $Pao_2 \leq 55$ mg Hg or $Sao_2 \leq 88\%$ taken during exercise for a patient whose awake, resting, room air Pao_2 is ≥ 56 mm Hg or $Sao_2 \geq 89\%$

    and

    b. There is evidence that the use of supplemental oxygen during exercise improves the hypoxemia that was demonstrated during exercise while breathing room air

Group II[b]:

$Pao_2 = 56{-}59$ mm Hg or $Sao_2 = 89\%$ if there is evidence of any of the following:

1. Dependent edema suggesting heart failure

2. P pulmonale on ECG (P wave > 3 mm in standard leads II, III, or aVF)

3. Hematocrit > 56%

[a]Centers for Medicare & Medicaid Services, 2003.

[b]Patients in this group must have a second oxygen test 3 mo after the initial oxygen setup.

— For most patients, a flow rate of 1 to 3 L achieves a $Pao_2 > 55$ mm Hg
— Medicare covers 80% of costs for patients who meet requirements (Table 5-2)
• Bronchodilators do not alter lung decline that is hallmark of the disease, but they do offer many patients an improvement in symptoms, exercise tolerance, and overall health (Table 5-3)
— Ipratropium bromide (2 to 4 puffs via metered dose inhaler every 6 hours) is first-line therapy because it is longer-acting and without sympathomimetic side effects
— Short-acting β_2-agonists (albuterol, metaproterenol) have a shorter onset of action and are less expensive
— At maximal doses, bronchodilation produced by β-agonists is equivalent to ipratropium, but with side effects of tremor, tachycardia, and hypokalemia
— Ipratropium and β_2-agonists together are more effective than either alone
— Long-acting β_2-agonists (formoterol, salmeterol, indacaterol, arformoterol, vilanterol) and anticholinergics (tiotropium, aclidinium, and umeclidinium) appear to achieve bronchodilation that is equivalent or superior to what is experienced with ipratropium, in addition to similar improvements on health status
• Oral theophylline is a third-line agent for patients who do not respond to ipratropium or β_2-agonists
• Corticosteroids
— COPD is generally not steroid-responsive; 10% to 20% of stable outpatients have a > 20% increase in FEV_1 compared with placebo
• Antibiotics improve outcomes slightly, when used to treat acute exacerbations, acute bronchitis, and to prevent acute exacerbations of chronic bronchitis
— Doxycycline (100 mg every 12 hours)
— Trimethoprim-sulfamethoxazole (160/800 mg every 12 hours)
— Cephalosporins (cefpodoxime 200 mg every 12 hours; cefprozil 500 mg every 12 hours)
— Macrolides (azithromycin 500 mg followed by 250 mg daily for 5 days)
— Fluoroquinolones (ciprofloxacin 500 mg every 12 hours)
— Amoxicillin-clavulanate (875/125 mg every 12 hours)

Table 5-3. Bronchodilator and anticholinergic medications for COPD.

Medication	Dosage Form	Adult Dose	Comments
Inhaled Long-Acting β_2-Agonists			**Should not be used for symptom relief or exacerbations.**
Salmeterol	DPI 50 µg/blister	1 blister every 12 h	• Decreased duration of protection against EIB may occur with regular use.
Formoterol	DPI 12 µg/single-use capsule	1 capsule every 12 h	• Decreased duration of protection against EIB may occur with regular use.
			• Each capsule is for single use only; additional doses should not be administered for at least 12 h.
			• Capsules should be used only with the Aerolizor™ inhaler and should not be taken orally.
Inhaled Short-Acting β_2-Agonists			
	MDI		
Albuterol CFC	90 µg/puff, 200 puffs/canister	2 puffs 5 min before exercise	• An increasing use or lack of expected effect indicates diminished control of COPD.
Albuterol HFA	90 µg/puff, 200 puffs/canister	2 puffs every 4–6 h as needed	• Not recommended for long-term daily treatment. Regular use exceeding 2 d/wk for symptom control (not prevention of EIB) indicates the need to step up therapy.
			• Differences in potency exist, but all products are essentially comparable on a per puff basis.
Pirbuterol CFC	200 µg/puff, 400 puffs/canister		• May double usual dose for mild exacerbations.
			• Should prime the inhaler by releasing four actuations prior to use.
Levalbuterol HFA	45 µg/puff, 200 puffs/canister		• Periodically clean HFA activator, as drug may block/plug orifice.
	Nebulizer Solution		• Nonselective agents (ie, epinephrine, isoproterenol, metaproterenol) are not recommended due to their potential for excessive cardiac stimulation, especially in high doses.
Albuterol	0.63 mg/3 mL 1.25 mg/3 mL 2.5 mg/3 mL 5 mg/mL (0.5%)	1.25–5 mg in 3 mL of saline every 4–8 h as needed	• May mix with budesonide inhalant suspension, cromolyn, or ipratropium nebulizer solutions. May double dose for severe exacerbations.
Levalbuterol (R-albuterol)	0.31 mg/3 mL 0.63 mg/3 mL 1.25 mg/0.5 mL 1.25 mg/3 mL	0.63 mg–1.25 mg every 8 h as needed	• Compatible with budesonide inhalant suspension. The product is a sterile-filled, preservative-free, unit dose vial.
Anticholinergics			**Should not be used for symptom relief or exacerbations. Use with inhaled corticosteroids.**
Tiotropium	DPI 18 µg/blister	1 blister daily	
Ipratropium HFA			
	MDI		
	17 µg/puff, 200 puffs/canister	2–3 puffs every 6 h	
	Nebulizer Solution		
	0.25 mg/mL (0.025%)	0.25 mg every 6 h	
Ipratropium with albuterol			
	MDI		
	18 µg/puff of ipratropium bromide and 90 µg/puff of albuterol 200 puffs/canister	2–3 puffs every 6 h	
	Nebulizer solution		
	0.5 mg/3 mL ipratropium bromide and 2.5 mg/3 mL albuterol	3 mL every 4–6 h	• Contains EDTA to prevent discolorations of the solution. This additive does not induce bronchospasm.
Methylxanthines			
Theophylline	Liquids, sustained-release tablets, and capsules	Starting dose 10 mg/kg/d up to 300 mg maximum; usual maximum dose 800 mg/d	• Adjust dosage to achieve serum concentration of 5–15 µg/mL at steady-state (at least 48 h on same dosage) • Due to wide interpatient variability in theophylline metabolic clearance, routine serum theophylline level monitoring is important.

EDTA, ethylenediaminetetraacetic acid; EIB, exercise-induced bronchospasm; HFA, hydrofluoroalkane; MDI, metered dose inhaler.

Adapted from National Asthma Education and Prevention Program. Expert Panel Report 3: Guidelines for the Diagnosis and Management of Asthma. National Institutes of Health Pub. No. 08-4051. Bethesda, MD, 2007. http://www.nhlbi.nih.gov/health-pro/guidelines/current/asthma-guidelines/.

— In patients subject to frequent exacerbations despite optimal medical therapy, azithromycin (daily or thrice weekly) and moxifloxacin (a 5-day course 1 week in 8 over 48 weeks) were modestly effective in clinical trials at reducing the frequency of exacerbations
- Opioids: severe dyspnea in spite of optimal management may warrant a trial of an opioid (eg, morphine 5 to 10 mg orally every 3 to 4 hours, oxycodone 5 to 10 mg orally every 4 to 6 hours, sustained-release morphine 10 mg orally once daily)
- Sedative-hypnotic drugs (diazepam 5 mg three times daily orally) may benefit very anxious patients with intractable dyspnea

Surgery
- Lung transplantation offers substantial improvement in pulmonary function and exercise performance; 2-year survival is 75%
- Lung volume reduction surgery in highly selected patients results in modest improvements in pulmonary function, exercise performance, and dyspnea; surgical mortality rates at experienced centers are 4% to 10%
- Bullectomy is used for palliation of dyspnea in patients with severe bullous emphysema; most commonly pursued when a single bulla occupies at least 30% to 50% of the hemithorax

Therapeutic Procedures
- Smoking cessation is the single most important goal
- Simply telling a patient to quit succeeds 5% of the time
- Behavioral approaches, ranging from clinician advice to intensive group programs, may improve cessation rates
- Pharmacologic therapy includes bupropion, nicotine replacement (transdermal patch, gum, lozenge, inhaler, or nasal spray), varenicline (a partial agonist of nicotinic acetylcholine receptors), and cytosine
- One trial showed electronic cigarettes to be noninferior to nicotine transdermal patches, though most pulmonologists do not recommend electronic cigarettes as a tobacco cessation aid
- Cough suppressants and sedatives should be avoided as routine measures
- Graded physical exercise programs
- Measure theophylline levels in hospitalized patients who have already been taking theophylline; it should not be started in the acute setting
- Noninvasive positive pressure ventilation
  — Reduces the need for intubation
  — Shortens ICU lengths of stay
  — May reduce the risk of health care-associated infection and antibiotic use

8. Outcomes

Complications
- Otherwise stable COPD may be made worse by
- Acute bronchitis
- Pneumonia
- Pulmonary thromboembolism
- Atrial dysrhythmias, such as atrial fibrillation, atrial flutter, and multifocal atrial tachycardia
- Concomitant left ventricular failure
- Pulmonary hypertension, cor pulmonale, and chronic respiratory failure are common in advanced disease
- Spontaneous pneumothorax occurs in a small fraction of emphysematous patients
- Hemoptysis may result from chronic bronchitis or bronchogenic carcinoma

Prevention
- Largely preventable by eliminating chronic exposure to tobacco smoke
- Smoking cessation slows the decline in FEV_1 in middle-age smokers with mild airways obstruction
- Vaccinations against influenza and pneumococcal infection

Prognosis

- Median survival of patients with $FEV_1 < 1$ L is 4 years
- Degree of dysfunction at presentation is the most important predictor of survival
- A multidimensional index (the BODE index), which includes body mass index (BMI), airway obstruction (FEV_1), dyspnea (Medical Research Council dyspnea score), and exercise capacity, predicts death and hospitalization better than FEV_1 alone

9. When to Refer and When to Admit

When to Refer

- COPD onset occurs before the age of 40
- Frequent exacerbations (2 or more a year) despite optimal treatment
- Severe or rapidly progressive COPD
- Symptoms disproportionate to the severity of airflow obstruction
- Need for long-term oxygen therapy
- Onset of comorbid illnesses (such as bronchiectasis, heart failure, or lung cancer)

When to Admit

- Severe symptoms or acute worsening that fails to respond to outpatient management
- Acute or worsening hypoxemia, hypercapnia, peripheral edema, or change in mental status
- Inadequate home care, or inability to sleep or maintain nutrition/hydration due to symptoms
- The presence of high-risk comorbid conditions

SUGGESTED REFERENCES

Leuppi JD et al. Short-term vs conventional glucocorticoid therapy in acute exacerbations of chronic obstructive pulmonary disease: the REDUCE randomized clinical trial. *JAMA*. 2013 Jun 5;309(21):2223–2231. [PMID: 23695200]

Qaseem A et al. Diagnosis and management of stable chronic obstructive pulmonary disease: a clinical practice guideline update from the American College of Physicians, American College of Chest Physicians, American Thoracic Society, and European Respiratory Society. *Ann Intern Med*. 2011 Aug 2;155(3):179–191. [PMID: 21810710]

Torpy JM et al. JAMA patient page. Chronic obstructive pulmonary disease. *JAMA*. 2012 Sep 26;308(12):1281. [PMID: 23011720]

Walker N et al. Cytisine versus nicotine for smoking cessation. *N Engl J Med*. 2014 Dec 18;371(25):2353–2362. [PMID: 25517706]

Walters JA et al. Systemic corticosteroids for acute exacerbations of chronic obstructive pulmonary disease. *Cochrane Database Syst Rev*. 2009 Jan 21;(1):CD001288. [PMID: 19160195]

Cough

6

A 32-year-old man presents to the urgent care clinic with 4 weeks of cough. He describes a recent illness that coincided with the onset of his cough in which he had nasal congestion, sore throat, fatigue, and myalgias. His other symptoms have since subsided, but his cough has continued. He denies any shortness of breath, fevers, or weight loss. He does not smoke cigarettes or use any illicit drugs. His vital signs are normal and his physical examination does not reveal any abnormalities.

LEARNING OBJECTIVES

▶ Learn the classification of cough
▶ Learn the clinical manifestations and objective findings that help differentiate the causes of cough
▶ Recognize when to pursue imaging and other diagnostic procedures in patients with cough
▶ Know the pulmonary and nonpulmonary causes of both acute and persistent cough
▶ Learn the treatments for the common causes of cough

QUESTIONS

1. What are the salient features of this patient's problem?
2. How do you think through his problem?
3. What are the key features, including essentials of diagnosis and general considerations, of cough?
4. What are the symptoms and signs of cough?
5. What is the differential diagnosis of cough?
6. What are laboratory, imaging, and procedural findings in cough?
7. What are the treatments for cough?
8. When should patients with cough be referred to a specialist or admitted to the hospital?

ANSWERS

1. Salient Features

Four week time course; recent viral illness with resolution of all symptoms except cough; no shortness of breath, fevers, weight loss; nonsmoker; normal vital signs and physical examination

2. How to Think Through

Cough is common and usually benign, but can be the presenting symptom of several serious illnesses. First, consider whether the patient has risk factors for a serious underlying cause of his cough. (Here, apparently none: he is young and a nonsmoker and has no reported chronic medical problems, immune deficiency, or recent travel.) Next, think through the serious causes of cough that one must never overlook. What features reassure us that he does not have pneumonia? (Absence of sputum, pleuritic chest pain, dyspnea, fever, hypoxia, tachycardia, or lung examination findings, eg, rales or egophony.) What features reassure us that he does not have cancer? (Absence of risk factors, weight loss, or hemoptysis.) What reassures us that he does not have tuberculosis? Restrictive lung disease, eg, interstitial lung disease? Cardiac disease? Next, consider the most likely diagnoses for the case. Does a duration of 4 weeks qualify as acute, subacute, or chronic cough? (Subacute.) Are there infectious etiologies that fit with this presentation? (Pertussis.) What is the most likely etiology? (Postinfectious bronchospasm, [or virus-induced wheezing], is common; a minimally productive cough persists for several weeks despite resolution of all other symptoms.)

How should he be counseled and treated? (The patient should be reassured that prolonged cough following a viral URI is common; bronchodilator therapy is effective for symptom control.) If his cough persists, what additional risk factor information should be gathered? (Explicit travel history, asthma history, occupational or other exposures, HIV risk factors.)

3. Key Features

Essentials of Diagnosis
- Inquire about
  — Age
  — Duration of cough
  — Dyspnea (at rest or with exertion)
  — Tobacco use history
- Vital signs (temperature, respiratory rate, heart rate)
- Chest examination findings

General Considerations
- Cough results from stimulation of mechanical or chemical afferent nerve receptors in the bronchial tree
- Cough illness syndromes are defined as acute (< 3 weeks), persistent (3–8 weeks), or chronic (> 8 weeks)
- Postinfectious cough lasting 3 to 8 weeks also called "subacute cough" to distinguish this distinct clinical entity from acute and chronic cough
- The prevalence of pertussis infection in adults with a cough lasting > 3 weeks is 20%, although exact prevalence is difficult to ascertain due to the limited sensitivity of diagnostic tests

4. Symptoms and Signs

Symptoms
- Timing and character of cough are usually not useful in establishing cause

- However, cough-variant asthma should be considered in adults with prominent nocturnal cough, and persistent cough with phlegm increases the patient's likelihood of chronic obstructive pulmonary disease (COPD)
- Acute cough syndromes
  — Most due to viral respiratory tract infections
  — Presence of post-tussive emesis or inspiratory whoop modestly increases the likelihood of pertussis, and absence of paroxysmal cough decreases the likelihood of pertussis in adolescents and adults with cough lasting > 1 week
  — Less common causes include heart failure (HF), hay fever (allergic rhinitis), and environmental factors
- Search for additional features of infection such as fever, nasal congestion, and sore throat
- Dyspnea (at rest or with exertion) may reflect a more serious condition
- Persistent cough is usually due to
  — Postnasal drip
  — Asthma
  — Gastroesophageal reflux disease (GERD)
  — Angiotensin-converting enzyme (ACE) inhibitor therapy
- Less common causes of persistent cough
  — Bronchogenic carcinoma
  — Chronic bronchitis
  — Bronchiectasis
  — Other chronic lung disease
  — HF
  — Pertussis infection, especially in adolescents and in selected geographic areas

Signs
- Signs of pneumonia
  — Tachycardia
  — Tachypnea
  — Fever
  — Rales
  — Decreased breath sounds
  — Fremitus
  — Egophony
- Signs of acute bronchitis: wheezing and rhonchi
- Signs of chronic sinusitis: postnasal drip, sore throat, facial pain
- Signs of COPD
  — Cough with phlegm production
  — Abnormal match test (inability to blow out a match from 10 inches away)
  — Maximum laryngeal height < 4 cm (measured from the sternal notch to the cricoid cartilage at end expiration)
- Signs of HF
  — Symmetric basilar rales
  — Elevated jugular venous pressure
  — Positive hepatojugular reflux

5. Differential Diagnosis

Acute Cough
- Viral upper respiratory infection or postviral infection cough (most common)
- Postnasal drip (allergic rhinitis)
- Pneumonia
- Pulmonary edema
- Pulmonary embolism
- Aspiration pneumonia

Persistent Cough
- Top three causes: postnasal drip, asthma, GERD
- Pulmonary infection
  — Postviral
  — Pertussis
  — Bronchiectasis
  — Eosinophilic bronchitis
  — Tuberculosis
  — Cystic fibrosis
  — *Mycobacterium avium* complex
  — *Mycoplasma, Chlamydia,* respiratory syncytial virus (underrecognized in adults)
- Pulmonary noninfectious
  — Asthma (cough-variant asthma)
  — COPD
  — ACE inhibitors
  — Environmental exposures (eg, cigarette smoking, air pollution)
  — Endobronchial lesion (eg, tumor)
  — Interstitial lung disease
  — Sarcoidosis
  — Chronic microaspiration
  — β-blockers causing asthma
- Nonpulmonary
  — GERD
  — Postnasal drip (allergic rhinitis)
  — Sinusitis
  — HF
  — Laryngitis
  — Ear canal or tympanic membrane irritation
  — Psychogenic or habit cough

6. Laboratory, Imaging, and Procedural Findings

Laboratory Tests
- Pulse oximetry or arterial blood gas measurement
- Peak expiratory flow rate or spirometry
- Serum C-reactive protein levels > 30 mg/dL likely improve diagnostic accuracy for pneumonia in adults with acute cough

Imaging Studies
- Acute cough: obtain chest radiograph if abnormal vital signs or chest examination; higher index of suspicion in elderly and immunocompromised persons
- Persistent or chronic cough: obtain chest radiograph if unexplained cough lasts > 3 to 8 weeks

Diagnostic Procedures
- Sinus CT scan for cough with postnasal drip
- Spirometry (if normal, possible methacholine challenge) for cough with wheezing or possible asthma, though pulmonary function tests are often normal in cough-variant asthma
- Esophageal pH monitoring for cough with GERD symptoms
- See Table 6-1
- Procedures should be reserved for patients with persistent cough who do not respond to therapeutic trials
- Pertussis detection by culture and polymerase chain reaction of nasopharyngeal swab

Table 6–1. Empiric treatments or tests for persistent cough.

Suspected Condition	Step 1 (Empiric Therapy)	Step 2 (Diagnostic Testing)
Postnasal drip	Therapy for allergy or chronic sinusitis	ENT referral; sinus CT scan
Asthma	β_2-agonist	Spirometry; consider methacholine challenge if normal
GERD	Proton-pump inhibitors	Esophageal pH monitoring

ENT, ear, nose, and throat; GERD, gastroesophageal reflux disease.

7. Treatments

Medications

Acute Cough

- Treatment should target
  — The underlying cause of the illness
  — The cough reflex itself
  — Any additional factors that exacerbate the cough
- Oseltamivir and zanamivir are equally effective (1 less day of illness) when initiated within 30 to 48 hours of onset of influenza
- Macrolide or doxycycline are first-line antibiotics for documented *Chlamydia* or *Mycoplasma* infection
- In patients diagnosed with acute bronchitis, inhaled β_2-agonist therapy reduces severity and duration of cough in some patients; antibiotics do not improve cough severity or duration in acute uncomplicated bronchitis
- Dextromethorphan has a modest benefit on the severity of cough due to acute respiratory tract infections
- Empiric treatment trial for postnasal drip (with antihistamines, decongestants, and/or nasal steroids) or asthma (with β2-agonist) or GERD (with proton-pump inhibitors [or H2-blockers]), when accompanying acute cough illness, can also be helpful
- Zinc lozenges > 75 mg/d, when initiated within 24 hours of symptom onset, may reduce the duration and severity of cold symptoms
- Vitamin C and echinacea are not effective in reducing the severity of acute cough illness after it develops

Persistent Cough

- If due to pertussis, macrolide antibiotic therapy to reduce transmission
  — Azithromycin, 500 mg on day 1, then 250 mg once daily for days 2 to 5
  — Clarithromycin, 500 mg twice daily for 7 days
  — Erythromycin, 250 mg four times daily for 14 days
- When pertussis infection has lasted > 7 to 10 days, antibiotic treatment does not affect the duration of cough—which can last up to 6 months
- Nebulized lidocaine therapy or oral codeine (15–60 mg orally 4 times daily) or morphine sulfate (5–10 mg orally twice daily) for idiopathic persistent cough

8. When to Refer and When to Admit

When to Refer

- Failure to control persistent cough following empiric treatment trials.
- Patients with recurrent symptoms should be referred to an otolaryngologist or a pulmonologist
- Adults needing Tdap vaccination to enable "cocooning" of at-risk individuals (eg, infants age < 1 year)

When to Admit

- Patient at high risk for tuberculosis for whom compliance with respiratory precautions is uncertain
- Need for urgent bronchoscopy, such as suspected foreign body
- Smoke or toxic fume inhalational injury
- Intractable cough despite treatment, when cough impairs gas exchange or in patients at high risk for barotraumas (eg, recent pneumothorax)

SUGGESTED REFERENCES

Benich JJ 3rd, et al. Evaluation of the patient with chronic cough. *Am Fam Physician*. 2011 Oct 15;84(8):887–892. [PMID: 22010767]

Broekhuizen BD et al. Undetected chronic obstructive pulmonary disease and asthma in people over 50 years with persistent cough. *Br J Gen Pract*. 2010 Jul;60(576):489–494. [PMID: 20594438]

Centers for Disease Control and Prevention (CDC). Updated recommendations for use of tetanus toxoid, reduced diphtheria toxoid, and acellular pertussis (Tdap) vaccine in adults aged 65 years and older—Advisory Committee on Immunization Practices (ACIP), 2012. MMWR Morb Mortal Wkly Rep. 2012 Jun 29;61(25):468–470. Erratum in: *MMWR Morb Mortal Wkly Rep*. 2012 Jul 13;61(27):515. [PMID: 22739778]

Centers for Disease Control and Prevention (CDC). Updated recommendations for use of tetanus toxoid, reduced diphtheria toxoid and acellular pertussis vaccine (Tdap) in pregnant women and persons who have or anticipate having close contact with an infant aged < 12 months—Advisory Committee on Immunization Practices (ACIP), 2011. *MMWR Morb Mortal Wkly Rep*. 2011 Oct 21;60(41):1424–1426. [PMID: 22012116]

Chang CC et al. Over-the-counter (OTC) medications to reduce cough as an adjunct to antibiotics for acute pneumonia in children and adults. *Cochrane Database Syst Rev*. 2014 Mar 10;3:CD006088. [PMID: 24615334]

Held U et al. Diagnostic aid to rule out pneumonia in adults with cough and feeling of fever. A validation study in the primary care setting. *BMC Infect Dis*. 2012 Dec 17;12:355. [PMID: 23245504]

Iyer VN et al. Chronic cough: an update. *Mayo Clin Proc*. 2013 Oct;88(10):1115–1126. [PMID: 24079681]

Johnstone KJ et al. Inhaled corticosteroids for subacute and chronic cough in adults. *Cochrane Database Syst Rev*. 2013 Mar 28;3:CD009305. [PMID: 23543575]

Kline JM et al. Pertussis: a reemerging infection. *Am Fam Physician*. 2013 Oct 15;88(8):507–514. Erratum in: *Am Fam Physician*. 2014 Mar 1;89(5):317. [PMID: 24364571]

Lim KG et al. Long-term safety of nebulized lidocaine for adults with difficult-to-control chronic cough: a case series. *Chest*. 2013 Apr;143(4):1060–1065. [PMID: 23238692]

van Vugt SF et al. Use of serum C reactive protein and procalcitonin concentrations in addition to symptoms and signs to predict pneumonia in patients presenting to primary care with acute cough: diagnostic study. *BMJ*. 2013 Apr 30;346:f2450. [PMID: 23633005]

Dyspnea

7

A 39-year-old woman presents with gradual onset of shortness of breath over the past 6 months, both at rest (when it is mild) and with exertion (when it can force her to stop activity to "catch her breath"). Prior to this problem, she has been healthy, with only two hospitalizations for uncomplicated spontaneous vaginal deliveries at ages 27 and 30. She does not smoke cigarettes and has no known allergies. On review of symptoms, she states that she has had no pleuritic or exertional chest pain and no cough or wheezing; sometimes, she has palpitations with activity. Over the past 1 year, she has had heavy menses, with periods that can last up to 6 to 7 days frequently soaking several pads per day. Two weeks ago, she saw her gynecologist who ordered a complete blood count that showed a hemoglobin 7.2 g/dL and hematocrit 21%. A pelvic ultrasound shows a large myomatous uterus. A chest x-ray was negative.

LEARNING OBJECTIVES

▶ Learn the clinical manifestations and objective findings of dyspnea that help differentiate its cause

▶ Understand the factors that predispose to the different causes of dyspnea

▶ Know the differential diagnosis of dyspnea, including the life-threatening causes that must be identified quickly

▶ Learn the ways that laboratory, imaging, and diagnostic procedures can help diagnose the cause of dyspnea

QUESTIONS

1. What are the salient features of this patient's problem?

2. How do you think through her problem?

3. What are the key features, including essentials of diagnosis and general considerations, of dyspnea?

4. What are the symptoms and signs of dyspnea?

5. What is the differential diagnosis of dyspnea?

6. What are the laboratory, imaging, and procedural findings in dyspnea?

7. What are the treatments for dyspnea?

8. What are the outcomes, including prevention and prognosis, of dyspnea?

9. When should patients with dyspnea be referred to a specialist or admitted to the hospital?

ANSWERS

1. Salient Features

Premenopausal woman; gradual onset of dyspnea; 6 months' duration; exertional; nonsmoker; no chest pain, cough, wheeze; heavy menses; severe anemia; normal chest x-ray

2. How to Think Through

Patients with subacute progressive dyspnea present an important diagnostic challenge. Primary pulmonary and primary cardiac problems should be looked for, but this case highlights another important cause: severe anemia. The absence of pleuritic chest pain, cough, wheezing, and history of smoking point away from most pulmonary etiologies, though interstitial lung disease could present in this insidious fashion. What are the key questions to elicit a possible cardiac etiology? (Chest pain, orthopnea, paroxysmal nocturnal dyspnea, syncope, peripheral edema, and palpitations.) The patient has palpitations, so an arrhythmia is plausible, but this symptom is not consistently associated with her dyspnea.

What noncardiac causes of dyspnea must therefore be considered? (Anemia, respiratory muscle weakness, methemoglobinemia, cyanide ingestion, carbon monoxide [CO] intoxication, metabolic acidosis, chronic pulmonary embolism, and psychogenic [panic or anxiety].) In the clinic setting, pulse oximetry, a proxy for the Pao_2, provides valuable information. What will her oxygen saturation likely show? (With anemia, it should be normal.)

How should she be managed? (Iron supplementation and prompt, elective myomectomy. Transfusion will likely be needed, especially in anticipation of surgical blood loss.)

3. Key Features

Essentials of Diagnosis

• Inquire about
  — Fever, cough, chest pain; onset, duration, severity, and periodicity of symptoms
  — Vital sign measurement and pulse oximetry
  — Cardiac and chest examination findings
  — Chest radiography findings; arterial blood gas measurement in selected patients

General Considerations

• Dyspnea is the subjective perception of uncomfortable breathing
• Can result from psychogenic origins or from conditions that
  — Increase the mechanical effort of breathing (eg, chronic obstructive pulmonary disease [COPD], restrictive lung disease, respiratory muscle weakness)
  — Produce compensatory tachypnea (eg, hypoxemia or acidosis)
• The following factors play a role in how and when dyspnea presents in patients:
  — Rate of onset
  — Previous dyspnea
  — Medications
  — Comorbidities
  — Psychological profile
  — Severity of underlying disorder

4. Symptoms and Signs

• Rapid onset, severe dyspnea suggests pneumothorax, pulmonary embolism, or increased left ventricular (LV) end-diastolic pressure
• Association with pleuritic chest pain may suggest pneumothorax, pulmonary embolism, pericarditis, or pleurisy from acute viral respiratory tract infection

Table 7-1. Clinical findings suggesting obstructive airways disease.

	Adjusted Likelihood Ratios	
	Factor Present	Factor Absent
> 40-pack-y smoking	11.6	0.9
Age ≥ 45 y	1.4	0.5
Maximum laryngeal height ≤ 4 cm	3.6	0.7
All three factors	58.5	0.3

Reproduced, with permission, from Straus SE et al. The accuracy of patient history, wheezing, and laryngeal measurements in diagnosing obstructive airway disease. CARE-COAD1 Group. Clinical Assessment of the Reliability of the Examination—Chronic Obstructive Airways Disease. *JAMA.* 2000;283(14):1853–1857.

- Pulmonary embolism should be suspected with risk factors for deep vein thrombosis such as immobilization or hospitalization, estrogen therapy, cancer, obesity, or lower extremity trauma
- Cough and fever suggest pulmonary disease, particularly infections, myocarditis, or pericarditis
- Wheezing suggests acute bronchitis, chronic obstructive pulmonary disease (COPD) (Table 7-1), asthma, foreign body, or vocal cord dysfunction
- Prominent dyspnea with no accompanying features suggests noncardiopulmonary causes such as anemia, metabolic acidosis, panic disorder, neuromuscular disorders, chronic pulmonary embolism, or other causes of impaired oxygen delivery (eg, methemoglobinemia, CO poisoning)
- Observation of respiratory pattern can suggest obstructive airway disease (pursed-lip breathing, accessory respiratory muscle use, barrel-shaped chest), asymmetric expansion (pneumothorax), or metabolic acidosis (deep Kussmaul respirations)
- Focal wheezing may suggest foreign body or bronchial obstruction
- Pulmonary hypertension or pulmonary embolism may have an accentuated pulmonic second heart sound (loud P2)
- Orthopnea (dyspnea that occurs in recumbency) and paroxysmal nocturnal dyspnea (shortness of breath that occurs abruptly 30 minutes to 4 hours after going to bed and is relieved by sitting or standing up) suggests cardiac disease and heart failure (HF); other findings suggestive of elevated LV end-diastolic pressure are summarized in Table 7-2

Table 7-2. Clinical findings suggesting increased left ventricular end-diastolic pressure.

Tachycardia
Systolic hypotension
Jugular venous distention (> 5–7 cm H$_2$O)[a]
Hepatojugular reflux (> 1 cm)[b]
Crackles, especially bibasilar
Third heart sound[c]
Lower extremity edema
Radiographic pulmonary vascular redistribution or cardiomegaly[a]

[a]These findings are particularly helpful.

[b]Proper abdominal compression for evaluating hepatojugular reflux requires > 30 s of sustained right upper quadrant abdominal compression.

[c]Cardiac auscultation of the patient at 45° angle in left lateral decubitus position doubles the detection rate of third heart sounds.

Modified, with permission, from Badgett RG et al. Can the clinical examination diagnose left-sided heart failure in adults? *JAMA.* 1997;277(21):1712–1719.

5. Differential Diagnosis

- Acute
  - Asthma, pneumonia, pulmonary edema, pneumothorax, pulmonary embolus, metabolic acidosis, acute respiratory distress syndrome, panic attack
- Pulmonary
  - Airflow obstruction (asthma, chronic obstructive pulmonary disease, upper airway obstruction), restrictive lung disease (interstitial lung disease, pleural thickening or effusion, respiratory muscle weakness, obesity), pneumonia, pneumothorax, pulmonary embolism, aspiration, acute respiratory distress syndrome
- Cardiac
  - Myocardial ischemia, HF, valvular obstruction, arrhythmia, cardiac tamponade
- Metabolic
  - Acidosis, hypercapnia, sepsis, CO poisoning
- Hematologic
  - Anemia, methemoglobinemia
- Psychiatric
  - Anxiety

6. Laboratory, Imaging, and Procedural Findings

Laboratory Tests

- Serum B-type natriuretic peptide (BNP or NT-proBNP) testing can be useful in distinguishing cardiac from noncardiac causes of dyspnea in the emergency department
  - Values < 300 ng/L rule out HF
  - Values for ruling in HF increase with age; > 450 ng/L for age < 50; > 900 ng/L for age 50 to 75; and > 1800 ng/L for age > 75
- Arterial blood gas measurement
- Hematocrit/hemoglobin, methemoglobin, or CO measurement, as indicated

Imaging Studies

- Chest radiograph is essential
  - Normal chest radiograph and physical examination suggests pulmonary embolism, *Pneumocystis jiroveci* infection, upper airway obstruction, foreign body, anemia, or metabolic acidosis, anemia, methemoglobinemia, CO poisoning
- High resolution chest CT can evaluate for pulmonary embolism, interstitial, and alveolar lung disease

Diagnostic Procedures

- Physical examination to include head, neck, chest, heart, and lower extremities
- Pulse oximetry at rest and with ambulation (not to supplant arterial blood gas and, when indicated, CO and methemoglobin measurements)
- Electrocardiogram
- Spirometry in patients with suspected obstructive or restrictive airway disease

7. Treatments

Medications

- Treatment should be aimed at the underlying cause (eg, transfusion and iron repletion for severe anemia due to blood loss; inhaled β_2-agonist, anticholinergic, and corticosteroid for asthma)
- Opioid therapy can relieve dyspnea that occurs in patients nearing the end of life

Therapeutic Procedures

- Supplemental oxygen for patients with hypoxemia; such supplementation in severe COPD with hypoxemia confers a mortality benefit
- Pulmonary rehabilitation in patients with COPD or interstitial pulmonary fibrosis

8. Outcomes

Prevention
• Smoking cessation can prevent many causes of dyspnea and slow the progression of COPD

Prognosis
• Depends on underlying cause

9. When to Refer and When to Admit

When to Refer
• Following acute stabilization, patients with advanced COPD should be referred to a pulmonologist
• Patients with HF or valvular heart disease should be referred to a cardiologist after acute stabilization
• Cyanide and CO poisoning should be managed in conjunction with a toxicologist

When to Admit
• Impaired gas exchange from any cause or high risk of pulmonary embolism pending definitive diagnosis
• Suspected methemoglobinemia, or cyanide or CO poisoning

SUGGESTED REFERENCES

Burri E et al. Value of arterial blood gas analysis in patients with acute dyspnea: an observational study. *Crit Care*. 2011;15(3):R145. [PMID: 21663600]

Jang TB et al. The predictive value of physical examination findings in patients with suspected acute heart failure syndrome. *Intern Emerg Med*. 2012 Jun;7(3):271–274. [PMID: 22094407]

Junker C et al. Are arterial blood gases necessary in the evaluation of acutely dyspneic patients? *Crit Care*. 2011 Aug 2;15(4):176. [PMID: 21892979]

Kline JA et al. Multicenter, randomized trial of quantitative pretest probability to reduce unnecessary medical radiation exposure in emergency department patients with chest pain and dyspnea. *Circ Cardiovasc Imaging*. 2014 Jan;7(1):66–73. [PMID: 24275953]

Lin RJ et al. Dyspnea in palliative care: expanding the role of corticosteroids. *J Palliat Med*. 2012 Jul;15(7):834–837. [PMID: 22385025]

Mastandrea P. The diagnostic utility of brain natriuretic peptide in heart failure patients presenting with acute dyspnea: a meta-analysis. *Clin Chem Lab Med*. 2013 Jun;51(6):1155–1165. [PMID: 23152414]

Parshall MB et al; American Thoracic Society Committee on Dyspnea. An official American Thoracic Society statement: update on the mechanisms, assessment, and management of dyspnea. *Am J Respir Crit Care Med*. 2012 Feb 15;185(4):435–452. [PMID: 22336677]

Shreves A et al. Emergency management of dyspnea in dying patients. *Emerg Med Pract*. 2013 May;15(5):1–20. [PMID: 23967787]

Smith TA et al. The use of non-invasive ventilation for the relief of dyspnoea in exacerbations of chronic obstructive pulmonary disease; a systematic review. *Respirology*. 2012 Feb;17(2):300–307. [PMID: 22008176]

Uronis H et al. Symptomatic oxygen for non-hypoxaemic chronic obstructive pulmonary disease. *Cochrane Database Syst Rev*. 2011 Jun 15;(6):CD006429. [PMID: 21678356]

8

Lung Cancer

A 73-year-old man presents to his primary care clinician with a new cough productive of blood. He reports gradual weight loss of approximately 15 pounds over the past 6 months. He has smoked two packs of cigarettes per day for the past 50 years. On physical examination, he has decreased breath sounds and dullness to percussion at the left lung base. His chest radiograph shows a left-sided pleural effusion and consolidation in the left lung.

LEARNING OBJECTIVES

▶ Learn the clinical manifestations and objective findings of lung cancer
▶ Understand the risk factors that predispose to lung cancer
▶ Know the differential diagnosis of lung cancer
▶ Learn the treatment for each type and stage of lung cancer
▶ Know the common paraneoplastic syndromes associated with lung cancer

QUESTIONS

1. What are the salient features of this patient's problem?
2. How do you think through his problem?
3. What are the key features, including essentials of diagnosis, general considerations, and demographics, of lung cancer?
4. What are the symptoms and signs of lung cancer?
5. What is the differential diagnosis of lung cancer?
6. What are the laboratory, imaging, and procedural findings in lung cancer?
7. What are the treatments for lung cancer?
8. What are the outcomes, including follow-up, complications, prevention, and prognosis, of lung cancer?
9. When should patients with lung cancer be referred to a specialist or admitted to the hospital?

ANSWERS

1. Salient Features

Older patient; new cough and hemoptysis; weight loss; heavy cigarette smoking history; dull lung base with likely malignant effusion; consolidation on chest radiograph

2. How to Think Through

Lung cancer is the leading cause of cancer-related death, has a high mortality rate at the time of detection, and is largely preventable. This patient presents with significant "red flag" features, including a 100-pack-year smoking history, hemoptysis, and weight loss. Other than primary lung cancer, what other disease processes could cause this presentation? (Tuberculosis, pneumonia, lung abscess, lymphoma, metastatic cancer.) What neurologic examination findings suggest complications of lung cancer? (Any mental status, cranial nerve, motor, sensory, or coordination abnormality may indicate brain metastasis; hoarseness or Horner syndrome may indicate compression of the recurrent laryngeal nerve or sympathetic ganglion by an apical [Pancoast] tumor.) What are the next steps in the evaluation of this patient? (CT scan to characterize tumor location, plan biopsy, begin staging, and plan possible surgery. Pathologic diagnosis is essential.) What imaging is needed for staging? (CT, PET/CT, and MRI scans are all used in staging; in addition to the chest, the brain and abdomen must be assessed.) In the treatment of primary lung cancer, surgery, chemotherapy, and radiation are employed, depending upon the cancer type and stage. If this patient is not a candidate for surgery or chemotherapy, what palliative therapies should be considered? (Thoracentesis, radiation including stereotactic body radiotherapy, oxygen, opioids for palliation of pain and dyspnea.)

3. Key Features

Essentials of Diagnosis

- New cough or change in chronic cough
- Dyspnea, hemoptysis, anorexia, weight loss
- Enlarging nodule or mass, persistent opacity, atelectasis, or pleural effusion on chest radiograph or CT scan
- Cytologic or histologic findings of lung cancer in sputum, pleural fluid, or biopsy specimen

General Considerations

- Leading cause of cancer deaths in both men and women
- Cigarette smoking causes 85% to 90% of lung cancers
- Small cell lung cancer (SCLC) (13% of lung cancer cases)
  — Bronchial origin, begins centrally, and infiltrates submucosally
  — Prone to early hematogenous spread
  — Is rarely amenable to resection
  — Has an aggressive course
- Non-small cell lung cancer (NSCLC)
  — Spreads more slowly
  — Early disease may be cured with resection
  — Histologic types
    ◦ Squamous cell carcinoma (22% of cases) arises from bronchial epithelium; it is usually centrally located and intraluminal
    ◦ Adenocarcinoma (42% of cases) arises from mucous glands as a peripheral nodule or mass
    ◦ Large cell carcinoma (2% of cases) is a heterogeneous group and presents as a central or peripheral mass
    ◦ Adenocarcinoma in situ (formerly bronchioloalveolar cell carcinoma) (2% of cases) arises from epithelial cells distal to the terminal bronchiole and spreads along preexisting alveolar structures (lepidic growth) without evidence of invasion

Demographics

- Median age at diagnosis in the United States is 70 years; it is unusual under age 40
- Environmental risk factors include
  — Tobacco smoke
  — Radon gas
  — Asbestos

— Metals
— Industrial carcinogens
- A familial predisposition is recognized
- Chronic obstructive pulmonary disease, pulmonary fibrosis, asbestosis, and sarcoidosis are associated with an increased risk of lung cancer

4. Symptoms and Signs

- Over 75% of patients are symptomatic at diagnosis
- Presentation depends on
  — Type and location of tumor
  — Extent of spread
  — Presence of distant metastases and any paraneoplastic syndromes
- Anorexia, weight loss, and asthenia in 55% to 90% of cases
- New or changed cough in up to 60%
- Hemoptysis in 5% to 30%
- Pain, often from bony metastases, in 25% to 40%
- Local spread may result in endobronchial obstruction and postobstructive pneumonia, effusions, or a change in voice due to recurrent laryngeal nerve involvement
- Superior vena cava (SVC) syndrome
- Horner syndrome
- Liver metastases are associated with asthenia and weight loss
- Possible presentation of brain metastases
  — Headache
  — Nausea and vomiting
  — Seizures
  — Dizziness
  — Altered mental status
- Paraneoplastic syndromes (Table 8-1) are not necessarily indicative of metastasis
  — Syndrome of inappropriate antidiuretic hormone secretion occurs in 10% to 15% of lung cancer (both NSCLC and SCLC) patients
  — Hypercalcemia occurs in 10% of SCLC patients

5. Differential Diagnosis

- Pneumonia
- Tuberculosis

Table 8-1. Paraneoplastic syndromes associated with lung cancer.

Hormone Excess or Syndrome	Non-Small Cell Lung Cancer	Small Cell Lung Cancer
Hypercalcemia	++	
Cushing syndrome	+	++
SIADH	++	++
Gonadotropin secretion	+	++
Lambert–Eaton myasthenia syndromes	+	++
Subacute cerebellar syndrome		++
Sensory motor peripheral neuropathy		++
Dermatomyositis	++	++
Acanthosis nigricans	+	
Hypertrophic osteoarthropathy	++	

+, reported associated; ++, strong association.

SIADH, syndrome of inappropriate antidiuretic hormone.

- Metastatic cancer to lung
- Benign pulmonary nodule or nodules
- Bronchial carcinoid tumor
- Lymphoma
- *Mycobacterium avium* complex infection
- Fungal pneumonia
- Sarcoidosis
- Foreign body aspiration (retained)

6. Laboratory, Imaging, and Procedural Findings

Laboratory Tests

- Tissue or cytology specimen is needed for diagnosis
- Sputum cytology is highly specific, but insensitive; yield is highest when lesions are in central airways
- Serum tumor markers are neither sensitive nor specific
- Complete blood cell count, serum electrolytes, calcium, creatinine, liver tests, lactate dehydrogenase, and albumin
- Pulmonary function tests are required in all NSCLC patients prior to surgery
  — Preoperative $FEV_1 \geq 2$ L is adequate to undergo surgery
  — Estimate of postresection FEV_1 is needed if < 2 L preresection
  — Postresection FEV_1 > 800 mL or > 40% predicted is associated with a low incidence of perioperative complications

Imaging Studies

- Nearly all patients have abnormal findings on chest radiograph or CT scan
  — Hilar adenopathy and mediastinal thickening (squamous cell)
  — Infiltrates, single or multiple nodules (bronchioloalveolar cell)
  — Central or peripheral masses (large cell)
  — Hilar and mediastinal abnormalities (small cell)
- Chest CT is the most important modality in staging to determine resectability
- An MRI of the brain to rule out brain metastases is important to stage patients who present with at least stage II disease
- PET imaging can help confirm no metastases in NSCLC patients who are candidates for surgical resection
- PET-CT scans are inadequate for evaluating brain metastases due to the high FDG uptake there

Diagnostic Procedures

- Thoracentesis can be diagnostic in the setting of malignant effusions (50%–65%)
- If pleural fluid cytology is nondiagnostic after two thoracenteses, thoracoscopy is preferred to blind pleural biopsy
- Fine-needle aspiration of palpable supraclavicular or cervical lymph nodes is frequently diagnostic
- Tissue diagnostic yield from bronchoscopy is 10% to 90%; electromagnetic navigational bronchoscopy allows approaches to small peripheral nodules
- Transthoracic needle biopsy has a sensitivity of 50% to 97%
- CT-guided FNA of peripheral nodules has diagnostic yields approaching 80% to 90%, but significant rates of pneumothorax (15%–30%), especially in those with emphysema
- Mediastinoscopy, video-assisted thoracoscopic surgery (VATS), or thoracotomy is necessary where less invasive techniques are not diagnostic

Staging

- NSCLC is staged with the TNM international staging system
  — Stages I and II disease may be cured surgically
  — Stage IIIA disease may benefit from surgery
  — Stages IIIB and IV disease does not benefit from surgery

Table 8-2. Treatment choices for lung cancer.

Non-small cell lung cancer	**Combination chemotherapy:** Cisplatin, vinorelbine or Cisplatin, etoposide or Paclitaxel, carboplatin or Cisplatin, gemcitabine (squamous histology) Cisplatin, pemetrexed (nonsquamous histology) All regimens with or without bevacizumab	Docetaxel, cetuximab, erlotinib (EGFR mutation positive), crizotinib (ALK mutation positive)
Small cell lung cancer	**Combination chemotherapy:** Cisplatin, etoposide or Carboplatin, pemetrexed or Gemcitabine, cisplatin	Irinotecan, cyclophosphamide, doxorubicin, vincristine, topotecan, gemcitabine, paclitaxel

7. Treatments

Medications
- Tables 8-2 and 8-3

Neoadjuvant chemotherapy in NSCLC
- Administration *in advance* of surgery or radiation therapy
- There is no consensus on the survival impact in stages I and II disease but it is widely used in stage IIIA and IIIB disease

Adjuvant chemotherapy in NSCLC
- Administration of drugs *after* surgery or radiation therapy
- Cisplatinum-containing therapy confers a 5% 5-year survival benefit in at least stage II disease and possibly a subset of stage IB disease; there is no benefit (and may be detrimental) in patients with poor performance status (Eastern Cooperative Oncology Group Score ≥ 2)
- Targeted therapies with tyrosine kinase inhibitors (erlotinib, gefitinib, crizotinib, ceritinib) can be helpful depending upon tumor molecular profile

Early stage NSCLC
- Stereotactic body radiotherapy is an option for those patients who are not candidates for surgery because of significant comorbidity or surgical contraindication

Stages IIIA and IIIB NSCLC
- Improved survival when treated with *concurrent* chemotherapy and radiation therapy in those cannot be treated surgically (compared with no therapy, radiation alone, or sequential chemotherapy and radiation)

Stages IIIB and IV NSCLC
- Increase in survival from 5 months to 7 to 11 months in those with good performance status who are treated with chemotherapy; platinum-based regimen is most often used
- Survival benefit with the addition of bevacizumab (antibody to vascular endothelial growth factor) to a platinum doublet regimen
- Erlotinib (epidermal growth factor receptor tyrosine kinase inhibitor) improves survival as second-line treatment for advanced NSCLC; especially effective in women, nonsmokers, Asians, adenocarcinoma and bronchioalveolar carcinoma histology

Chemotherapy in SCLC
- 80% to 90% response to cisplatin/etoposide in limited stage disease (50%–76% complete response)
- 60% to 80% response to cisplatin/etoposide in extensive disease (15%–20% complete response)
- Remissions last a median of 6 to 8 months
- Median survival is 3 to 4 months after recurrence

Surgery
- Resection of solitary brain metastases
  — Does not improve survival
  — May improve quality of life in combination with radiation therapy

Table 8-3. Chemotherapeutic agents for lung cancer: Dosage and toxicity.

Chemotherapeutic Agent	Usual Adult Dosage	Acute Toxicity	Delayed Toxicity
Alkylating Agents—Nitrogen Mustards			
Cyclophosphamide (Cytoxan)	500–1000 mg/m^2 intravenously every 3 wk; 100 mg/m^2/d orally for 14 d every 4 wk; various doses	Nausea and vomiting	Myelosuppression, hemorrhagic cystitis, alopecia, cardiotoxicity with high-dose therapy
Alkylating Agents—Platinum Analogs			
Carboplatin (Paraplatin)	Area under the curve (AUC)-based dosing uses Calvert equation [Dose (mg) = AUC × (GFR + 25)] AUC = 2–7 mg/mL/min every 2–4 wk	Nausea, and vomiting	Myelosuppression, electrolyte disturbances, peripheral neuropathy, nephrotoxicity, hypersensitivity reaction
Cisplatin (Platinol)	50–100 mg/m^2 intravenously every 3–4 wk; 20 mg/m^2/d intravenously for 5 d every 3 wk; various doses	Severe nausea and vomiting	Myelosuppression, electrolyte disturbances, peripheral neuropathy, nephrotoxicity, hypersensitivity reaction
Antimetabolites—Folate Antagonists			
Pemetrexed (Alimta)	500 mg/m^2 intravenously every 3 wk	Nausea, vomiting, diarrhea, rash	Myelosuppression, fatigue, mucositis
Antimetabolites—Pyrimidine Analogs			
Gemcitabine (Gemzar)	1000–1250 mg/m^2 intravenously on days 1, 8, 15 every 4 wk	Nausea, rash, flu-like symptoms, fever, diarrhea	Myelosuppression, edema, elevated transaminases
Antimicrotubules—Vinca Alkaloids			
Vincristine (Oncovin)	0.5–1.4 mg/m^2 intravenously every 3 wk; various doses; maximum single dose usually limited to 2 mg	Constipation, nausea	Peripheral neuropathy, alopecia
Vinorelbine (Navelbine)	25–30 mg/m^2 intravenously every week	Nausea, vomiting	Myelosuppression, peripheral neuropathy, fatigue
Antimicrotubules—Taxanes			
Docetaxel (Taxotere)	60–100 mg/m^2 intravenously every 3 wk	Nausea, vomiting, diarrhea, hypersensitivity reaction	Myelosuppression, asthenia, peripheral neuropathy, alopecia, edema, fatigue, mucositis
Paclitaxel (Taxol)	135–175 mg/m^2 intravenously every 3 wk; 50–80 mg/m^2 intravenously weekly; various doses	Diarrhea, nausea, vomiting, hypersensitivity reaction	Myelosuppression, peripheral neuropathy, alopecia, mucositis, arthralgia
Paclitaxel protein-bound (Abraxane)	100–250 mg/m^2 on days 1, 8, 15 every 3–4 wk; 260 mg/m^2 intravenously every 3 weeks	Nausea, vomiting, diarrhea	Myelosuppression, peripheral neuropathy, asthenia
Enzyme Inhibitors—Anthracyclines			
Doxorubicin (Adriamycin)	45–75 mg/m^2 intravenously every 3 wk; various doses	Nausea, vomiting, diarrhea, red/orange discoloration of urine	Myelosuppression, mucositis, alopecia, cardiotoxicity (cardiomyopathy with heart failure–dose related)
Enzyme Inhibitors—Topoisomerase Inhibitors			
Etoposide (VePesid)	50–100 mg/m^2 intravenously for 3–5 d every 3 wk	Nausea, vomiting, diarrhea, hypersensitivity reaction, fever, hypotension	Myelosuppression, alopecia, fatigue
Etoposide phosphate (Etopophos)	35–100 mg/m^2 intravenously for 3–5 d every 3–4 wk		
Irinotecan (Camptosar)	180 mg/m^2 intravenously every other week; various doses	Diarrhea, cholinergic syndrome, nausea, vomiting	Myelosuppression, alopecia, asthenia
Topotecan (Hycamtin)	1.5 mg/m^2 intravenously for 5 d every 3 wk; 2.3 mg/m^2 orally for 5 d every 3 wk	Nausea, vomiting, diarrhea	Myelosuppression, alopecia, asthenia
Targeted Therapy—Monoclonal Antibodies			
Bevacizumab (Avastin)	5–15 mg/kg intravenously every 2–3 wk	Infusion-related reaction	Hypertension, proteinuria, wound healing complications, gastrointestinal perforation, hemorrhage
Cetuximab (Erbitux)	Loading dose 400 mg/m^2 intravenously maintenance dose 250 mg/m^2 intravenously weekly	Infusion-related reaction, nausea, diarrhea	Acneiform skin rash, hypomagnesemia, asthenia, paronychial inflammation, dyspnea
Targeted Therapy—Tyrosine Kinase Inhibitors			
Crizotinib (Xalkori)	250 mg orally twice daily	Nausea, vomiting, diarrhea, constipation	Vision disorder, edema, elevated transaminases, fatigue
Erlotinib (Tarceva)	100–150 mg orally once daily without food	Diarrhea, nausea, vomiting	Acneiform skin rash, fatigue, anorexia, dyspnea

NSCLC
- Stages I and II are treated with surgical resection where possible
- Stage IIIA disease should be treated with multimodal protocols
- Selected patients with stage IIIB who undergo resection after multimodal therapy have shown long-term survival
- Patients with stage IV disease are treated palliatively

Therapeutic Procedures
- Radiation therapy is used as part of multimodal regimens in NSCLC
- Intraluminal radiation (brachytherapy) is an alternative approach to endobronchial disease
- Palliative care
  - Pain control at the end of life is essential
  - External-beam radiation therapy is used to control
    - Dyspnea
    - Hemoptysis
    - Pain from bony metastases
    - Obstruction from SVC syndrome
    - Solitary brain metastases

8. Outcomes

Follow-Up
- Depends on type and stage of cancer as well as the patient's functional status and comorbid conditions

Complications
- SVC syndrome
- Paraneoplastic syndromes
- Venous thrombosis
- Postobstructive pneumonia

Prevention
- Smoking cessation
- Screening current and former heavy smokers with annual low-dose helical CT scans has been shown to improve mortality rates for lung cancer and is recommended by the USPSTF; studies on the cost-effectiveness of screening are ongoing

Prognosis
- Table 8-4
- The overall 5-year survival rate is approximately 17%
- Predictors of survival
  - Type of tumor (SCLC vs NSCLC)
  - Molecular typing
  - Stage of the tumor
  - Patient's performance status, including weight loss in the past 6 months

9. When to Refer and When to Admit

When to Refer
- All patients deserve an evaluation by a multidisciplinary lung cancer evaluation and treatment program
- A palliative care specialist should be involved in advanced disease care

When to Admit
- Respiratory distress, altered mental status, pain control

Table 8-4. Approximate survival rates following treatment for lung cancer.[a]

Non-Small Cell Lung Cancer: Mean 5-y Survival Following Resection		
Stage	Clinical TNM Staging (%)	Pathologic TNM Staging (%)
IA (T1a/T1b,N0M0)	50–80	73
IB (T2aN0M0)	47	58
IIA (T1a/T1b,N1M0)	36	46
IIB (T2bN1M0, T3N0M0)	26	36
IIIA (T1/T2,N2M0, T3,N1/N2,M0, T4,N0/N1,M0)	19	24
IIIB (T4N2M0, Any T,N3, M0)	7	9
IV (Any T, Any N, M1a/M1b)	2	13
Small Cell Lung Cancer: Survival Following Chemotherapy		
Stage	Mean 2-y Survival (%)	Median Survival (mo)
Limited	20–40	15–20
Extensive	5	8–13

[a]Independent of therapy, generally not surgical patients.

Data from multiple sources. Modified and reproduced, with permission, from Tsim S et al. Staging of non-small-cell lung cancer (NSCLC): a review. *Respir Med*. 2010 Dec;104(12):1767–1774; Goldstraw P et al. The IASLC Lung Cancer Staging Project: proposals for the revision of the TNM stage groupings in the forthcoming (seventh) edition of the TNM Classification of malignant tumours. *J Thorac Oncol*. 2007 Aug;2(8):706–714; and Van Meerbeeck JP et al. Small-cell lung cancer. *Lancet*. 2011 Nov 12;378(9804):1741–1755.

SUGGESTED REFERENCES

Gould MK. Clinical practice. Lung-cancer screening with low-dose computed tomography. *N Engl J Med*. 2014 Nov 6;371(19):1813–1820. [PMID: 25372089]

Hornbech K et al. Current status of pulmonary metastasectomy. *Eur J Cardiothorac Surg*. 2011 Jun;39(6):955–962. [PMID: 21115259]

Hornbech K et al. Outcome after pulmonary metastasectomy: analysis of 5 years consecutive surgical resections 2002–2006. *J Thorac Oncol*. 2011 Oct;6(10):1733–1740. [PMID: 21869715]

Howington JA et al. Treatment of stage I and II non-small cell lung cancer: diagnosis and management of lung cancer, 3rd ed: American College of Chest Physicians evidence-based clinical practice guidelines. *Chest*. 2013 May;143(5 suppl):e278S–e313S. [PMID: 23649443]

Jett JR et al. Treatment of small cell lung cancer: diagnosis and management of lung cancer, 3rd ed: American College of Chest Physicians evidence-based clinical practice guidelines. *Chest*. 2013 May;143(5 suppl):e400S–19S. [PMID: 23649448]

Pfannschmidt J et al. Surgical intervention for pulmonary metastases. *Dtsch Arztebl Int*. 2012 Oct;109(40):645–651. [PMID: 23094000]

Ramnath N et al. Treatment of stage III non-small cell lung cancer: diagnosis and management of lung cancer, 3rd ed: American College of Chest Physicians evidence-based clinical practice guidelines. *Chest*. 2013 May;143(5 suppl):e314S–e340S. [PMID: 23649445]

Silvestri GA et al. The stage classification of lung cancer: diagnosis and management of lung cancer, 3rd edition: American College of Chest Physicians evidence-based clinical practice guidelines. *Chest*. 2013 May;143(5 suppl):e191S–e210S. [PMID: 23649438]

Socinski MA et al. Treatment of stage IV non-small cell lung cancer: diagnosis and management of lung cancer, 3rd ed: American College of Chest Physicians evidence-based clinical practice guidelines. *Chest*. 2013 May;143(5 suppl):e341S–e368S. [PMID: 23649446]

9

Pharyngitis

A 19-year-old girl presents to her primary care clinic complaining of a sore throat for 2 days. She also reports a fever, which reached 38.4°C yesterday. She denies cough. A friend at her place of employment has also had similar symptoms. On physical examination, her neck reveals tender anterior cervical lymphadenopathy, and her tonsils are inflamed and exudative.

LEARNING OBJECTIVES

▶ Learn the clinical manifestations and objective findings of pharyngitis and how to distinguish group A β-hemolytic streptococcal (GABHS) infections
▶ Learn the Centor criteria for group A beta-hemolytic streptococcus infection and how they relate to the clinical diagnosis and rapid streptococcal tests
▶ Understand the public health concerns regarding pharyngitis
▶ Know the differential diagnosis of pharyngitis including acute HIV infection
▶ Learn the treatment for pharyngitis and the complications that it prevents

QUESTIONS

1. What are the salient features of this patient's problem?
2. How do you think through her problem?
3. What are the key features, including essentials of diagnosis, general considerations, and demographics, of pharyngitis?
4. What are the symptoms and signs of pharyngitis?
5. What is the differential diagnosis of pharyngitis?
6. What are laboratory findings in pharyngitis?
7. What are the treatments for pharyngitis?
8. What are the outcomes, including follow-up, complications, and prognosis, of pharyngitis?
9. When should patients with pharyngitis be referred to a specialist or admitted to the hospital?

ANSWERS

1. Salient Features

Young age; sick contact; 4/4 Centor criteria: sore throat; fever, lack of cough, cervical adenopathy, exudative tonsils

2. How to Think Through

Assessment of acute pharyngitis in adults requires the clinician to separate viral pharyngitis from probable group A β-hemolytic streptococcus infection, while remaining vigilant for more serious causes of sore throat. Why is it important to identify and treat GABHS pharyngitis? (Risk of subsequent rheumatic fever and glomerulonephritis.) How many Centor criteria are present in this patient? (4 of 4 diagnostic criteria: fever, absence of cough, tender cervical lymphadenopathy, tonsillar exudate.) Were a rapid strep test to be negative in this case, what would be the appropriate management strategy? (Antibiotic therapy in a patient with 4 of 4 the Centor criteria is reasonable regardless of the rapid test result.)

What other important infectious diseases present with pharyngitis in young adults and must be considered? (Lemierre syndrome [*Fusobacterium necrophorum*], acute HIV infection, gonococcal pharyngitis, infectious mononucleosis [Epstein–Barr virus, EBV], and cytomegalovirus infection.) Were infectious mononucleosis a consideration, what antibiotic should be avoided due to the high frequency of associated rash? (Ampicillin.)

If she provides a history of a recent high-risk sexual encounter, should she receive an HIV antibody test now? (No. Detectable antibodies take between 3 weeks and 2 months to form in the majority of infected patients. An HIV viral load nucleic acid test would be more appropriate.)

3. Key Features

Essentials of Diagnosis
- Sore throat
- Fever
- Anterior cervical adenopathy
- Tonsillar exudate
- Focus is to treat group A β-hemolytic streptococcus infection to prevent rheumatic sequelae

General Considerations
- Group A β-hemolytic streptococci (*Streptococcus pyogenes*) are the most common bacterial cause of exudative pharyngitis
- The main concern is to determine whether the cause is GABHS, because of the complications of rheumatic fever and glomerulonephritis
- A second public health policy concern is to reduce the extraordinary cost (in both dollars and the development of antibiotic-resistant *Streptococcus pneumoniae* in the United States) associated with unnecessary antibiotic use
- About one-third of patients with infectious mononucleosis have secondary streptococcal tonsillitis requiring treatment
- Ampicillin should routinely be avoided if mononucleosis is suspected because it commonly induces a rash

Demographics
- Pharyngitis and tonsillitis account for > 10% of all office visits to primary care clinicians and 50% of outpatient antibiotic use

4. Symptoms and Signs
- Centor diagnostic criteria for group A β-hemolytic streptococcus infection
  — Fever > 38°C
  — Tender anterior cervical adenopathy
  — Lack of cough
  — Pharyngotonsillar exudate
- Sore throat may be severe, with odynophagia, tender adenopathy, and a scarlatiniform rash
- Hoarseness, cough, and coryza are not suggestive of group A β-hemolytic streptococcus infection

- Marked lymphadenopathy and a shaggy white–purple tonsillar exudate, often extending into the nasopharynx, suggest mononucleosis, especially if present in a young adult

5. Differential Diagnosis

- Viral pharyngitis
- EBV/infectious mononucleosis
- Primary HIV infection
- Candidiasis
- Necrotizing ulcerative gingivostomatitis (Vincent fusospirochetal disease)
- Retropharyngeal abscess
- Diphtheria
- *Neisseria gonorrhoeae*
- *Mycoplasma*
- Anaerobic streptococci
- *Corynebacterium haemolyticum*
- Epiglottitis

6. Laboratory Findings

Laboratory Tests

- The presence of the 4 Centor diagnostic criteria strongly suggests GABS
- When 3 of the 4 Centor criteria are present, there is an intermediate likelihood of GABHS
- When 2 or 3 Centor criteria are present, throat cultures or rapid antigen detection testing of a throat swab should be obtained
- When 0 or 1 Centor criterion is present, GABS infection is unlikely; throat culture or rapid antigen detection testing of a throat swab is not necessary
- A single-swab throat culture is 90% to 95% sensitive and the rapid antigen detection testing (RADT) is 90% to 99% sensitive for GABHS
- With about 90% sensitivity, lymphocyte to white blood cell ratios of > 35% suggest EBV infection and not tonsillitis
- Consider HIV antibody or viral load testing for acute HIV infection

7. Treatments

- Patients with 0 or 1 Centor criterion should not receive antibiotics
- Patients with 2 or 3 Centor criteria whose throat cultures or rapid antigen detection testing show positive results should receive antibiotic treatment
- Patients who have 4 Centor criteria can receive empiric therapy without throat culture or rapid antigen detection testing

Medications

- Benzathine penicillin intramuscular injection
  - 1.2 million units once is optimal but painful
  - Use for noncompliant patients
- Oral antibiotics
  - Penicillin V potassium (250 mg three times daily or 500 mg twice daily orally for 10 days) or cefuroxime axetil (250 mg twice daily orally, 5–10 days)
  - Efficacy of 5-day penicillin V is similar to 10-day course: 94% clinical response, 84% eradication
  - Erythromycin (500 mg four times daily orally) or azithromycin (500 mg once daily orally for 3 days) for penicillin-allergic patients
  - Macrolide antibiotics have been reported to be successful in shorter duration regimens
  - Cephalosporins more effective than penicillin for bacterial cure (eg, cefpodoxime and cefuroxime for 5 days)
- Analgesic, anti-inflammatory drugs (aspirin, acetaminophen, corticosteroids)

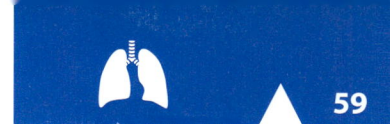

- Treatment failure
  — Second course with the same drug
  — Penicillin alternatives: cephalosporins (eg, cefuroxime), dicloxacillin, amoxicillin-clavulanate
  — Erythromycin resistance (failure rates of ~25%) increasing
  — With severe penicillin allergy, avoid cephalosporins; cross-reaction common ($\geq 8\%$)

Surgery
- Remove tonsils in cases of recurrent abscess

Therapeutic Procedures
- Saltwater gargling may be soothing
- Anesthetic gargles and lozenges (eg, benzocaine) for additional symptomatic relief
- Avoidance of contact sports in mononucleosis (risk of splenic rupture)

8. Outcomes

Follow-Up
- Patients who have had rheumatic fever should be treated with a continuous course of antimicrobial prophylaxis (erythromycin, 250 mg twice daily orally, or penicillin G, 500 mg once daily orally) for at least 5 years

Complications
- Low (10%–20%) incidence of treatment failures (positive culture after treatment despite symptomatic resolution) and recurrences
- Rheumatic myocarditis
- Glomerulonephritis
- Scarlet fever
- Local abscess formation

Prognosis
- Streptococcal pharyngitis usually resolves after 1 week
- Spontaneous resolution of symptoms without treatment still leaves the risk of rheumatic complications

9. When to Refer and When to Admit

When to Refer
- Peritonsillar abscess

When to Admit
- Occasionally, odynophagia is so intense that hospitalization for intravenous hydration and antibiotics is necessary
- Suspected or known epiglottitis

SUGGESTED REFERENCES

Alweis R et al. An initiative to improve adherence to evidence-based guidelines in the treatment of URIs, sinusitis, and pharyngitis. *J Community Hosp Intern Med Perspect*. 2014 Feb 17;4. [PMID: 24596644]

Hayward G et al. Corticosteroids as standalone or add-on treatment for sore throat. *Cochrane Database Syst Rev*. 2012 Oct 17;10:CD008268. [PMID: 23076943]

Kociolek LK et al. In the clinic. Pharyngitis. *Ann Intern Med*. 2012 Sep 4;157(5):ITC3-1–16. [PMID: 22944886]

Randel A; Infectious Disease Society of America. IDSA updates guideline for managing group A strep-tococcal pharyngitis. *Am Fam Physician*. 2013 Sep 1;88(5):338–340. [PMID: 24010402]

van Driel ML et al. Different antibiotic treatments for group A streptococcal pharyngitis. *Cochrane Database Syst Rev*. 2010 Oct 6;(10):CD004406. [PMID: 20927734]

Weber R. Pharyngitis. *Prim Care*. 2014 Mar;41(1):91–98. [PMID: 24439883]

10

Pneumonia

A 67-year-old man with a history of alcoholism presents with a 2-day history of fevers, chills, rigors, shortness of breath, and a cough productive of dark yellow sputum. He had a recent binge of alcohol use that ended 2 days before admission, and he woke up with these symptoms. On physical examination, his temperature is 39.5°C, his respiratory rate is 30/min, and he is in moderate respiratory distress. His lower right lung field has inspiratory crackles on auscultation. Laboratory testing reveals a white blood cell count of 16,000/μL. A chest radiograph shows focal consolidation in the right middle and lower lobes.

LEARNING OBJECTIVES

▶ Learn the clinical manifestations and objective findings of pneumonia and how to distinguish community-acquired from hospital-acquired pneumonia
▶ Know which diagnostic tests are helpful for the diagnosis of pneumonia and which can guide treatment
▶ Understand the factors that predispose to pneumonia and the ways to prevent the disease
▶ Know the differential diagnosis of pneumonia
▶ Learn the treatments for pneumonia by patient risk factors

QUESTIONS

1. What are the salient features of this patient's problem?
2. How do you think through his problem?
3. What are the key features, including essentials of diagnosis and general considerations, of pneumonia?
4. What are the symptoms and signs of pneumonia?
5. What is the differential diagnosis of pneumonia?
6. What are laboratory, imaging, and procedural findings in pneumonia?
7. What are the treatments for pneumonia?
8. What are the outcomes, including follow-up, complications, prognosis, and prevention, of pneumonia?
9. When should patients with pneumonia be referred to a specialist or admitted to the hospital?

ANSWERS

1. Salient Features

History of alcoholism predisposing to aspiration; fever and chills; rigors; shortness of breath; cough with purulent sputum; tachypnea; consolidation on examination and radiograph; leukocytosis

2. How to Think Through

Pneumonia is a clinical diagnosis in which symptoms, examination, WBC, and chest radiograph are all considered. While these all point to a diagnosis of pneumonia in this case, what other etiologies are plausible? (Aspiration pneumonitis, lung neoplasm, lung abscess, acute respiratory distress syndrome [ARDS], bronchitis, tuberculosis, pulmonary embolism, heart failure, atelectasis, drug reactions.) What are the next diagnostic steps? (Blood cultures; arterial blood gases.)

Pathogens and outcomes vary with epidemiological risk factors. This patient likely has community-acquired pneumonia (CAP), but recent exposure to health care settings and immune status (including HIV testing) should be assessed. His alcoholism may indicate other substance abuse, both of which increase the risk of tuberculosis. What pathogens are most likely in this case? (The acuity of his illness is most consistent with "typical" bacterial pneumonia from *Streptococcus pneumoniae*, *Haemophilus influenzae*, and *Klebsiella pneumoniae*. "Atypical" pneumonia, eg, *Mycoplasma pneumoniae*, is less likely in patients admitted to the hospital. But empiric antibiotic coverage for both types may be important. Although *Staphylococcus aureus* pneumonia is uncommon, it is associated with morbidity, so coverage for it may be appropriate with severe disease, and for patients requiring intensive care.) If this patient responds to antibiotic treatment within the first 2 to 3 days, its duration should be 7 days for most pathogens.

3. Key Features

Essentials of Diagnosis

- Fever or hypothermia, tachypnea, cough with or without sputum, dyspnea, chest discomfort, sweats, or rigors (or both)
- Bronchial breath sounds or inspiratory crackles on chest auscultation
- Leukocytosis
- Purulent sputum
- Parenchymal opacity on chest radiograph
- CAP occurs outside of the hospital or within 48 hours of hospital admission in a patient not residing in a long-term care facility
- Hospital-acquired pneumonia (HAP) occurs more than 48 hours after admission to the hospital or other health care facility and excludes any infection present at the time of admission
- Ventilation-associated pneumonia (VAP) develops in a mechanically ventilated patient more than 48 hours after endotracheal intubation
- Health care-associated pneumonia (HCAP) occurs in community members whose extensive contact with health care has changed their risk for virulent and drug-resistant organisms

General Considerations

- The most deadly infectious disease in the United States and the eighth leading cause of death overall
- Mortality rate is 10% to 12% among hospitalized patients
- Prospective studies fail to identify the cause in 40% to 60% of cases, although bacteria are more commonly identified than viruses
- The most common bacterial pathogens in CAP
  - *Streptococcus pneumoniae* (two-thirds of cases)
  - *Haemophilus influenzae*

  — *Mycoplasma pneumonia*
  — *Chlamydophila pneumoniae*
  — *Staphylococcus aureus*
  — *Neisseria meningitidis*
  — *Moraxella catarrhalis*
  — *Klebsiella pneumoniae*
- Common viral causes
  — Influenza
  — Respiratory syncytial virus
  — Adenovirus
  — Parainfluenza virus
- Most common organisms in HAP
  — *S aureus* (both methicillin-sensitive *S aureus* and methicillin-resistant *S aureus*)
  — *Pseudomonas aeruginosa*
  — Gram-negative rods including non-extended spectrum β-lactamase (ESBL)-producing and ESBL-producing (*Enterobacter* species, *K pneumoniae*, and *Escherichia coli*)
- Organisms seen in VAP
  — *Acinetobacter* species
  — *Stenotrophomonas maltophilia*
- Assessment of epidemiologic risk factors may help in diagnosing pneumonia due to the following
  — *Chlamydophila psittaci* (psittacosis)
  — *Coxiella burnetii* (Q fever)
  — *Francisella tularensis* (tularemia)
  — Endemic fungi (*Blastomyces, Coccidioides,* and *Histoplasma*)
  — Sin Nombre virus (hantavirus pulmonary syndrome)

4. Symptoms and Signs

- Acute or subacute onset of fever, cough with or without sputum, and dyspnea
- Rigors, sweats, chills, pleurisy, chest discomfort, and hemoptysis are common
- Fatigue, anorexia, headache, myalgias, and abdominal pain can be present
- Physical findings include
  — Fever or hypothermia
  — Tachypnea
  — Tachycardia
  — Arterial oxygen desaturation
- Altered breath sounds or rales are common
- Dullness to percussion may be observed if lobar consolidation or a parapneumonic effusion is present
- Symptoms may be more nonspecific in HAP and VAP; however, two or more clinical findings (fever, leukocytosis, and purulent sputum) in the setting of a new or progressive pulmonary opacity on chest radiograph are approximately 70% sensitive and 75% specific for the diagnosis of VAP

5. Differential Diagnosis

- Aspiration pneumonia or pneumonitis
- *Pneumocystis jirovecii* pneumonia (PCP)
- Acute respiratory distress syndrome (ARDS)
- Bronchitis
- Lung abscess or obstructing neoplasm
- Tuberculosis
- Pulmonary emboli
- Myocardial infarction

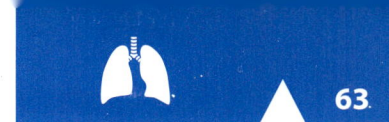

- Heart failure
- Sarcoidosis
- Interstitial lung disease
- Hypersensitivity pneumonitis
- Bronchiolitis, cryptogenic (bronchiolitis obliterans) organizing pneumonitis
- Drug reactions
- Pulmonary hemorrhage
- Atelectasis

6. Laboratory, Imaging, and Procedural Findings

Laboratory Tests
- Sputum Gram stain
  - Neither sensitive nor specific for *Str pneumonia*, the most common cause of CAP
  - Usefulness lies in broadening initial coverage, most commonly to cover *S aureus* (including community-acquired methicillin-resistant strains) or Gram-negative rods (Table 10-1)
- Urinary antigen assays for *Legionella pneumophila* and *Str pneumoniae*
  - At least as sensitive and specific as sputum Gram stain and culture
  - Results are available immediately and are not affected by early initiation of antibiotic therapy
    - Positive tests may allow narrowing of initial antibiotic coverage
    - Indications for urinary antigen assay for *Legionella pneumophilia*
      - Active alcohol use
      - Travel within 2 weeks
      - Pleural effusion
      - ICU admission

Table 10-1. Selected pneumonias: organisms, Gram stain appearance, clinical settings, and complications.

Organism; Appearance on Gram-Stained Smear of Sputum	Clinical Settings	Complications
Streptococcus pneumoniae (pneumococcus). Gram-positive diplococci	Chronic cardiopulmonary disease; follows upper respiratory tract infection	Bacteremia, meningitis, endocarditis, pericarditis, empyema
Haemophilus influenzae. Pleomorphic gram-negative coccobacilli	Chronic cardiopulmonary disease; follows upper respiratory tract infection	Empyema, endocarditis
Staphylococcus aureus. Plump gram-positive cocci in clumps	Residence in chronic care facility, health care-associated, influenza epidemics; cystic fibrosis, bronchiectasis, injection drug use	Empyema, cavitation
Klebsiella pneumoniae. Plump gram-negative encapsulated rods	Alcoholism, diabetes mellitus; health care-associated	Cavitation, empyema
Escherichia coli. Gram-negative rods	Health care-associated; rarely, community-acquired	Empyema
Pseudomonas aeruginosa. Gram-negative rods	Health care-associated; cystic fibrosis, bronchiectasis	Cavitation
Anaerobes. Mixed flora	Aspiration, poor dental hygiene	Necrotizing pneumonia, abscess, empyema
Mycoplasma pneumoniae. PMNs and monocytes; no bacteria	Young adults; summer and fall	Skin rashes, bullous myringitis; hemolytic anemia
Legionella species. Few PMNs; no bacteria	Summer and fall; exposure to contaminated construction site, water source, air conditioner; community-acquired or health care-associated	Empyema, cavitation, endocarditis, pericarditis
Chlamydophila pneumoniae. Nonspecific	Clinically similar to *M pneumoniae*, but prodromal symptoms last longer (up to 2 wk). Sore throat with hoarseness common. Mild pneumonia in teenagers and young adults	Reinfection in older adults with underlying COPD or heart failure may be severe or even fatal
Moraxella catarrhalis. Gram-negative diplococci	Preexisting lung disease; elderly; corticosteroid or immunosuppressive therapy	Rarely, pleural effusions and bacteremia
Pneumocystis jiroveci. Nonspecific	AIDS, immunosuppressive or cytotoxic drug therapy, cancer	Pneumothorax, respiratory failure, ARDS, death

ARDS, acute respiratory distress syndrome; COPD, chronic obstructive pulmonary disease.

○ Indications for urinary antigen assay for *Str pneumoniae*
  • Leukopenia
  • Asplenia
  • Active alcohol use
  • Chronic severe liver disease
  • Pleural effusion
  • ICU admission
• Rapid influenza testing
  — Has intermediate sensitivity but high specificity
  — Positive tests may reduce unnecessary antibacterial use and lead to isolation of hospitalized patients
• All hospitalized patients should have the following tests
  — Complete blood count with differential
  — Chemistry panel (including serum glucose, electrolytes, urea nitrogen, creatinine, bilirubin, and liver enzymes)
  — Arterial blood gases to assess severity of illness
• HIV testing should be done in all adult patients, no longer just those with risk factors
• Additional microbiologic testing, including preantibiotic sputum and blood cultures, has been standard practice for patients who require hospitalization
• Blood cultures identify the pathogen in up to 20% of cases of HAP

Imaging Studies
• Chest radiograph can confirm the diagnosis and detect associated lung diseases
• Findings range from patchy airspace opacities to lobar consolidation with air bronchograms to diffuse alveolar or interstitial opacities
• Clearing of opacities can take 6 weeks or longer

Diagnostic Procedures
• Sputum induction and fiberoptic bronchoscopy are reserved for patients who cannot provide expectorated samples or who may have *P jirovecii* or *Mycobacterium tuberculosis* pneumonia
• Serologic assays, polymerase chain reaction tests, specialized culture tests, and other new diagnostic tests for organisms such as viruses, *Legionella*, *M pneumoniae*, and *C pneumoniae* may be performed when these diagnoses are suspected
• Thoracentesis with pleural fluid analysis should be performed in all patients with effusions
• Procalcitonin
  — A calcitonin precursor released in response to bacterial toxins and inhibited by viral infections
  — Measurement allows clinicians to reduce both initial administration of antibiotics and the duration of antibiotic therapy in CAP
  — Holds promise as a noninvasive strategy to distinguish bacterial pneumonia from noninfectious causes of fever with pulmonary infiltrates in hospitalized patients
• Endotracheal aspiration and fiberoptic bronchoscopy with lavage or use of a protected specimen brush are used most commonly in patients with VAP
• A recent trial using quantitative culture of bronchoalveolar lavage or protected specimen brush samples in suspected VAP
  — Reduced antibiotic use
  — Shortened the duration of organ dysfunction
  — Decreased mortality

7. Treatments

Medications
• See Table 10-2 for dosages of recommended empiric antibiotics for CAP by setting of care
• See Table 10-3 for dosages of recommended empiric antibiotics for HAP, VAP, or HCAP

Table 10-2. Recommended empiric antibiotics for community-acquired pneumonia.

Outpatient management

1. For previously healthy patients who have not taken antibiotics within the last 3 mo:

   a. A macrolide (clarithromycin, 500 mg orally twice a day; or azithromycin, 500 mg orally as a first dose and then 250 mg orally daily for 4 d, or 500 mg orally daily for 3 d).

or

   b. Doxycycline, 100 mg orally twice a day.

2. For patients with such comorbid medical conditions as chronic heart, lung, liver, or renal disease; diabetes mellitus; alcoholism; malignancy; asplenia; immunosuppressant conditions or use of immunosuppressive drugs; or use of antibiotics within the previous 3 mo (in which case, an alternative from a different antibiotic class should be selected):

   a. A respiratory fluoroquinolone (moxifloxacin, 400 mg orally daily; gemifloxacin, 320 mg orally daily; levofloxacin, 750 mg orally daily).

or

   b. A macrolide (as above) plus a β-lactam (amoxicillin, 1 g orally three times a day; amoxicillin-clavulanate, 2 g orally twice a day are preferred to cefpodoxime, 200 mg orally twice a day; cefuroxime, 500 mg orally twice a day).

3. In regions with a high rate (> 25%) of infection with high-level (MIC ≥ 16 μg/mL) macrolide-resistant *Streptococcus pneumoniae*, consider use of alternative agents listed above in (2) for patients without comorbidities.

Inpatient management not requiring intensive care

1. A respiratory fluoroquinolone

   a. See above for oral therapy.

   b. For intravenous therapy, moxifloxacin, 400 mg daily; levofloxacin, 750 mg daily; ciprofloxacin, 400 mg every 8–12 h;

or

2. A macrolide *plus* a β-lactam

   a. See above for oral therapy.

   b. For intravenous therapy, ampicillin, 1–2 g every 4–6 h; cefotaxime, 1–2 g every 4–12 h; ceftriaxone, 1–2 g every 12–24 h.

Inpatient management requiring intensive care

1. Azithromycin (500 mg orally as a first dose and then 250 mg orally daily for 4 d, or 500 mg orally daily for 3 d) or a respiratory fluoroquinolone *plus* an intravenous antipneumococcal β-lactam (cefotaxime, ceftriaxone, or ampicillin-sulbactam, 1.5–3 g every 6 h).

2. For patients allergic to β-lactam antibiotics, a fluoroquinolone *plus* aztreonam (1–2 g every 6–12 h).

3. For patients at risk for *Pseudomonas* infection

   a. An antipneumococcal, antipseudomonal β-lactam (piperacillin-tazobactam, 3.375–4.5 g every 6 h; cefepime, 1–2 g twice a day; imipenem, 0.5–1 g every 6–8 h; meropenem, 1 g every 8 h) *plus* ciprofloxacin (400 mg every 8–12 h) or levofloxacin (750 mg daily).

or

   b. An antipneumococcal, antipseudomonal β-lactam (piperacillin-tazobactam, 3.375–4.5 g every 6 h; cefepime, 1–2 g twice a day; imipenem, 0.5–1 g every 6–8 h; meropenem, 1 g every 8 h) *plus* an aminoglycoside (gentamicin, tobramycin, amikacin, all weight-based dosing administered daily adjusted to appropriate trough levels) *plus* azithromycin or a respiratory fluoroquinolone.

4. For patients at risk for methicillin-resistant *Staphylococcus aureus* infection, add vancomycin (interval dosing based on renal function to achieve serum tough concentration 15–20 μg/mL) or linezolid (600 mg twice a day).

MIC, minimum inhibitory concentration.

Adapted, with permission of Oxford University Press, from Mandell LA et al. Infectious Diseases Society of America/American Thoracic Society consensus guidelines on the management of community-acquired pneumonia in adults. *Clin Infect Dis*. 2007;44:S27–S72. [PMID: 17278083]

- See Table 10-4 for drugs of first choice and alternatives by suspected or proved microbial pathogen
- Outpatient therapy
  — For previously healthy patients with no recent use of antibiotics: a macrolide (clarithromycin or azithromycin) *or* doxycycline
  — In patients at risk for drug resistance:
    › A respiratory fluoroquinolone (eg, moxifloxacin, gemifloxacin, or levofloxacin) *or*
    › A macrolide plus a β-lactam (high-dose amoxicillin and amoxicillin-clavulanate are preferred to cefpodoxime and cefuroxime)

Table 10-3. Recommended empiric antibiotics for hospital-acquired, ventilator-associated, or health care-associated pneumonias.

When there is low risk for multiple drug-resistant pathogens, use *one* of the following:
Ceftriaxone, 1–2 g intravenously every 12–24 h
Gemifloxacin, 320 mg orally daily
Moxifloxacin, 400 mg orally or intravenously daily
Levofloxacin, 750 mg orally or intravenously daily
Ciprofloxacin, 400 mg intravenously every 8–12 h
Ampicillin-sulbactam, 1.5–3 g intravenously every 6 h
Piperacillin-tazobactam 3.375–4.5 g intravenously every 6 h
Ertapenem, 1 g intravenously daily
When there is higher risk for multiple drug-resistant pathogens, use one agent from each of the following categories:
1. Antipseudomonal coverage
a. Cefepime, 1–2 g intravenously twice a day or ceftazidime, 1–2 g intravenously every 8 h
b. Imipenem, 0.5–1 g intravenously every 6–8 h or meropenem, 1 g intravenously every 8 h
c. Piperacillin-tazobactam, 3.375–4.5 g intravenously every 6 h
d. For penicillin allergic patients, aztreonam, 1–2 g intravenously every 6–12 h
2. A second antipseudomonal agent
a. Levofloxacin, 750 mg intravenously daily or ciprofloxacin, 400 mg intravenously every 8–12 h
b. Intravenous gentamicin, tobramycin, amikacin, all weight-based dosing administered daily adjusted to appropriate trough levels
3. Coverage for MRSA if appropriate with either
a. Intravenous vancomycin (interval dosing based on renal function to achieve serum trough concentration 15–20 μg/mL)
or
b. Linezolid, 600 mg intravenously twice a day

MRSA, methicillin-resistant *Staphylococcus aureus*.

Adapted with permission of the American Thoracic Society. Copyright © American Thoracic Society. American Thoracic Society, Infectious Diseases Society of America. Guidelines for the management of adults with hospital-acquired, ventilator-associated and healthcare-associated pneumonia. *Am J Respir Crit Care Med*. 2005;171(4):388–416. [PMID: 15699079]

Table 10-4. Drugs of choice for suspected or proved microbial pathogens causing pneumonia, 2014.[a]

Suspected or Proved Etiologic Agent	Drug(s) of First Choice	Alternative Drug(s)
Gram-positive cocci		
Streptococcus pneumoniae[g] (pneumococcus)	Penicillin[f]	An erythromycin,[c] a cephalosporin,[h] vancomycin, clindamycin, azithromycin, clarithromycin, a tetracycline,[d] respiratory fluoroquinolones[b]
Staphylococcus, methicillin-resistant	Vancomycin	TMP-SMZ,[e] doxycycline, minocycline, linezolid, daptomycin, quinupristin-dalfopristin, tigecycline, televancin
Staphylococcus, non-penicillinase-producing	Penicillin[f]	A cephalosporin,[h] clindamycin
Staphylococcus, penicillinase-producing	Penicillinase-resistant penicillin[j]	Vancomycin, a cephalosporin,[h] clindamycin, amoxicillin-clavulanic acid, ampicillin-sulbactam, piperacillin-tazobactam, TMP-SMZ[e]
Gram-negative cocci		
Moraxella catarrhalis	Cefuroxime, a fluoroquinolone[b]	Cefotaxime, ceftriaxone, cefuroxime axetil, an erythromycin,[c] a tetracycline,[d] azithromycin, amoxicillin-clavulanic acid, clarithromycin, TMP-SMZ[e]
Gram-negative rods		
Acinetobacter	Imipenem, meropenem	Tigecycline, ertapenem, minocycline, doxycycline, aminoglycosides,[i] colistin
Prevotella, oropharyngeal strains	Clindamycin	Metronidazole

(continued)

Table 10-4. Drugs of choice for suspected or proved microbial pathogens causing pneumonia, 2014.[a] (continued)

Suspected or Proved Etiologic Agent	Drug(s) of First Choice	Alternative Drug(s)
Escherichia coli	Cefotaxime, ceftriaxone,	Imipenem[m] or meropenem,[m] aminoglycosides,[j] a fluoroquinolone,[b] aztreonam, ticarcillin-clavulanate, ampicillin-sulbactam, piperacillin-tazobactam
Haemophilus (respiratory infections, otitis)	TMP-SMZ[e]	Doxycycline, azithromycin, clarithromycin, cefotaxime, ceftriaxone, cefuroxime, cefuroxime axetil, ampicillin-clavulanate
Klebsiella[k]	A cephalosporin	TMP-SMZ,[e] aminoglycoside,[j] imipenem[k] or meropenem,[k] a fluoroquinolone,[b] aztreonam, ticarcillin-clavulanate, ampicillin-sulbactam, piperacillin-tazobactam
Legionella species (pneumonia)	Azithromycin, or fluoroquinolones[b] ± rifampin	Doxycycline ± rifampin
Pseudomonas aeruginosa	Piperacillin-tazobactam or ceftazidime or cefepime, or imipenem or meropenem or doripenem ± aminoglycoside[j]	Ciprofloxacin (or levofloxacin) ± piperacillin-tazobactam; ciprofloxacin (or levofloxacin) ± ceftazidime; ciprofloxacin (or levofloxacin) ± cefepime; piperacillin-tazobactam + tobramycin; ceftazidime + tobramycin; cefepime + tobramycin; meropenem (imipenem, doripenem) + tobramycin
Acid-fast rods		
Mycobacterium tuberculosis[l]	Isoniazid (INH) + rifampin + pyrazinamide ± ethambutol	Streptomycin
Mycobacterium avium complex	Clarithromycin or azithromycin + ethambutol ± rifabutin	Amikacin, ciprofloxacin
Nocardia	TMP-SMZ[e]	Minocycline, imipenem or meropenem, linezolid
Mycoplasmas		
Mycoplasma pneumoniae	Clarithromycin or azithromycin or doxycycline	A fluoroquinolone,[b] erythromycin[c]
Chlamydiae		
C psittaci	Doxycycline	Chloramphenicol
C pneumoniae	Doxycycline[d]	Erythromycin,[c] clarithromycin, azithromycin, a fluoroquinolone[b,m]

[a]Adapted, with permission, from *Treat Guide Med Lett*. 2010;6(94):43–52.

[b]Fluoroquinolones include ciprofloxacin, ofloxacin, levofloxacin, moxifloxacin, and others. Gemifloxacin, levofloxacin, and moxifloxacin have the best activity against Gram-positive organisms, including penicillin-resistant *Str pneumoniae* and methicillin-sensitive *S aureus*. Activity against enterococci and *S epidermidis* is variable.

[c]Erythromycin estolate is best absorbed orally but carries the highest risk of hepatitis; erythromycin stearate and erythromycin ethylsuccinate are also available.

[d]All tetracyclines have similar activity against most microorganisms. Minocycline (most likely to have *S aureus* activity), doxycycline, and tetracycline have increased activity against *S aureus*.

[e]TMP-SMZ is a mixture of 1 part trimethoprim and 5 parts sulfamethoxazole.

[f]Penicillin G is preferred for parenteral injection; penicillin V for oral administration—to be used only in treating infections due to highly sensitive organisms.

[g]Infections caused by isolates with intermediate resistance may respond to high doses of penicillin, cefotaxime, or ceftriaxone. Infections caused by highly resistant strains should be treated with vancomycin. Many strains of penicillin-resistant pneumococci are resistant to macrolides, cephalosporins, tetracyclines, and TMP-SMZ.

[h]Most intravenous cephalosporins (with the exception of ceftazidime) have good activity against gram-positive cocci.

[i]Parenteral nafcillin or oxacillin; oral dicloxacillin, cloxacillin, or oxacillin.

[j]Aminoglycosides—gentamicin, tobramycin, amikacin, netilmicin—should be chosen on the basis of local patterns of susceptibility.

[k]Extended β-lactamase-producing isolates should be treated with a carbapenem.

[l]Resistance is common and susceptibility testing should be done.

[m]Ciprofloxacin has inferior antichlamydial activity compared with levofloxacin or ofloxacin.

Key: ±, alone or combined with.

— In regions where there is a high incidence of macrolide-resistant *Str pneumoniae*, patients with no comorbidities may receive a respiratory fluoroquinolone or the combination of a β-lactam added to a macrolide as initial therapy

• First-line therapy in hospitalized patients
  — Fluoroquinolone (eg, moxifloxacin, gemifloxacin, or levofloxacin) *or*
  — The combination of a macrolide (clarithromycin or azithromycin) plus a β-lactam (cefotaxime, ceftriaxone, or ampicillin)

- Patients in intensive care unit
  — Azithromycin or a fluoroquinolone (moxifloxacin, gemifloxacin, or levofloxacin) plus an antipneumococcal β-lactam (cefotaxime, ceftriaxone, or ampicillin–sulbactam)
- In hospitalized patients at risk for *Pseudomonas* infection
  — Use an antipneumococcal, antipseudomonal β-lactam (piperacillin-tazobactam, cefepime, imipenem, and meropenem) plus ciprofloxacin or levofloxacin
  — The above antipneumococcal β-lactam plus an aminoglycoside (gentamicin, tobramycin, and amikacin)
- HAP or VAP patients require empiric coverage for both *Pseudomonas* and methicillin-resistant *S aureus* (vancomycin).
- Data from a large trial assessing treatment outcomes in VAP suggest that 8 days of antibiotics is as good as 15 days, except in cases caused by *P aeruginosa*

8. Outcomes

Follow-Up
- Chest radiograph 6 weeks after therapy

Complications
- Parapneumonic effusion—simple or complicated
- Empyema
- Sepsis
- Respiratory failure or ARDS, or both
- Pneumatocele
- Lung abscess
- Focal bronchiectasis

Prognosis
- Excellent for CAP with appropriate antimicrobial and supportive care
- HAP is the second most common cause of infection among hospital inpatients and is the leading cause of hospital death due to infection with mortality rates ranging from 20% to 50%

Prevention
- Polyvalent pneumococcal vaccine
  — Can prevent or lessen the severity of pneumococcal infections
  — Indications are age ≥ 65 or any chronic illness increasing the risk of CAP
- Influenza vaccine
  — Effective at preventing primary influenza pneumonia and secondary bacterial pneumonia
  — Given annually to patients who are age ≥ 65, are residents of long-term care facilities, have cardiopulmonary disease, or were recently hospitalized with chronic metabolic disorders
- Hospitalized patients who would benefit from vaccine should receive it in hospital
- Pneumococcal and influenza vaccines can be given simultaneously and may be administered as soon as the patient has stabilized
- Sucralfate use for gastric ulcer prophylaxis (rather than H_2-receptor antagonists or proton-pump inhibitors) may reduce the incidence of VAP
- Hand washing in patient care areas

9. When to Refer and When to Admit

When to Refer
- Extensive disease
- Seriously ill patient, particularly in the setting of comorbid conditions (eg, liver disease)
- Progression of disease or failure to improve on antibiotics

When to Admit
- Failure of outpatient therapy, including inability to maintain oral intake and medications
- Exacerbations of underlying disease that would benefit from hospitalization

SUGGESTED REFERENCES

Bartlett JG. Anaerobic bacterial infection of the lung. *Anaerobe*. 2012 Apr;18(2):235–239. [PMID: 22209937]

Desai H et al. Pulmonary emergencies: pneumonia, acute respiratory distress syndrome, lung abscess, and empyema. *Med Clin North Am*. 2012 Nov;96(6):1127–1148. [PMID: 23102481]

Kwong JC et al. New aspirations: the debate on aspiration pneumonia treatment guidelines. *Med J Aust*. 2011 Oct 3;195(7):380–381. [PMID: 21978335]

Madaras-Kelly KJ et al. Guideline-based antibiotics and mortality in healthcare-associated pneumonia. *J Gen Intern Med*. 2012 Jul;27(7):845–852. [PMID: 22396110]

Mandell LA et al. Infectious Diseases Society of America/American Thoracic Society consensus guidelines on the management of community-acquired pneumonia in adults. *Clin Infect Dis*. 2007 Mar 1;44(Suppl 2):S27–S72. [PMID: 17278083]

Marik PE. Aspiration syndromes: aspiration pneumonia and pneumonitis. *Hosp Pract (Minneap)*. 2010 Feb;38(1):35–42. [PMID: 20469622]

Restrepo MI et al. Severe community-acquired pneumonia. *Infect Dis Clin North Am*. 2009 Sep;23(3):503–520. [PMID: 19665080]

Richards G et al. CURB-65, PSI, and APACHE II to assess mortality risk in patients with severe sepsis and community acquired pneumonia in PROWESS. *J Intensive Care Med*. 2011 Jan–Feb;26(1):34–40. [PMID: 21341394]

Waterer GW et al. Management of community-acquired pneumonia in adults. *Am J Respir Crit Care Med*. 2011 Jan 15;183(2):157–164. [PMID: 20693379]

Watkins RR et al. Diagnosis and management of community-acquired pneumonia in adults. *Am Fam Physician*. 2011 Jun 1;83(11):1299–1306. [PMID: 21661712]

11

Pulmonary Embolism

A 57-year-old man undergoes total knee replacement for severe degenerative joint disease. Four days after surgery, he develops acute onset of shortness of breath and right-sided pleuritic chest pain. He is now in moderate respiratory distress with a respiratory rate of 28/min, heart rate of 120 bpm, and blood pressure of 110/70 mm Hg. Oxygen saturation is 88% on room air. Lung examination is normal. Cardiac examination reveals tachycardia but is otherwise unremarkable. The right lower extremity is postsurgical, healing well, with 2+ pitting edema, calf tenderness, erythema, and warmth; the left leg is normal.

LEARNING OBJECTIVES

▶ Learn the common and uncommon clinical manifestations and objective findings of pulmonary embolism

▶ Know the options for diagnosing pulmonary embolism

▶ Understand the factors that predispose to pulmonary embolism

▶ Know the differential diagnosis of pulmonary embolism

▶ Learn the treatment options and duration for pulmonary embolism

QUESTIONS

1. What are the salient features of this patient's problem?

2. How do you think through his problem?

3. What are the key features, including essentials of diagnosis and general considerations, of pulmonary embolism?

4. What are the symptoms and signs of pulmonary embolism?

5. What is the differential diagnosis of pulmonary embolism?

6. What are laboratory and imaging findings in pulmonary embolism?

7. What are the treatments for pulmonary embolism?

8. What are the outcomes, including complications, prevention, and prognosis, of pulmonary embolism?

9. When should patients with pulmonary embolism be referred to a specialist or admitted to the hospital?

ANSWERS

1. Salient Features

Recent surgery; acute shortness of breath; pleuritic chest pain; tachypnea and tachycardia; hypoxia and oxygen desaturation; symptoms and signs of deep venous thrombosis (DVT) with unilateral calf tenderness; and edema

2. How to Think Through

This patient has sudden onset dyspnea, chest pain, tachypnea, hypoxemia, and tachycardia. What diagnoses are in the differential for this clinical scenario? (Myocardial infarction, pneumothorax, cardiac tamponade, pulmonary embolism [PE].) What features make PE more likely than the other diagnoses? (Pleuritic quality, normal lung and heart examination, postsurgical setting.) After attending to the management priorities of this unstable patient (supplemental oxygen, IV access), what are the immediate diagnostic priorities? (ECG, chest x-ray.) If the ECG shows sinus tachycardia and the chest x-ray shows clear lung fields, how should the possibility of PE be evaluated? (Helical CT scan.) Is there a role for a D-dimer test? (No. This test is best used for intermediate probability scenarios. The clinical prediction rule for pulmonary embolism score [Modified Wells Criteria] in this case is 9 [see Table 11-2 and Figure 11-1].) The CT scan shows extensive bilateral pulmonary emboli. How will you decide if this is a "massive" or "submassive" PE? Why is this distinction important? ("Massive PE" indicates hemodynamic compromise and cardiogenic shock and is treated by thrombolysis. Its benefits in "submassive" PE are less clear.) How might you better assess right heart strain in this case, given that the BP is likely below baseline, but the patient is not in shock? (Echocardiogram.) What is the treatment you should initiate regardless of the thrombolysis decision? (Heparin or LMWH.) Is a workup for thrombophilia indicated? (The surgery and stasis are more likely than an inherited or acquired thrombophilia to be the cause of this "provoked" PE so a workup for other causes of hypercoagulability is not needed.) What is the typical duration of anticoagulation therapy for "provoked" VTE? (6 months.)

3. Key Features

Essentials of Diagnosis

- Predisposition to venous thrombosis, usually of the lower extremities
- Usually dyspnea, chest pain, hemoptysis, or syncope

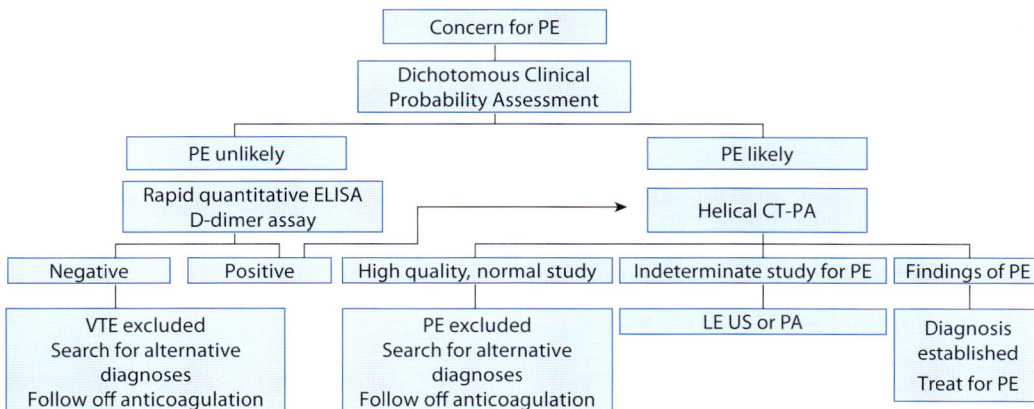

Figure 11-1. D-dimer and helical CT-PA based diagnostic algorithm for PE. CT-PA, CT pulmonary angiogram; PE, pulmonary embolism; ELISA, enzyme-linked immunosorbent assay; VTE, venous thromboembolic disease; LE US, lower extremity venous ultrasound for deep venous thrombosis; PA, pulmonary angiogram. (Reproduced, with permission, from van Belle A, et al. Effectiveness of managing suspected pulmonary embolism using an algorithm combining clinical probability, D-dimer testing, and computed tomography. *JAMA.* 2006;295(2):172–179.)

- Tachypnea and a widened alveolar–arterial PO_2 difference
- Elevated rapid D-dimer and characteristic defects on CT arteriogram of the chest, ventilation-perfusion lung scan, or pulmonary angiogram

General Considerations

- Third most common cause of death in hospitalized patients
- Most cases are not recognized antemortem: < 10% with fatal emboli receive specific treatment
- Pulmonary thromboembolism (PE) and DVT are manifestations of the same disease, with the same risk factors
  — Immobility (bed rest, stroke, and obesity)
  — Hyperviscosity (polycythemia)
  — Increased central venous pressures (low cardiac output, pregnancy)
  — Vessel damage (prior DVT, orthopedic surgery, and trauma)
  — Hypercoagulable states, either acquired or inherited
- Pulmonary thromboemboli most often originate in deep veins of the lower extremities
- PE develops in 50% to 60% of patients with proximal lower extremity DVT; 50% of these events are asymptomatic
- Hypoxemia results from vascular obstruction leading to dead space ventilation, right-to-left shunting, and decreased cardiac output
- Other types of pulmonary emboli
  — Fat embolism
  — Air embolism
  — Amniotic fluid embolism
  — Septic embolism (eg, endocarditis)
  — Tumor embolism (eg, renal cell carcinoma)
  — Foreign body embolism (eg, talc in injection drug use)
  — Parasite egg embolism (schistosomiasis)

4. Symptoms and Signs

- Clinical findings depend on the size of the embolus and the patient's preexisting cardio-pulmonary status
- Dyspnea occurs in 75% to 85% and chest pain in 65% to 75% of patients
- Tachypnea is the only sign reliably found in > 50% of patients
- In the Prospective Investigation of Pulmonary Embolism Diagnosis (PIOPED) study, 97% of patients had **at least one** of the following
  — Dyspnea
  — Tachypnea
  — Chest pain with breathing
- See Table 11-1

5. Differential Diagnosis

- Myocardial infarction (heart attack)
- Pneumonia
- Pericarditis
- Heart failure
- Pleuritis (pleurisy)
- Pneumothorax
- Pericardial tamponade

6. Laboratory and Imaging Findings

Laboratory Tests

- ECG is abnormal in 70% of patients
  — Sinus tachycardia and nonspecific ST-T changes are the most common findings

Table 11-1. Frequency of specific symptoms and signs in patients at risk for pulmonary thromboembolism.

	UPET[a] PE + (n = 327)	PIOPED I[b] PE + (n = 117)	PIOPED I[b] PE − (n = 248)
Symptoms			
Dyspnea	84%	73%	72%
Respirophasic chest pain	74%	66%	59%
Cough	53%	37%	36%
Leg pain	Nr	26%	24%
Hemoptysis	30%	13%	8%
Palpitations	Nr	10%	18%
Wheezing	Nr	9%	11%
Anginal pain	14%	4%	6%
Signs			
Respiratory rate ≥ 16 UPET, ≥ 20 PIOPED I	92%	70%	68%
Crackles (rales)	58%	51%	40%[c]
Heart rate ≥ 100/min	44%	30%	24%
Fourth heart sound (S$_4$)	Nr	24%	13%[c]
Accentuated pulmonary component of second heart sound (S$_2$P)	53%	23%	13%[c]
T ≥ 37.5°C UPET, ≥ 38.5°C PIOPED	43%	7%	12%
Homans sign	Nr	4%	2%
Pleural friction rub	Nr	3%	2%
Third heart sound (S$_3$)	Nr	3%	4%
Cyanosis	19%	1%	2%

Nr, not reported; PE+, confirmed diagnosis of pulmonary embolism; PE−, diagnosis of pulmonary embolism ruled out.

[a]Data from the Urokinase-Streptokinase Pulmonary Embolism Trial, as reported in Bell WR, et al. The clinical features of submassive and massive pulmonary emboli. *Am J Med*. 1977;62(3):355–360. [PMID: 842555]

[b]Data from patients enrolled in the PIOPED I study, as reported in Stein PD et al. Clinical, laboratory, roentgenographic, and electrocardiographic findings in patients with acute pulmonary embolism and no preexisting cardiac or pulmonary disease. *Chest*. 1991;100(3):598–603. [PMID: 1909617]

[c]P < .05 comparing patients in the PIOPED I study.

- Acute respiratory alkalosis, hypoxemia, and widened arterial–alveolar O$_2$ gradient (A–a DO$_2$), but these findings are not diagnostic (Table 11-2)
- Using a D-dimer threshold between 300 and 500 ng/mL (300 and 500 μg/L), a rapid ELISA has shown a sensitivity for venous thromboembolism of 95% to 97% and a specificity of 45%

Imaging Studies
- Chest radiograph—most common findings
  — Atelectasis
  — Infiltrates
  — Pleural effusions
  — Westermark sign is focal oligemia with a prominent central pulmonary artery
  — Hampton hump is a pleural-based area of increased intensity from intraparenchymal hemorrhage
- Lung scanning (V/Q scan)
  — A normal scan can exclude PE
  — A high-probability scan is sufficient to make the diagnosis in most cases
  — Indeterminate scans are common and do not further refine clinical pretest probabilities

Table 11-2. Clinical prediction rule for pulmonary embolism (PE).

Variable	Points
Clinical symptoms and signs of deep venous thrombosis (DVT) (leg swelling and pain with palpation of deep veins)	3.0
Alternative diagnosis less likely than PE	3.0
Heart rate > 100 beats/min	1.5
Immobilization for more than 3 d or surgery in previous 4 wk	1.5
Previous PE or DVT	1.5
Hemoptysis	1.0
Cancer (with treatment within past 6 mo or palliative care)	1.0
Three-tiered clinical probability assessment	**Score**
High	> 6.0
Moderate	2.0–6.0
Low	< 2.0
Dichotomous clinical probability assessment	**Score**
PE likely	> 4.0
PE unlikely	< or = 4.0

Data from Wells PS, et al. Derivation of a simple clinical model to categorize patients probability of pulmonary embolism: increasing the models utility with the SimpliRED D-dimer. *Thromb Haemost.* 2000;83(3):416–420. [PMID: 10744147]

- Helical CT arteriography is supplanting V/Q scanning as the initial diagnostic study
  — It requires administration of intravenous radiocontrast dye but is otherwise noninvasive
  — It is very sensitive for the detection of thrombus in the proximal pulmonary arteries but less so in the segmental and subsegmental arteries
- Venous thrombosis studies
  — Lower extremity venous Doppler ultrasonography is the test of choice in most centers
  — Diagnosing DVT establishes the need for treatment and may preclude invasive testing in patients in whom there is a high suspicion for PE
- In the setting of a nondiagnostic V/Q scan, negative serial DVT studies over 2 weeks predict a low risk (< 2%) of subsequent DVT over the next 6 weeks
- Pulmonary angiography is the reference standard for the diagnosis of PE
  — Invasive, but safe—minor complications in < 5%
  — Role in the diagnosis of PE controversial, but generally used when there is a high clinical probability and negative noninvasive studies
- MRI is a research tool for the diagnosis of PE
- Integrated approach is used (Figure 11-1)

7. Treatments

Medications
- See Table 11-3.
- Full anticoagulation with heparin should begin with the diagnostic evaluation in patients with a moderate to high clinical likelihood of PE and no contraindications
- Once the diagnosis of proximal DVT or PE is established, it is critical to ensure adequate therapy
- LMWHs are as effective as unfractionated heparin
  — Administered in dosages determined by body weight once or twice daily without the need for coagulation monitoring
  — Subcutaneous administration appears to be as effective as the intravenous route

Table 11-3. Initial anticoagulation for venous thromboembolism.[a]

Anticoagulant	Dose/Frequency	Clinical Scenario					Comment
		DVT, Lower Extremity	DVT, Upper Extremity	PE	VTE, with Concomitant Severe Renal Impairment[b]	VTE, Cancer-Related	
Unfractionated Heparin							
Unfractionated heparin	80 units/kg IV bolus then continuous IV infusion of 18 units/kg/h	×	×	×	×		Bolus may be omitted if risk of bleeding is perceived to be elevated. Maximum bolus, 10000 units. Requires aPTT monitoring. Most patients: begin warfarin at time of initiation of heparin
	330 units/kg SC × 1 then 250 units/kg SC q12h	×					Fixed-dose; no aPTT monitoring required
LMWH and Fondaparinux							
Enoxaparin[c]	1 mg/kg SC q12h	×	×	×			Most patients: begin warfarin at time of initiation of LMWH
	1.5 mg/kg SC once daily		×				
Dalteparin[c]	200 units/kg SC once daily for first month	×	×	×	×		Cancer: administer LMWH for ≥ 3–6 mo; reduce dose to 150 units/kg after first month of treatment
Fondaparinux	5–10 mg SC once daily (see Comment)	×	×	×			Use 7.5 mg for body weight 50–100 kg; 10 mg for body weight > 100 kg
Novel Oral Anticoagulants							
Rivaroxaban	15 mg orally twice daily for first 3 wk then 20 mg orally every bedtime						

DVT, deep venous thrombosis; IV, intravenously; PE, pulmonary embolism; SC, subcutaneously; VTE, venous thromboembolic disease (includes DVT and PE).

Note: An "×" denotes appropriate use of the anticoagulant.

[a]Obtain baseline hemoglobin, platelet count, aPTT, PT/INR, creatinine, urinalysis, and hemoccult prior to initiation of anticoagulation. *Anticoagulation is contraindicated in the setting of active bleeding.*

[b]Defined as creatinine clearance < 30 mL/min.

[c]Body weight < 50 kg: reduce dose and monitor anti-Xa levels.

- Warfarin
  - Initial dose: 2.5 to 10 mg/d
  - Usually requires 5 to 7 days to become therapeutic; therefore, heparin is generally continued for 5 days
  - Maintenance therapy usually requires 2 to 15 mg/d
  - Contraindicated in pregnancy; LMWHs are safe alternatives
- New (novel) oral anticoagulants such as the factor Xa inhibitors (eg, rivaroxaban) are alternatives to warfarin
- Guidelines for the duration of full anticoagulation
  - 3 months of anticoagulation after a first episode provoked by a surgery or a transient nonsurgical risk factor
  - 6–12 months for unprovoked or recurrent episode with a low to moderate risk of bleeding
  - 6 months for an initial episode with a reversible risk factor
  - 12 months after an initial, idiopathic episode
  - 6 to 12 months to indefinitely in patients with irreversible risk factors or recurrent disease
- Thrombolytic therapy accelerates resolution of thrombi when compared with heparin, but does not improve mortality
  - Carries 10-fold greater risk of intracranial hemorrhage compared with heparin (0.2%–2.1%)
  - Indicated in patients who are hemodynamically unstable while on heparin

Table 11-4. Pharmacologic prophylaxis of VTE in selected clinical scenarios.[a]

Anticoagulant	Dose	Frequency	Clinical Scenario	Comment
Enoxaparin	40 mg	Once daily	Most medical inpatients and critical care patients	—
			Surgical patients (moderate risk for VTE)	Consider continuing for 4 wk total duration for cancer surgery and high-risk medical patients
			Abdominal/pelvic cancer surgery	
		Twice daily	Bariatric surgery	Higher doses may be required
	30 mg	Twice daily	Orthopedic surgery[b]	Give for at least 10 d. For THR, TKA, or HFS, consider continuing up to 1 mo after surgery in high-risk patients
			Major trauma	Not applicable to patients with isolated lower extremity trauma
			Acute spinal cord injury	—
Dalteparin	2500 units	Once daily	Most medical inpatients	—
			Abdominal surgery (moderate risk for VTE)	Give for 5–10 d
	5000 units	Once daily	Orthopedic surgery[b]	First dose = 2500 units. Give for at least 10 d. For THR, TKA, or HFS, consider continuing up to 1 mo after surgery in high-risk patients
			Abdominal surgery (higher risk for VTE)	Give for 5–10 d
			Medical inpatients	—
Fondaparinux	2.5 mg	Once daily	Orthopedic surgery[b]	Give for at least 10 d. For THR, TKA or HFS, consider continuing up to 1 mo after surgery in high-risk patients
Rivaroxaban	10 mg	Once daily	Orthopedic surgery—total hip and total knee replacement	Give for 12 d following THR; give for 35 d following THR
Apixaban	2.5 mg orally	Twice daily	following hip or knee replacement surgery	Give for 12 d following total knee replacement; give for 35 d following total hip replacement
Unfractionated heparin	5000 units	Three times daily	Higher VTE risk with low bleeding risk	Includes gynecologic surgery for malignancy and urologic surgery, medical patients with multiple risk factors for VTE
	5000 units	Twice daily	Hospitalized patients at intermediate risk for VTE Patients with epidural catheters Patients with severe kidney disease[c]	Includes gynecologic surgery (moderate risk) LMWHs usually avoided due to risk of spinal hematoma LMWHs contraindicated
Warfarin	(variable)	Once daily	Orthopedic surgery[b]	Titrate to goal INR = 2.5. Give for at least 10 d. For high-risk patients undergoing THR, TKA, or HFS, consider continuing up to 1 mo after surgery

HFS, hip fracture surgery; LMWH, low-molecular-weight heparin; THR, total hip replacement; TKA, total knee arthroplasty; VTE, venous thromboembolic disease.

[a]All regimens administered subcutaneously, except for warfarin.

[b]Includes TKA, THR, and HFS.

[c]Defined as creatinine clearance < 30 mL/min.

- Inferior venal caval (IVC) interruption (IVC filters) may be indicated when a significant contraindication to anticoagulation exists or when recurrence occurs despite adequate anticoagulation
- IVC filters decrease the short-term incidence of PE, but increase the long-term rate of recurrent DVT; thus, provision should be made at insertion for their subsequent removal

Surgery
- Pulmonary embolectomy is an emergency procedure with a high mortality rate performed at few centers

Therapeutic Procedures
- Catheter devices that fragment and extract thrombus have been used on small numbers of patients
- Platelet counts should be monitored for the first 14 days of UFH due to the risk of immune-mediated thrombocytopenia
- Warfarin has interactions with many drugs

8. Outcomes

Complications
- Immune-mediated thrombocytopenia occurs in 3% of patients taking UFH
- Hemorrhage is the major complication of anticoagulation with heparin: risk of any hemorrhage is 0% to 7%; risk of fatal hemorrhage is 0% to 2%
- Risk of hemorrhage with warfarin therapy is 3% to 4% per patient year, but correlates with INR
- Chronic thromboembolic pulmonary hypertension occurs in about 1% of patients; selected patients may benefit from pulmonary endarterectomy

Prevention
- See Table 11-4

Prognosis
- Overall prognosis depends on the underlying disease rather than the thromboembolic event
- Death from recurrent PE occurs in only 3% of cases; 6 months of anticoagulation therapy reduces the risk of recurrent thrombosis and death by 80% to 90%
- Perfusion defects resolve in most survivors

9. When to Refer and When to Admit

When to Refer
- All patients evaluated for or diagnosed with a PE should be evaluated by an expert (typically a pulmonologist, hematologist, or internist)

When to Admit
- Patients with an acute PE should be admitted for stabilization, initiation of therapy, evaluation of cause of PE, and education

SUGGESTED REFERENCES

American College of Emergency Physicians Clinical Policies Subcommittee on Critical Issues in the Evaluation and Management of Adult Patients Presenting to the Emergency Department With Suspected Pulmonary Embolism; Fesmire FM et al. Critical issues in the evaluation and management of adult patients presenting to the emergency department with suspected pulmonary embolism. *Ann Emerg Med.* 2011 Jun;57(6):628–652.e75. [PMID: 21621092]

Burns SK, et al. Diagnostic imaging and risk stratification of patients with acute pulmonary embolism. *Cardiol Rev.* 2012 Jan–Feb;20(1):15–24. [PMID: 22143281]

Goldhaber SZ, et al. Pulmonary embolism and deep vein thrombosis. *Lancet.* 2012 May 12;379(9828):1835–1846. [PMID: 22494827]

Jaff MR, et al. American Heart Association Council on Cardiopulmonary, Critical Care, Perioperative and Resuscitation; American Heart Association Council on Peripheral Vascular Disease; American Heart Association Council on Arteriosclerosis, Thrombosis and Vascular Biology. Management of massive and submassive pulmonary embolism, iliofemoral deep vein thrombosis, and chronic thromboembolic pulmonary hypertension: a scientific statement from the American Heart Association. *Circulation*. 2011 Apr 26;123(16):1788–1830. [PMID: 21422387]

Kearon C, et al. Antithrombotic therapy for VTE disease: Antithrombotic Therapy and Prevention of Thrombosis, 9th ed: American College of Chest Physicians Evidence-Based Clinical Practice Guideline. *Chest*. 2012 Feb;141(2 Suppl):e419S–e494S. [PMID: 22315268]

Lucassen W, et al. Clinical decision rules for excluding pulmonary embolism: a meta-analysis. *Ann Intern Med*. 2011 Oct 4;155(7):448–460. [PMID: 21969343]

Merrigan JM, et al. JAMA patient page. Pulmonary embolism. *JAMA*. 2013 Feb 6;309(5):504. [PMID: 23385279]

Sinusitis (Bacterial)

A 25-year-old man presents to the urgent care clinic with 3 weeks of facial pain and pressure. He describes the pain as a right-sided fullness and tenderness over his cheek. He has yellow-green drainage from his nose along with subjective fevers, halitosis, and malaise. He felt as though he was getting better 1 week ago, but then his symptoms returned worse than before. On physical examination, his right maxillary sinus is tender to palpation and percussion.

LEARNING OBJECTIVES

▶ Learn the clinical manifestations and objective findings of sinusitis for the various sinuses
▶ Understand how to differentiate between viral and bacterial sinusitis
▶ Know the differential diagnosis of sinusitis
▶ Learn the diagnostic imaging modalities for sinusitis and when to use them
▶ Know the first- and second-line treatments for sinusitis, and patient factors that may help guide choice of agent

QUESTIONS

1. What are the salient features of this patient's problem?
2. How do you think through his problem?
3. What are the key features, including essentials of diagnosis, general considerations, and demographics, of sinusitis?
4. What are the symptoms and signs of sinusitis?
5. What is the differential diagnosis of sinusitis?
6. What are laboratory, imaging, and procedural findings in sinusitis?
7. What are the treatments for sinusitis?
8. What are the outcomes, including complications and prognosis, of sinusitis?
9. When should patients with sinusitis be referred to a specialist or admitted to the hospital?

ANSWERS

1. Salient Features

Unilateral facial pain, pressure, and fullness; purulent drainage; fevers and halitosis; partial resolution with subsequent worsening; tender maxillary sinus on examination

2. How to Think Through

Sinus pressure and nasal discharge accompanied by headache, cough, or subjective fever are a common constellation of findings in sinusitis. The majority of such presentations are due to viral rhinosinusitis, are self-limited, and are treated symptomatically. The two main tasks for the clinician are to determine the likelihood of a bacterial cause of the sinusitis and rule out serious complications of sinusitis. What are the elements of the clinical history associated with bacterial sinusitis? (Unilateral facial pain, purulent drainage, fevers, associated dental pain, partial resolution followed by worsening symptoms—so-called "double worsening"—and duration of > 7 days.) What are the common organisms implicated in bacterial sinusitis? (*Streptococcus pneumoniae*, other streptococci, *Haemophilus influenzae*; possibly *Staphylococcus aureus* or *Moraxella catarrhalis*.) What are the "red flags" for a serious complication of acute sinusitis? (Eye involvement—proptosis, vision change—altered mental status, and facial erythema concerning for cellulitis. Immune compromise should heighten vigilance for such complications.) When should one consider sinus imaging or referral to an otolaryngologist for nasal endoscopy? (Patients who receive appropriate antibiotic treatment and have no improvement at 4 weeks.) What are first-line antibiotics for treatment of acute bacterial sinusitis? (Amoxicillin, trimethoprim-sulfamethoxazole [TMP-SMZ], doxycycline.) What are the symptomatic treatments? (Oral decongestant; possibly intranasal decongestant but for ≤ 3 days. Intranasal steroid spray and intranasal saline wash.)

3. Key Features

Essentials of Diagnosis
- Purulent yellow-green nasal discharge or expectoration
- Facial pain or pressure over the affected sinus or sinuses
- Nasal obstruction
- Acute onset of symptoms (between 1 and 4 weeks' duration)
- Associated symptoms, including cough, malaise, fever, and headache

General Considerations
- Usually results from impaired mucociliary clearance and obstruction of the ostiomeatal complex, or sinus "pore"
- Edematous mucosa causes obstruction of the complex, resulting in the accumulation of mucous secretion in the sinus cavity that becomes secondarily infected by bacteria
- The typical pathogens are the same as those that cause acute otitis media
  — *S pneumoniae*
  — Other streptococci
  — *H influenzae*
  — Less commonly, *S aureus* and *M catarrhalis*
- About 25% of healthy asymptomatic individuals may, if sinus aspirates are cultured, harbor these bacteria
- Discolored nasal discharge and poor response to decongestants suggest sinusitis

Demographics
- Uncommon compared with viral rhinitis, but still affects nearly 20 million Americans annually

4. Symptoms and Signs
- Major symptoms
  — Purulent nasal drainage
  — Nasal obstruction/congestion
  — Facial pain/pressure
  — Altered smell
  — Cough
  — Fever

- Minor symptoms
  — Headache
  — Otalgia
  — Halitosis
  — Dental pain
  — Fatigue
- More specific signs and symptoms may be related to the affected sinuses
- Maxillary sinusitis
  — Unilateral facial fullness, pressure, and tenderness over the cheek
  — Pain may refer to the upper incisor and canine teeth
  — May result from dental infection, and tender teeth should be carefully examined for abscess
  — Bacterial rhinosinusitis can be distinguished from viral rhinitis when symptoms last > 10 days after onset or worsen within 10 days after initial improvement
  — Nonspecific symptoms include fever, malaise, halitosis, headache, hyposmia, and cough
- Ethmoid sinusitis
  — Usually accompanied by maxillary sinusitis; the symptoms of maxillary sinusitis generally predominate
  — Pain and pressure over the high lateral wall of the nose between the eyes that may radiate to the orbit
- Sphenoid sinusitis
  — Usually seen in the setting of pansinusitis, or infection of all the paranasal sinuses on at least one side
  — The patient may complain of a headache "in the middle of the head" and often points to the vertex
- Frontal sinusitis
  — May cause pain and tenderness of the forehead
  — This is most easily elicited by palpation of the orbital roof just below the medial end of the eyebrow
- Hospital-acquired sinusitis
  — May present without any symptoms in head and neck
  — Common source of fever in critically ill patients
  — Often associated with prolonged presence of nasogastric or, rarely, nasotracheal tube
  — Pansinusitis on side of tube commonly seen on imaging studies

5. Differential Diagnosis

- Upper respiratory tract infection
- Viral rhinitis
- Allergic rhinitis
- Nasal polyposis
- Dental abscess
- Rhinocerebral mucormycosis
- Otitis media
- Pharyngitis
- Dacryocystitis
- Paranasal sinus cancer

6. Laboratory, Imaging, and Procedural Findings

Laboratory Tests

- Diagnosis usually made on clinical grounds alone

Imaging Studies

- May be helpful when clinically based criteria are difficult to evaluate, when patient does not respond to appropriate therapy after 4 to 12 weeks, or when symptoms or signs of more serious infection (eg, mucormycosis [*Rhizopus, Mucor, Absidia, Cunninghamella* sp]) are noted

- Noncontrast coronal CT scans
  — More cost-effective and provide more information than conventional sinus films
  — Provide a rapid and effective means to assess all of the paranasal sinuses, to identify areas of greater concern (such as bony dehiscence, periosteal elevation or maxillary tooth root exposure within the sinus), and to direct therapy
- Routine sinus series radiographs
  — Not cost-effective
- Magnetic resonance imaging (MRI) with gadolinium
  — Useful if malignancy, intracranial extension, or opportunistic infection is suspected
  — MRI is better at distinguishing tumor from fluid and inflammation, and can also show bone destruction

Procedures
- Nasal endoscopy is indicated when symptoms persist longer than 4 to 12 weeks

7. Treatments

Medications

Criteria for Antibiotic Therapy
- Symptoms lasting more than 10 days
- Severe symptoms, including fever, facial pain, and periorbital swelling

First-line Antibiotic Therapy
- Amoxicillin, 1000 mg three times daily orally for 7 to 10 d
- TMP-SMZ
  — 160/800 mg twice daily orally for 7 to 10 days
  — Suitable in penicillin allergy
- Doxycycline
  — 200 mg once daily orally ×1 day, then 100 mg twice daily orally thereafter for 7 to 10 days
  — Suitable in penicillin allergy
- Broad-spectrum antibiotics given for hospital-acquired infections

First-line Therapy after Recent Antibiotic Use
- Levofloxacin, 500 mg once daily orally for 10 days
- Amoxicillin-clavulanate, 875/125 mg twice daily orally for 10 days

Second-line Antibiotic Therapy
- Amoxicillin-clavulanate
  — 1000/62.5 mg two extended-release tablets twice daily orally for 10 days
  — Consider if no improvement after 3 days of first-line therapy
- Moxifloxacin
  — 400 mg once daily orally for 10 days
  — Consider if no improvement after 3 days of first-line therapy

Decongestants
- For symptom improvement, use oral or nasal decongestants or both
  — Oral pseudoephedrine, 30 to 120 mg/dose, up to 240 mg/d
  — Nasal oxymetazoline, 0.05%, or xylometazoline, 0.05% to 0.1%, one or two sprays in each nostril every 6 to 8 hours for up to 3 days

Intranasal corticosteroids
- High-dose mometasone furoate (200 mcg each nostril twice daily) for 21 days
  — All clinical practice guidelines recommend using intranasal corticosteroids
  — Non–FDA-labeled indication

Therapeutic Procedures
- For hospital-acquired sinusitis
  — Remove nasogastric tube
  — Improve nasal hygiene (saline sprays, humidification of supplemental nasal oxygen, nasal decongestants)

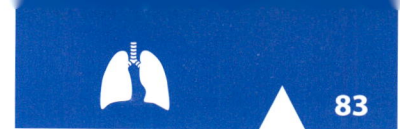

— Endoscopic or transantral cultures (particularly in HIV-infected or other immuno-compromised patients or in complicated cases) may help direct antibiotic therapy

8. Outcomes

Complications

- Orbital cellulitis and abscess
- Osteomyelitis
- Intracranial extension
- Cavernous sinus thrombosis

Prognosis

- 40% to 69% of untreated patients will improve symptomatically within 2 weeks

9. When to Refer and When to Admit

When to Refer

- Failure of acute bacterial rhinosinusitis to resolve after an adequate course of oral antibiotics may necessitate referral to an otolaryngologist for evaluation
- Nasal endoscopy and CT scan are indicated when symptoms persist > 4 to 12 weeks
- Any patient with suspected extension of disease outside the sinuses should be evaluated urgently by an otolaryngologist and imaging

When to Admit

- Facial swelling and erythema indicative of facial cellulitis
- Proptosis
- Vision change or gaze abnormality indicative of orbital cellulitis
- Abscess or cavernous sinus involvement
- Mental status changes suggestive of intracranial extension
- Immunocompromised status
- Failure to respond to appropriate first-line treatment or symptoms persisting longer than 4 weeks

SUGGESTED REFERENCES

Bhattacharyya N et al. Patterns of care before and after the adult sinusitis clinical practice guideline. *Laryngoscope*. 2013 Jul;123(7):1588–1591. [PMID: 23417327]
Hayward G et al. Intranasal corticosteroids in management of acute sinusitis: a systematic review and meta-analysis. *Ann Fam Med*. 2012 May–Jun;10(3):241–249. [PMID: 22585889]
Lemiengre MB et al. Antibiotics for clinically diagnosed acute rhinosinusitis in adults. *Cochrane Database Syst Rev*. 2012 Oct 17;10:CD006089. [PMID: 23076918]
Meltzer EO et al. Rhinosinusitis diagnosis and management for the clinician: a synopsis of recent consensus guidelines. *Mayo Clin Proc*. 2011 May;86(5):427–443. [PMID: 21490181]

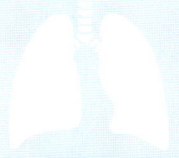

Heart/Hypertension/Lipid Disorders

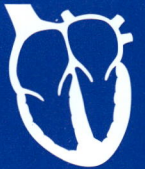

13 Acute Myocardial Infarction

A 71-year-old man presents to the emergency room with a sudden onset of substernal chest pain 1 hour ago. He describes the pain as a heavy pressure sensation that radiates down both arms and that is 10/10 in intensity. He states that his pain started while he was walking around his yard and is better, but not resolved, with rest. His past medical history is significant for diabetes mellitus. He has smoked 1 pack of cigarettes per day for the past 50 years. His mother died of a myocardial infarction (MI) at age 56. On heart examination, you hear an S_4 gallop and on lung examination, bibasilar fine crackles. An electrocardiogram (ECG) is performed showing 3-mm ST-segment elevations in leads II, III, and aVF.

LEARNING OBJECTIVES

► Learn the clinical manifestations and objective findings of acute MI
► Know the differential diagnosis of the chest pain associated with acute MI
► Learn the medical and procedural treatments for acute MI
► Understand the complications of acute MI
► Know how to prevent acute MI

QUESTIONS

1. What are the salient features of this patient's problem?
2. How do you think through his problem?
3. What are the key features, including essentials of diagnosis and general considerations, of acute MI?
4. What are the symptoms and signs of acute MI?
5. What is the differential diagnosis of acute MI?
6. What are laboratory, imaging, and procedural findings in acute MI?
7. What are the treatments for acute MI?
8. What are the outcomes, including follow-up, complications, prevention, and prognosis, of acute MI?
9. When should patients with acute MI be referred to a specialist or admitted to the hospital?

ANSWERS

1. Salient Features

Advanced age; sudden onset of substernal chest pain radiating to arms; pain worse with exertion; cardiac risk factors of diabetes mellitus, smoking, and family history; S_4 gallop and crackles consistent with pulmonary edema; ECG with ST elevations in an inferior distribution

2. How to Think Through

Acute coronary syndrome (ACS) captures the continuum of unstable angina, non–ST-elevation MI (NSTEMI), and ST-elevation MI (STEMI), all of which result from ischemia to the myocardium due to a thrombus at a site of coronary atherosclerosis. There are other causes of MI, but ACS is the most common. This patient presents with typical chest pain, meaning substernal, pressure-like or squeezing, related to exertion, and relieved by rest or nitroglycerin. Radiation to both arms also correlates strongly with cardiac chest pain. To evaluate a patient with chest pain, we first determine the likelihood of ACS as its cause, then stratify the patient's risk for mortality to ensure timely intervention in high-risk patients. Here, the history alone strongly suggests ACS. The patient is immediately deemed to be high risk due to the ST elevations on ECG. Were the ECG to show ST depressions, would management as a high-risk patient still be warranted? (Yes. Evidence of new heart failure [HF] confers high risk.)

What medications should be administered after diagnosis? (Aspirin; $P2Y_{12}$ inhibitors [eg, prasugrel, ticagrelor, or clopidogrel]; unfractionated heparin, enoxaparin, or fondaparinux [if not undergoing percutaneous coronary intervention (PCI)]; glycoprotein IIb/IIIa inhibitors [eg, abciximab].) Should he receive a β-blocker? (No. Evidence of new HF is a relative contraindication.) Should he receive nitroglycerin or morphine? (No. His inferior ST-segment-elevation MI may be affecting the right ventricle, making him preload dependent and nitroglycerin or opiates could result in hypotension. Right-sided ECG leads could help with the diagnosis.) If the hospital lacks facilities for cardiac catheterization, how should he be managed? (If transfer to another facility for PCI within 90 minutes of first medical contact is not possible, and barring contraindications, fibrinolytic therapy should be given.)

3. Key Features

Essentials of Diagnosis

- Sudden but not instantaneous development of prolonged (> 30 minutes) anterior chest discomfort (sometimes felt as "gas" or pressure)
- Sometimes painless, masquerading as acute HF, syncope, stroke, or shock
- ECG: ST-segment elevation or new left bundle branch block occur with STEMI; new right bundle branch block in STEMI is a poor prognostic sign; ECG may show ST depressions or no changes in NSTEMI
- Immediate reperfusion treatment is warranted in STEMI
  — PCI within 90 minutes of first medical contact is the goal and is superior to fibrinolytic therapy
  — If PCI is unavailable within 90 minutes, fibrinolytic therapy within 30 minutes of hospital presentation is the goal, and reduces mortality if given within 12 hours of onset of symptoms; fibrinolysis is harmful in NSTEMI and unstable angina
- An early invasive strategy of reperfusion with PCI may be indicated in NSTEMI, depending on clinical factors

General Considerations

- Acute MI results, in most cases, from an occlusive coronary thrombus at the site of a preexisting (though not necessarily severe) atherosclerotic plaque
- More rarely, may result from prolonged vasospasm, inadequate myocardial blood flow (eg, hypotension), or excessive metabolic demand
- Very rarely, may be caused by embolic occlusion, vasculitis, aortic root or coronary artery dissection, or aortitis
- Cocaine use may cause MI and should be considered in young individuals without risk factors

4. Symptoms and Signs

- Recent onset of angina pectoris or alteration in the pattern of angina or chest pressure, squeezing, or "indigestion"
- Pain characteristics
  — Similar to angina in location and radiation but more severe
  — Usually occurs at rest, often in the early morning
  — Builds rapidly
  — Minimally responsive to sublingual nitroglycerin or oral opioids
- Associated symptoms
  — Diaphoresis
  — Weakness
  — Apprehensiveness
  — Aversion to lying quietly
  — Light-headedness
  — Syncope
  — Dyspnea
  — Orthopnea
  — Cough
  — Wheezing
  — Nausea and vomiting
  — Abdominal bloating
- Thirty-three percent of patients do not experience chest pain, especially older patients, women, and patients with diabetes mellitus
- Of all deaths due to MI, ~50% occur before the patient reaches the hospital, usually of ventricular fibrillation
- Marked bradycardia (inferior infarction) or tachycardia (increased sympathetic activity, low cardiac output, or arrhythmia) may occur
- Jugular venous distention indicates right atrial hypertension, often from RV infarction or elevated LV filling pressures
- Soft heart sounds may indicate LV dysfunction
- S_4 is common; S_3 indicates significant LV dysfunction
- Mitral regurgitation murmur usually indicates papillary muscle dysfunction or, rarely, rupture
- Pericardial friction rubs are uncommon in the first 24 hours but may appear later
- Edema is usually not present
- Cyanosis and cold temperature indicate low output
- Peripheral pulses should be noted, since later shock or emboli may alter the examination

5. Differential Diagnosis

Unstable angina without MI
- Aortic dissection
- Pulmonary embolism
- Tension pneumothorax
- Pericarditis
- Esophageal rupture
- Stress cardiomyopathy (Tako-Tsubo cardiomyopathy or apical ballooning syndrome)

6. Laboratory, Imaging, and Procedural Findings

Laboratory Tests
- Troponin I, troponin T, and quantitative creatine kinase (CK-MB) elevations as early as 4 to 6 hours after onset; almost always abnormal by 8 to 12 hours
- High-sensitivity troponin assays
  — When positive, help enable myocardial infarction to be detected earlier
  — When negative, may be useful in excluding myocardial infarction in patients with chest pain

- Troponins may remain elevated for 5 to 7 days and are therefore less useful for the evaluation of suspected early reinfarction

Imaging Studies

- Chest radiograph: signs of HF, often lagging behind the clinical findings
- Echocardiography: assesses global and regional LV function, wall motion
- Doppler echocardiography: can diagnose postinfarction mitral regurgitation or ventricular septal defect
- Thallium-201 or technetium scintigraphy: does not distinguish recent from old MI

Diagnostic Procedures

- ECG
  - Extent of abnormalities, especially the sum of the total amount of ST-segment deviation, is a good indicator of extent of acute infarction and risk of subsequent adverse events
  - The classic evolution of changes is from peaked ("hyperacute") T waves, to ST-segment elevation, to Q wave development, to T wave inversion; this may occur over a few hours to several days
  - The evolution of new Q waves (> 30 milliseconds in duration and 25% of the R wave amplitude) is diagnostic, but Q waves do not occur in 30% to 50% of acute infarctions (non-Q wave infarctions)
- Cardiac catheterization and coronary angiography can demonstrate coronary artery occlusions and allow PCI
- Echocardiography or left ventriculography can demonstrate akinesis or dyskinesis and measure ejection fraction
- Swan-Ganz hemodynamic measurements can be invaluable in managing suspected cardiogenic shock

7. Treatments

Medications

- Aspirin
  - All patients with definite or suspected acute MI should receive aspirin at a dose of 162 mg or 325 mg at once, regardless of whether fibrinolytic therapy is being considered or the patient has been taking aspirin
  - Chewable aspirin provides more rapid blood levels
- Statin
  - Atorvastatin 80 mg orally should be given initially and continued once daily, based on the benefits seen in the PROVE IT-TIMI 22 and MIRACL trials
- $P2Y_{12}$ inhibitor (eg, prasugrel, ticagrelor, or clopidogrel)
  - Given to patients with a definite aspirin allergy
  - $P2Y_{12}$ inhibitors, in combination with aspirin, have been shown to be beneficial to patients with acute STEMI
  - Guidelines call for a $P2Y_{12}$ inhibitor to be added to aspirin to all patients with STEMI, regardless of whether reperfusion is given, and continued for at least 14 days, and generally for 1 year
  - Prasugrel and ticagrelor are preferred; both have shown superior outcomes compared to clopidogrel
  - All patients who receive a coronary stent should be discharged with both aspirin and a $P2Y_{12}$ inhibitor
- Prasugrel
  - Dose is 60 mg orally on day 1, then 10 mg daily
  - In the TRITON study, prasugrel was shown to be of greater benefit than clopidogrel in reducing thrombotic events in the subgroup of patients with STEMI, including a 50% reduction in stent thrombosis
  - Contraindicated in patients with history of stroke or who are older than age 75 years

- Ticagrelor
  — Dose is 150 mg orally on day 1, then 90 mg twice daily
  — In the PLATO trial, ticagrelor was shown to be of greater benefit than clopidogrel in reducing cardiovascular death, myocardial infarction, and stroke as well as in reducing stent thrombosis
- Clopidogrel
  — Loading dose of 600 mg orally (or 300 mg) results in faster onset of action than standard 75 mg maintenance dose
- Nitroglycerin
  — Agent of choice for continued or recurrent ischemic pain and is useful in lowering BP or relieving pulmonary congestion
- Morphine sulfate, 4 to 8 mg intravenously, or meperidine, 50 to 75 mg intravenously, if nitroglycerin alone does not relieve pain
- Enoxaparin reduced death and MI at day 30 (compared with unfractionated heparin) at the expense of a modest increase in bleeding
  — Give as a 30-mg intravenous bolus and 1 mg/kg every 12 hours for patients under age 75 years
  — Give with no bolus and 0.75 mg/kg intravenously every 12 hours for patients age ≥ 75 years
- Fondaparinux reduced death and reinfarction (compared with unfractionated heparin when indicated, otherwise placebo) with less bleeding
  — Dose: 2.5 mg once daily subcutaneously
  — Not recommended as sole anticoagulant during PCI due to risk of catheter thrombosis
- Fibrinolytic therapy (Table 13-1)
  — Reduces mortality and limits infarct size in patients with acute MI associated with ST-segment elevation (defined as ≥ 0.1 mV in two inferior or lateral leads or two contiguous precordial leads), or with left bundle branch block
  — Greatest benefit occurs if initiated within the first 3 hours, when up to a 50% reduction in mortality rate can be achieved
  — The magnitude of benefit declines rapidly thereafter, but a 10% relative mortality reduction can be achieved up to 12 hours after the onset of chest pain
  — *Fibrinolytic therapy should not be used in NSTEMI or unstable angina*

Table 13-1. Fibrinolytic therapy for acute myocardial infarction.

	Alteplase; Tissue Plasminogen Activator (t-PA)	Reteplase	Tenecteplase (TNK-t-PA)	Streptokinase[a]
Source	Recombinant DNA	Recombinant DNA	Recombinant DNA	Group C Streptococcus
Half-life	5 min	15 min	20 min	20 min
Usual dose	100 mg	20 units	40 mg	1.5 million units
Administration	Initial bolus of 15 mg, followed by 50 mg infused over the next 30 min and 35 mg over the following 60 min	10 units as a bolus over 2 min, repeated after 30 min	Single weight-adjusted bolus, 0.5 mg/kg	750,000 units over 20 min followed by 750,000 units over 40 min
Anticoagulation after infusion	Aspirin, 325 mg daily; heparin, 5000 units as bolus, followed by 1000 units per h infusion, subsequently adjusted to maintain PTT 1.5–2 times control	Aspirin, 325 mg; heparin as with t-PA	Aspirin, 325 mg daily	Aspirin, 325 mg daily; there is no evidence that adjunctive heparin improves outcome following streptokinase
Clot selectivity	High	High	High	Low
Fibrinogenolysis	+	+	+	+++
Bleeding	+	+	+	+
Hypotension	+	+	+	+++
Allergic reactions	0	0	+	++
Reocclusion	10% to 30%	—	5% to 20%	5% to 20%

PTT, partial thromboplastin time.
[a]Not available in the United States.

- Glycoprotein IIb/IIIa inhibitors, specifically abciximab, have been shown to reduce major thrombotic events, and possibly mortality, for patients undergoing primary PCI

Therapeutic Procedures

- ST elevation connotes an acute total coronary occlusion with transmural ischemia and infarction and thus warrants immediate reperfusion therapy
- NSTEMI connotes subendocardial ischemia and infarction and may be treated with an early conservative or early invasive approach with cardiac catheterization and PCI (see Table 13-2)
- In patients with cardiogenic shock, early catheterization and percutaneous or surgical revascularization are the preferred management and have been shown to reduce mortality
- For patients who have received fibrinolytic therapy but will undergo angiography in the first day or two, the early benefits of a P2Y$_{12}$ inhibitor need to be weighed against the

Table 13-2. Indications for catheterization and percutaneous coronary intervention.[a]

Acute coronary syndromes (unstable angina and non-ST elevation MI)	
Class I	Early invasive strategy for any of the following high-risk indicators:
	Recurrent angina/ischemia at rest or with low-level activity
	Elevated troponin
	ST-segment depression
	Recurrent ischemia with evidence of HF
	High-risk stress test result
	EF < 40%
	Hemodynamic instability
	Sustained ventricular tachycardia
	PCI within 6 mo
	Prior CABG
	In the absence of these findings, either an early conservative or early invasive strategy
Class IIa	Early invasive strategy for patients with repeated presentations for ACS despite therapy
Class III	Extensive comorbidities in patients in whom benefits of revascularization are not likely to outweigh the risks
	Acute chest pain with low likelihood of ACS
Acute MI after fibrinolytic therapy (2013 ACCF/AHA guidelines)	
Class I	Cardiogenic shock or acute severe heart failure that develops after initial presentation
	Intermediate or high-risk findings on predischarge noninvasive ischemia testing
	Spontaneous or easily provoked myocardial ischemia
Class IIa	Failed reperfusion or reocclusion after fibrinolytic therapy
Class IIa	Stable[b] patients after successful fibrinolysis, before discharge and ideally between 3 and 24 h

[a]Class I indicates treatment is useful and effective, IIa indicates weight of evidence is in favor of usefulness/efficacy, class IIb indicates weight of evidence is less well established, and class III indicates intervention is not useful/effective and may be harmful. Level of evidence A recommendations are derived from large-scale randomized trials, and B recommendations are derived from smaller randomized trials or carefully conducted observational analyses.

[b]Although individual circumstances will vary, clinical stability is defined by the absence of low output, hypotension, persistent tachycardia, apparent shock, high-grade ventricular or symptomatic supraventricular tachyarrhythmias, and spontaneous recurrent ischemia.

ACCF/AHA, American College of Cardiology Foundation/American Heart Association; ACS, acute coronary syndrome; AMI, acute myocardial infarction; CABG, coronary artery bypass grafting; HF, heart failure; EF, ejection fraction; LVEF, left ventricular ejection fraction; MI, myocardial infarction; PCI, percutaneous coronary intervention.

Source: O'Gara PT et al. 2013 ACCF/AHA guideline for the management of ST-elevation myocardial infarction: a report of the American College of Cardiology Foundation/American Heart Association Task Force on Practice Guidelines. *Circulation*. 2013;127.

necessary delay in bypass surgery for approximately 5 days for those patients found to require surgical revascularization
- Patients with continued circulatory compromise after revascularization may need ventricular support

8. Outcomes

Follow-Up
- For nonhypotensive patients with low ejection fractions, large infarctions, or clinical evidence of HF, start angiotensin-converting enzyme (ACE) inhibitor on first postinfarction day; titrate and continue long term
- Patients with recurrent ischemic pain prior to discharge should undergo catheterization and, if indicated, revascularization

Complications
- Myocardial dysfunction, HF, hypotension, cardiogenic shock
- Postinfarction ischemia
- Sinus bradycardia, sinus tachycardia
- Supraventricular premature beats
- Atrial fibrillation, ventricular fibrillation
- Ventricular premature beats
- Ventricular tachycardia
- Accelerated idioventricular rhythm
- Right bundle branch block (RBBB) or left bundle branch block (LBBB) or fascicular blocks
- Second- or third-degree AV block
- Rupture of a papillary muscle, interventricular septum, or LV free wall
- LV aneurysm
- Pericarditis, Dressler syndrome
- Mural thrombi

Prevention
- Smoking cessation
- Treat hyperlipidemia
- Control HBP
- β-blockers
- Antiplatelet agents
- Exercise training and cardiac rehabilitation programs

Prognosis
- Killip classification classifies HF in patients with acute MI and has powerful prognostic value
  — Class I is absence of rales and S_3
  — Class II is rales that do not clear with coughing over one-third or less of the lung fields or presence of an S_3
  — Class III is rales that do not clear with coughing over more than one-third of the lung fields
  — Class IV is cardiogenic shock (rales, hypotension, and signs of hypoperfusion)

9. When to Refer and When to Admit

When to Refer
- Following an acute MI, all patients should be referred to a cardiologist

When to Admit
- All patients with possible acute MI should be admitted to the Coronary Care Unit

SUGGESTED REFERENCES

Armstrong PW et al. STREAM Investigative Team. Fibrinolysis or primary PCI in ST-segment elevation myocardial infarction. *N Engl J Med*. 2013 Apr 11;368(15):1379–1387. [PMID: 23473396]

O'Gara PT et al. 2013 ACCF/AHA guideline for the management of ST-elevation myocardial infarction: executive summary: a report of the American College of Cardiology Foundation/American Heart Association Task Force on Practice Guidelines: developed in collaboration with the American College of Emergency Physicians and Society for Cardiovascular Angiography and Interventions. *Catheter Cardiovasc Interv*. 2013 Jul 1;82(1):E1–E27. [PMID: 23299937]

Shahzad A et al. HEAT-PPCI trial investigators. Unfractionated heparin versus bivalirudin in primary percutaneous coronary intervention (HEAT-PPCI): an open-label, single centre, randomised controlled trial. *Lancet*. 2014 Nov 22;384(9957):1849–1858. [PMID: 25002178]

Sinnaeve P et al. ASSENT-2 Investigators. One-year follow-up of the ASSENT-2 trial: a double-blind, randomized comparison of single-bolus tenecteplase and front-loaded alteplase in 16,949 patients with ST-elevation acute myocardial infarction. *Am Heart J*. 2003 Jul;146(1):27–32. [PMID: 12851604]

Steg PG et al. ESC Guidelines for the management of acute myocardial infarction in patients presenting with ST-segment elevation: the Task Force on the management of ST-segment elevation acute myocardial infarction of the European Society of Cardiology (ESC). *Eur Heart J*. 2012 Oct;33(20): 2569–2619. [PMID: 22922416]

Tamis-Holland JE et al. Highlights from the 2013 ACCF/AHA guidelines for the management of ST-elevation myocardial infarction and beyond. *Clin Cardiol*. 2014 Apr;37(4):252–259. [PMID: 24523153]

Torpy JM et al. JAMA patient page. Myocardial infarction. *JAMA*. 2008 Jan 30;299(4):476. [PMID: 18230786]

14

Aortic Regurgitation

A 64-year-old man presents to the clinic with a 3-month history of worsening shortness of breath. He finds that he becomes short of breath after walking one block or one flight of stairs. He awakens at night gasping for breath and has to prop himself up with pillows in order to sleep. On physical examination, his blood pressure is 190/60 mm Hg and his pulses are hyperdynamic. His apical impulse is displaced to the left and downward. On physical examination, there are rales over both lower lung fields. There are two distinct cardiac murmurs: a high-pitched, early diastolic murmur loudest at the left lower sternal border and a diastolic rumble heard at the apex. Chest x-ray film shows cardiomegaly and pulmonary edema, and an echocardiogram shows severe aortic regurgitation (AR) with a dilated and hypertrophied left ventricle (LV).

LEARNING OBJECTIVES

▶ Learn the clinical manifestations, objective findings, and unique physical examination characteristics of AR

▶ Understand the factors that predispose to AR and the most common causes of AR

▶ Know the differential diagnosis of AR

▶ Learn the treatments for AR including in which patients surgery is indicated

▶ Understand the risks and benefits of aortic replacement surgery

▶ Know the difference between chronic and acute AR

QUESTIONS

1. What are the salient features of this patient's problem?

2. How do you think through his problem?

3. What are the key features, including essentials of diagnosis and general considerations, of AR?

4. What are the symptoms and signs of AR?

5. What is the differential diagnosis of AR?

6. What are laboratory, imaging, and procedural findings in AR?

7. What are the treatments for AR?

8. What is the outcome, including prognosis, of AR?

9. When should patients with AR be referred to a specialist?

ANSWERS

1. Salient Features

Progressive shortness of breath on exertion; paroxysmal nocturnal dyspnea, orthopnea, pulmonary edema, and cardiomegaly indicating heart failure; wide pulse pressure; hyperdynamic or "water hammer" pulses; early diastolic murmur and diastolic rumble at apex (Austin Flint murmur); LV hypertrophy and dilation; echocardiogram is diagnostic

2. How to Think Through

Recognition of the symptoms of clinical heart failure (HF) is essential. This patient complains of dyspnea on exertion, paroxysmal nocturnal dyspnea, and orthopnea. Can a clinician generally distinguish between systolic, diastolic, and valvular dysfunction based on symptoms? (Not reliably.) The findings of pulmonary rales support the diagnosis of HF and the murmurs suggest a valvular cause. The systolic murmur at the left upper sternal border suggests aortic stenosis (AS) while the apical diastolic rumble suggests AR (with Austin Flint murmur). What data in the case help determine whether AR or AS is the clinically significant problem? (The wide pulse pressure and high systolic blood pressure are characteristic of AR, and not of AS. In AS, the carotid pulse is diminished and delayed [pulsus parvus et tardus], while here it is hyperdynamic.) What other examination findings could further clarify this? (The wide pulse pressure can manifest as a Corrigan pulse ["water hammer" pulse], pulsatile uvula, and other findings.) What underlying processes cause AR? (Rheumatic heart disease, congenitally bicuspid valve, infective endocarditis, hypertension, cystic medial necrosis, Marfan syndrome, aortic dissection, ankylosing spondylitis, reactive arthritis.)

Echocardiography is the key to diagnosis and to monitoring progression of AR. Imaging by contrast CT may be indicated to assess aortic root diameter or ascending aneurysm. How should this patient be managed? (Blood pressure control with afterload reduction can decrease regurgitation. This patient is symptomatic and elective valve replacement is indicated.)

3. Key Features

Essentials of Diagnosis
- Usually asymptomatic until middle age, then presents with left-sided HF or chest pain
- Wide pulse pressure
- Hyperactive, enlarged LV
- Diastolic murmur along the left sternal border
- ECG shows left ventricular hypertrophy (LVH); radiograph shows LV dilation
- Echocardiography with Doppler is diagnostic

General Considerations
- Rheumatic heart disease as a cause is less common since the advent of antibiotics
- Nonrheumatic causes now predominate
  — Congenitally bicuspid valve
  — Infective endocarditis
  — Hypertension
  — Marfan syndrome
  — Aortic dissection
  — Ankylosing spondylitis
  — Reactive arthritis (formerly Reiter syndrome)
  — Aortic root disease

- Rarely, AR is atherosclerotic in nature
- LVH occurs from both an increased preload and afterload; the LVH in AR is often greater than in AS or mitral regurgitation
- Afterload reduction may be beneficial if there is evidence for systolic BP elevation
- Surgery indicated for symptoms, EF < 55%, LV end-systolic dimension > 5.0 cm, or LV end-diastolic dimension > 6.5 cm

4. Symptoms and Signs

- High-pitched, decrescendo aortic diastolic murmur along the left sternal border; no change with respiration
- Hyperactive, enlarged LV
- Wide pulse pressure with peripheral signs
  — Water-hammer pulse or Corrigan pulse: rapid rise and fall with an elevated systolic and low diastolic pressure
  — Quincke pulses: pulsatile nail beds
  — Duroziez sign: to and fro murmur over a partially compressed peripheral artery, commonly the femoral
  — Musset sign: head bob with each pulse
  — Hill sign: leg systolic pressure > 40 mm Hg higher than arm
- Angina pectoris or atypical chest pain may occasionally be present
- Associated coronary artery disease and syncope are less common than in aortic stenosis
- Exertional dyspnea and fatigue are the most frequent symptoms, but paroxysmal nocturnal dyspnea and pulmonary edema may also occur
- Symptoms and signs are determined by how quickly regurgitation develops
- Chronic AR is usually slowly progressive and asymptomatic until middle age
- In acute AR, such as in infective endocarditis or aortic dissection, pulmonary edema and LV failure manifest rapidly, and the LV dilation does not occur
- Extra volume in the LV is handled poorly in acute AR, and surgery is often required urgently
- The diastolic murmur of acute regurgitation is shorter and may be minimal in intensity, making clinical diagnosis difficult

5. Differential Diagnosis

- Aortic dissection
- Graham Steel murmur (pulmonary insufficiency secondary to pulmonary hypertension)
- Mitral stenosis
- Tricuspid stenosis
- Dock's murmur of stenotic left anterior descending artery

6. Laboratory, Imaging, and Procedural Findings

Laboratory Tests
- Serum brain natriuretic peptide (BNP) may be an early sign of LV dysfunction

Imaging Studies
- Chest radiograph: cardiomegaly with LV prominence and sometimes aortic dilation
- Doppler echocardiography
  — Confirms the diagnosis
  — Estimates severity of regurgitation
- Annual echocardiographic assessments of LV size and function are critical in determining the timing of valve replacement when the aortic regurgitation is severe
- Computed tomography (CT) or magnetic resonance imaging (MRI)
  — Can estimate aortic root size
  — Can exclude ascending aneurysm

Table 14-1. When to operate in chronic severe aortic regurgitation (AR).

Indication for Surgery	Class and Level of Evidence (LOE)
Symptomatic	Class 1 LOE B
Asymptomatic	
Abnormal LVEF < 50%	CLASS 1 LOE B
Undergoing other heart surgery	CLASS 1 LOE C
Normal LVEF, but LVESD > 50 mm	CLASS 2a LOE B
Moderate AR and other heart surgery	CLASS 2a LOE C
Normal LVEF, but LVEDD > 65 mm	CLASS 2b LOE C

LVEDD, left ventricular end-diastolic dimension; LVEF, left ventricular ejection fraction; LVESD, left ventricular end-systolic dimension.

Diagnostic Procedures
- ECG shows LV hypertrophy
- Cardiac catheterization
  — Can help quantify severity
  — Can evaluate the coronary and aortic root anatomy preoperatively

7. Treatments
- See Table 14-1

Medications
- Medications that decrease afterload can reduce regurgitation severity
  — Current recommendations advocate afterload reduction only when there is associated systolic hypertension (systolic BP > 140 mm Hg)
- Angiotensin receptor blockers (ARBs)
  — Preferred over β-blockers as additions to medical therapy in patients with Marfan disease
  — Reduce aortic stiffness (by blocking TGF-β) and slow the rate of aortic dilation

Surgery
- Elective surgery is indicated
  — Once AR causes symptoms
  — Before symptoms emerge for those who have an ejection fraction < 50% or increasing end-systolic or end-diastolic LV volume
  — For asymptomatic ascending aneurysm indicated when maximal dimension > 5.0 cm (> 4.5 cm in patients with Marfan syndrome)
- Urgent surgery is indicated in acute AR (usually due to endocarditis or dissection)
- Mechanical valves last longer than tissue valves, but require anticoagulation

8. Outcome

Prognosis
- Operative mortality is usually 3% to 5%
- Following surgery the LV size usually decreases and LV function generally improves

9. When to Refer
- Patients with audible AR should be seen, at least initially, by a cardiologist and decision made as to how often the patient needs follow-up
- Patients with a dilated aortic root should be monitored by a cardiologist, since imaging studies other than the chest radiograph or echocardiogram may be required to decide surgical timing

SUGGESTED REFERENCES

Bonow RO. Chronic mitral regurgitation and aortic regurgitation: have indications for surgery changed? *J Am Coll Cardiol.* 2013 Feb 19;61(7):693–701. [PMID: 23265342]

Brooke BS et al. Angiotensin II blockade and aortic-root dilation in Marfan's syndrome. *N Engl J Med.* 2008 Jun 26;358(26):2787–2795. [PMID: 18579813]

Elder DH et al. The impact of renin-angiotensin-aldosterone system blockade on heart failure outcomes and mortality in patients identified to have aortic regurgitation: a large population study. *J Am Coll Cardiol.* 2011 Nov 8;58(20):2084–2091. [PMID: 22051330]

Nishimura RA et al. 2014 AHA/ACC guideline for the management of patients with valvular heart disease: executive summary: a report of the American College of Cardiology/American Heart Association Task Force on Practice Guidelines. *J Am Coll Cardiol.* 2014 Jun 10;63(22):2438–2488. Erratum in: *J Am Coll Cardiol.* 2014 Jun 10;63(22):2489. [PMID: 24603192]

Vahanian A et al; Joint Task Force on the Management of Valvular Heart Disease of the European Society of Cardiology (ESC); European Association for Cardio-Thoracic Surgery (EACTS). Guidelines on the management of valvular heart disease (version 2012). *Eur Heart J.* 2012 Oct;33(19):2451–2496. [PMID: 22922415]

Aortic Stenosis

15

A 52-year-old man is brought to the emergency department after a syncopal episode. He was running in the park when he suddenly lost consciousness. He denies any premonitory symptoms, and had no symptoms or deficits upon regaining consciousness. For the last several weeks, however, he had had substernal chest pressure associated with exercise. He had no shortness of breath, dyspnea on exertion, orthopnea, or paroxysmal nocturnal dyspnea. As a child, he was told he had a heart murmur, but this was never further evaluated. He has no relevant family history and does not smoke, drink alcohol, or use drugs. On examination, his blood pressure is 110/90 mm Hg, heart rate 95 beats/min, respiratory rate 15/min, and oxygen saturation 98%. The carotid pulse is weak and delayed in character. Cardiac examination reveals a laterally displaced and sustained apical impulse, a grade 3/6 midsystolic crescendo–decrescendo murmur, loudest at the base and radiating to the neck, and an S4 gallop. The lungs are clear to auscultation. There is no lower extremity edema. An electrocardiogram shows left ventricular hypertrophy.

LEARNING OBJECTIVES

▶ Learn the clinical manifestations and objective findings of aortic stenosis (AS)

▶ Understand the factors that predispose to AS in both middle-aged and elderly patients

▶ Know the differential diagnosis of AS

▶ Learn the options for treatment of AS including percutaneous valvular replacement

▶ Know which patients require surgical intervention and the risks associated with surgical procedures

QUESTIONS

1. What are the salient features of this patient's problem?

2. How do you think through his problem?

3. What are the key features, including essentials of diagnosis and general considerations, of AS?

4. What are the symptoms and signs of AS?

5. What is the differential diagnosis of AS?

6. What are laboratory, imaging, and procedural findings in AS?

7. What are the treatments for AS?

8. What is the outcome, including prognosis, of AS?

9. When should patients with AS be referred to a specialist or admitted to the hospital?

ANSWERS

1. Salient Features

Syncope without prodrome or postictal period; angina pectoris; no signs of heart failure (as yet); narrow pulse pressure; pulsus parvus (weak) et tardus (late); systolic murmur at the base radiating to the carotids; an S4 gallop and electrocardiogram suggest left ventricular hypertrophy; lack of atherosclerotic risk factors, middle age, and history of childhood murmur.

2. How to Think Through

With this patient's recent exertional substernal chest pressure, followed by sudden syncope, what diagnoses are most likely? (Coronary artery disease with threshold angina, followed by acute myocardial infarction [MI], causing transient ventricular arrhythmia and syncope.) This case, though, reminds us of the importance of maintaining a broad differential diagnosis, and of the physical examination. The radiation of the murmur to the neck establishes this as AS, as opposed to the more common aortic sclerosis. The diminished and delayed carotid artery pulse is a crucial finding, indicating that the murmur is due to severe AS. Why does he have a laterally displaced and sustained apical impulse? (Left ventricular hypertrophy [LVH] due to a high pressure gradient across the aortic valve.) Given his childhood murmur, what risk factor likely predisposed this patient to AS? (Bicuspid aortic valve.) What are the next steps in his management? (Cardiac enzymes to rule out MI; echocardiography to characterize the problem and to assess the aortic root; consultations to discuss surgical versus percutaneous aortic valve replacement. With no major comorbidities, he will likely be a candidate for surgery.)

3. Key Features

Essentials of Diagnosis
- Diminished and delayed carotid pulses (pulsus parvus et tardus)
- Soft, absent, or paradoxically split S2
- Harsh systolic murmur, classically crescendo–decrescendo, along the left sternal border, often radiating to the neck and sometimes associated with a thrill
- ECG with LVH; calcified valve on radiography
- Echocardiography is diagnostic
- Visual observation of immobile aortic valve plus a valve area of < 1.0 cm² define severe disease; low gradient but severe AS can thus be recognized.

General Considerations
- In middle-aged persons congenital bicuspid valve is the most common cause, and is usually asymptomatic until middle or old age
- May be accompanied by dilated ascending aorta or coarctation of the aorta
- In the elderly valvular degeneration caused by progressive valvular calcification (sclerosis precedes stenosis)
  — About 25% of patients age > 65 and 35% of those age > 70 have evidence of aortic sclerosis
  — About 10% to 20% of these will progress to hemodynamically significant AS over 10 to 15 years
  — Risk factors are the same as for atherosclerosis—hypertension, hypercholesterolemia, smoking
- In developed countries, AS is most common valve lesion requiring surgery
- Much more frequent in men, smokers, and patients with hypercholesterolemia and hypertension

- Pathologically, calcific AS likely contributed to by the same process as atherosclerosis
- Surgery is typically indicated for patients who are symptomatic, or severe disease that is asymptomatic, or if patient is undergoing heart surgery for other reasons
- Surgical risk is typically low; percutaneous valve replacement may be an option for high-risk patients
- Coronary artery disease is present in over one-third

4. Symptoms and Signs

- Diminished and delayed carotid pulses
- Soft, absent, or paradoxically split S2
- Harsh systolic murmur, classically crescendo–decrescendo
  — Sometimes with thrill along left sternal border, often radiating to the neck
  — May be louder at apex in older patients and resemble mitral regurgitation (Gallavardin phenomenon)
  — Ejection click may be present
  — With increasing severity the murmur often peaks later in systole, eventually obliterating the second heart sound
- With bicuspid valve, usually asymptomatic until middle or old age
  — Always check for an associated coarctation of the aorta
  — Many persons have a dilated root due to intrinsic root disease (cystic medial necrosis)
- Left ventricular (LV) hypertrophy, which progresses over time and may lead to myocardial dysfunction
- Patients may present with LV heart failure, angina pectoris, or syncope—all tend to occur with exertion
- Angina is due to underperfusion of the endocardium
- Syncope
  — Occurs with exertion as the LV pressures rises, stimulating the LV baroreceptors to cause peripheral vasodilation
  — This vasodilation results in need for increased stroke volume, which increases the LV systolic pressure again, creating a cycle of vasodilation and stimulation of the baroreceptors that eventually results in a drop in blood pressure, as the stenotic valve prevents further increase in stroke volume
  — Less commonly may be due to arrhythmias
- Sudden death is rare without premonitory symptoms
- The 2014 AHA/ACC guidelines defined severe aortic stenosis to include those with very severe disease and those with severe AS but lower aortic gradients due to low flow (low output/stroke volume) (see Table 15-1)

5. Differential Diagnosis

- Other causes for angina or chest pain, eg, coronary artery disease, coronary vasospasm, and pulmonary embolism

Table 15-1. Summary of 2014 AHA/ACC guideline definitions of severe aortic stenosis.

Category of Severe Aortic Stenosis[a]	Properties
High gradient	> 4.0 m/s Doppler jet velocity > 40 mm Hg mean gradient
Super severe	> 5.0 m/s Doppler jet velocity > 55 mm Hg mean gradient
Low flow	Reduced LVEF (< 50%) Normal LVEF (> 50%)

[a]All categories of severe aortic stenosis have abnormal systolic opening of the aortic valve and an aortic valve area < 1.0 cm^2.

LVEF, left ventricular ejection fraction.

- Other causes of syncope, eg, cardiac arrhythmia, vasovagal syncope, and seizure
- Other causes of heart failure
- Systolic murmur of a different cause
- Pulmonary hypertension
- Aortic sclerosis without stenosis
- Coarctation of the aorta

6. Laboratory, Imaging, and Procedural Findings

Laboratory Tests
- Brain natriuretic peptide (BNP) may be useful in diagnosis and prognostication of heart failure due to AS

Imaging Studies
- Chest radiography or fluoroscopy shows calcified valve and may show enlarged cardiac silhouette
- Doppler echocardiography
  — Usually diagnostic
  — Can estimate the aortic valve gradient
  — In low flow states, the aortic valve gradient may underestimate the stenosis; valve area can be used in patients with normal LVEF, exercise or pharmacologic stress to increase the cardiac output can diagnose low flow aortic stenosis in patients with reduced LVEF

Diagnostic Procedures
- ECG usually shows LV hypertrophy
- Cardiac catheterization
  — Provides confirmatory data of stenosis, though not needed if echocardiography is diagnostic
  — Assesses hemodynamics
  — Excludes concomitant coronary artery disease prior to surgery

7. Treatments
- See Table 15-2 and Figure 15-1.

Medications
- Medical treatment may stabilize heart failure, but surgical intervention is definitive
- Lipid lowering therapy has not shown to slow progression of AS, though longer-term studies are pending
- Control of systemic hypertension is important to reduce excess afterload

Therapeutic Procedures and Surgery
- Table 15-2 outlines the ACCF/ACC guidelines for surgical indications in aortic stenosis
- Balloon valvuloplasty has a small role in young and adolescent patients, but ineffective long-term in adults and is only used as a temporizing measure
- Type of prosthetic valve depends on patient age and risk of anticoagulation with warfarin
- Pericardial valves appear to last longer than porcine valves; neither require warfarin
- Mechanical valves have longest life, but require warfarin therapy; use of valve-in-valve procedures for bioprosthetic valves may decrease mechanical valve use
- Patients with bicuspid aortic valves may have coincident aortic root dilatation that may require replacement, especially if the dimension exceeds 5.0 cm
- Transcutaneous aortic valve replacement (TAVR) using either the FDA-approved Edwards-Sapien or CoreValve device is being performed widely through a number of implantation routes, and trials of other device brands are ongoing
- TAVR can also be used in a valve-in-valve procedure for patients with prosthetic valve stenosis (regardless of whether in the aortic, mitral, tricuspid, or pulmonary position)
- Table 15-3 outlines recommendations for the use of TAVR

Table 15-2. 2014 ACCF/ACC guidelines for surgical indications in aortic stenosis.

Recommendations	COR	LOE
AVR is recommended in symptomatic patients with severe AS (stage D)	I	B
AVR is recommended for asymptomatic patients with severe AS (stage C2 or D) and LVEF < 50%	I	B
AVR is indicated for patients with severe AS (stage C or D) when undergoing other cardiac surgery	I	B
AVR is reasonable for asymptomatic patients with very severe AS (aortic velocity ≥ 5 m/s) (stage C2) and low surgical risk	IIa	B
AVR is reasonable in asymptomatic patients (stage C1) with severe AS and an abnormal exercise test	IIa	B
AVR is reasonable in symptomatic patients with low-flow/low-gradient severe AS with reduced LVEF (stage S1) with a low-dose dobutamine stress study that shows an aortic velocity ≥ 4 m/s (or mean gradient ≥ 40 mm Hg) with a valve area ≤ 1.0 cm² at any dobutamine dose	IIa	B
AVR is reasonable for patients with moderate AS (stage B) (velocity 3.0–3.9 m/s) who are undergoing other cardiac surgery	IIa	C
AVR may be considered for asymptomatic patients with severe AS (stage C1) and rapid disease progression and low surgical risk	IIb	C
AVR may be considered in symptomatic patients who have low-flow/low-gradient severe AS (stage S2) who are normotensive and have an LVEF ≥ 50% if clinical, hemodynamic, and anatomic data support valve obstruction as the most likely cause of symptoms	IIb	C

AS, aortic stenosis; AVR, aortic valve replacement; COR, class of recommendation; LOE, level of evidence; LVEF, left ventricular ejection fraction; N/A, not applicable.

Reproduced, with permission, from Nishimura RA et al. 2014 AHA/ACC Guideline for the Management of Patients With Valvular Heart Disease: A Report of the American College of Cardiology/American Heart Association Task Force on Practice Guidelines. *Circulation.* 2014 Jun 10;129(23):e521–e643. [PMID: 24589853]

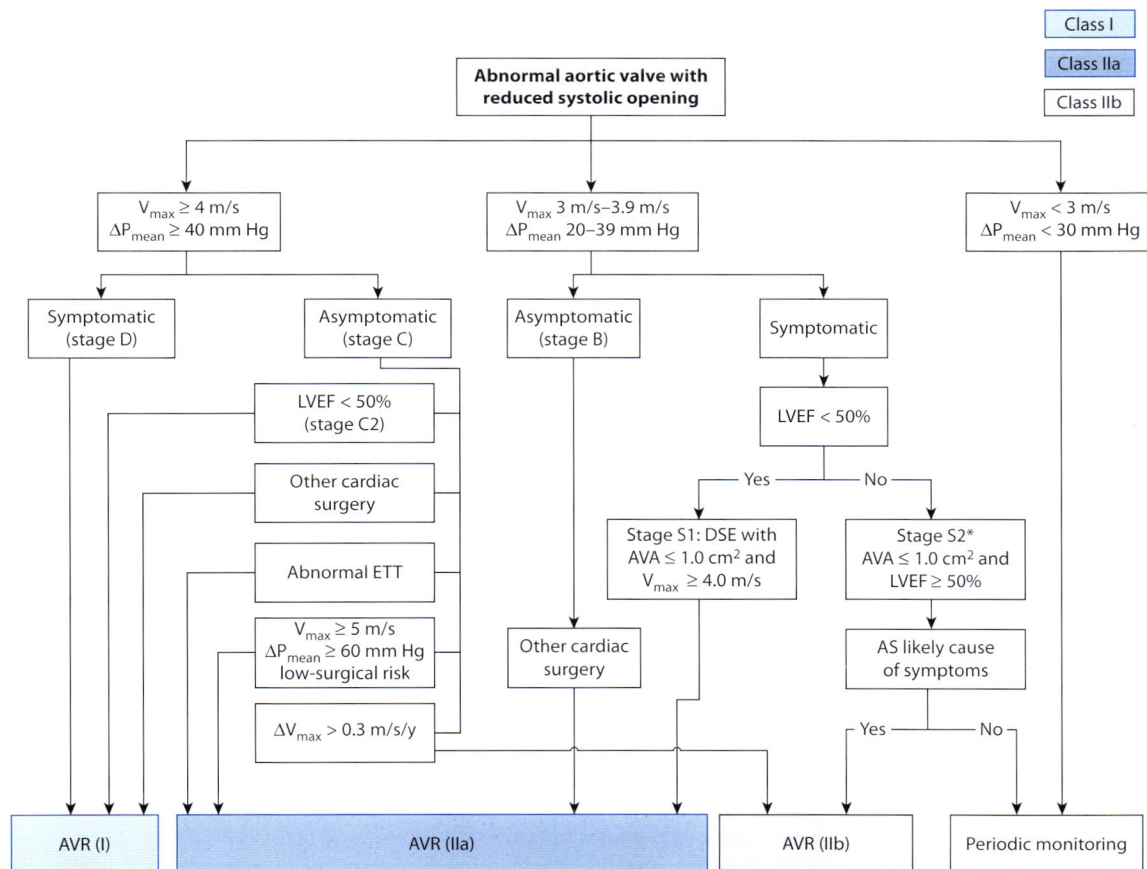

*AVR should be considered with stage S2 AS only if valve obstruction is the most likely cause of symptoms, stroke volume index is < 35 mL/m², indexed AVA is ≤ 0.6 cm²/m² and data are recorded when the patient is normotensive (systolic BP < 140 mm Hg).
AS, aortic stenosis; AVA, aortic valve area; AVR, aortic valve replacement; BP, blood pressure; DSE, dobutamine stress echocardiography; ETT, exercise treadmill test; LVEF, left ventricular ejection fraction; ΔP_mean, mean pressure gradient; V_max, maximum velocity.

Figure 15–1. Algorithm for the management of aortic valve stenosis. (Reproduced, with permission from, Nishimura RA et al. 2014 AHA/ACC Guideline for the Management of Patients With Valvular Heart Disease: A Report of the American College of Cardiology/American Heart Association Task Force on Practice Guidelines. *Circulation.* 2014 Jun 10;129(23):e521–e643. [PMID: 24589853])

Table 15-3. Recommendations for use of TAVR.

Recommendations	COR	LOE
Surgical AVR is recommended in patients who meet indication for AVR with low or intermediate surgical risk	I	A
TAVR is recommended in patients who meet an indication for AVR for AS who have a prohibitive surgical risk and a predicted post-TAVR survival > 12 mo	I	B
For patient in whom TAVR or high-risk surgical AVR is being considered, members of a Heart Valve Team should collaborate closely to provide optimal patient care	I	C
TAVR is a reasonable alternative to surgical AVR for AS in patients who meet indication for AVR and who have high surgical risk	IIa	B
Percutaneous aortic balloon dilation may be considered as a bridge to surgical or transcatheter AVR in severely symptomatic patients (NYHA class III–IV) with severe AS	IIb	C
TAVR is not recommended in patients in whom the existing comorbidities would preclude the expected benefit from correction of AS	III: No benefit	B

AS, aortic stenosis; AVR, aortic valve replacement; COR, class of recommendation; LOE, level of evidence; N/A, not applicable; NYHA. New York Heart Association; TVAR, transcatheter aortic valve replacement.

Reproduced, with permission, from Nishimura RA et al. 2014 AHA/ACC Guideline for the Management of Patients With Valvular Heart Disease: A Report of the American College of Cardiology/American Heart Association Task Force on Practice Guidelines. *Circulation*. 2014 Jun 10;129(23): e521–e643. [PMID: 24589853]

8. Outcome

Prognosis

- After onset of heart failure, angina pectoris, or syncope, the mortality rate without surgery is 50% within 3 years
- Surgical mortality rate is low (2%–5%), even in the elderly
- TAVR significantly reduces mortality in patients who cannot undergo surgical AVR

9. When to Refer and When to Admit

When to Refer

- All patients with symptomatic AS or symptoms suggestive of AS should be seen by a cardiologist
- All patients with evidence for mild to moderate AS should be seen by a cardiologist for evaluation and to determine frequency of follow-up

When to Admit

- Patients with an indication for surgical replacement

SUGGESTED REFERENCES

Goel SS et al. Severe aortic stenosis and coronary artery disease—implications for management in the transcatheter aortic valve replacement era: a comprehensive review. *J Am Coll Cardiol*. 2013 Jul 2;62(1):1–10. [PMID: 23644089]

Herrmann HC et al. Predictors of mortality and outcomes of therapy in low-flow severe aortic stenosis: a Placement of Aortic Transcatheter Valves (PARTNER) trial analysis. *Circulation*. 2013 Jun 11;127(23):2316–2326. [PMID: 23661722]

Holmes DR Jr et al. 2012 ACCF/AATS/SCAI/STS expert consensus document on transcatheter aortic valve replacement. *J Am Coll Cardiol*. 2012 Mar 27;59(13):1200–1254. [PMID: 22300974]

Lindman BR et al. Current management of calcific aortic stenosis. *Circ Res*. 2013 Jul 5;113(2):223–237. [PMID: 23833296]

Nishimura RA et al. 2014 AHA/ACC guideline for the management of patients with valvular heart disease: executive summary: a report of the American College of Cardiology/American Heart Association Task Force on Practice Guidelines. *J Am Coll Cardiol*. 2014 Jun 10;63(22):2438–2488. Erratum in: *J Am Coll Cardiol*. 2014 Jun 10;63(22):2489. [PMID: 24603192]

Puskas J et al; PROACT Investigators. Reduced anticoagulation after mechanical aortic valve replacement: interim results from the prospective randomized on-X valve anticoagulation clinical trial randomized Food and Drug Administration investigational device exemption trial. *J Thorac Cardiovasc Surg*. 2014 Apr;147(4):1202–1210. [PMID: 24512654]

Vahanian A et al; Joint Task Force on the Management of Valvular Heart Disease of the European Society of Cardiology (ESC); European Association for Cardio-Thoracic Surgery (EACTS). Guidelines on the management of valvular heart disease (version 2012). *Eur Heart J*. 2012 Oct;33(19):2451–2496. [PMID: 22922415]

Webb JG et al. Transcatheter aortic valve replacement for bioprosthetic aortic valve failure: the valve-in-valve procedure. *Circulation*. 2013 Jun 25;127(25):2542–2550. [PMID: 23797741]

Chest Pain

A 55-year-old man presents to clinic complaining of chest pain. He states that for the last 5 months he has noted intermittent substernal chest pressure radiating to the left arm. The pain occurs primarily when exercising vigorously and is relieved with rest. He denies associated shortness of breath, nausea, vomiting, or diaphoresis. He has a medical history significant for hypertension and hyperlipidemia. He is taking atenolol for high blood pressure and is eating a low-cholesterol diet. His family history is notable for a father who died of a myocardial infarction at age 56 years. He has a 50-pack-year smoking history and is currently trying to quit. His physical examination is within normal limits with the exception of his blood pressure, which is 145/95 mm Hg, with a heart rate of 75 beats/min.

LEARNING OBJECTIVES

▶ Learn the important historical features that need to be obtained in a patient with chest pain

▶ Understand the factors that predispose to certain causes of chest pain

▶ Know the possible causative organ systems and differential diagnosis of chest pain

▶ Learn the characteristic symptoms and signs that suggest the cause of chest pain

▶ Know which diagnostic tests can be helpful in distinguishing the causes of chest pain

QUESTIONS

1. What are the salient features of this patient's problem?

2. How do you think through his problem?

3. What are the key features, including essentials of diagnosis and general considerations, of chest pain?

4. What are the symptoms and signs of chest pain?

5. What is the differential diagnosis of chest pain?

6. What are laboratory, imaging, and procedural findings in chest pain?

7. What are the treatments for chest pain?

8. When should patients with chest pain be referred to a specialist or admitted to the hospital?

ANSWERS

1. Salient Features

Middle-aged man; intermittent pain with exercise and relieved with rest; substernal location with radiation to the arm; risk factors: hyperlipidemia, hypertension, family history, cigarette smoking; normal vital signs; overall picture is suggestive of stable angina pectoris

2. How to Think Through

When evaluating a patient with chest pain in the primary care setting, one first determines if the pain is acute in onset (or progressive) with features concerning for acute coronary syndrome, pulmonary emboli, aortic dissection, pneumothorax, or another process warranting emergent care. The majority of patients with chest pain, however, do not require emergent evaluation. Thus, separation of serious from benign causes is an essential skill. This patient's chest pain has characteristics of typical angina—it is located substernally, related to exertion, radiating to the arm, and relieved with rest. Risk factors for coronary artery disease (CAD) are weighed alongside the history, examination, and electrocardiogram (ECG). What are the major CAD risk factors? (Age, sex, family history, tobacco use, diabetes mellitus, hypertension, low high-density lipoprotein [HDL] cholesterol, elevated non-HDL cholesterol.)

Could this be aortic stenosis? (Based on the history alone, it could. Cardiac auscultation and assessment of the carotid pulses will help rule this in or out.) Other causes such as esophageal spasm or musculoskeletal pain are possible, but the symptoms, long smoking history, and family history, confer a high pretest probability of CAD. While there are several noninvasive testing options for CAD, all involve a stressor (exercise or pharmacologic), and a detector (ECG, echocardiogram, nuclear medicine). Is medical therapy indicated at this point? (Yes: aspirin, statin, β-blocker and nitroglycerin should all be considered, given the high suspicion for CAD.)

3. Key Features

Essentials of Diagnosis

- Inquire about
  - Chest pain onset, character, location/size, duration, periodicity, and exacerbators
  - Presence of shortness of breath
- Vital signs
- Chest and cardiac examination findings
- ECG
- Cardiac biomarkers

General Considerations

- Chest pain is a common symptom and can occur as a result of cardiovascular, pulmonary/pleural, esophageal/gastrointestinal, musculoskeletal, or psychiatric/anxiety disorders
- Life-threatening causes of chest pain include acute coronary syndromes (ACS), pericarditis, aortic dissection, pulmonary emboli, pneumonia, and esophageal perforation
- Inflammatory conditions predisposing patients to coronary artery disease include HIV, systemic lupus erythematosus, and rheumatoid arthritis
- Risk factors for pulmonary emboli from venous thromboembolism include cancer, trauma, recent surgery, immobilization or hospitalization, pregnancy, oral contraceptives, heart failure (HF), chronic obstructive pulmonary disease (COPD), and family or personal history of thrombosis

4. Symptoms and Signs

- Symptoms and signs vary with etiology; each cause has typical symptoms, but may present atypically
- Myocardial ischemia typical pain:
  - Dull, aching; retrosternal or left precordial, poorly localized
  - Described as "pressure," "tightness," "squeezing," or "gas," lasting 5 to 20 minutes or longer

— Symptoms that progress or occur at rest may be unstable angina
— Up to one-third have no chest pain
— May radiate to throat, jaw, shoulders, inner arms, upper abdomen, or back
— Precipitated by exertion or stress, relieved by rest or nitroglycerin
— May be accompanied by dizziness, nausea, diaphoresis, and anxiety such as a feeling of impending doom
— Elderly may complain of fatigue instead of chest pain
— Pleuritic chest pain is usually not myocardial ischemia
— Pointing to location of pain with one finger is correlated with nonischemic chest pain
— See Table 16-1
• Pericarditis pain is typically greater supine than upright and may increase with respiration, coughing, or swallowing
• Aortic dissection: abrupt onset, tearing pain, radiates to the back
• Pulmonary emboli: wide-ranging presentations—assessment relies on thrombosis risk and associated symptoms and signs using a validated scoring system
• Esophageal perforation: usually recent medical procedures or severe vomiting/retching
• Physical examination can provide clues, but cannot rule out diagnoses such as ACS or aortic dissection
— Vital signs, including pulse oximetry, and cardiopulmonary examination are important for assessing this symptom's urgency

Table 16-1. Likelihood ratios (LRs) for clinical features associated with acute myocardial infarction.

Clinical Feature	LR+ (95% CI)
History	
Chest pain that radiates to the left arm	2.3 (1.7–3.1)
Chest pain that radiates to the right shoulder	2.9 (1.4–3.0)
Chest pain that radiates to both arms	7.1 (3.6–14.2)
Pleuritic chest pain	0.2 (0.2–0.3)
Sharp or stabbing chest pain	0.3 (0.2–0.5)
Positional chest pain	0.3 (0.2–0.4)
Chest pain reproduced by palpation[a]	0.2–0.41
Nausea or vomiting	1.9 (1.7–2.3)
Diaphoresis	2.0 (1.9–2.2)
Physical examination	
Systolic blood pressure ≤ 80 mm Hg	3.1 (1.8–5.2)
Pulmonary crackles	2.1 (1.4–3.1)
Third heart sound	3.2 (1.6–6.5)
Electrocardiogram	
Any ST-segment elevation (≥ 1 mm)	11.2 (7.1–17.8)
Any ST-segment depression	3.2 (2.5–4.1)
Any Q wave	3.9 (2.7–7.7)
Any conduction defect	2.7 (1.4–5.4)
New ST-segment elevation (≥ 1 mm)[a]	5.7–53.91
New ST-segment depression[a]	3.0–5.21
New Q wave[a]	5.3–24.81
New conduction defect	6.3 (2.5–15.7)

[a]Heterogenous studies do not allow for calculation of a point estimate.

Adapted, with permission, from Panju AA et al. The rational clinical examination. Is this patient having a myocardial infarction? *JAMA.* 1998 Oct 14;280(14):1256–1263.

— ACS may have diaphoresis, hypotension, S3 or S4 gallop, pulmonary crackles, or elevated JVP
— Reproducibility with palpation suggests musculoskeletal cause, though 15% of patients with ACS may have this chest wall tenderness
— Aortic dissection can result in differential blood pressures, pulse amplitude deficits, and new diastolic murmurs
— Cardiac friction rub with patient sitting forward suggests pericarditis; must rule out tamponade
— Subcutaneous emphysema suggests esophageal perforation
— Normal physical examination may be seen in pulmonary emboli, anxiety disorder, or musculoskeletal disease

5. Differential Diagnosis

- Emergency/don't miss
  — Myocardial ischemia
  — Pericarditis
  — Aortic dissection
  — Pulmonary emboli
  — Tension pneumothorax
  — Esophageal rupture
- Cardiovascular
  — Myocardial ischemia (angina or ACS)
  — Pericarditis
  — Aortic stenosis
  — Aortic dissection
  — Pulmonary emboli
  — Cardiomyopathy
  — Myocarditis
  — Mitral valve prolapse
  — Pulmonary hypertension
  — Hypertrophic obstructive cardiomyopathy (HOCM)
  — Carditis (eg, acute rheumatic fever)
  — Aortic insufficiency
  — Right ventricular hypertrophy
- Pulmonary
  — Pneumonia
  — Pleuritis
  — Bronchitis
  — Pneumothorax
  — Tumor
- Gastrointestinal
  — Esophageal rupture
  — Gastroesophageal reflux disease (GERD)
  — Esophageal spasm
  — Mallory–Weiss tear
  — Peptic ulcer disease
  — Biliary disease
  — Pancreatitis
  — Functional gastrointestinal pain
- Musculoskeletal
  — Cervical or thoracic disk disease or arthritis
  — Shoulder arthritis
  — Costochondritis (anterior chest wall syndrome or Tietze syndrome)
  — Subacromial bursitis

- Other
  - Anxiety or panic attack
  - Herpes zoster
  - Breast disorders
  - Chest wall tumors
  - Thoracic outlet syndrome
  - Mediastinitis

6. Laboratory, Imaging, and Procedural Findings

Laboratory Tests
- Cardiac biomarkers including cardiac troponin I for suspected ACS
- D-dimer test, if negative, can rule out pulmonary emboli in patients with low clinical probability

Imaging Studies
- Chest radiography, especially useful when shortness of breath accompanies chest pain
- CT scanning is method of choice for diagnosis of esophageal perforation, aortic dissection
- CT angiography with helical or multidetector imaging is the preferred test for pulmonary emboli
- Ventilation-perfusion scanning for pulmonary emboli may be used if the patient cannot tolerate CT scan or associated contrast
- CT angiography with multidetector imaging
- Enables diagnosis (or exclusion) of coronary artery disease, ACS, and pulmonary emboli (so-called "triple rule-out")
- However, test involves both radiation and contrast exposure

Diagnostic Procedures
- ECG is warranted in most patients; normal ECG does not rule out ACS or other diagnoses
- Exercise stress testing (ETT)
- Exercise stress testing with perfusion imaging when patient with chest pain has cardiovascular risk factors and normal ECG and ETT
- Pulmonary angiogram, though infrequently used, is the gold standard for diagnosis of pulmonary emboli

7. Treatments

Medications
- Treatment must be guided by underlying etiology
  - Short-acting PRN nitroglycerin, daily aspirin, β-blocker, long-acting nitrate, statin for stable angina pectoris
  - Empiric trial of high-dose proton-pump inhibitor therapy has been reported to improve symptoms in patients with noncardiac chest pain of unknown etiology
- Antidepressants may have modest benefit in reducing noncardiac chest pain
- A meta-analysis of 15 trials suggested psychological interventions (especially cognitive-behavioral) may have modest-to-moderate benefit
- Hypnotherapy may have some benefit

8. When to Refer and When to Admit

When to Refer
- Patients with poorly controlled noncardiac chest pain to a pain specialist
- Patients with sickle-cell anemia and recurrent thrombosis should be referred to a hematologist

When to Admit
- Failure to adequately exclude life-threatening causes of chest pain (eg, ACS, aortic dissection, pulmonary emboli, esophageal rupture)

- Pain control for rib fractures that impair gas exchange
- High risk of pulmonary embolism and a positive sensitive D-dimer test
- TIMI score of ≥ 1, abnormal electrocardiogram and abnormal 0- and 2-hour troponin tests

SUGGESTED REFERENCES

Ayloo A et al. Evaluation and treatment of musculoskeletal chest pain. *Prim Care*. 2013 Dec;40(4): 863–887, viii. [PMID: 24209723]

Bandstein N et al. Undetectable high-sensitivity cardiac troponin T level in the emergency department and risk of myocardial infarction. *J Am Coll Cardiol*. 2014 Jun 17;63(23):2569–2578. [PMID: 24694529]

Collinson P et al. Comparison of contemporary troponin assays with the novel biomarkers, heart fatty acid binding protein and copeptin, for the early confirmation or exclusion of myocardial infarction in patients presenting to the emergency department with chest pain. *Heart*. 2014 Jan;100(2):140–145. [PMID: 24270743]

Hoffmann U et al; ROMICAT-II Investigators. Coronary CT angiography versus standard evaluation in acute chest pain. *N Engl J Med*. 2012 Jul 26;367(4):299–308. [PMID: 22830462]

Holly J et al. Prospective evaluation of the use of the Thrombolysis In Myocardial Infarction score as a risk stratification tool for chest pain patients admitted to an ED observation unit. *Am J Emerg Med*. 2013 Jan;31(1):185–189. [PMID: 22944539]

Kisely SR et al. Psychological interventions for symptomatic management of non-specific chest pain in patients with normal coronary anatomy. *Cochrane Database Syst Rev*. 2012 Jun 13;6:CD004101. [PMID: 22696339]

Kosowsky JM. Approach to the ED patient with "low risk" chest pain. *Emerg Med Clin North Am*. 2011 Nov;29(4):721–727. [PMID: 22040703]

McConaghy JR et al. Outpatient diagnosis of acute chest pain in adults. *Am Fam Physician*. 2013 Feb 1;87(3):177–182. [PMID: 23418761]

Ranasinghe AM et al. Acute aortic dissection. *BMJ*. 2011 Jul 29;343:d4487. [PMID: 21803810]

Rogers IS et al. Usefulness of comprehensive cardiothoracic computed tomography in the evaluation of acute undifferentiated chest discomfort in the emergency department (CAPTURE). *Am J Cardiol*. 2011 Mar 1;107(5):643–650. [PMID: 21247533]

Scheuermeyer FX et al. Safety and efficiency of a chest pain diagnostic algorithm with selective outpatient stress testing for emergency department patients with potential ischemic chest pain. *Ann Emerg Med*. 2012 Apr;59(4):256–264. [PMID: 22221842]

Than M et al. A 2-hour diagnostic protocol for possible cardiac chest pain in the emergency department: a randomized clinical trial. *JAMA Intern Med*. 2014 Jan;174(1):51–58. [PMID: 24100783]

Dyslipidemia

17

A 47-year-old man presents to his primary care clinician for a routine checkup. The patient denies any symptoms, but is worried about his weight and diet, which consists of many saturated fats. On physical examination his blood pressure is 153/102 mm Hg and his body habitus reveals a large amount of abdominal obesity. Blood tests reveal a serum total cholesterol level of 220 mg/dL, a triglyceride level of 321 g/dL, a high-density lipoprotein (HDL) cholesterol level of 24 mg/dL, a low-density lipoprotein (LDL) of 132 mg/dL, and a hemoglobin A_{1c} of 6.2%.

LEARNING OBJECTIVES

▶ Learn the clinical manifestations and objective findings of dyslipidemia and the criteria for the diagnosis of the metabolic syndrome

▶ Understand the factors that predispose to dyslipidemia and how to recognize those patients who may have a familial genetic lipid disorder

▶ Know the causes of cholesterol and triglyceride lipid abnormalities

▶ Learn the treatments for dyslipidemia and their side effects

▶ Know which patients need screening for dyslipidemia

QUESTIONS

1. What are the salient features of this patient's problem?

2. How do you think through his problem?

3. What are the key features, including essentials of diagnosis, general considerations, and demographics, of dyslipidemia?

4. What are the symptoms and signs of dyslipidemia?

5. What is the differential diagnosis of dyslipidemia?

6. What are laboratory findings in dyslipidemia?

7. What are the treatments for dyslipidemia?

8. What are the outcomes, including complications and prognosis, of dyslipidemia?

9. When should patients with lipid abnormalities be referred to a specialist?

ANSWERS

1. Salient Features

Obese man; large waist circumference, elevated blood pressure, elevated triglycerides, low HDL cholesterol, and insulin resistance consistent with the metabolic syndrome

2. How to Think Through

Serum LDL and HDL cholesterol, along with triglycerides, are important markers of risk for coronary artery disease (CAD). Elevated LDL cholesterol is associated with increased CAD, and LDL is the primary target of lipid-lowering therapies. This patient has a different, but equally important, pattern of dyslipidemia: low HDL and elevated triglycerides. The degree to which these abnormalities are independent predictors of CAD is debated, because they so often travel with other metabolic abnormalities, collectively termed the metabolic syndrome. What are the elements of this syndrome? (Large waist circumference, elevated blood pressure, elevated triglycerides, low serum HDL, and insulin resistance.)

What other secondary causes of hypertriglyceridemia should be considered? (Alcoholism, hypothyroidism, nephrotic syndrome, familial disorders of triglyceride metabolism, and medications [eg, corticosteroids].) What is an important complication of elevated triglycerides and is this patient likely to experience this complication? (Pancreatitis, which typically occurs with levels greater than 2000 mg/dL; this patient's triglyceride level is not high enough to cause pancreatitis.)

Should he receive targeted therapy to lower his triglycerides? (Not necessarily.) Weight loss and reduction of CAD risk factors known to improve outcomes is the primary treatment strategy for dyslipidemia. The first interventions should be diet, exercise, blood pressure control, and a statin medication. Targeted triglyceride-lowering therapies are recommended for patients with levels above 500 mg/dL. What medications lower triglycerides? (Fibric acid derivatives [eg, gemfibrozil, fenofibrate].) What downside might there be to prescribing nicotinic acid for this patient? (Worsened glucose intolerance.)

3. Key Features

Essentials of Diagnosis

- Elevated serum total cholesterol or LDL cholesterol, low serum HDL cholesterol, or elevated serum triglycerides
- Usually asymptomatic
- In severe cases associated with metabolic abnormalities, superficial lipid deposition occurs

General Considerations

- Cholesterol and triglycerides are the two main circulating lipids
- Elevated levels of LDL cholesterol are associated with increased risk of atherosclerotic heart disease
- High levels of HDL cholesterol are associated with lower risk of atherosclerotic heart disease
- The exact mechanism by which LDL and HDL affect atherosclerosis is not fully delineated
- Familial genetic disorders are an uncommon, but often lethal, cause of elevated cholesterol
- Familial genetic disorders should be considered in patients who have onset of atherosclerosis in their 20s or 30s

Demographics

- Dyslipidemia is more common in men than women before age 50
- More common in women than men after age 50
- More common in whites and Hispanics than among blacks

- Up to 25% of Americans have the metabolic syndrome that consists of
  — Large waist circumference
  — Elevated blood pressure
  — Elevated serum triglycerides
  — Low serum HDL cholesterol
  — Elevated serum glucose (insulin resistance)

4. Symptoms and Signs

- Dyslipidemia is usually asymptomatic
- Extremely high levels of chylomicrons or very low-density lipoprotein (VLDL) particles are associated with eruptive xanthomas
- Very high LDL levels are associated with tendinous xanthomas
- Very high triglycerides (> 2000 mg/dL) are associated with lipemia retinalis (cream-colored vessels in the fundus)

5. Differential Diagnosis

Hypercholesterolemia (elevated serum cholesterol)
- Hypothyroidism
- Diabetes mellitus
- Cushing syndrome
- Obstructive liver disease
- Nephrotic syndrome
- Chronic kidney disease
- Anorexia nervosa
- Familial, eg, familial hypercholesterolemia
- Drugs
  — Oral contraceptives
  — Thiazides (short-term effect)
  — β-blockers (short-term effect)
  — Corticosteroids
  — Cyclosporine
- Idiopathic

Hypertriglyceridemia (elevated serum triglycerides)
- Alcohol intake
- Obesity
- Metabolic syndrome
- Diabetes mellitus
- Chronic renal insufficiency
- Pregnancy
- Lipodystrophy, eg, protease inhibitor therapy
- Familial
- Drugs
  — Oral contraceptives
  — Thiazides (short-term effect)
  — β-blockers (short-term effect)
  — Corticosteroids
  — Bile-acid binding resins
  — Isotretinoin

6. Laboratory Findings

- Screen for lipid disorders in
  — Patients with coronary heart disease (CHD), diabetes mellitus, peripheral vascular disease, aortic aneurysm, cerebrovascular disease, chronic renal insufficiency, heart failure, or a family history of premature CHD

Table 17-1. Indications for high-intensity and moderate-intensity statins: Recommendations of the 2013 ACC/AHA Guidelines.

Indications	Treatment Recommendation
Presence of clinical atherosclerotic cardiovascular disease	High-intensity statin or moderate-intensity statin if over age 75
Primary elevation of LDL cholesterol ≥ 190 mg/dL (> 4.91 mmol/L)	High-intensity statin
Age 40–75 Presence of diabetes LDL ≥ 70 mg/dL (≥ 1.81 mmol/L)	Moderate-intensity statin or high-intensity statin if 10-year CVD risk > 7.5%
Age 40–75 No clinical atherosclerotic cardiovascular disease or diabetes LDL 70–189 mg/dL (1.81–4.91 mmol/L) Estimated 10-year CVD risk ≥ 7.5%	Treat with moderate- to high-intensity statin

ACC/AHA, American College of Cardiology/American Heart Association; CVD, cardiovascular disease; HDL, high-density lipoprotein; LDL, low-density lipoprotein.

— Persons aged 20 years only if there is increased risk of CHD
— Men without increased risk, beginning at age 35 years
• Obtain fasting serum total cholesterol, HDL cholesterol, and triglyceride levels
— LDL cholesterol is estimated by the following formula: LDL cholesterol = (Total cholesterol) − (HDL cholesterol) − (Triglycerides/5)
• Serum thyroid-stimulating hormone to screen for hypothyroidism
• Other tests only as indicated by symptoms and signs suggestive of a secondary cause
• LDL cholesterol is classified into five categories
— Optimal, < 100 mg/dL
— Near optimal, 100 to 129 mg/dL
— Borderline high, 130 to 159 mg/dL
— High, 160 to 189 mg/dL
— Very high, ≥ 190 mg/dL

7. Treatments

Medications
• Choice of whether to initiate drug therapy should be based on overall risk of cardiovascular events, using a risk calculator such as the Framingham calculator or the AHA/ACC CV Risk Calculator, and LDL cholesterol level
• Indications for high-intensity and moderate-intensity statins have been formulated by the American Heart Association and American College of Cardiology (Table 17-1)
• Treatment guidelines no longer recommend treating to a goal LDL level, but rather selecting a statin intensity for each given risk level (Table 17-2)
• HMG-CoA reductase inhibitors (statins, eg, atorvastatin, fluvastatin, lovastatin, pitavastatin, pravastatin, rosuvastatin, and simvastatin)
— Potent impact on reducing LDL
— Minimal impact on increasing HDL
— Best data for reducing coronary events, mortality
• Niacin
— Moderate impact on reducing LDL and increasing HDL
— Reduces triglycerides and has mortality benefit
— High rates of intolerance (flushing), which can be improved with use of extended-release niacin and concomitant aspirin use
• Bile acid binding resins (eg, cholestyramine, colestipol, and colesevelam)
— Moderate impact on reducing LDL
— Minimal impact on increasing HDL
— Reduce coronary events but not mortality

Table 17-2. Effects of selected lipid-modifying drugs.

Drug	Lipid-Modifying Effects			Initial Daily Dose	Maximum Daily Dose
	LDL	HDL	Triglyceride		
Atorvastatin (Lipitor)	−25% to −40%	+5%–10%	↓↓	10 mg once	80 mg once
Cholestyramine (Questran, others)	−15% to −25%	+5%	±	4 g twice a day	24 g divided
Colesevelam (WelChol)	−10% to −20%	+10%	±	625 mg, 6–7 tablets once	625 mg, 6–7 tablets once
Colestipol (Colestid)	−15% to −25%	+5%	±	5 g twice a day	30 g divided
Ezetimibe (Zetia)	−20%	+5%	±	10 mg once	10 mg once
Fenofibrate (Tricor, others)	−10% to −15%	+15% to +25%	↓↓	48 mg once	145 mg once
Fenofibric acid (Trilipix)	−10% to −15%	+15% to +25%	↓↓	45 mg once	135 mg once
Fluvastatin (Lescol)	−20% to −30%	+5% to +10%	↓	20 mg once	40 mg once
Gemfibrozil (Lopid, others)	−10% to −15%	+15% to +20%	↓↓	600 mg once	1200 mg divided
Lovastatin (Mevacor, others)	−25% to −40%	+5% to +10%	↓	10 mg once	80 mg divided
Niacin (OTC, Niaspan)	−15% to −25%	+25% to +35%	↓↓	100 mg once	3 g to 4.5 g divided
Pitavastatin (Livalo)	−30% to −40%	+10% to +25%	↓↓	2 mg once	4 mg once
Pravastatin (Pravachol)	−25% to −40%	+5% to +10%	↓	20 mg once	80 mg once
Rosuvastatin (Crestor)	−40% to −50%	+10% to 15%	↓↓	10 mg once	40 mg once
Simvastatin (Zocor, others)	−25% to −40%	+5% to +10%	↓↓	5 mg once	80 mg once

HDL, high-density lipoprotein; LDL, low-density lipoprotein; OTC, over the counter; ±, variable; others, indicates availability of less-expensive generic preparations.

- — Mainly gastrointestinal side effects; can block the absorption of fat-soluble vitamins
- — Safe in pregnancy
- Fibric acid derivatives (eg, gemfibrozil, fenofibrate)
  - — Moderate impact on reducing LDL and increasing HDL
  - — Reduce triglycerides
  - — Reduce coronary events but not mortality
  - — Side effects increased when taken with statins
- When treating with statins, there is no evidence that combination with other classes of agents leads to better outcomes and such combination may increase side effects, even if cholesterol levels are reduced

Therapeutic Procedures
- For hypercholesterolemia, low-fat diets may produce a moderate (5%–10%) decrease in LDL cholesterol
- More restricted, plant-based diets may lower LDL cholesterol substantially more
- Low-fat diet may also lower HDL cholesterol
- Substituting monounsaturated fats for saturated fats can lower LDL without affecting HDL
- In diabetics, control of hyperglycemia can improve lipid profile, particularly triglycerides
- Exercise and moderate alcohol consumption can increase HDL levels
- For hypertriglyceridemia, primary therapy is dietary, including reducing alcohol, fatty food and excess dietary carbohydrate intake; and controlling hyperglycemia in diabetics

8. Outcomes

Follow-Up
- Fasting lipid panel 3 to 6 months after initiation of therapy
- Annual or biannual screening depending on risk factors
- Monitoring for side effects of therapy, such as liver enzyme elevation or myopathy in those on statins

Complications
- Atherosclerotic: myocardial infarction, stroke, and other vascular diseases
- Nonatherosclerotic: xanthomas and pancreatitis
- Metabolic syndrome patients are at increased risk for cardiovascular events
- Very high triglyceride levels (fasting serum triglycerides greater than 2000 mg/dL) increase the risk of pancreatitis

9. When to Refer and When to Admit

When to Refer
- Refer patients to a lipid specialist who have
  — Extremely high serum LDL cholesterol or triglyceride, or extremely low serum HDL cholesterol
  — Striking family history of hyperlipidemia or premature atherosclerosis
  — Known genetic lipid disorders

When to Admit
- Acute pancreatitis related to hypertriglyceridemia

SUGGESTED REFERENCES

Berglund L et al. Evaluation and treatment of hypertriglyceridemia: an Endocrine Society clinical practice guideline. *J Clin Endocrinol Metab*. 2012 Sep;97(9):2969–2989. [PMID: 22962670]

Eckel RH et al. 2013 AHA/ACC Guideline on Lifestyle Management to Reduce Cardiovascular Risk: a report of the American College of Cardiology/American Heart Association Task Force on Practice Guidelines. *Circulation*. 2014 Jun 24;129(25 suppl 2):S76–S99. [PMID: 24222015]

Kavousi M et al. Comparison of application of the ACC/AHA guidelines, Adult Treatment Panel III guidelines, and European Society of Cardiology guidelines for cardiovascular disease prevention in a European cohort. *JAMA*. 2014 Apr 9;311(14):1416–1423. [PMID: 24681960]

Keaney JF Jr et al. A pragmatic view of the new cholesterol treatment guidelines. *N Engl J Med*. 2014 Jan 16;370(3):275–278. [PMID: 24283199]

Krumholz HM. Target cardiovascular risk rather than cholesterol concentration. *BMJ*. 2013 Nov 27;347:f7110. [PMID: 24284344]

Lavigne PM et al. The current state of niacin in cardiovascular disease prevention: a systematic review and meta-regression. *J Am Coll Cardiol*. 2013 Jan 29;61(4):440–446. [PMID: 23265337]

Nordestgaard BG et al. Triglycerides and cardiovascular disease. *Lancet*. 2014 Aug 16;384(9943):626–635. [PMID: 25131982]

Pencina MJ et al. Application of new cholesterol guidelines to a population-based sample. *N Engl J Med*. 2014 Apr 10;370(15):1422–1431. [PMID: 24645848]

Rader DJ et al. HDL and cardiovascular disease. *Lancet*. 2014 Aug 16;384(9943):618–625. [PMID: 25131981]

Rees K et al. "Mediterranean" dietary pattern for the primary prevention of cardiovascular disease. *Cochrane Database Syst Rev*. 2013 Aug 12;8:CD009825. [PMID: 23939686]

Ridker PM. LDL cholesterol: controversies and future therapeutic directions. *Lancet*. 2014 Aug 16;384(9943):607–617. [PMID: 25131980]

Ridker PM et al. A trial-based approach to statin guidelines. *JAMA*. 2013 Sep 18;310(11):1123–1124. [PMID: 23942579]

Schaefer EW et al. Management of severe hypertriglyceridemia in the hospital: a review. *J Hosp Med*. 2012 May–Jun;7(5):431–438. [PMID: 22128096]

Singh A et al. What should we do about hypertriglyceridemia in coronary artery disease patients? *Curr Treat Options Cardiovasc Med*. 2013 Feb;15(1):104–117. [PMID: 23109123]

Sniderman AD et al. The severe hypercholesterolemia phenotype: clinical diagnosis, management, and emerging therapies. *J Am Coll Cardiol*. 2014 May 20;63(19):1935–1947. [PMID: 24632267]

Stone NJ et al. 2013 ACC/AHA guideline on the treatment of blood cholesterol to reduce atherosclerotic cardiovascular risk in adults: a report of the American College of Cardiology/American Heart Association Task Force on Practice Guidelines. *J Am Coll Cardiol*. 2014 Jul 1;63(25 pt B):2889–2934. [PMID: 24239923]

Stone NJ et al. Treatment of blood cholesterol to reduce atherosclerotic cardiovascular disease risk in adults: synopsis of the 2013 American College of Cardiology/American Heart Association cholesterol guideline. *Ann Intern Med*. 2014 Mar 4;160(5):339–343. [PMID: 24474185]

Wang X et al. Cholesterol levels and risk of hemorrhagic stroke: a systematic review and meta-analysis. *Stroke*. 2013 Jul;44(7):1833–1839. [PMID: 23704101]

Heart Failure

18

A 75-year-old man with a history of coronary artery disease (CAD) and multiple previous myocardial infarctions (MIs) presents to his primary care clinician with increasing shortness of breath. The patient's exercise tolerance has gone from walking 10 blocks without stopping to needing to catch his breath after walking across the room. He can no longer lie flat at night and uses 4 pillows to prop himself up in bed. On physical examination, he has bilateral crackles halfway up his lung fields, his jugular venous pulsations are elevated, and his lower extremities have pitting edema.

LEARNING OBJECTIVES

► Learn the clinical manifestations and objective findings of left- and right-sided heart failure
► Understand the causes of heart failure
► Know the differential diagnosis heart failure
► Learn the treatment for systolic and diastolic heart failure
► Know which patients need consideration for advanced therapies for heart failure such as implantable defibrillators and inotropic agents

QUESTIONS

1. What are the salient features of this patient's problem?

2. How do you think through his problem?

3. What are the key features, including essentials of diagnosis, and general considerations of heart failure?

4. What are the symptoms and signs of heart failure?

5. What is the differential diagnosis of heart failure?

6. What are laboratory, imaging, and procedural findings in heart failure?

7. What are the treatments for heart failure?

8. What are the outcomes, including follow-up, complications, prevention, and prognosis, of heart failure?

9. When should patients with heart failure be referred to a specialist or admitted to the hospital?

ANSWERS

1. Salient Features

Elderly man with CAD and previous MI; shortness of breath; orthopnea; lung crackles from left-sided failure; elevated jugular venous pressure (JVP) and lower extremity edema from right-sided failure

2. How to Think Through

Heart failure (HF) is a prevalent, important syndrome. Prompt diagnosis and effective management improve morbidity, mortality, and quality of life. As in this case, HF diagnosis typically begins with a complaint of undifferentiated dyspnea on exertion. This patient also describes orthopnea. What additional symptoms should be elicited? (Exertional chest pain, paroxysmal nocturnal dyspnea, lower extremity edema, syncope or presyncope, palpitations.)

What cardiac pathologies can produce HF and the physical examination signs found in this patient? (Impaired systolic function, impaired diastolic function, arrhythmia, congenital heart disease, and valvular disease.) What physical examination sign should be present with palpation of the chest? (Enlarged, sustained, displaced point of maximal impulse [PMI] at the apex.) Once a diagnosis of HF is made, the underlying cause should be identified. In this case, the patient has known CAD, and an echocardiogram or nuclear imaging study may show wall motion abnormalities consistent with ischemia or infarction.

What medication classes improve mortality in heart failure with reduced ejection fraction and should be added if not already part of his regimen? (ACE inhibitor, β-blocker, and aldosterone receptor blocker, angiotensin receptor; neprilysin inhibitors are under investigation.) A loop diuretic should be started for symptomatic relief immediately following assessment of electrolytes and renal function.

If this patient proves to have an ejection fraction of less than 35%, what other interventions might help? (Implantable cardiac defibrillator improves mortality. Biventricular pacing can significantly improve symptoms and systolic function in some patients.)

3. Key Features

Essentials of Diagnosis

- Left ventricular (LV) failure
  — Due to systolic or diastolic dysfunction
  — Predominant symptoms are those of low cardiac output and congestion including dyspnea
- Right ventricular (RV) failure
  — Usually secondary to LV failure
  — Predominant symptoms are those of fluid overload
- Assessment of LV function is a crucial part of diagnosis and management
- Optimal management of chronic heart failure includes combination medical therapies such as ACE inhibitors, aldosterone antagonists, and β-blockers

General Considerations

- Heart failure (HF) occurs as a result of depressed contractility with fluid retention and/or impaired cardiac output, or diastolic dysfunction with fluid retention
- Acute exacerbations of chronic HF are caused by patient nonadherence to or alterations in therapy, excessive salt and fluid intake, arrhythmias, excessive activity, pulmonary emboli, intercurrent infection, progression of the underlying disease
- High-output HF is caused by thyrotoxicosis, beriberi, severe anemia, arteriovenous shunting, and Paget disease
- Systolic dysfunction is caused by MI, ethanol abuse, long-standing hypertension, viral myocarditis (including HIV), Chagas disease, and idiopathic dilated cardiomyopathy

- Diastolic dysfunction is associated with abnormal filling of a "stiff" LV caused by chronic hypertension, LV hypertrophy, and diabetes

4. Symptoms and Signs

- Symptoms of diastolic dysfunction are often difficult to distinguish clinically from those of systolic dysfunction
- LV failure
  — Exertional dyspnea progressing to orthopnea and then dyspnea at rest
  — Paroxysmal nocturnal dyspnea
  — Chronic nonproductive cough (often worse in recumbency)
  — Nocturia
  — Fatigue and exercise intolerance
- RV failure
  — Anorexia
  — Nausea
  — Right upper quadrant pain due to chronic passive congestion of the liver and gut
- Tachycardia, hypotension, reduced pulse pressure, cold extremities, and diaphoresis
- Long-standing severe HF: cachexia or cyanosis
- Physical examination findings in LV HF
  — Crackles at lung bases, pleural effusions and basilar dullness to percussion, expiratory wheezing, and rhonchi
  — Parasternal lift, an enlarged and sustained LV impulse, a diminished first heart sound
  — S_3 gallop
  — S_4 gallop in diastolic dysfunction
- Physical examination findings in RV HF
  — Elevated JVP, abnormal pulsations, such as regurgitant v waves
  — Tender or nontender hepatic enlargement, hepatojugular reflux, and ascites
  — Peripheral pitting edema sometimes extending to the thighs and abdominal wall

5. Differential Diagnosis

- Chronic obstructive pulmonary disease (COPD)
- Pneumonia
- Cirrhosis
- Peripheral venous insufficiency
- Nephrotic syndrome

6. Laboratory, Imaging, and Procedural Findings

Laboratory Tests

- Obtain complete blood cell count, blood urea nitrogen, serum electrolytes, creatinine, thyroid-stimulating hormone, ferritin
- Electrocardiogram (ECG) to look for
  — Arrhythmia
  — MI
  — Nonspecific changes, including low-voltage, intraventricular conduction delay; LV hypertrophy; and repolarization changes
- "B-type" natriuretic peptide (BNP)
  — Elevation is a sensitive indicator of symptomatic (diastolic or systolic) HF but may be less specific, especially in older patients, women, and patients with COPD
  — Adds to clinical assessment in differentiating dyspnea due to HF from noncardiac causes
  — Evidence from trials shows benefit from using BNP to guide therapy in heart failure with reduced ejection fraction, but practice guidelines do not yet recommend

Imaging Studies
- Chest radiograph shows
  - Cardiomegaly
  - Dilation of the upper lobe veins
  - Perivascular or interstitial edema
  - Alveolar fluid
  - Bilateral or right-sided pleural effusions
- Echocardiography can assess
  - Ventricular size and function
  - Valvular abnormalities
  - Pericardial effusions
  - Intracardiac shunts
  - Segmental wall motion abnormalities
- Radionuclide angiography and cardiac MRI: measure LV ejection fraction and assess regional wall motion
- Stress imaging: indicated if ECG abnormalities or suspected myocardial ischemia

Diagnostic Procedures
- ECG helps rule out
  - Valvular lesions
  - Myocardial ischemia
  - Arrhythmias
  - Alcohol- or drug-induced myocardial depression
  - Intracardiac shunts
  - High-output states
  - Hyperthyroidism and hypothyroidism
  - Medications
  - Hemochromatosis
  - Sarcoidosis
  - Amyloidosis
- Left heart catheterization
  - To exclude significant valvular disease
  - To delineate presence and extent of CAD
- Right heart catheterization: to select and monitor therapy in patients not responding to standard therapy

7. Treatments

Medications
- **Systolic dysfunction:** a diuretic and an angiotensin-converting enzyme (ACE) inhibitor (or angiotensin receptor blocker [ARB]) with subsequent addition of a β-blocker and aldosterone blocker (if tolerated)
- Diuretics (Table 18-1)
- Thiazide
  - Loop
  - Thiazide and loop
  - Thiazide and spironolactone
- Aldosterone blockers (Table 18-1)
  - Spironolactone, 25 mg once daily orally (may decrease to 12.5 mg or increase to 50 mg depending on kidney function, K^+, and symptoms)
  - Eplerenone, 25 to 50 mg once daily orally
- ACE inhibitors (Table 18-2): start at low doses and titrate to higher dosages; proved effective in clinical trials over 1 to 3 months; eg, to
  - Captopril, 50 mg three times daily orally
  - Enalapril, 10 mg twice daily orally
  - Lisinopril, 20 mg once daily orally

Table 18-1. Diuretics.

Drugs	Proprietary Names	Initial Oral Doses	Dosage Range	Adverse Effects	Comments
Thiazides and loop diuretics					
Hydrochlorothiazide	Esidrix, Microzide	12.5 or 25 mg once daily	12.5–50 mg once daily	$\downarrow$ K$^+$, $\downarrow$ Mg^{2+}, $\uparrow$ Ca^{2+}, $\downarrow$ Na$^+$, $\uparrow$ uric acid, $\uparrow$ glucose, $\uparrow$ LDL cholesterol, $\uparrow$ triglycerides; rash, erectile dysfunction	Low dosages effective in many patients without associated metabolic abnormalities; metolazone more effective with concurrent kidney disease; indapamide does not alter serum lipid levels
Chlorthalidone	Thalitone	12.5 or 25 mg once daily	12.5–50 mg once daily		
Metolazone	Zaroxolyn	1.25 or 2.5 mg once daily	1.25–5 mg once daily		
Indapamide	Lozol	2.5 mg once daily	2.5–5 mg once daily		
Furosemide	Lasix	20 mg twice daily	40–320 mg in 2 or 3 doses	Same as thiazides, but higher risk of excessive diuresis and electrolyte imbalance. Increases calcium excretion	Furosemide: Short duration of action a disadvantage; should be reserved for patients with kidney disease or fluid retention. Poor antihypertensive
Ethacrynic acid	Edecrin	50 mg once daily	50–100 mg once or twice daily		
Bumetanide	Bumex	0.25 mg twice daily	0.5–10 mg in 2 or 3 doses		
Torsemide	Demadex	2.5 mg once daily	5–10 mg once daily		Torsemide: Effective blood pressure medication at low dosage
Aldosterone receptor blockers					
Spironolactone	Aldactone	12.5 or 25 mg once daily	12.5–100 mg once daily	Hyperkalemia, metabolic acidosis, gynecomastia	Can be useful add-on therapy in patients with refractory hypertension
Amiloride	Midamor	5 mg once daily	5–10 mg once daily		
Eplerenone	Inspra	25 mg once daily	25–100 mg once daily		
Combination products					
Hydrochlorothiazide and triamterene	Dyazide (25/50 mg); Maxzide (25/37.5 mg; 50/75 mg)	1 tab once daily	1 or 2 tabs once daily	Same as thiazides plus GI disturbances, hyperkalemia rather than hypokalemia, headache; triamterene can cause kidney stones and kidney dysfunction; spironolactone causes gynecomastia. Hyperkalemia can occur if this combination is used in patients with advanced kidney disease or those taking ACE inhibitors	Use should be limited to patients with demonstrable need for a potassium-sparing agent
Hydrochlorothiazide and amiloride	Moduretic (50/5 mg)	½ tab once daily	1 or 2 tabs once daily		
Hydrochlorothiazide and spironolactone	Aldactazide (25/25 mg; 50/50 mg)	1 tab [25/25 mg] once daily	1 or 2 tabs once daily		

ACE, angiotensin-converting enzyme; GI, gastrointestinal; LDL, low-density lipoprotein.

- ARBs (Table 18-2) for ACE-intolerant patients
- ARB valsartan (titrated to a dose of 160 mg twice daily) added to ACE inhibitor therapy reduced composite of death or hospitalization for HF
- β-Blockers (Table 18-3): in stable patients, start at low doses and titrate gradually to higher doses with great care; eg, to
  — Carvedilol, started at 3.125 mg twice daily orally, increased to 6.25, 12.5, and 25 mg twice daily at intervals of ~2 weeks
  — Metoprolol extended-release, started at 12.5 or 25 mg once daily, increased to 50, 75, 100, 150, and 200 mg at intervals of ~2 weeks or longer
- Digoxin
  — Oral maintenance dose ranges from 0.125 mg three times weekly to 0.5 mg daily
  — May induce ventricular arrhythmias, especially when hypokalemia or myocardial ischemia is present
- Anticoagulation: for patients with LV HF associated with atrial fibrillation or large recent (within 3–6 months) MI
- Angiotensin receptor–neprilysin inhibitors are in the process of FDA approval and reduce the risk of death and hospitalization in patients with heart failure and reduced ejection fraction
- Ivabradine
  — Not approved for use in the United States
  — Approved by the European Medicines Agency for use in patients with a heart rate ≥ 75 beats/min

Table 18-2. Renin and ACE inhibitors and angiotensin II receptor blockers.

Drug	Proprietary Name	Initial Oral Dosage	Dosage Range	Adverse Effects	Comments
Renin inhibitors					
Aliskiren	Tekturna	150 mg once daily	150–300 mg once daily	Angioedema, hypotension, hyperkalemia. Contraindicated in pregnancy	Probably metabolized by CYP3A4. Absorption is inhibited by high-fat meal
Aliskiren and HCTZ	Tekturna HCT	150 mg/12.5 mg once daily	150 mg/12.5 mg–300 mg/25 mg once daily		
ACE inhibitors					
Benazepril	Lotensin	10 mg once daily	5–40 mg in 1 or 2 doses	Cough, hypotension, dizziness, kidney dysfunction, hyperkalemia, angioedema; taste alteration and rash (may be more frequent with captopril); rarely, proteinuria, blood dyscrasia. Contraindicated in pregnancy	More fosinopril is excreted by the liver in patients with renal dysfunction (dose reduction may or may not be necessary). Captopril and lisinopril are active without metabolism. Captopril, enalapril, lisinopril, and quinapril are approved for heart failure
Benazepril and HCTZ	Lotensin HCT	5 mg/6.25 mg once daily	5 mg/6.25 mg to 20 mg/25 mg		
Benazepril and amlodipine	Lotrel	10 mg/2.5 mg once daily	10 mg/2.5 mg to 40 mg/10 mg		
Captopril	Capoten	25 mg twice daily	50–450 mg in 2 or 3 doses		
Captopril and HCTZ	Capozide	25 mg/15 mg twice daily	25 mg/15 mg to 50 mg/25 mg		
Enalapril	Vasotec	5 mg once daily	5–40 mg in 1 or 2 doses		
Enalapril and HCTZ	Vaseretic	5 mg/12.5 mg once daily	5 mg/12.5 mg to 10 mg/25 mg		
Fosinopril	Monopril	10 mg once daily	10–80 mg in 1 or 2 doses		
Fosinopril and HCTZ	Monopril HCT	10 mg/12.5 mg once daily	10 mg/12.5 mg to 20 mg/12.5 mg		
Lisinopril	Prinivil, Zestril	5–10 mg once daily	5–40 mg once daily		
Lisinopril and HCTZ	Prinzide or Zestoretic	10 mg/12.5 mg once daily	10 mg/12.5 mg to 20 mg/12.5 mg to 20 mg/25 mg		
Moexipril	Univasc	7.5 mg once daily	7.5–30 mg in 1 or 2 doses		
Moexipril and HCTZ	Uniretic	7.5 mg/12.5 mg once daily	7.5 mg/12.5 mg to 15 mg/25 mg		
Perindopril	Aceon	4 mg once daily	4–16 mg in 1 or 2 doses		
Quinapril	Accupril	10 mg once daily	10–80 mg in 1 or 2 doses		
Quinapril and HCTZ	Accuretic	10 mg/12.5 mg once daily	10 mg/12.5 mg to 20 mg/25 mg		
Ramipril	Altace	2.5 mg once daily	2.5–20 mg in 1 or 2 doses		
Trandolapril	Mavik	1 mg once daily	1–8 mg once daily		
Trandolapril and verapamil	Tarka	2 mg/180 mg ER once daily	2 mg/180 mg ER to 8 mg/480 mg ER		
Angiotensin II receptor blockers					
Candesartan cilexetil	Atacand	16 mg once daily	8–32 mg once daily	Hyperkalemia, kidney dysfunction, rare angioedema. Combinations have additional side effects. Contraindicated in pregnancy	Losartan has a very flat dose-response curve. Valsartan and irbesartan have wider dose-response ranges and longer durations of action. Addition of low-dose diuretic (separately or as combination pills) increases the response
Candesartan cilexetil/HCTZ	Atacand HCT	16 mg/12.5 mg once daily	32 mg/12.5 mg once daily		
Eprosartan	Teveten	600 mg once daily	400–800 mg in 1–2 doses		
Eprosartan/HCTZ	Teveten HCT	600 mg/12.5 mg once daily	600 mg/12.5 mg to 600 mg/25 mg once daily		
Irbesartan	Avapro	150 mg once daily	150–300 mg once daily		
Irbesartan and HCTZ	Avalide	150 mg/12.5 mg once daily	150–300 mg irbesartan once daily		
Losartan	Cozaar	50 mg once daily	25–100 mg in 1 or 2 doses		
Losartan and HCTZ	Hyzaar	50 mg/12.5 mg once daily	50 mg/12.5 mg to 100 mg/25 mg tablets once daily		
Olmesartan	Benicar	20 mg once daily	20–40 mg once daily		
Olmesartan and HCTZ	Benicar HCT	20 mg/12.5 mg once daily	20 mg/12.5 mg to 40 mg/25 mg once daily		
Olmesartan and amlodipine	Azor	20 mg/5 mg once daily	20 mg/5 mg to 40 mg/10 mg		

(continued)

Table 18-2. Renin and ACE inhibitors and angiotensin II receptor blockers. (continued)

Drug	Proprietary Name	Initial Oral Dosage	Dosage Range	Adverse Effects	Comments
Olmesartan and amlodipine and HCTZ	Tribenzor	20 mg/5 mg/12.5 mg once daily	20 mg/5 mg/12.5 mg to 40 mg/10 mg/25 mg once daily		
Telmisartan	Micardis	40 mg once daily	20–80 mg once daily		
Telmisartan and HCTZ	Micardis HCT	40 mg/12.5 mg once daily	40 mg/12.5 mg to 80 mg/25 mg once daily		
Telmisartan and amlodipine	Twynsta	40 mg/5 mg once daily	40 mg/5 mg to 80 mg/10 mg once daily	Hyperkalemia, kidney dysfunction, rare angioedema. Combinations have additional side effects. Contraindicated in pregnancy	Losartan has a very flat dose-response curve. Valsartan and irbesartan have wider dose-response ranges and longer durations of action. Addition of low-dose diuretic (separately or as combination pills) increases the response
Valsartan	Diovan	80 mg once daily	80–320 mg once daily		
Valsartan and HCTZ	Diovan HCT	80 mg/12.5 mg once daily	80–320 mg valsartan once daily		
Valsartan and amlodipine	Exforge	160 mg/5 mg once daily	160 mg/5 mg–320 mg/10 mg once daily		
Other combination products					
Aliskiren and valsartan	Valturna	150 mg/160 mg once daily	150 mg/160 mg to 300 mg/320 mg once daily	Angioedema, hypotension, hyperkalemia. Contraindicated in pregnancy	
Amlodipine/HCTZ/valsartan	Exforge HCT	5 mg/12.5 mg/160 mg once daily	10 mg/25 mg/320 mg up to once daily	Angioedema, hypotension, hyperkalemia. Contraindicated in pregnancy	

ACE, angiotensin-converting enzyme; HCTZ, hydrochlorothiazide.

— Class IIa recommendation by European guidelines for patients in sinus rhythm with heart rate $\geq$ 70 beats/min, EF $\leq$ 35%, and persisting symptoms despite treatment with an evidence-based dose of β-blocker (or maximum tolerated dose below that), ACE inhibitor (or ARB), and an aldosterone antagonist (or ARB)

• **Heart failure with preserved ejection fraction:** diuretics, rigorous blood pressure control

Surgery
• Coronary revascularization appears warranted for some patients with HF, including those with more severe angina or left main coronary disease or selected patients with less-severe symptoms
• Bypass surgery provides more complete revascularization than angioplasty
• Cardiac transplantation for advanced HF
• Implantable defibrillators for chronic HF and ischemic or nonischemic cardiomyopathy with ejection fraction < 35%
• Biventricular pacing (resynchronization) for patients with moderate to severe systolic HF and LV dyssynchrony
• Resynchronization therapy is indicated for patients with
  — Class II, III, and ambulatory class IV heart failure
  — EF $\leq$ 35%
  — LBBB pattern with QRS duration of $\geq$ 120 ms

Therapeutic Procedures
• Moderate salt restriction (2.0–2.5 g sodium or 5–6 g salt per day)
• Temporary restriction of activity

8. Outcomes
Follow-Up
• Monitor patients taking diuretics and ACE inhibitors for hypokalemia, acute kidney injury
• Case management, home monitoring of weight and clinical status, and patient adjustment of diuretics can prevent rehospitalizations

Table 18-3. β-Adrenergic blocking agents.

Drug	Proprietary Name	Initial Oral Dosage	Dosage Range	Special Properties					Comments[d]
				β₁ Selectivity[a]	ISA[b]	MSA[c]	Lipid Solubility	Renal vs Hepatic Elimination	
Acebutolol	Sectral	400 mg once daily	200–1200 mg in 1 or 2 doses	+	+	+	+	H > R	Positive ANA; rare LE syndrome; also indicated for arrhythmias. Doses > 800 mg have β₁ and β₂ effects
Atenolol	Tenormin	25 mg once daily	25–100 mg once daily	+	0	0	0	R	Also indicated for angina pectoris and post-MI. Doses > 100 mg have β₁ and β₂ effects
Betaxolol	Kerlone	10 mg once daily	10–40 mg once daily	+	0	0	+	H > R	
Bisoprolol and hydrochlorothiazide	Ziac	2.5 mg/6.25 mg once daily	2.5 mg/6.25 mg to 10 mg/6.25 mg once daily	+	0	0	0	R = H	Low-dose combination approved for initial therapy. Bisoprolol also effective for heart failure
Carvedilol	Coreg	6.25 mg twice daily	12.5–50 mg in 2 doses	0	0	0	+++	H > R	α: β-Blocking activity 1:9; may cause orthostatic symptoms; effective for heart failure. Nitric oxide potentiating vasodilatory activity
Labetalol	Normodyne, Trandate	100 mg twice daily	200–2400 mg in 2 doses	0	0/+	0	++	H	α: β-blocking activity 1:3; more orthostatic hypotension, fever, hepatotoxicity
Metoprolol	Lopressor	50 mg twice daily	50–200 mg twice daily	+	0	+	+++	H	Also indicated for angina pectoris and post-MI. Approved for heart failure. Doses > 100 mg have β₁ and β₂ effects
	Toprol XL (SR preparation)	25 mg once daily	25–400 mg once daily						
Metoprolol and hydrochlorothiazide	Lopressor HCT	50 mg/25 mg once daily	50 mg/25 mg– 200 mg/50 mg	+	0	+	+++	H	
Nadolol	Corgard	20 mg once daily	20–320 mg once daily	0	0	0	0	R	
Nebivolol	Bystolic	5 mg once daily	40 mg once daily	+	0	0	++	H	Nitric oxide potentiating vasodilatory activity
Penbutolol	Levatol	20 mg once daily	20–80 mg once daily	0	+	0	++	R > H	
Pindolol	Visken	5 mg twice daily	10–60 mg in 2 doses	0	++	+	+	H > R	In adults, 35% renal clearance
Propranolol	Inderal	20 mg twice daily	40–640 mg in 2 doses	0	0	++	+++	H	Once-daily SR preparation also available. Also indicated for angina pectoris and post-MI
Timolol	Blocadren	5 mg twice daily	10–60 mg in 2 doses	0	0	0	++	H > R	Also indicated for post-MI. 80% hepatic clearance

ANA, antinuclear antibody; ISA, intrinsic sympathomimetic activity; LE, lupus erythematosus; MI, myocardial infarction; MSA, membrane-stabilizing activity; SR, sustained release; 0, no effect; +, some effect; ++, moderate effect; +++, most effect.

[a]Agents with β₁ selectivity are less likely to precipitate bronchospasm and decreased peripheral blood flow in low doses, but selectivity is only relative.

[b]Agents with ISA cause less resting bradycardia and lipid changes.

[c]MSA generally occurs at concentrations greater than those necessary for β-adrenergic blockade. The clinical importance of MSA by β-blockers has not been defined.

[d]Adverse effects of all β-blockers: bronchospasm, fatigue, sleep disturbance and nightmares, bradycardia and atrioventricular block, worsening of heart failure, cold extremities, gastrointestinal disturbances, erectile dysfunction, triglycerides, ↓ HDL cholesterol, rare blood dyscrasias.

Complications

- Myocardial ischemia in patients with underlying CAD
- Asymptomatic and symptomatic arrhythmias, especially nonsustained ventricular tachycardia
- Sudden death and unexplained syncope

Prevention

- Antihypertensive therapy
- Antihyperlipidemic therapy
- Treat valvular lesions (aortic stenosis and mitral and aortic regurgitation) early

Prognosis

- HF carries a poor prognosis with both reduced and preserved ejection fraction
- Five-year mortality is approximately 50%
- Mortality rates vary from < 5% per year in those with no or few symptoms to > 30% per year in those with severe and refractory symptoms
- Higher mortality is related to
  — Older age
  — Lower left ventricular ejection fraction
  — More severe symptoms
  — Renal insufficiency
  — Diabetes

9. When to Refer and When to Admit

When to Refer

- Patients with new symptoms of HF not explained by an obvious cause should be referred to a cardiologist

When to Admit

- Patients with unexplained new or worsened symptoms, or positive cardiac biomarkers concerning for acute myocardial necrosis
- Patients with hypoxia, fluid overload, or pulmonary edema not readily resolved in outpatient setting

SUGGESTED REFERENCES

Brignole M et al. 2013 ESC Guidelines on cardiac pacing and cardiac resynchronization therapy: the Task Force on cardiac pacing and resynchronization therapy of the European Society of Cardiology (ESC). Developed in collaboration with the European Heart Rhythm Association (EHRA). *Eur Heart J.* 2013 Aug;34(29):2281–2329. [PMID: 23801822]

Ezekowitz JA et al. Standardizing care for acute decompensated heart failure in a large megatrial: the approach for the Acute Studies of Clinical Effectiveness of Nesiritide in Subjects with Decompensated Heart Failure (ASCEND-HF). *Am Heart J.* 2009 Feb;157(2):219–228. [PMID: 19185628]

Hunt SA et al. 2009 focused update incorporated into the ACC/AHA 2005 Guidelines for the Diagnosis and Management of Heart Failure in Adults: a report of the American College of Cardiology Foundation/American Heart Association Task Force on Practice Guidelines: developed in collaboration with the International Society for Heart and Lung Transplantation. *Circulation.* 2009 Apr 14;119(14):e391–e479. [PMID: 19324966]

McMurray JJ et al. ESC guidelines for the diagnosis and treatment of acute and chronic heart failure 2012: the Task Force for the Diagnosis and Treatment of Acute and Chronic Heart Failure 2012 of the European Society of Cardiology. *Eur J Heart Fail.* 2012 Aug;14(8):803–869. [PMID: 22828712]

Pitt B et al; TOPCAT Investigators. Spironolactone for heart failure with preserved ejection fraction. *N Engl J Med.* 2014 Apr 10;370(15):1383–1392. [PMID: 24716680]

Troughton RW et al. Effect of B-type natriuretic peptide-guided treatment of chronic heart failure on total mortality and hospitalization: an individual patient meta-analysis. *Eur Heart J.* 2014 Jun 14;35(23):1559–1567. [PMID: 24603309]

Velazquez EJ et al; STICH Investigators. Coronary-artery bypass surgery in patients with left ventricular dysfunction. *N Engl J Med.* 2011 Apr 28;364(17):1607–1616. [PMID: 21463150]

19 Hypertension

A 56-year-old African American man presents to the clinic for a routine physical examination. On arrival, he is noted to have a blood pressure (BP) of 160/90 mm Hg, which you verify after he has sat for 20 minutes in the examination room. You look back in his record and see that during his last two visits he has had BPs of 154/91 and 161/89 mm Hg. He denies any symptoms. He also denies any recent caffeine or other stimulant use.

LEARNING OBJECTIVES

▶ Learn the classification and clinical manifestations of hypertension
▶ Understand the identifiable causes of hypertension, including the causes of hypertension resistant to treatment
▶ Know the differential diagnosis of hypertension
▶ Learn which laboratory tests are recommended for evaluation for patients newly diagnosed with hypertension
▶ Learn the treatments for hypertension, including modifications for compelling disease-specific indications

QUESTIONS

1. What are the salient features of this patient's problem?
2. How do you think through his problem?
3. What are the key features, including essentials of diagnosis, general considerations, and demographics, of hypertension?
4. What are the symptoms and signs of hypertension?
5. What is the differential diagnosis of hypertension?
6. What laboratory tests are indicated in hypertension?
7. What are the treatments for hypertension?
8. What are the outcomes, including follow-up and complications, of hypertension?
9. When should patients with hypertension be referred to a specialist or admitted to the hospital?

ANSWERS

1. Salient Features

Elevated BP on multiple occasions and after resting; African American race; no temporary cause

2. How to Think Through

Is this patient's hypertension likely primary or secondary? (Primary.) What are some causes of secondary hypertension? What prescription and OTC medications and other substances might cause hypertension? (Nonsteroidal anti-inflammatory drugs [NSAIDs], oral contraceptives, sympathomimetics.) What dietary and lifestyle factors most impact BP? (Weight loss, dietary sodium reduction, moderation of alcohol consumption.) In the absence of other comorbidities, what would be your first choice antihypertensive agent? Is the patient likely to need more than one medication? (A thiazide diuretic such as HCTZ would be first line; with two out of three readings > 160 mm Hg, this is stage 2 hypertension and multiple agents will likely be necessary.) How would you assess for end-organ damage? (Serum creatinine and blood urea nitrogen, urinalysis, ECG.) What evidence might you find on cardiac and ophthalmic examination, standard laboratory studies, urinalysis, or electrocardiogram (ECG)? (Loud cardiac A2; flame hemorrhages and arteriovenous nicking; elevated serum creatinine; proteinuria; left ventricular hypertrophy.)

What is the treatment goal for systolic BP in this patient? (< 140 mm Hg.) If this patient's BP did not achieve the treatment goal despite therapy with an angiotensin-converting enzyme (ACE) inhibitor, β-blocker, and a calcium channel blocker, would of the patient's BP be characterized as "resistant hypertension"? (No. Resistant hypertension criteria mandate a regimen of ≥ 3 agents *including a diuretic*. A thiazide diuretic should generally be the first or second agent.)

3. Key Features

Essentials of Diagnosis
• Usually asymptomatic
• In severe hypertension, occipital headache at awakening and blurry vision may occur

General Considerations
• Mild-to-moderate hypertension is nearly always asymptomatic
• Severe hypertension is usually due to
  — Parenchymal renal disease
  — Endocrine abnormalities
    ◦ Primary hyperaldosteronism
    ◦ Cushing syndrome
    ◦ Pheochromocytoma
  — Renal artery stenosis
  — Abrupt cessation of antihypertensive medications ("rebound")
  — Medication or illicit drug use
• Adequate blood pressure control reduces the incidence of acute coronary syndrome by 20% to 25%, stroke by 30% to 35%, and heart failure by 50%
• Figure 19-1 provides an approach to the expedited assessment and diagnosis of patients with hypertension
• Table 19-1 summarizes potential identifiable causes of hypertension
• Resistant hypertension is defined as failure to reach BP control in patients adherent to full doses of a 3-drug regimen (including a diuretic)
• Table 19-2 summarizes reasons for failure to reach BP control

Demographics
• About 71 million Americans are hypertensive
• Half of those affected are uncontrolled
• 36% of those that are uncontrolled are unaware of their condition
• 60% of patients who are being treated for hypertension are controlled
• Incidence of hypertension increases with age and varies by sex and ethnicity
  — More men than women in early life
  — More women than men later in life
  — More common in African Americans (up to 25%)

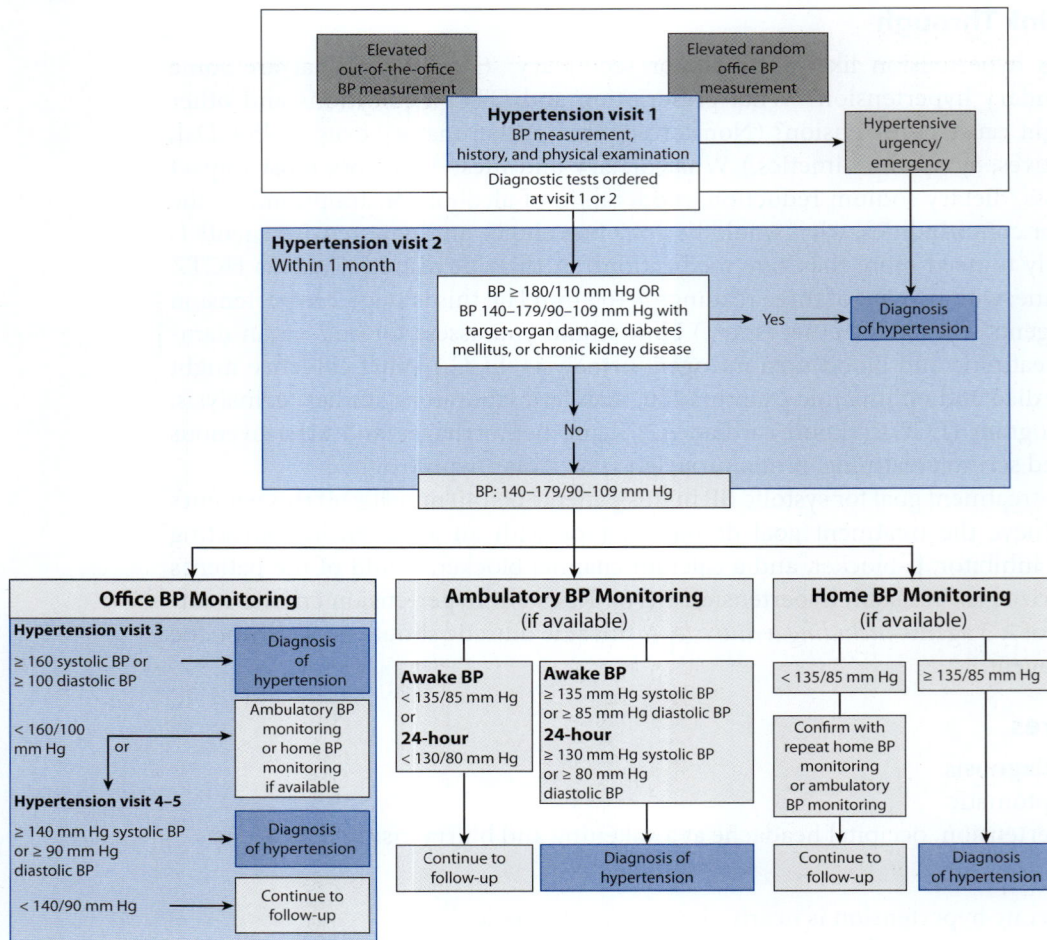

Figure 19-1. The Canadian Hypertension Education Program expedited assessment and diagnosis of patients with hypertension: Focus on validated technologies for blood pressure (BP) assessment. (Reprinted, with permission, from the Canadian Hypertension Education Program. The 2012 Canadian Hypertension Education Program recommendations for the management of hypertension: blood pressure management, diagnosis, assessment of risk, and therapy.)

4. Symptoms and Signs

- Usually asymptomatic
- Headaches are the most common symptom but are nonspecific
- Elevated BP
- Loud A_2 on cardiac examination
- Retinal arteriolar narrowing with "silver-wiring," arteriovenous nicking
- Flame-shaped retinal hemorrhages

Table 19-1. Identifiable causes of hypertension.

Sleep apnea
Drug-induced or drug-related
Chronic kidney disease
Primary aldosteronism
Renovascular disease
Long-term corticosteroid therapy and Cushing syndrome
Pheochromocytoma
Coarctation of the aorta
Thyroid or parathyroid disease

Data from Chobanian AV et al. The Seventh Report of the Joint National Committee on Prevention, Detection, Evaluation, and Treatment of High Blood Pressure: the JNC 7 report. *JAMA.* 2003;289(19):2560–2572.

Table 19-2. Causes of resistant hypertension.

Improper blood pressure measurement
Volume overload and pseudotolerance
Excess sodium intake
Volume retention from kidney disease
Inadequate diuretic therapy
Drug-induced or other causes
Nonadherence
Inadequate doses
Inappropriate combinations
Nonsteroidal anti-inflammatory drugs; cyclooxygenase-2 inhibitor
Cocaine, amphetamines, other illicit drugs
Sympathomimetics (decongestants, anorectics)
Oral contraceptives
Adrenal steroids
Cyclosporine and tacrolimus
Erythropoietin
Licorice (including some chewing tobacco)
Selected over-the-counter dietary supplements and medicines (eg, ephedra, ma huang, bitter orange)
Associated conditions
Obesity
Excess alcohol intake
Identifiable causes of hypertension (see Table 19-1)

Data from Chobanian AV et al. The Seventh Report of the Joint National Committee on Prevention, Detection, Evaluation, and Treatment of High Blood Pressure: the JNC 7 report. *JAMA*. 2003;289(19):2560–2572.

5. Differential Diagnosis

Primary (Essential) Hypertension
- "White-coat" hypertension
- BP cuff too small

Secondary Hypertension
- See Table 19-1
- Adrenal
  - Primary hyperaldosteronism
  - Cushing syndrome
  - Pheochromocytoma
- Renal
  - Chronic kidney disease
  - Renal artery stenosis (atherosclerotic or fibromuscular dysplasia)
- Other
  - Oral contraceptives
  - Alcohol
  - NSAIDs
  - Pregnancy associated
  - Hypercalcemia
  - Hyperthyroidism
  - Obstructive sleep apnea
  - Obesity
  - Coarctation of the aorta
  - Acromegaly
  - Increased intracranial pressure
  - Cocaine or amphetamine use

6. Laboratory Tests

- Urinalysis
- Serum creatinine, blood urea nitrogen
- Serum potassium

- Fasting blood glucose
- Cholesterol
- Hemoglobin
- Serum uric acid
- ECG
- When a secondary cause is suspected, consider
  — Chest radiograph
  — ECG
  — Plasma metanephrine levels
  — Plasma aldosterone concentration, plasma renin activity
  — Urine electrolytes

7. Treatments

- The blood pressure goals for most patients should be SBP < 140 mm Hg and diastolic BP (DBP) < 90 mm Hg
- The JNC 8 guidelines suggested that nondiabetic patients age 60 years or older have a goal of a SBP < 150 mm Hb and DBP < 90 mm Hg, though most clinical guidelines still suggest a goal of SBP < 140 mm Hg and DBP < 90 mm Hg in patients age 60–80 years
- Elderly patients (older than age 80 years) should be treated with more moderation; a goal of SBP < 150 mm Hg and DBP < 90 mm Hg may be more reasonable

Medications

- Initiation of drug therapy based on level of BP, cardiovascular risk factors, presence of target-organ damage (Table 19-3), and demographic considerations (Table 19-4)
- Major risk factors include
  — Smoking
  — Dyslipidemia
  — Diabetes mellitus
  — Age > 60 years
  — Family history of cardiovascular disease

Table 19-3. Cardiovascular risk factors.

Major risk factors
Hypertension[a]
Cigarette smoking
Obesity (BMI ≥ 30)[a]
Physical inactivity
Dyslipidemia[a]
Diabetes mellitus[a]
Microalbuminuria or estimated GFR < 60 mL/min
Age (> 55 years for men, > 65 years for women)
Family history of premature cardiovascular disease (men < 55 years or women < 65 years)
Target-organ damage
Heart
Left ventricular hypertrophy
Angina or prior myocardial infarction
Prior coronary revascularization
Heart failure
Brain
Stroke or transient ischemic attack
Chronic kidney disease
Peripheral arterial disease
Retinopathy

[a]Components of the metabolic syndrome.

BMI indicates body mass index calculated as weight in kilograms divided by the square of height in meters; GFR, glomerular filtration rate.

Data from Chobanian AV et al. The Seventh Report of the Joint National Committee on Prevention, Detection, Evaluation, and Treatment of High Blood Pressure: the JNC 7 report. *JAMA.* 2003 May 21; 289(19):2560–2572.

Table 19-4. Choice of antihypertensive agent based on demographic considerations.[a,b]

	Black, All Ages	All Others, Age < 55 Years	All Others, Age > 55 Years
First-line	CCB or diuretic	ACE or ARB[c] or CCB or diuretic[d]	CCB or diuretic[e]
Second-line	ACE or ARB[c] or vasodilating β-blocker[f]	Vasodilating β-blocker[f]	ACE or ARB or vasodilating β-blocker[f]
Alternatives	α-Agonist or α-antagonist[g]	α-Agonist or α-antagonist	α-Agonist or α-antagonist[g]
Resistant hypertension	Aldosterone receptor blocker	Aldosterone receptor blocker	Aldosterone receptor blocker

ACE, angiotensin-converting enzyme; ARB, angiotensin II receptor blocker; CCB, calcium channel blocker.

[a]Compelling indications may alter the selection of an antihypertensive drug.

[b]Start with full dose of one agent, or lower doses of combination therapy. In stage 2 hypertension, consider initiating therapy with a fixed dose combination.

[c]Women of childbearing age should avoid ACE and ARB or discontinue as soon as pregnancy is diagnosed.

[d]The adverse metabolic effects of thiazide diuretics and β-blockers should be considered in younger patients but may be less important in the older patient.

[e]For patients with significant renal impairment, use loop diuretic instead of thiazide.

[f]There are theoretical advantages in the use of vasodilating β-blockers such as carvedilol and nebivolol.

[g]α-Antagonists may precipitate or exacerbate orthostatic hypotension in the elderly.

- Figure 19-2: British Hypertension Society algorithm for diagnosis and treatment of hypertension
- Diuretics: Table 19-5
- β-Adrenergic blocking agents: Table 19-6
- ACE inhibitors and angiotensin receptor blockers: Table 19-7

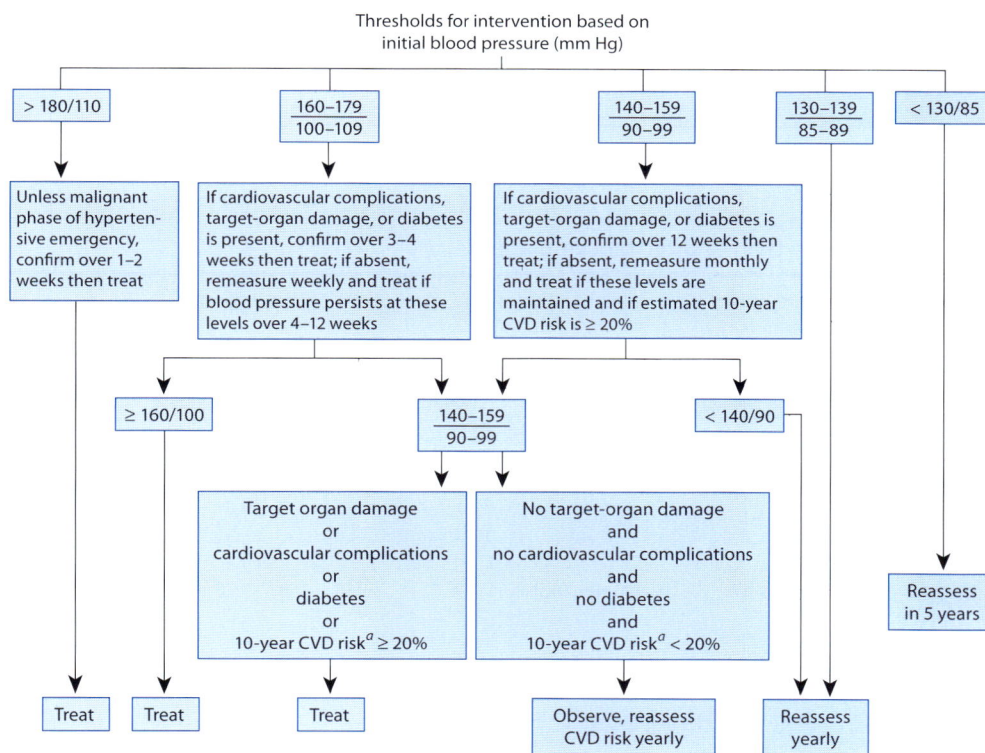

Figure 19-2. British Hypertension Society algorithm for diagnosis and treatment of hypertension, incorporating total cardiovascular risk in deciding which "prehypertensive" patients to treat. CVD, cardiovascular disease. CVD risk chart available at qrisk.org. (Reproduced, with permission, from Guidelines for management of hypertension: report of the Fourth Working Party of the British Hypertension Society, 2004-BHS IV. *J Hum Hypertens*. 2004 Mar;18(3):139–185.)

Table 19-5. Antihypertensive drugs: Diuretics (In descending order of preference).

Drugs	Proprietary Names	Initial Oral Doses	Dosage Range	Adverse Effects	Comments
Thiazides and related diuretics					
HCTZ	Esidrix, Microzide	12.5 or 25 mg once daily	12.5–50 mg once daily	$\downarrow$ K+, $\downarrow$ Mg^{2+}, $\uparrow$ Ca^{2+}, $\downarrow$ Na^{+}, $\uparrow$ uric acid, $\uparrow$ glucose, $\uparrow$ LDL cholesterol, $\uparrow$ triglycerides; rash, erectile dysfunction	Low dosages effective in many patients without associated metabolic abnormalities; metolazone more effective with concurrent kidney disease; indapamide does not alter serum lipid levels
Chlorthalidone	Thalitone	12.5 or 25 mg once daily	12.5–50 mg once daily		
Metolazone	Zaroxolyn	1.25 or 2.5 mg once daily	1.25–5 mg once daily		
Indapamide	Lozol	2.5 mg once daily	2.5–5 mg once daily		
Loop diuretics					
Furosemide	Lasix	20 mg twice daily	40–320 mg in 2 or 3 doses	Same as thiazides, but higher risk of excessive diuresis and electrolyte imbalance. Increases calcium excretion	Furosemide: Short duration of action a disadvantage; should be reserved for patients with kidney disease or fluid retention. Poor antihypertensive
Ethacrynic acid	Edecrin	50 mg once daily	50–100 mg once or twice daily		
Bumetanide	(generic)	0.25 mg twicedaily	0.5–10 mg in 2 or 3 doses		
Torsemide	Demadex	2.5 mg once daily	5–10 mg once daily		Torsemide: Effective blood pressure medication at low dosage
Aldosterone receptor blockers					
Spironolactone	Aldactone	12.5 or 25 mg once daily	12.5–100 mg once daily	Hyperkalemia, metabolic acidosis, gynecomastia	Can be useful add-on therapy in patients with refractory hypertension
Amiloride	(generic)	5 mg once daily	5–10 mg once daily		
Eplerenone	Inspra	25 mg once daily	25–100 mg once daily		
Combination products					
HCTZ and triamterene	Dyazide, Maxzide (25/37.5 mg)	1 tab once daily	1 or 2 tabs once daily	Same as thiazides plus GI disturbances, hyperkalemia rather than hypokalemia, headache; triamterene can cause kidney stones and kidney dysfunction; spironolactone causes gynecomastia. Hyperkalemia can occur if this combination is used in patients with advanced kidney disease or those taking ACE inhibitors	Use should be limited to patients with demonstrable need for a potassium-sparing agent
HCTZ and amiloride	(generic) (50/5 mg)	½ tab once daily	1 or 2 tabs once daily		
HCTZ and spironolactone	Aldactazide (25/25 mg)	1 tab (25/25 mg) once daily	1-4 tabs once daily		

ACE, angiotensin-converting enzyme; GI, gastrointestinal; LDL, low-density lipoprotein.

Table 19-6. Antihypertensive drugs: β-adrenergic blocking agents.

Drug	Proprietary Name	Initial Oral Dosage	Dosage Range	Special Properties					Comments[d]
				β$_1$ Selectivity[a]	ISA[b]	MSA[c]	Lipid Solubility	Renal vs Hepatic Elimination	
Acebutolol	Sectral	400 mg once daily	200–1200 mg in 1 or 2 doses	+	+	+	+	H > R	Positive ANA; rare LE syndrome; also indicated for arrhythmias. Doses > 800 mg have β$_1$ and β$_2$ effects
Atenolol	Tenormin	25 mg once daily	25–100 mg once daily	+	0	0	0	R	Also indicated for angina pectoris and post-MI. Doses > 100 mg have β$_1$ and β$_2$ effects
Atenolol/ chlorthalidone	Tenoretic	50 mg/25 mg once daily	50/25–100/25 mg once daily	+	0	0	0	R	
Betaxolol	Kerlone	10 mg once daily	10–40 mg once daily	+	0	0	+	H > R	
Bisoprolol	Zebeta	5 mg once daily	5–20 mg once daily	+	0	0	0	R = H	Bisoprolol also effective for heart failure

(continued)

Table 19-6. Antihypertensive drugs: β-adrenergic blocking agents. (continued)

Drug	Proprietary Name	Initial Oral Dosage	Dosage Range	β₁ Selectivity[a]	ISA[b]	MSA[c]	Lipid Solubility	Renal vs Hepatic Elimination	Comments[d]
Bisoprolol and HCT	Ziac	2.5 mg/6.25 mg once daily	2.5 mg/6.25 mg to 10 mg/25 mg once daily	+	0	0	0	R = H	Low-dose combination approved for initial therapy.
Carvedilol	Coreg Coreg CR	6.25 mg twice daily 20 mg ER once daily	12.5–50 mg in 2 doses 20–80 mg ER once daily	0	0	0	+++	H > R	α: β-blocking activity 1:9; may cause orthostatic symptoms; effective for heart failure. Nitric oxide potentiating vasodilatory activity
Labetalol	Trandate	100 mg twice daily	200–2400 mg in 2 doses	0	0/+	0	++	H	α: β-blocking activity 1:3; more orthostatic hypotension, fever, hepatotoxicity
Metoprolol	Lopressor	50 mg twice daily	50–200 mg twice daily	+	0	+	+++	H	Also indicated for angina pectoris and post-MI. Approved for heart failure. Doses > 100 mg have β₁ and β₂ effects
	Toprol - XL (SR preparation)	25 mg once daily	25–400 mg once daily						
Metoprolol and HCTZ	Lopressor HCT	50 mg/25 mg once daily	50 mg/25 mg to 200 mg/50 mg	+	0	+	+++	H	
Nadolol	Corgard	20 mg once daily	20–320 mg once daily	0	0	0	0	R	
Nadolol and bendroflumethiazide	Corzide	40 mg/5 mg once daily	40 mg/5 mg– 80 mg/ 5 mg once daily						
Nebivolol	Bystolic	5 mg once daily	40 mg once daily	+	0	0	++	H	Nitric oxide potentiating vasodilatory activity
Penbutolol	Levatol	20 mg once daily	20–80 mg once daily	0	+	0	++	R > H	
Pindolol	Visken	5 mg twice daily	10–60 mg in 2 doses	0	++	+	+	H > R	In adults, 35% renal clearance
Propranolol	Inderal Inderal LA InnoPran XL	20 mg twice daily 80 mg ER once daily 80 mg ER once nightly	40–640 mg in 2 doses 120–640 mg ER once daily 80–120 mg ER once nightly	0	0	++	+++	H	Also indicated for angina pectoris and post-MI
Propranolol and HCTZ	(Generic)	40 mg/25 mg twice daily	80 mg/25 mg twice daily	0	0	++	+++	H	
Timolol	Blocadren	5 mg twice daily	10–60 mg in 2 doses	0	0	0	++	H > R	Also indicated for post-MI. 80% hepatic clearance

ANA, antinuclear antibody; HCTZ, hydrochlorothiazide; ISA, intrinsic sympathomimetic activity; LE, lupus erythematosus; MI, myocardial infarction; MSA, membrane-stabilizing activity; SR, sustained release; 0, no effect; +, some effect; ++, moderate effect; +++, most effect.

[a]Agents with β₁ selectivity are less likely to precipitate bronchospasm and decreased peripheral blood flow in low doses, but selectivity is only relative.

[b]Agents with ISA cause less resting bradycardia and lipid changes.

[c]MSA generally occurs at concentrations greater than those necessary for β-adrenergic blockade. The clinical importance of MSA by β-blockers has not been defined.

[d]Adverse effects of all β-blockers: bronchospasm, fatigue, sleep disturbance and nightmares, bradycardia and atrioventricular block, worsening of heart failure, cold extremities, gastrointestinal disturbances, erectile dysfunction, triglycerides, ↓ HDL cholesterol, rare blood dyscrasias.

Table 19-7. Antihypertensive drugs: Renin and ACE inhibitors and angiotensin II receptor blockers.

Drug	Proprietary Name	Initial Oral Dosage	Dosage Range	Adverse Effects	Comments
Renin inhibitors					
Aliskiren	Tekturna	150 mg once daily	150–300 mg once daily	Angioedema, hypotension, hyperkalemia. Contraindicated in pregnancy	Probably metabolized by CYP3A4. Absorption is inhibited by high-fat meal
Aliskiren and HCTZ	Tekturna HCT	150 mg/12.5 mg once daily	150 mg/12.5 mg to 300 mg/25 mg once daily		
Aliskiren and amlodipine	Tekamlo	150 mg/5 mg once daily	150 mg/5 mg–300 mg/10 mg once daily		
ACE inhibitors					
Azilsartan	Edarbi	40 mg once daily	40–80 mg once daily	Cough, hypotension, dizziness, kidney dysfunction, hyperkalemia, angioedema; taste alteration and rash (may be more frequent with captopril); rarely, proteinuria, blood dyscrasia. Contraindicated in pregnancy	More fosinopril is excreted by the liver in patients with renal dysfunction (dose reduction may or may not be necessary). Captopril and lisinopril are active without metabolism. Captopril, enalapril, lisinopril, and quinapril are approved for heart failure
Benazepril	Lotensin	10 mg once daily	5–40 mg in 1 or 2 doses		
Benazepril and HCTZ	Lotensin HCT	5 mg/6.25 mg once daily	5 mg/6.25 mg to 20 mg/25 mg		
Benazepril and amlodipine	Lotrel	10 mg/2.5 mg once daily	10 mg/2.5 mg to 40 mg/10 mg		
Captopril	Capoten	25 mg twice daily	50–450 mg in 2 or 3 doses		
Captopril and HCTZ	Capozide	25 mg/15 mg twice daily	25 mg/15 mg to 50 mg/25 mg		
Enalapril	Vasotec	5 mg once daily	5–40 mg in 1 or 2 doses		
Enalapril and HCTZ	Vaseretic	5 mg/12.5 mg once daily	5 mg/12.5 mg to 10 mg/25 mg		
Fosinopril	Monopril	10 mg once daily	10–80 mg in 1 or 2 doses		
Fosinopril and HCTZ	Monopril HCT	10 mg/12.5 mg once daily	10 mg/12.5 mg to 20 mg/12.5 mg		
Lisinopril	Prinivil, Zestril	5–10 mg once daily	5–40 mg once daily		
Lisinopril and HCTZ	Prinzide or Zestoretic	10 mg/12.5 mg once daily	10 mg/12.5 mg to 20 mg/12.5 mg to 20 mg/25 mg		
Moexipril	Univasc	7.5 mg once daily	7.5–30 mg in 1 or 2 doses		
Moexipril and HCTZ	Uniretic	7.5 mg/12.5 mg once daily	7.5 mg/12.5 mg to 15 mg/25 mg		
Perindopril	Aceon	4 mg once daily	4–16 mg in 1 or 2 doses		
Perindopril and amlodipine	Coveram	4 mg/5 mg once daily	8 mg/10 mg once daily		
Quinapril	Accupril	10 mg once daily	10–80 mg in 1 or 2 doses		
Quinapril and HCTZ	Accuretic	10 mg/12.5 mg once daily	10 mg/12.5 mg to 20 mg/25 mg		
Ramipril	Altace	2.5 mg once daily	2.5–20 mg in 1 or 2 doses		
Trandolapril	Mavik	1 mg once daily	1–8 mg once daily		
Trandolapril and verapamil	Tarka	2 mg/180 mg ER once daily	2 mg/180 mg ER to 8 mg/480 mg ER		
Angiotensin II receptor blockers					
Azilsartan and HCTZ	Edarbychlor	40 mg/12.5 mg once daily	40 mg/12.5–40 mg/25 mg once daily	Hyperkalemia, kidney dysfunction, rare angioedema. Combinations have additional side effects. Contraindicated in pregnancy	Losartan has a very flat dose-response curve. Valsartan and irbesartan have wider dose-response ranges and longer durations of action. Addition of low-dose diuretic (separately or as combination pills) increases the response
Candesartan cilexitil	Atacand	16 mg once daily	8–32 mg once daily		
Candesartan cilexitil and HCTZ	Atacand HCT	16 mg/12.5 mg once daily	32 mg/12.5 mg once daily		
Eprosartan	Teveten	600 mg once daily	400–800 mg in 1–2 doses		
Eprosartan/HCTZ	Teveten HCT	600 mg/12.5 mg once daily	600 mg/12.5 mg to 600 mg/25 mg once daily		
Irbesartan	Avapro	150 mg once daily	150–300 mg once daily		
Irbesartan and HCTZ	Avalide	150 mg/12.5 mg once daily	150–300 mg irbesartan once daily		
Losartan	Cozaar	50 mg once daily	25–100 mg in 1 or 2 doses		
Losartan and HCTZ	Hyzaar	50 mg/12.5 mg once daily	50 mg/12.5 mg to 100 mg/25 mg tablets once daily		
Olmesartan	Benicar	20 mg once daily	20–40 mg once daily		
Olmesartan and HCTZ	Benicar HCT	20 mg/12.5 mg once daily	20 mg/12.5 mg to 40 mg/25 mg once daily		

(continued)

Table 19-7. Antihypertensive drugs: Renin and ACE inhibitors and angiotensin II receptor blockers. (continued)

Drug	Proprietary Name	Initial Oral Dosage	Dosage Range	Adverse Effects	Comments
Olmesartan and amlodipine	Azor	20 mg/5 mg once daily	20 mg/5 mg to 40 mg/10 mg	Hyperkalemia, kidney dysfunction, rare angioedema. Combinations have additional side effects. Contraindicated in pregnancy	Losartan has a very flat dose-response curve. Valsartan and irbesartan have wider dose-response ranges and longer durations of action. Addition of low-dose diuretic (separately or as combination pills) increases the response
Olmesartan and amlodipine and HCTZ	Tribenzor	20 mg/5 mg/12.5 mg once daily	20 mg/5 mg/12.5 mg to 40 mg/10 mg/25 mg once daily		
Telmisartan	Micardis	40 mg once daily	20–80 mg once daily		
Telmisartan and HCTZ	Micardis HCT	40 mg/12.5 mg once daily	40 mg/12.5 mg to 80 mg/25 mg once daily		
Telmisartan and amlodipine	Twynsta	40 mg/5 mg once daily	40 mg/5 mg to 80 mg/10 mg once daily		
Valsartan	Diovan	80 mg once daily	80–320 mg once daily		
Valsartan and HCTZ	Diovan HCT	80 mg/12.5 mg once daily	80–320 mg valsartan once daily		
Valsartan and amlodipine	Exforge	160 mg/5 mg once daily	160 mg/5 mg to 320 mg/10 mg once daily		
Other combination products					
Aliskiren and amlodipine and HCTZ	Amturnide	150 mg/5 mg/12.5 mg once daily	150 mg/5 mg/12.5 mg–300 mg/10 mg/25 mg once daily	Angioedema, hypotension, hyperkalemia. Contraindicated in pregnancy	
Aliskiren and valsartan	Valturna	150 mg/160 mg once daily	150 mg/160 mg to 300 mg/320 mg once daily		
Amlodipine and Valsartan and HCTZ	Exforge HCT	5 mg/160 mg/12.5 mg once daily	10 mg/320 mg/25 mg once daily		

ACE, angiotensin-converting enzyme; HCTZ, hydrochlorothiazide.

- Calcium channel blocking agents: Table 19-8
- α-Adrenergic blockers, vasodilators, centrally acting agents: Table 19-9

Therapeutic Procedures
- Table 19-10: Lifestyle modifications to manage hypertension
- Dietary changes (dietary approaches to stop hypertension [DASH] diet): high in fruits and vegetables, low fat, low salt (< 2 g of sodium per day)
- Weight reduction
- Alcohol restriction
- Salt reduction
- Adequate potassium intake
- Adequate calcium intake
- Increase physical activity
- Smoking cessation
- Aggressive risk factor management, including use of a statin, should be considered in all patients with hypertension
- Choice of antihypertensive medications is determined by the presence of compelling indications (see Table 19-11)
- Treatment strategies for persons with diabetics and hypertension and patients with chronic renal disease
  — Include ACE inhibitors or angiotensin receptor blockers as part of regimen
  — Some patients with high risk for stroke may benefit from a lower target BP of < 130/80 mm Hg
- In the absence of compelling indications, choice of antihypertensive regimen is guided by demographics and synergy (see Figure 19-3)

Table 19-8. Antihypertensive drugs: Calcium channel blocking agents.

Drug	Proprietary Name	Initial Oral Dosage	Dosage Range	Special Properties			Adverse Effects	Comments
				Peripheral Vasodilation	Cardiac Automaticity and Conduction	Contractility		
Nondihydropyridine agents								
Diltiazem	Cardizem LA Cardizem CD Cartia XT Dilacor XR Diltia CD Diltia XT Tiazac Taztia XT	90 mg twice daily 180 mg ER once daily 180 or 240 mg ER once daily 180 or 240 mg ER once daily 180 or 240 mg ER once daily 180 or 240 mg ER once daily 120 or 240 mg ER once daily 120 or 180 mg ER once daily	180—360 mg in 2 doses 180—360 mg ER once daily 180—480 mg ER once daily 180—540 mg ER once daily 180—480 mg ER once daily 180—540 mg ER once daily 120—540 mg ER once daily 120—540 mg ER once daily	++	↓↓	↓↓	Edema, headache, bradycardia, GI disturbances, dizziness, AV block, heart failure, urinary frequency	Also approved for angina
Verapamil	Calan Calan SR Verelan Verelan PM	80 mg three times daily 180 mg ER once daily 120 or 240 mg ER once daily 100 or 200 mg ER once daily	80—480 mg in 3 divided doses 180—480 mg ER in 1 or 2 doses 240—480 mg ER once daily 100—400 mg ER once daily	++	↓↓↓	↓↓↓	Same as diltiazem but more likely to cause constipation and heart failure	Also approved for angina and arrhythmias
Dihydropyridines								
Amlodipine	Norvasc	2.5 mg once daily	2.5—10 mg once daily	+++	↓/0	↓/0	Edema, dizziness, palpitations, flushing, headache, hypotension, tachycardia, GI disturbances, urinary frequency, worsening of heart failure (may be less common with felodipine, amlodipine) Myopathy, hepatotoxicity, edema with amlodipine and atorvastatin	Amlodipine, nicardipine, and nifedipine also approved for angina
Amlodipine and atorvastatin	Caduet	2.5 mg/10 mg once daily	10 mg /80 mg once daily	+++	↓/0	↓/0		
Felodipine	Plendil	5 mg ER once daily	5—10 mg ER once daily	+++	↓/0	↓/0		
Isradipine	DynaCirc	2.5 mg twice daily	2.5—5 mg twice daily	+++	↓/0	↓		
Nicardipine	Cardene Cardene SR	20 mg three times daily 30 mg twice daily	20—40 mg three times daily 30—60 mg twice daily	+++	↓/0	↓		
Nifedipine	Adalat CC Afeditab CR Nifediac CC Nifedical XL Procardia XL	30 mg ER once daily 30 mg ER once daily 30 mg ER once daily 30 mg ER once daily 30 or 60 mg ER once daily	30—120 mg once daily 30—90 mg ER once daily 30—90 ER mg once daily 30—120 mg ER once daily 30—120 mg ER once daily	+++	↓	↓↓		
Nisoldipine	Sular	17 mg once daily	17—34 mg daily	+++	↓/0	↓		

AV, atrioventricular; GI, gastrointestinal.

8. Outcomes

Follow-Up
- Frequent visits until BP is controlled
- Once controlled, visits can be infrequent, with limited follow-up laboratory tests
- Lipid monitoring every year
- ECG every 2 to 4 years, depending on initial ECG

Complications
- Stroke
- Dementia
- Myocardial infarction
- Heart failure

Table 19-9. α-Adrenoceptor blocking agents, sympatholytics, and vasodilators.

Drug	Proprietary Names	Initial Dosage	Dosage Range	Adverse Effects	Comments
α-Adrenoceptor blockers					
Doxazosin	Cardura Cardura XL	1 mg at bedtime 4 mg ER once daily	1–16 mg once daily 4–8 mg ER once daily	Syncope with first dose; postural hypotension, dizziness, palpitations, headache, weakness, drowsiness, sexual dysfunction, anticholinergic effects, urinary incontinence; first-dose effects may be less with doxazosin	May ↑ HDL and ↓ LDL cholesterol. May provide short-term relief of obstructive prostatic symptoms. Less effective in preventing cardiovascular events than diuretics
Prazosin	Minipress	1 mg at bedtime	2–20 mg in 2 or 3 doses		
Terazosin	Hytrin	1 mg at bedtime	1–20 mg in 1 or 2 doses		
Central sympatholytics					
Clonidine	Catapres Catapres TTS (transdermal patch) Nexiclon XR (suspension)	0.1 mg twice daily 0.1 mg/day patch weekly 0.17 mg ER once daily	0.2–0.6 mg in 2 doses 0.1–0.3 mg/day patch weekly 0.17–0.52 mg ER once daily	Sedation, dry mouth, sexual dysfunction, headache, bradyarrhythmias; side effects may be less with guanfacine. Contact dermatitis with clonidine patch. Methyldopa also causes hepatitis, hemolytic anemia, fever	"Rebound" hypertension may occur even after gradual withdrawal. A 0.09 mg /mL ER oral suspension is available. Its initial dose should be given at bedtime
Clonidine and chlorthalidone	Clorpres	0.1 mg/15 mg 1to 3 times daily	0.1 mg/15 mg to 0.3 mg/15 mg		
Guanabenz	Wytensin	4 mg twice daily	8–64 mg in 2 doses		
Guanfacine	Tenex	1 mg once daily	1–3 mg once daily		
Methyldopa	Aldochlor	250 mg twice daily	500–2000 mg in 2 doses		Methyldopa should be avoided in favor of safer agents
Peripheral neuronal antagonists					
Reserpine	(Generic)	0.05 mg once daily	0.05–0.25 mg once daily	Depression (less likely at low dosages, ie, < 0.25 mg), night terrors, nasal stuffiness, drowsiness, peptic disease, gastrointestinal disturbances, bradycardia	
Direct vasodilators					
Hydralazine	Apresoline	25 mg twice daily	50–300 mg in 2–4 doses	GI disturbances, tachycardia, headache, nasal congestion, rash, LE-like syndrome	May worsen or precipitate angina
Minoxidil	(Generic)	5 mg once daily	10–40 mg once daily	Tachycardia, fluid retention, headache, hirsutism, pericardial effusion, thrombocytopenia	Should be used in combination with β-blocker and diuretic

GI, gastrointestinal; LE, lupus erythematosus.

Table 19-10. Lifestyle modifications to manage hypertension.[a]

Modification	Recommendation	Approximate Systolic BP Reduction, Range
Weight reduction	Maintain normal body weight (BMI, 18.5–24.9)	5–20 mm Hg/10 kg weight loss
Adopt DASH eating plan	Consume a diet rich in fruits, vegetables, and low-fat dairy products with a reduced content of saturated fat and total fat	8–14 mm Hg
Dietary sodium reduction	Reduce dietary sodium intake to no more than 100 mEq/d (2.4 g sodium or 6 g sodium chloride)	2–8 mm Hg
Physical activity	Engage in regular aerobic physical activity such as brisk walking (at least 30 min/d, most days of the week)	4–9 mm Hg
Moderation of alcohol consumption	Limit consumption to no more than two drinks per day (1 oz or 30 mL ethanol [eg, 24 oz beer, 10 oz wine, or 3 oz 80-proof whiskey]) in most men and no more than one drink per day in women and lighter-weight persons	2–4 mm Hg

BMI, body mass index calculated as weight in kilograms divided by the square of height in meters; BP, blood pressure; DASH, Dietary Approaches to Stop Hypertension.

[a]For overall cardiovascular risk reduction, stop smoking. The effects of implementing these modifications are dose and time dependent and could be higher for some individuals.

Data from Chobanian AV et al. The Seventh Report of the Joint National Committee on Prevention, Detection, Evaluation, and Treatment of High Blood Pressure: the JNC 7 report. *JAMA.* 2003;289(19):2560–72.

Table 19-11. Clinical trial and guideline basis for compelling indications for individual drug classes.[a]

High-Risk Conditions with Compelling Indication[b]	Recommended Drugs						Clinical Trial Basis
	Diuretic	β-Blockers	ACE Inhibitors	ARB	CCB	Aldosterone Antagonist	
Heart failure	•	•	•	•		•	ACC/AHA Heart Failure Guideline, MERIT-HF, COPERNICUS, CIBIS, SOLVD, AIRE, TRACE, ValHEFT, RALES
Post-myocardial infarction		•	•			•	ACC/AHA Post-MI Guideline, BHAT, SAVE, Capricorn, EPHESUS
High coronary disease risk	•	•	•		•		ALLHAT, HOPE, ANBP2, LIFE, CONVINCE
Diabetes mellitus	•	•	•	•	•		NKF-ADA Guideline, UKPDS, ALLHAT
Chronic kidney disease			•	•			NKF Guideline, Captopril Trial, RENAAL, IDNT, REIN, AASK
Recurrent stroke prevention	•		•				PROGRESS

AASK, African American Study of Kidney Disease and Hypertension; ACC/AHA, American College of Cardiology/American Heart Association; ACE, angiotensin converting enzyme; AIRE, Acute Infarction Ramipril Efficacy; ALLHAT, Antihypertensive and Lipid-Lowering Treatment to Prevent Heart Attack Trial; ANBP2, Second Australian National Blood Pressure Study; ARB, angiotensin receptor blocker; BHAT, β-Blocker Heart Attack Trial; CCB, calcium channel blocker; CIBIS, Cardiac Insufficiency Bisoprolol Study; CONVINCE, Controlled Onset Verapamil Investigation of Cardiovascular End Points; COPERNICUS, Carvedilol Prospective Randomized Cumulative Survival Study; EPHESUS, Eplerenone Post-acute Myocardial Infarction Heart Failure Efficacy and Survival Study; HOPE, Heart Outcomes Prevention Evaluation Study; IDNT, Irbesartan Diabetic Nephropathy Trial; LIFE, Losartan Intervention For Endpoint Reduction in Hypertension Study; MERIT-HF, Metoprolol CR/XL Randomized Intervention Trial in Heart Failure; NKF-ADA, National Kidney Foundation–American Diabetes Association; PROGRESS, Perindopril Protection Against Recurrent Stroke Study; RALES, Randomized Aldactone Evaluation Study; REIN, Ramipril Efficacy in Nephropathy Study; RENAAL, Reduction of Endpoints in Noninsulin-Dependent Diabetes Mellitus with the Angiotensin II Antagonist Losartan Study; SAVE, Survival and Ventricular Enlargement Study; SOLVD, Studies of Left Ventricular Dysfunction; TRACE, Trandolapril Cardiac Evaluation Study; UKPDS, United Kingdom Prospective Diabetes Study; ValHEFT, Valsartan Heart Failure Trial.

[a]Compelling indications for antihypertensive drugs are based on benefits from outcome studies or existing clinical guidelines; the compelling indication is managed in parallel with the blood pressure.

[b]Conditions for which clinical trials demonstrate benefit of specific classes of antihypertensive drugs.

Data from Chobanian AV et al. The Seventh Report of the Joint National Committee on Prevention, Detection, Evaluation, and Treatment of High Blood Pressure: the JNC 7 report. *JAMA*. 2003;289(19):2560–72.

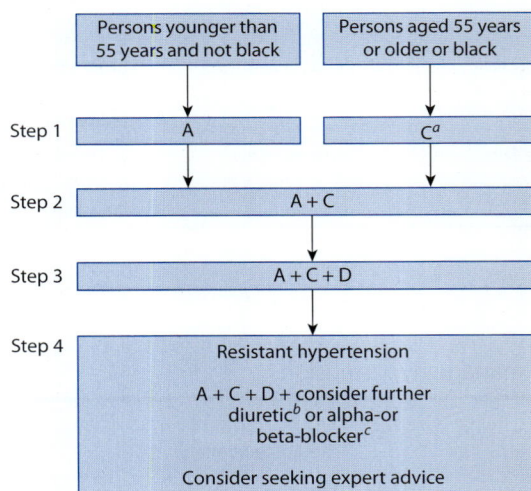

Figure 19-3. Hypertension treatment guidelines from the United Kingdom's National Institute for Health and Care Excellence. Guidelines identify angiotensin-converting enzyme (ACE) inhibitors, angiotensin receptor blockers (ARBs), or calcium channel blockers (CCB) as first-line medications and suggest a sequence of escalating drug therapy depending on blood pressure response. As noted, the choice of the initial agent is influenced by patient demographics. In Step 4, higher doses of thiazide-type diuretics may be used as long as serum potassium levels exceed 4.5 mmol/L. A, ACE inhibitor or ARB; C, calcium channel blocker; D, diuretic, thiazide-like. (Modified, with permission, from the 2013 hypertension guidelines published by the National Institute for Health and Care Excellence. https://www.nice.org.uk/guidance/cg127/evidence/cg127-hypertension-full-guideline3)

- Retinal vasculopathy
- Aortic dissection
- Kidney disease, including proteinuria and nephrosclerosis

9. When to Refer and When to Admit

When to Refer

- If BP remains uncontrolled after three concurrent medications
- If patient has uncontrolled BP and symptoms and signs of end-organ damage
- Younger patients with stage 1 or greater hypertension

When to Admit

- Consider hospitalization if the patient has very high BP and symptoms and signs of a hypertensive emergency, including
  — Severe headache
  — Neurologic symptoms
  — Chest pain
  — Altered mental status
  — Acutely worsening renal failure

SUGGESTED REFERENCES

Brook RD et al. American Heart Association Professional Education Committee of the Council for High Blood Pressure Research, Council on Cardiovascular and Stroke Nursing, Council on Epidemiology and Prevention, and Council on Nutrition, Physical Activity. Beyond medications and diet: alternative approaches to lowering blood pressure: a scientific statement from the American Heart Association. *Hypertension*. 2013 Jun;61(6):1360–1383. [PMID: 23608661]

Carter BL et al. Efficacy and safety of nighttime dosing of antihypertensives: review of the literature and design of a pragmatic clinical trial. *J Clin Hypertens (Greenwich)*. 2014 Feb;16(2):115–121. [PMID: 24373519]

Dasgupta K et al. The 2014 Canadian Hypertension Education Program recommendations for blood pressure measurement, diagnosis, assessment of risk, prevention, and treatment of hypertension. *Can J Cardiol*. 2014 May;30(5):485–501. [PMID: 24786438]

Howard G et al. Racial differences in the impact of elevated systolic blood pressure on stroke risk. *JAMA Intern Med*. 2013 Jan 14;173(1):46–51. [PMID: 23229778]

James PA et al. 2014 evidence-based guideline for the management of high blood pressure in adults: report from the panel members appointed to the Eighth Joint National Committee (JNC 8). *JAMA*. 2014 Feb 5;311(5):507–520. [PMID: 24352797]

Lipsitz LA. A 91-year-old woman with difficult-to-control hypertension: a clinical review. *JAMA*. 2013 Sep 25;310(12):1274–1280. [PMID: 24065014]

McCormack T et al. Management of hypertension in adults in primary care: NICE guideline. *Br J Gen Pract*. 2012 Mar;62(596):163–164. [PMID: 22429432]

Stern HR. The new hypertension guidelines. *J Clin Hypertens (Greenwich)*. 2013 Oct;15(10):748–751. [PMID: 24088284]

Textor SC. Secondary hypertension: renovascular hypertension. *J Am Soc Hypertens*. 2014 Dec;8(12):943–945. [PMID: 25492839]

20

Mitral Regurgitation

A 58-year-old man presents to the emergency department with 20 minutes of crushing substernal chest pain and marked shortness of breath. Physical examination shows inspiratory crackles over the lower three-fourth of both lung fields, basilar dullness to percussion, a hyperdynamic left ventricular (LV) impulse, brisk carotid upstroke, pansystolic murmur at the apex, which radiates into the axilla, and a S3 gallop. An electrocardiogram (ECG) shows ST-segment elevations in leads II, III, aVF. Chest radiograph shows Kerley B lines and bilateral pleural effusions, consistent with acute pulmonary edema. Doppler echocardiography shows severe mitral regurgitation and transesophageal echocardiography revealed a posterior mitral leaflet prolapsing into the left atrium (LA) and dyskinesis of basal lateral wall segment of the LV. The patient was diagnosed as having a posterolateral myocardial infarction with acute mitral regurgitation resulting from papillary muscle ischemia and rupture.

LEARNING OBJECTIVES

▶ Learn the clinical manifestations and objective findings of acute and chronic mitral regurgitation
▶ Understand the causes that predispose to mitral regurgitation
▶ Know the differential diagnosis of mitral regurgitation
▶ Learn the treatment for mitral regurgitation depending upon the cause

QUESTIONS

1. What are the salient features of this patient's problem?
2. How do you think through his problem?
3. What are the key features, including essentials of diagnosis and general considerations, of mitral regurgitation?
4. What are the symptoms and signs of mitral regurgitation?
5. What is the differential diagnosis of mitral regurgitation?
6. What are the laboratory, imaging, and procedural findings in mitral regurgitation?
7. What are the treatments for mitral regurgitation?

8. What is the outcome, including prognosis, of mitral regurgitation?

9. When should patients with mitral regurgitation be referred to a specialist?

ANSWERS

1. Salient Features

Crushing chest pain; shortness of breath; crackles and dullness to percussion with chest radiograph indicating acute pulmonary edema; hyperdynamic LV, brisk carotid upstroke, and S3 gallop; pansystolic murmur at apex radiating to the axilla; ECG with inferior ST elevations indicating myocardial infarction; echocardiography is diagnostic

2. How to Think Through

Given this patient's initial presentation, physical examination and ECG, how should the problem be framed? (ST-elevation myocardial infarction [MI] with clinical evidence of acute left heart failure.) What complications of acute MI can lead to acute heart failure? (LV myocardial dysfunction, rupture of the septum or LV free wall with tamponade, arrhythmia, and acute valvular dysfunction.) What examination findings suggest that acute mitral regurgitation is the cause of heart failure in this case? (The character of the murmur in the setting of inferior myocardial infarction on ECG.)

In the setting of acute MI, true rupture of the papillary muscles is much less common than papillary muscle dysfunction (due to ischemia) or displacement (due to LV dilation). With dysfunction or displacement causing mild to moderate mitral regurgitation, angiography and percutaneous revascularization are often the first steps, and the mitral regurgitation generally resolves with reperfusion. Echocardiography in this case, however, reveals posterior mitral leaflet prolapsing into the LA. (In papillary muscle rupture, sometimes the free ends of the muscle can be visualized as well.) What would be the optimum intervention to address the mitral regurgitation, as well as the wall motion abnormalities of the LV? (Emergent coronary artery bypass grafting with mitral valve repair; valve replacement may be necessary, though repair is preferred when possible.)

3. Key Features

Essentials of Diagnosis
- The cause of mitral regurgitation determines the clinical presentation
- May be asymptomatic for many years (or for life) or may cause left-sided heart failure
- Pansystolic murmur at the apex, radiating into the axilla; associated with an S3 gallop when regurgitant volume is great
- ECG shows LA abnormality or atrial fibrillation and left ventricular hypertrophy (LVH); chest radiograph shows LA and LV enlargement
- Echocardiographic findings are diagnostic and can help decide when to operate

General Considerations
- Mitral regurgitation results from
  — Ischemia at base or rupture of papillary muscle (myocardial ischemia or infarction or infection [endocarditis])
  — Displacement of papillary muscles (dilated cardiomyopathy)
  — Excessive length of chordae or myxomatous degeneration of leaflets (mitral valve prolapse)
  — Noncontraction of annulus (annular calcification)
  — Scarring (rheumatic fever, calcific invasion)
- Places a volume load on heart (increased preload), but reduces afterload, resulting in enlarged LV and initial increase in ejection fraction (EF)
- Over time, myocardial contractile function is reduced and EF drops
- Calculated regurgitant orifice areas ≤ 40 mm^2 by echocardiogram are considered severe

- For chronic primary mitral regurgitation, surgery is generally indicated for symptomatic patients or when the LV EF is < 60% or the echocardiographic LV end-systolic dimension is ≥ 40 mm
- In asymptomatic patients with severe mitral regurgitation without left ventricular dysfunction, surgery may be indicated if it is likely the mitral valve can be successfully repaired instead of replaced

4. Symptoms and Signs

- Pansystolic murmur at the apex, radiating into the axilla in most
- Patients with mitral valve prolapsed may have a murmur only after the mitral click
- The murmur may be difficult to hear in those patients with very severe mitral regurgitation, especially if it develops acutely
- Often associated with an S3
- Hyperdynamic LV impulse
- Brisk carotid upstroke
- May be asymptomatic for many years (or life)
- When regurgitation develops acutely, left atrial pressure rises abruptly, leading to pulmonary edema if severe
- When regurgitation progresses more slowly, exertional dyspnea and fatigue worsen gradually over many years
- Chronic LA and LV enlargement and may result in subsequent atrial fibrillation and LV dysfunction
- Systemic embolization occurs but is relatively unusual compared with other conditions causing atrial fibrillation

5. Differential Diagnosis

- Aortic stenosis
- Aortic sclerosis
- Tricuspid regurgitation
- Hypertrophic obstructive cardiomyopathy (HOCM)
- Atrial septal defect
- Ventricular septal defect

6. Laboratory, Imaging, and Procedural Findings

Laboratory Tests

- B-type natriuretic peptide (BNP) is useful in the early identification of LV dysfunction in the presence of mitral regurgitation
  — Asymptomatic patients with BNP values > 105 pg/mL are at higher risk for developing heart failure

Imaging

- Chest radiograph shows left atrial and ventricular enlargement
- Doppler echocardiography
  — Confirms the diagnosis, etiology and estimates severity by a variety of methods
  — Used for measuring LV function and LV end-systolic and diastolic sizes
  — Should be done at least yearly in patients with severe mitral regurgitation (stage C1) but preserved LV dimensions
- Transesophageal echocardiography
  — May reveal the cause and better identify candidates for valvular repair
  — Important in diagnosis of endocarditis
- Coronary angiography is often indicated to determine the presence of coronary artery disease before valve surgery in all men ≥ 40 years and in menopausal women with risk factors
- CT angiography may be sufficient to rule out coronary artery disease (CAD) in younger patients without symptoms of CAD

- Exercise hemodynamics with either Doppler echocardiography or cardiac catheterization may be useful when the symptoms do not fit the anatomic severity of mitral regurgitation
- Cardiac magnetic resonance imaging (MRI) may be useful if searching for specific causes of dilated cardiomyopathy such as amyloid or myocarditis, or if assessment of myocardial viability is needed prior to deciding if coronary artery bypass grafting should be added to mitral valve repair

Diagnostic Procedures
- ECG shows left atrial abnormality or atrial fibrillation and LV hypertrophy
- Coronary angiography is often indicated (especially after age 45) to determine the presence of CAD before valve surgery

7. Treatments

Medications
- Vasodilators may be used to stabilize acute mitral regurgitation while awaiting for surgery by decreasing the systemic vascular resistance and therefore reducing the amount of regurgitant flow
- Afterload reduction in chronic mitral regurgitation is controversial; β-blockade may be beneficial

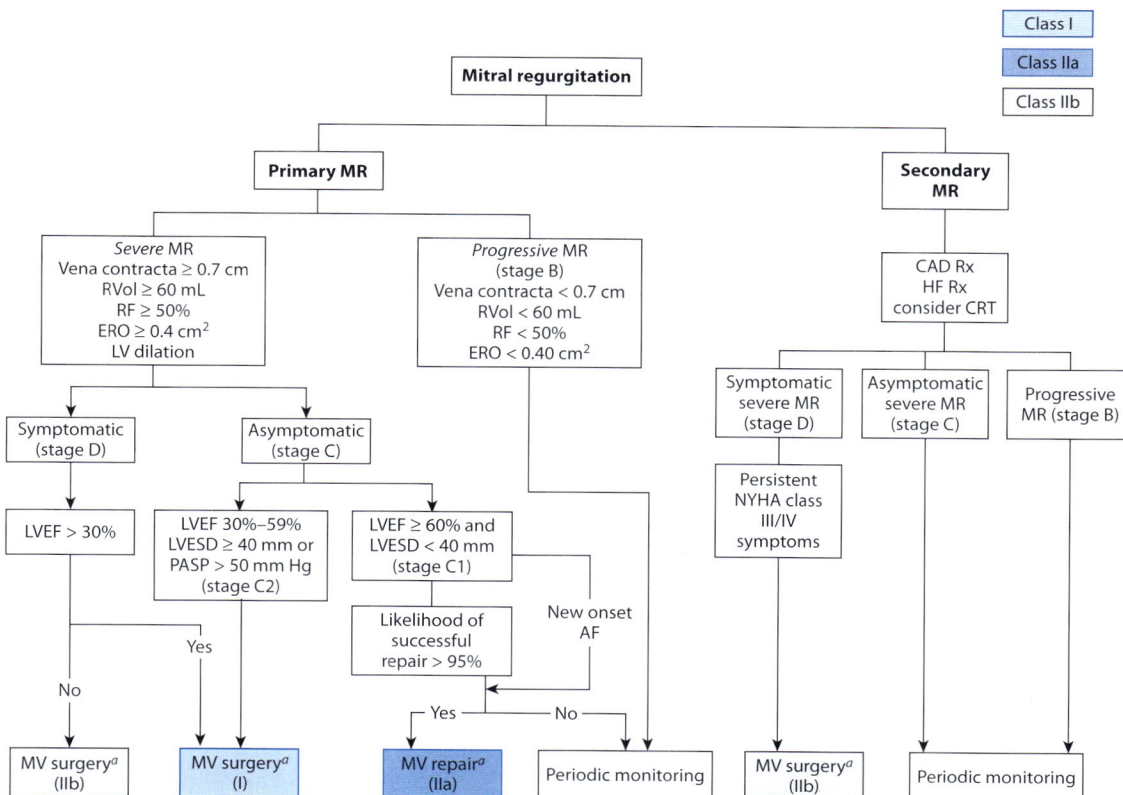

^{a}Mitral valve repair preferred over MVR when possible.
AF, atrial fibrillation; CAD, coronary artery disease; CRT, cardiac resynchronization therapy; ERO, effective regurgitant orifice; HF, heart failure; LV, left ventricular; LVEF, left ventricular ejection fraction; LVESD, left ventricular end-systolic dimension; MR, mitral regurgitation, MV, mitral valve; MVR, mitral valve replacement; NYHA, New York Heart association; PASP, pulmonary artery systolic pressure; RF, regurgitant fraction; R Vol, regurgitant volume; Rx, prescription.

Figure 20-1. The 2014 AHA/ACC guidelines for intervention in mitral regurgitation. (Reproduced with permission from Nishimura RA et al. *2014 AHA/ACC Guideline for the Management of Patients With Valvular Heart Disease: A Report of the American College of Cardiology/American Heart Association Task Force on Practice Guidelines. Circulation.* 2014 Jun 10;129(23):e521–e643. [PMID: 24589853]

Surgery

- Acute mitral regurgitation resulting from endocarditis, myocardial infarction, and ruptured chordae tendineae often requires emergent surgery
- Chronic mitral regurgitation usually requires surgery when symptoms develop or in asymptomatic patients when the LV end-systolic dimension is ≥ 40 mm or EF is < 60%
- Calculated regurgitant orifice areas ≤ 40 mm^2 by echocardiogram are considered severe
- Surgical valve repair
  — Preferred in mitral prolapse and in some with endocarditis
  — Essentially all patients who undergo valve repair also get mitral annular rings placed
  — Also used in patients with cardiomyopathy
- Mitral valve replacement uses mechanical or bioprosthetic valves
- See Figure 20-1.

Therapeutic Procedures

- Patients with cardiomyopathy may improve with cardiac resynchronization therapy from a biventricular pacemaker; guidelines recommend biventricular pacing prior to surgical repair in those patients with have functional MR due to cardiomyopathy.
- Percutaneous, cathetered based interventions for mitral valve repair and replacement have been developed and continue to be explored, including
  — Mitral clipping devices to create a double orifice valve and reduce regurgitation
  — Catheters to reduce the mitral annular area
  — Devices to reduce the septal-lateral ventricular size and consequently the mitral orifice size
  — Transcatheter stented valves for valve replacement
  — Percutaneous approaches tend to be reserved for patients in whom surgical risk is excessive or are otherwise not candidates for surgery

8. Outcome

Prognosis

- When mitral regurgitation is due to papillary muscle dysfunction, it may subside as the ischemia is treated, the infarction heals or the LV dilation diminishes

9. When to Refer

- All patients with more than mild mitral regurgitation should be referred to a cardiologist for an evaluation. Serial examinations and echocardiograms (usually yearly) should be obtained, and referral made if there is any increase in the LV end-systolic dimensions, a fall in the EF to < 60%, pulmonary hypertension, new atrial fibrillation, or any symptoms

SUGGESTED REFERENCES

Ahmed MI et al. A randomized controlled phase IIb trial of beta(1)-receptor blockade for chronic degenerative mitral regurgitation. *J Am Coll Cardiol.* 2012 Aug 28;60(9):833–838. [PMID: 22818065]

Mauri L et al; EVEREST II Investigators. 4-year results of a randomized controlled trial of percutaneous repair versus surgery for mitral regurgitation. *J Am Coll Cardiol.* 2013 Jul 23;62(4):317–328. [PMID: 23665364]

Nishimura RA et al. 2014 AHA/ACC guideline for the management of patients with valvular heart disease: executive summary: a report of the American College of Cardiology/American Heart Association Task Force on Practice Guidelines. *J Am Coll Cardiol.* 2014 Jun 10;63(22):2438–2488. Erratum in: J Am Coll Cardiol. 2014 Jun 10;63(22):2489. [PMID: 24603192]

Suri RM et al. Association between early surgical intervention vs watchful waiting and outcomes for mitral regurgitation due to flail mitral valve leaflets. *JAMA.* 2013 Aug 14;310(6):609–616. [PMID: 23942679]

Vahanian A et al; Joint Task Force on the Management of Valvular Heart Disease of the European Society of Cardiology (ESC); European Association for Cardio-Thoracic Surgery (EACTS). Guidelines on the management of valvular heart disease (version 2012). *Eur Heart J.* 2012 Oct;33(19):2451–2496. [PMID: 22922415]

Whitlow PL et al; EVEREST II Investigators. Acute and 12-month results with catheter-based mitral valve leaflet repair: The EVEREST II (Endovascular Valve Edge-to-Edge Repair) High Risk Study. *J Am Coll Cardiol.* 2012 Jan 10;59(2):130–139. [PMID: 22222076]

Mitral Stenosis

21

A 45-year-old woman presents with shortness of breath and irregular heartbeat. Over the past 2 weeks, she has become easily "winded" with minor activities. She has noted a fast heartbeat and, on occasion, a pounding sensation in her chest. She has a childhood history of being ill for several weeks after a severe sore throat. On physical examination, her pulse rate is noted to be 120 to 130 beats/min and her rhythm, irregularly irregular. She has distended jugular venous pulses and rales at the bases of both lung fields. On cardiac examination, in addition to the irregularly irregular rhythm, there is a soft low-pitched diastolic decrescendo murmur, heard best at the apex in the left lateral decubitus position. An electrocardiogram (ECG) shows atrial fibrillation as well as evidence of left atrial enlargement.

LEARNING OBJECTIVES

▶ Learn the clinical manifestations and objective findings of mitral stenosis depending on disease severity

▶ Understand the factors and patient history that predispose to mitral stenosis

▶ Know the differential diagnosis of mitral stenosis

▶ Learn the treatments for mitral stenosis and how to choose between different surgical options

▶ Know the mortality risk of valve replacement and valvuloplasty

QUESTIONS

1. What are the salient features of this patient's problem?

2. How do you think through her problem?

3. What are the key features, including essentials of diagnosis and general considerations, of mitral stenosis?

4. What are the symptoms and signs of mitral stenosis?

5. What is the differential diagnosis of mitral stenosis?

6. What are imaging and procedural findings in mitral stenosis?

7. What are the treatments for mitral stenosis?

8. What are the outcomes, including prevention and prognosis, of mitral stenosis?

9. When should patients with mitral stenosis be referred to a specialist?

ANSWERS

1. Salient Features

Dyspnea; palpitations and irregularly irregular heartbeat with atrial fibrillation on ECG; possible rheumatic fever as a child; tachycardia; jugular venous distension and pulmonary edema; diastolic decrescendo murmur at the apex in the left lateral decubitus position; left atrial enlargement

2. How to Think Through

Evaluation of palpitations becomes more pressing when it is associated with signs of hemodynamic compromise, such as light-headedness, syncope, or dyspnea. Based on the irregularly irregular pulse, atrial fibrillation is likely, and is confirmed on the ECG. Physical examination shows evidence of left heart failure, with pulmonary edema and jugular venous distention. What clinical scenarios might explain the subacute onset of heart failure in the setting of atrial fibrillation? (New onset atrial fibrillation alone may cause inefficient forward flow. New onset atrial fibrillation also occurs commonly in diastolic heart failure; with declining ejection fraction in systolic heart failure, leading to left atrial dilation and then to atrial fibrillation; and with mitral valve disease, especially mitral stenosis.) The diastolic murmur suggests mitral stenosis. A careful history may reveal a decrease in activity level over the past months, as the mitral stenosis progressed.

Given that the patient is symptomatic, should electrical or chemical cardioversion be performed immediately? (No. There is a high risk of systemic embolization in patients with symptoms of atrial fibrillation for > 48 hours, and patients with mitral stenosis have an even higher risk. We also do not yet know the etiology of her symptoms, which could be from atrial fibrillation, severe mitral stenosis, or a combination of factors.) How should she be managed? (Initially, rate control and diuresis are likely to improve her symptoms. Echocardiography can confirm and characterize the valve area and gradient. Anticoagulation with warfarin for stroke prevention in valvular atrial fibrillation is important. Cardiology and cardiac surgery consultations can help decide between percutaneous versus surgical repair.)

3. Key Features

Essentials of Diagnosis

- Exertional dyspnea, orthopnea, and paroxysmal nocturnal dyspnea when the stenosis becomes severe
- Symptoms often precipitated by onset of atrial fibrillation or pregnancy
- Prominent mitral first sound, opening snap (usually), and apical diastolic rumble
- ECG shows left atrium (LA) abnormality and, commonly, atrial fibrillation
- Echocardiography/Doppler is diagnostic
- Intervention indicated for symptoms or evidence of pulmonary hypertension. Most symptomatic patients have a valve area < 1.5 cm^2

General Considerations

- Underlying rheumatic heart disease in almost all patients (although history of rheumatic fever is often absent)
- May also occur due to congenital disease, calcification of the annulus invading the leaflets, or prosthetic valve annular ring mismatch

4. Symptoms and Signs

- An opening snap following A$_2$ due to stiff mitral valve
- Interval between opening snap and aortic closure sound is long when the left atrial pressure is low but shortens as left atrial pressure rises and approaches the aortic diastolic pressure
- Low-pitched diastolic decrescendo murmur, described as a rumble, at apex with the patient in left decubitus position, increased by brief exercise

- Mild to Moderate stenosis (valve area 1.5–1.0 cm^2): LA pressure and cardiac output may be essentially normal; patient may be asymptomatic or have dyspnea and fatigue with exertion, especially with tachycardia
- Severe stenosis (valve area < 1.0 cm^2): pulmonary hypertension, dyspnea, fatigue, right-sided heart failure, orthopnea, paroxysmal nocturnal dyspnea, and occasional hemoptysis
- Sudden increase in heart rate may precipitate pulmonary edema
- Paroxysmal or chronic atrial fibrillation develops in ~50% to 80%, may precipitate dyspnea or pulmonary edema
- May be accompanied by mitral regurgitation; if a regurgitant murmur is audible, valve replacement is usually required
- Mitral stenosis may be present for a lifetime with few symptoms, or it may become severe over a few years

5. Differential Diagnosis

- Mitral valve prolapse
- Atrial myxoma
- Cor triatriatum (congenital atrial anomaly)

6. Imaging and Procedural Findings

Imaging Studies

- Doppler echocardiography confirms diagnosis and quantifies severity by assigning 1 to 4 points to each of four observed parameters, with 1 being the least involvement and 4 the greatest
  — Mitral leaflet thickening
  — Mitral leaflet mobility
  — Submitral scarring
  — Commissural calcium

Diagnostic Procedures

- ECG typically shows left atrial abnormality and, often, atrial fibrillation
- Cardiac catheterization to detect valve, coronary, or myocardial disease, usually done only after a decision to intervene has been made

7. Treatments

Medications

- Control heart rate to allow for more diastolic filling of the left ventricle (LV)
- Once atrial fibrillation occurs, provide lifelong anticoagulation with warfarin, even if sinus rhythm is restored (newer oral anticoagulants are not yet approved for stroke prevention in valvular atrial fibrillation)

Surgery

- Intervention to relieve stenosis indicated for symptoms (eg, pulmonary edema, decline in exercise capacity) or evidence of pulmonary hypertension
- Surgical valve replacement is done in combined stenosis and regurgitation or when the mitral valve is significantly distorted and calcified
- Women of childbearing age with moderate to severe mitral stenosis should have the condition corrected prior to becoming pregnant if possible; third trimester surgery or balloon valvuloplasty is also possible
- See Figure 21-1.

Therapeutic Procedures

- Attempt conversion of atrial fibrillation with appropriate anticoagulation and imaging prior to procedure
- Percutaneous balloon valvuloplasty can be done when there is no significant mitral regurgitation

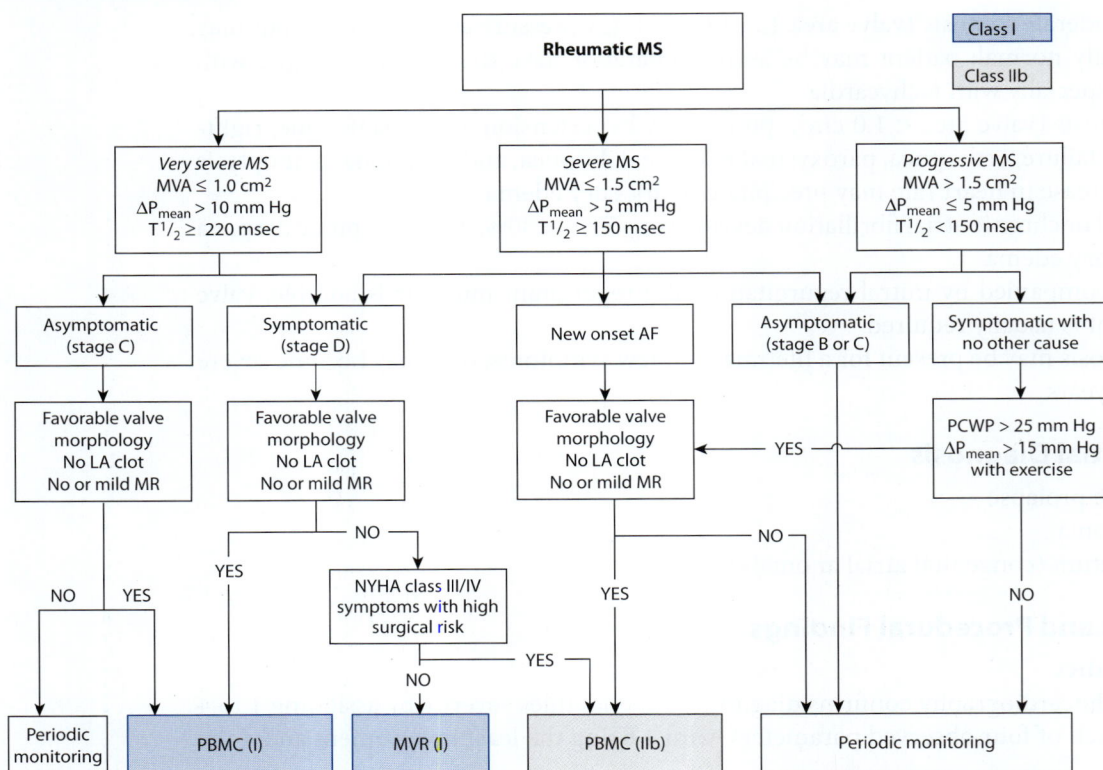

AF, atrial fibrillation; LA, left atrial; MR, mitral regurgitation; MS, mitral stenosis; MVA, mitral valve area; MVR, mitral valve replacement; NYHA, New York Heart Association; PBMC, percutaneous balloon mitral commissurotomy; PCWP, pulmonary capillary wedge pressure; ΔP_{mean}, mean pressure gradient; $T^1/_2$, half-life.

Figure 21–1. The 2014 AHA/ACC guidelines for intervention in mitral stenosis. (Reproduced, with permission, from Nishimura RA et al. 2014 AHA/ACC guideline for the management of patients with valvular heart disease: a report of the American College of Cardiology/American Heart Association Task Force on Practice Guidelines. *Circulation.* 2014 Jun 10;129(23):e521–e643. [PMID: 24589853])

8. Outcomes

Prevention
- Endocarditis prophylaxis is indicated for patients with prosthetic valves

Prognosis
- Percutaneous mitral valvuloplasty has a mortality rate of < 0.5% and a morbidity rate of 3% to 5%
- Operative mortality rate is ~1% to 3% for valve replacement

9. When to Refer

- Patients with mitral stenosis should be monitored with yearly examinations and echocardiograms, and should be ordered more frequently as the severity of obstruction increases
- All patients should initially be seen by a cardiologist, who can then decide how often the patient needs follow-up

SUGGESTED REFERENCES

Nishimura RA et al. 2014 AHA/ACC guideline for the management of patients with valvular heart disease: executive summary: a report of the American College of Cardiology/American Heart Association Task Force on Practice Guidelines. *J Am Coll Cardiol.* 2014 Jun 10;63(22):2438–2488. Erratum in: *J Am Coll Cardiol.* 2014 Jun 10;63(22):2489. [PMID: 24603192]

Vahanian A et al; Joint Task Force on the Management of Valvular Heart Disease of the European Society of Cardiology (ESC); European Association for Cardio-Thoracic Surgery (EACTS). Guidelines on the management of valvular heart disease (version 2012). *Eur Heart J.* 2012 Oct;33(19):2451–2496. [PMID: 22922415]

Shock

22

A young woman is brought to the emergency department by ambulance after a severe motor vehicle accident. She is unconscious. Her blood pressure is 64/40 mm Hg; heart rate is 150 beats/min. She has been intubated and is being hand-ventilated. There is no evidence of head trauma. The pupils are 2 mm and reactive. She withdraws to pain. Cardiac examination reveals no murmurs, gallops, or rubs. The lungs are clear to auscultation. The abdomen is tense, with decreased bowel sounds. The extremities are cool and clammy, with thready pulses.

LEARNING OBJECTIVES

► Learn the clinical manifestations and objective findings of shock
► Learn a classification for the different types of shock
► Understand the factors that predispose to each type of shock
► Learn the treatment for shock

QUESTIONS

1. What are the salient features of this patient's problem?
2. How do you think through her problem?
3. What are the key features, including essentials of diagnosis and general considerations, of shock?
4. What are the symptoms and signs of shock?
5. What are laboratory, imaging, and procedural findings in shock?
6. What are the treatments for shock?
7. What is the outcome, including prognosis, of shock?

ANSWERS

1. Salient Features

Trauma; tachycardia and hypotension; altered mental status; tense abdomen in the setting of trauma, suggesting internal bleeding; cool extremities suggesting high systemic vascular resistance (SVR); suspicion of hypovolemia due to blood loss

2. How to Think Through

Because of the urgency and confusion that accompany a presentation such as this, reliance on protocols is essential, and unequivocally improves outcomes. Begin with the ABCDE algorithm, with primary and secondary head-to-toe evaluation. In this case, the evaluation according to protocol reveals hypotension and evidence of poor perfusion—the definition of "shock"—and a rigid abdomen with no other obvious sources blood loss. What are the immediate management priorities? (Intravenous [IV] access with rapid fluid resuscitation, blood type and cross-match, central line and arterial line placement, initiation of pressor agents.) What are the immediate diagnostic priorities? (Electrocardiogram [ECG], chest X-ray, and abdominal imaging.) How might the tense abdomen explain the patient's blood pressure? (Blood loss in the peritoneal space with hypovolemia and compression of the IVC limiting venous return.) To avoid focusing on hypovolemic shock as the only etiology, what else might cause or contribute to shock in this patient? (Traumatic aortic dissection, cardiac tamponade, tension pneumothorax, other bleeding source, and underlying adrenal insufficiency.) What are the other major classes of shock? (Cardiogenic, obstructive, and distributive [septic, anaphylactic, and neurogenic].) What end-organ effects of poor perfusion can one evaluate and monitor during resuscitation? (Mental status; urine output; ECG evidence of cardiac ischemia and arrhythmia; peripheral perfusion with pulses, skin temperature, color, and capillary refill.)

3. Key Features

Essentials of Diagnosis
- Hypotension; tachycardia; oliguria; altered mental status; cool, clammy extremities
- Peripheral hypoperfusion and impaired oxygen delivery

General Considerations
- Can be classified as
  — Hypovolemic
  — Cardiogenic
  — Obstructive
  — Distributive, including septic, anaphylactic, neurogenic, and other
- Hypovolemic
  — Results from decreased intravascular volume secondary to loss of blood or fluids and electrolytes
  — A loss of > 15% in intravascular volume can result in hypotension and progressive tissue hypoxia
- Cardiogenic
  — Results from cardiac failure with the resultant inability of the heart to maintain adequate tissue perfusion
  — Clinical definition: evidence of tissue hypoxia due to decreased cardiac output (cardiac index < 2.2 L/min/m^2) in the presence of adequate intravascular volume
  — Most often caused by myocardial infarction but can also be due to cardiomyopathy, myocardial contusion, valvular incompetence or stenosis, or arrhythmias
- Obstructive
  — Results from acute decrease in cardiac output due to cardiac tamponade, tension pneumothorax, or massive pulmonary embolism
- Distributive
  — Causes include sepsis (most common), systemic inflammatory response syndrome produced by severe pancreatitis or burns, anaphylaxis, trauma, or ischemia
  — Reduction in SVR results in inadequate cardiac output and tissue hypoperfusion despite normal circulatory volume.
  — Septic shock
    ○ Gram-positive or gram-negative organisms most common cause, with a growing incidence of multidrug-resistant organisms

  ○ Polymicrobial infections are almost as likely
  ○ Incidence of sepsis caused by fungal organisms is increasing, but remains less than that for bacterial infections
— Anaphylactic is caused by an immunoglobulin-E-mediated allergic response.
— Neurogenic is typically caused by spinal cord injury or epidural or spinal anesthetic agents, but pain, gastric dilation, or fright may induce reflex vagal parasympathetic stimulation, which results in hypotension, bradycardia, and syncope
— Adrenal insufficiency can result in acute adrenal crisis

4. Symptoms and Signs

- Hypotension
- Weak or thready peripheral pulses
- Cold or mottled extremities
- Splanchnic vasoconstriction may lead to oliguria, bowel ischemia, and hepatic dysfunction
- Mentation may be normal or altered (eg, restlessness, agitation, confusion, lethargy, or coma)
- Hypovolemic
  — Jugular venous pressure is low
  — Narrow pulse pressure indicative of reduced stroke volume
- Cardiogenic
  — Jugular venous pressure is elevated
  — Global hypoperfusion with oliguria
  — Altered mental status
  — Cool extremities
  — May be evidence of pulmonary edema in the setting of left-sided heart failure and evidence of ECG changes
- Obstructive
  — Central venous pressure (CVP) may be elevated
- Distributive
  — Hyperdynamic heart sounds
  — Warm extremities
  — Wide pulse pressure indicative of large stroke volume
  — Septic
    ○ Evidence of infection in the setting of persistent hypotension
    ○ Evidence of organ hypoperfusion, such as in lactic acidosis, decreased urinary output, or altered mental status despite adequate volume resuscitation
  — Anaphylactic
    ○ Evidence of allergen exposure
  — Neurogenic
    ○ Evidence of central nervous system (CNS) injury and persistent hypotension despite adequate volume resuscitation

5. Laboratory, Imaging, and Procedural Findings

Laboratory Tests

- Complete blood count
- Serum electrolytes
- Serum glucose
- Serum lactate levels
- Coagulation parameters
- Type and cross-match
- Arterial blood gas determinations
- Blood cultures

Imaging Studies
- Chest radiograph
- Transesophageal echocardiography shows
  - Reduced left ventricular filling in hypovolemic and obstructive shock
  - Enlarged left ventricle in cardiogenic shock

Diagnostic Procedures
- ECG
- Arterial line should be placed for blood pressure and arterial oxygen monitoring
- Foley catheter should be inserted to monitor urinary output
- Pulmonary artery catheter
  - Can distinguish cardiogenic from septic shock
  - Can monitor effects of volume resuscitation or pressor medications
- CVP
  - < 5 mm Hg suggests hypovolemia
  - > 18 mm Hg suggests volume overload, cardiac failure, tamponade, or pulmonary hypertension
- Cardiac index
  - < 2 L/min/m^2 indicates need for inotropic or ventricular support
  - 4 L/min/m^2 in a hypotensive patient is consistent with early septic shock
- SVR
  - Low (< 800 dynes $\times$ s/cm^{-5}) in septic and neurogenic shock
  - High (> 1500 dynes $\times$ s/cm^{-5}) in hypovolemic and cardiogenic shock

6. Treatments

Volume Replacement
- Critical in initial management of shock
- Hemorrhagic shock
  - Rapid infusions of type-specific or type O negative packed red blood cells (PRBC) or whole blood, which also provides extra volume and clotting factors
  - Each unit of PRBC or whole blood is expected to raise the hematocrit by 3%
- Hypovolemic shock secondary to dehydration: rapid boluses of isotonic crystalloid, usually in 1 L increments
- Cardiogenic shock in absence of fluid overload: requires smaller fluid challenges usually in increments of 250 mL
- Septic shock
  - Usually requires large volumes of fluid for resuscitation
  - Use of unwarmed fluids can produce hypothermia, which can lead to hypothermia-induced coagulopathy; warming fluids before administration can avoid this complication
  - Early goal-directed therapy uses a set protocol for the treatment of septic shock by adjusting the use of fluids, vasopressors, inotropes, and blood transfusions to meet hemodynamic targets (MAP > 65 mmHg, CVP 8–12mm Hg, ScvO$_2$ > 70%,) and provides a significant mortality benefit

Medications
- Norepinephrine
  - Generally used for vasodilatory shock
  - Initial dosage: 1 to 2 μg/min as an intravenous infusion, titrated to maintain the mean arterial blood pressure of at least 65 mm Hg
  - Usual maintenance dosage: 2 to 4 μg/min (maximum dose is 30 μg/min)
  - Patients with refractory shock may require dosages of 10 to 30 μg/min
- Epinephrine
  - Treatment of choice in anaphylactic shock
  - Initial dosage: 0.1 to 0.5 mg of 1:1000 solution subcutaneously or intramuscularly every 5 to 15 minutes as needed or 0.1 to 0.25 mg of 1:10 000 solution intravenously every 5 to 15 minutes as needed

— Maximum dosage: 1 mg/dose
— May be used in severe shock and during acute resuscitation
— Initial dosage: 1 μg/min as a continuous intravenous infusion
— Usual dosage: 2 to 10 μg/min intravenously
• Dopamine
— Low doses (2–5 μg/kg/min) stimulate dopaminergic and β-agonist receptors, producing increased glomerular filtration, heart rate, and contractility
— With higher doses (> 10 μg/kg/min), α-adrenergic effects predominate, resulting in peripheral vasoconstriction
— Maximum dose is typically 50 μg/kg/min
— Should only be used as an alternative to norepinephrine in select patients with septic shock, including those with significant bradycardia or low potential for tachyarrhythmias
• Phenylephrine can be used as a first-line agent for hyperdynamic septic shock when
— There is low systemic venous resistance but high cardiac output, which can manifest as hypotension with warm extremities
— Dysrhythmias or tachycardias prevent the use of agents with β-adrenergic activity
• Vasopressin
— Used as an adjunctive therapy to catecholamine vasopressors in the treatment of distributive or vasodilatory shock
— Used as a second-line agent in refractory septic or anaphylactic shock
— Role as an initial vasopressor warrants further study
• Dobutamine
— Increases contractility and decreases afterload
— Used for patients with low cardiac output and high pulmonary capillary wedge pressure (PCWP) but who do not have hypotension
— Can be added to a vasopressor if
  ◦ There is reduced myocardial function (decreased cardiac output and elevated PCWP)
  ◦ Signs of hypoperfusion are present despite adequate volume resuscitation and an adequate mean arterial pressure
— Initial dose: 0.1–0.5 μg/kg/min as a continuous intravenous infusion, which can be titrated every few minutes as needed to achieve a hemodynamic effect; usual dosage range is 2–20 μg/kg/min intravenously
— Tachyphylaxis can occur after 48 hours from the downregulation of β-adrenergic receptors
• Amrinone or milrinone
— Can be substituted for dobutamine
— Increase cyclic AMP levels and increase cardiac contractility, bypassing the β-adrenergic receptor
— Vasodilation is a side effect of both
• Low-dose corticosteroids
— The Corticosteroid Therapy of Septic Shock (CORTICUS) study demonstrated that low-dose hydrocortisone (50 mg intravenously every 6 hours for 5 days and then tapered over 6 days) did not improve survival in patients with septic shock, either overall or in patients who had relative adrenal insufficiency
— Meta-analyses of multiple smaller trials of corticosteroids in patients with septic shock demonstrated that when shock was poorly responsive to fluid resuscitation and vasopressors, low-dose hydrocortisone (300 mg/d or less in divided doses) increased the mean arterial pressure but did not show a mortality benefit
• Activated protein C (drotrecogin alpha) was proven ineffective in decreasing mortality sepsis and has been withdrawn from the market
• Broad-spectrum antibiotics are administered in septic shock
• Sodium bicarbonate may be given for severed acidosis to patients with sepsis of any etiology and to those with lactic acidosis

Surgery

- Transcutaneous or transvenous pacing or placement of an intra-arterial balloon pump for cardiogenic shock
- Emergent revascularization by percutaneous angioplasty or coronary artery bypass surgery appears to improve long-term outcome

Therapeutic Procedures

- IV access and fluid resuscitation should be instituted along with cardiac monitoring and assessment of hemodynamic parameters such as blood pressure and heart rate
- Treatment is directed at maintaining a
  — CVP of 8 to 12 mm Hg
  — Mean arterial pressure of 65 to 90 mm Hg
  — Cardiac index of 2 to 4 L/min/m²
  — Central venous oxygen saturation > 70%
- Pulmonary artery catheter is most useful in managing cardiogenic shock
- Central venous catheter may be adequate in other types of shock
- In obstructive shock, pericardiocentesis or pericardial window, chest tube placement, or catheter-directed thrombolytic therapy can be lifesaving
- Urgent hemodialysis or continuous venovenous hemofiltration may be indicated for maintenance of fluid and electrolyte balance during acute kidney injury resulting from shock
- Lactate clearance of > 10% can be used as a potential substitute for central venous oxygen saturation ($ScvO_2$) criteria if $ScvO_2$ monitoring is not available

7. Outcome

Prognosis

- Septic shock mortality is 20% to 50%

SUGGESTED REFERENCES

Annane D et al; COIITSS Study Investigators. Corticosteroid treatment and intensive insulin therapy for septic shock in adults: a randomized controlled trial. *JAMA*. 2010 Jan 27;303(4):341–348. [PMID: 20103758]

Asfar P et al; SEPSISPAM Investigators. High versus low blood-pressure target in patients with septic shock. *N Engl J Med*. 2014 Apr 24;370(17):1583–1593. [PMID: 24635770]

Caironi P et al; ALBIOS Study Investigators. Albumin replacement in patients with severe sepsis or septic shock. *N Engl J Med*. 2014 Apr 10;370(15):1412–1421. [PMID: 24635772]

De Backer D et al; SOAP II Investigators. Comparison of dopamine and norepinephrine in the treatment of shock. *N Engl J Med*. 2010 Mar 4;362(9):779–789. [PMID: 20200382]

Dellinger RP et al; Surviving Sepsis Campaign Guidelines Committee including the Pediatric Subgroup. Surviving Sepsis Campaign: international guidelines for management of severe sepsis and septic shock: 2012. *Crit Care Med*. 2013 Feb;41(2):580–637. [PMID: 23353941]

Patel GP et al. Efficacy and safety of dopamine versus norepinephrine in the management of septic shock. *Shock*. 2010 Apr;33(4):375–380. [PMID: 19851126]

Patel GP et al. Systemic steroids in severe sepsis and septic shock. *Am J Respir Crit Care Med*. 2012 Jan 15;185(2):133–139. [PMID: 21680949]

Peake SL et al; ARISE Investigators; ANZICS Clinical Trials Group. Goal-directed resuscitation for patients with early septic shock. *N Engl J Med*. 2014 Oct 16;371(16):1496–1506. [PMID: 25272316]

Prondzinsky R et al. Intra-aortic balloon counterpulsation in patients with acute myocardial infarction complicated by cardiogenic shock: the prospective, randomized IABP SHOCK Trial for attenuation of multiorgan dysfunction syndrome. *Crit Care Med*. 2010 Jan;38(1):152–160. [PMID: 19770739]

Rivers E et al. Early goal-directed therapy in the treatment of severe sepsis and septic shock. *N Engl J Med*. 2001 Nov;345(19):1368–1377. [PMID: 11794169]

Russell JA et al; VASST Investigators. Vasopressin versus norepinephrine infusion in patients with septic shock. *N Engl J Med*. 2008 Feb 28;358(9):877–887. [PMID: 18305265]

Sprung CL et al. Hydrocortisone therapy for patients with septic shock. *N Engl J Med*. 2008 Jan;358(2):111–124. [PMID: 18184957]

Thiele H et al; IABP-SHOCK II Trial Investigators. Intraaortic balloon support for myocardial infarction with cardiogenic shock. *N Engl J Med*. 2012 Oct 4;367(14):1287–1296. [PMID: 22920912]

Yealy DM et al; ProCESS Investigators. A randomized trial of protocol-based care for early septic shock. N Engl J Med. 2014 May 1;370(18):1683–1693. [PMID: 24635773]

Hematologic Disorders

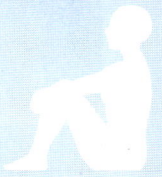

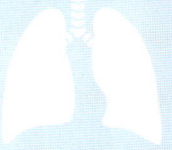

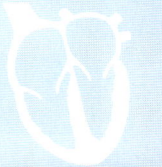

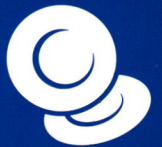

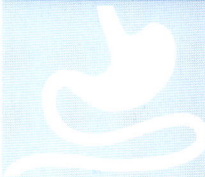

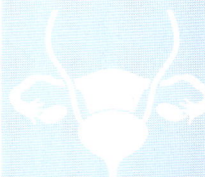

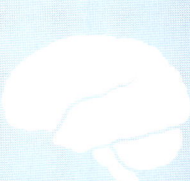

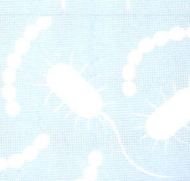

23

Hypercoagulable States

A 23-year-old woman presents to the emergency department with a chief complaint of acute onset of shortness of breath. It is associated with right-sided chest pain, which increases with inspiration. She denies fever, chills, cough, or other respiratory symptoms. She has had no lower extremity swelling. She has not been ill, bedridden, or immobile for prolonged periods. Her medical history is notable for an episode about 2 years ago of deep venous thrombosis (DVT) in the right lower extremity while taking oral contraceptives. She has been otherwise healthy and is currently taking no medications. The family history is notable for a father who died of a pulmonary embolus (PE). On physical examination she appears anxious and in mild respiratory distress. She is tachycardiac to 110 bpm, with a respiratory rate of 20/min. She has no fever, and her blood pressure is stable. The remainder of the physical examination is normal. Chest x-ray film is normal. Ventilation–perfusion (V–Q) scan reveals a high probability of PE. Given her history of DVT, a hypercoagulable state is suspected.

LEARNING OBJECTIVES

▶ Learn the clinical manifestations and objective findings that may suggest a hypercoagulable state

▶ Understand the different types of hypercoagulable states and the factors that predispose to them

▶ Know the differential diagnosis of a patient who has a hypercoagulable state

▶ Understand how to diagnose hypercoagulable states, including presence of a lupus anti-coagulant

▶ Learn the treatment for hypercoagulable states with single and recurrent thrombosis

QUESTIONS

1. What are the salient features of this patient's problem?

2. How do you think through her problem?

3. What are the key features, including essentials of diagnosis and general considerations, of hypercoagulable states?

4. What are the symptoms and signs of hypercoagulable states?

5. What is the differential diagnosis of hypercoagulable states?

6. What are laboratory and imaging findings in hypercoagulable states?

7. What are the treatments for hypercoagulable states?

8. What are the outcomes, including complications and prevention, of hypercoagulable states?

9. When should patients with hypercoagulable states be referred to a specialist or admitted to the hospital?

ANSWERS

1. Salient Features

Young woman; acute onset shortness of breath; pleuritic chest pain; personal and family history of DVT; tachycardia; respiratory distress; normal chest x-ray; PE on V–Q scan

2. How to Think Through

When a patient presents with acute chest pain or dyspnea, the likelihood of PE is framed in terms of pretest probability. In this case, the pleuritic quality of the chest pain, tachycardia, absence of another likely cause of her symptoms, and history of prior DVT, confer a high pretest probability of PE. She should be treated with heparin immediately, even before confirmation with computed tomography (CT)-angiography or V–Q scan.

When a removable risk factor for DVT or PE is identified, an evaluation for inherited causes of thrombophilia is often not performed, and anticoagulation is short term. What are examples of major, removable risk factors? (Immobility, cancer, recent surgery, or injury to a blood vessel wall.) In this case, the patient's prior DVT was likely considered to be provoked, given her use of an oral contraceptive. The history of PE in her father, however, suggests an inherited cause, and a complete evaluation at that point would have been appropriate. What are some components of a thrombophilia evaluation? (Prothrombin time [PT]; activated partial thromboplastin time [aPTT]; activated protein C resistance; and antithrombin [AT], protein C, and protein S levels; testing for lupus anticoagulant.) With a second episode that was unprovoked, together with her family history, lifelong anticoagulation is indicated, regardless of the results of a thrombophilia evaluation. The evaluation is important for other reasons, including fertility implications and guidance for her family members.

3. Key Features

Essentials of Diagnosis

- Recurrent thrombosis, often in the venous (eg, deep veins of the legs) or sometimes in the arterial circulation
- Personal or family history of clotting, presence of systemic disease, or no provoking factor associated with thrombosis are clues to a hypercoagulable state
- Pregnancy complications, specifically pregnancy losses after the first trimester, with the antiphospholipid syndrome
- Prolonged clotting times in some diseases

General Considerations

- Hypercoagulable states may be inherited or acquired
- Inherited causes
  — Activated protein C resistance (Factor V Leiden)
  — Protein C deficiency
  — Protein S deficiency
  — AT deficiency
  — Hyperprothrombinemia (prothrombin 20212AG mutation)
  — Hyperhomocysteinemia

— Dysfibrogenemia

— Abnormal plasminogen

- Activated protein C resistance (Factor V Leiden) is the most common inherited hypercoagulable state; the trait is found in ~3% of American men and in 20% to 40% of patients with unprovoked venous thrombosis. Activated protein C-resistant patients who are heterozygote have a fivefold increased thrombosis risk; homozygotes have a 30-fold increased risk

- Protein C deficiency is common; up to 1 of every 200 individuals in the population in a heterozygote; type I deficiency refers to individuals with decreased levels of protein C; type II deficiency denotes cases with normal protein C levels but low protein C activity

- Protein S deficiency is an uncommon and also heterogeneous disorder; type I deficiency refers to cases with low free and total protein S levels, type II deficiency (least common) refers to an abnormally functioning protein S; type III deficiency refers to only low levels of free protein S

- Homozygous protein C or protein S deficiencies are the most severe, causing thrombosis early in life that is often fatal

- Antithrombin (AT) deficiency is less common (about 1 in 2000 cases in the general population have one of the more than 100 mutations reported) but it causes a 10-fold increased risk of thrombosis; type I defects involve a parallel decrease in antigen and activity, type II defects involve a dysfunctional molecule that has normal or near-normal antigen levels but decreased activity

- Hyperprothrombinemia is due to a mutation in the 20210AG region of the prothrombin gene associated with elevated plasma prothrombin (factor II) levels; it is probably the second most common hereditary hypercoagulable state. Affected individuals are usually heterozygotes and have a threefold higher risk of thrombosis

- Acquired causes and risk factors

  — Immobility: bedrest (especially postoperative), stroke, obesity

  — Cancer

  — Inflammatory disorders, eg, ulcerative colitis

  — Myeloproliferative disorder, eg, polycythemia vera causing hyperviscosity or essential thrombocytosis

  — Estrogens (oral contraceptives, hormone replacement)

  — Pregnancy (increased central venous pressures)

  — Heparin-induced thrombocytopenia

  — Lupus anticoagulant

  — Nephrotic syndrome

  — Paroxysmal nocturnal hemoglobinuria

  — Heart failure, low cardiac output

  — Acute illness with disseminated intravascular coagulation (DIC)

- Lupus anticoagulants, one of the range of antiphospholipid antibodies, prolong clotting times by binding phospholipid associated proteins, which are necessary components of coagulation reactions

- Lupus anticoagulants were named because of their increased prevalence among patients with connective tissue disease; however, they may occur in individuals with underlying infection, inflammation, or malignancy, or in asymptomatic patients

- Primary antiphospholipid syndrome (APS) is diagnosed in patients who have

  — Venous or arterial occlusions

  — Recurrent fetal loss

  — Thrombocytopenia in the presence of persistent antiphospholipid antibodies but not other features of systemic lupus erythematosus (SLE)

- Catastrophic APS

  — Occurs in < 1% of patients with antiphospholipid antibodies

  — Leads to diffuse thromboses, thrombotic microangiopathy, and multiorgan system failure

- Patients with nephrotic syndrome, particularly those with membranous nephropathy, have urinary losses of AT, protein C, and protein S, along with increased platelet activation, and are thus prone to renal vein thrombosis, PE, and DVT
- Patients with a thrombosis and history of recurrent thrombosis; serious thrombosis; family history of thrombosis; or young patients without risk factors should be evaluated for hypercoagulable states
- Similarly, patients without thrombosis (DVT or PE) who have systemic lupus erythematosus, recurrent spontaneous abortions, or a relative with an inherited hypercoagulable state should be evaluated for hypercoagulable states

4. Symptoms and Signs

- May present with DVT—pain, swelling, redness of the limb with normal pulses, extremity perfusion
- May present with pulmonary emboli (PE) with or without obvious DVT—acute onset shortness of breath, hypoxemia, tachycardia, and chest pain
- In addition to DVT and PE, thrombotic events may occur in either the arterial or venous circulations and include
  — Cerebrovascular accidents
  — Budd–Chiari syndrome
  — Cerebral sinus vein thrombosis
  — Myocardial infarction
  — Digital infarction
- With lupus anticoagulants, increased risk of thrombosis but despite the name, no increased bleeding
- Antiphospholipid syndrome (APS) is often asymptomatic until a thrombotic event or a pregnancy loss occurs
- Other symptoms and signs often attributed to the APS include
  — Mental status changes
  — Livedo reticularis
  — Skin ulcers
  — Microangiopathic nephropathy
  — Cardiac valvular dysfunction—typically mitral regurgitation—due to Libman–Sacks endocarditis
- Pregnancy losses associated with APS include
  — Three or more unexplained consecutive spontaneous abortions prior to 10 weeks' gestation
  — One or more unexplained deaths of a morphologically normal fetus after 10 weeks gestation
  — Preterm delivery at less than 34 weeks' gestation due to preeclampsia or placental insufficiency

5. Differential Diagnosis

- Acquired causes of hypercoagulability
  — Immobility: bedrest (especially postoperative), stroke, obesity
  — Cancer
  — Inflammatory disorders, eg, ulcerative colitis
  — Myeloproliferative disorder, eg, polycythemia vera causing hyperviscosity or essential thrombocytosis
  — Estrogens (oral contraceptives, hormone replacement)
  — Pregnancy (increased central venous pressures)
  — Heparin-induced thrombocytopenia
  — Lupus anticoagulant
  — Nephrotic syndrome

— Paroxysmal nocturnal hemoglobinuria
— Disseminated intravascular coagulation
— Heart failure, low cardiac output
- Inherited causes of hypercoagulability
  — Activated protein C resistance (Factor V Leiden)
  — Protein C deficiency
  — Protein S deficiency
  — AT deficiency
  — Hyperprothrombinemia (prothrombin 20210AG mutation)
  — Hyperhomocysteinemia
  — Dysfibrogenemia
  — Abnormal plasminogen
- Catastrophic APS has a broad differential diagnosis, including
  — Sepsis
  — Pulmonary-renal syndromes
  — Systemic vasculitis
  — Disseminated intravascular coagulation
  — Thrombotic thrombocytopenic purpura
- DVT: cellulitis, trauma, superficial thrombophlebitis, venous insufficiency
- PE: MI, pneumothorax, thoracic aneurysmal rupture, pneumonia, pleuritic infection or inflammation, chest wall trauma, asthma, or COPD exacerbation

6. Laboratory and Imaging Findings

Laboratory Tests

- Complete blood count, including platelet count, and coagulation studies (PT/INR, and aPTT) to look for abnormalities
- Assays and polymerase chain reaction (PCR) are available to measure activated protein C resistance; AT, protein C, and protein S levels
- Three types of antiphospholipid antibodies are believed to contribute to the antiphospholipid syndrome:
  — Anticardiolipin antibodies
    ○ Anticardiolipin IgG or IgM antibodies are typically measured with enzyme immunoassays
  — A lupus anticoagulant that prolongs the partial thromboplastin time test in vitro
    ○ Although the lupus anticoagulant is detected by a prolongation of the PTT in vitro, paradoxically it is associated with a thrombotic tendency rather than a bleeding risk
    ○ The Russell viper venom time (RVVT) is more sensitive test for the lupus anticoagulant. A prolonged RVVT indicates the presence of the lupus anticoagulant
    ○ Prolonged aPTT that does not correct completely on mixing study
      - A mixing study takes the patient's blood and mixes it with plasma known to contain clotting factors
      - If the clotting time corrects, the patient's blood was factor deficient
      - If the clotting time does not fully correct, the patient's blood contains an anticoagulant that interferes with the clotting factors' activity
  — An antibody causing a "biologic false-positive test" for syphilis
    ○ In the "biologic false-positive" variant of the antiphospholipid antibody, the rapid plasma reagin (RPR) is (falsely) positive, but specific antitreponemal assays are negative
- In pregnancy
  — At least one of the following antiphospholipid antibodies is detectable
    ○ Lupus anticoagulant
    ○ Anticardiolipin antibodies
    ○ Anti-β_2-glycoprotein I antibodies

- The diagnosis of APS requires two positive antiphospholipid antibody test results at least 12 weeks apart since transient positive results can occur
- Specialized testing for lupus anticoagulant confirmation
  — Hexagonal phase phospholipid neutralization assay
  — Dilute Russell viper venom time
  — Platelet neutralization assays

Imaging Studies

- Patients with symptoms or signs of DVT should receive ultrasound with Doppler to assess lower extremity venous system
- Patients with symptoms or signs of pulmonary embolism may be diagnosed with helical chest CT scanning or lung ventilation–perfusion scanning

7. Treatments

Medications

- In patients with hypercoagulable states, anticoagulation with warfarin or heparin in standard doses and duration for most patients with first thrombosis
- Unfractionated heparin therapy is difficult to monitor in lupus anticoagulant because of the in vitro prolongation of the aPTT in that condition; therefore, low-molecular-weight heparin (LMWH) is preferred
- New (or noval) oral anticoagulants (NOACs) have a predictable dose effect, few drug–drug interactions, rapid onset of action, and freedom from laboratory monitoring. Dabigatran, rivaroxaban, and apixaban are approved for treatment of acute DVT and PE. While rivaroxaban and apixaban can be used as monotherapy immediately following diagnosis, patients who will be treated with dabigatran must first receive 5 to 10 days of parenteral anticoagulation then transition to the oral agent. When compared to warfarin and LMWH, the NOACs are all noninferior with respect to prevention of recurrent VTE and both rivaroxaban and apixaban boast a lower bleeding risk.
- Agent selection for acute treatment of VTE should be individualized; consider kidney function, concomitant medications, ability to use LMWH bridge therapy, cost, and adherence
- In patients with catastrophic APS, a three-pronged approach is taken in the acute setting
  — Intravenous heparin
  — High doses of corticosteroids
  — Either intravenous immune globulin or plasmapheresis
- Patients with major removable or reversible risk factors for hypercoagulation typically receive 3 to 6 months of anticoagulation therapy
- If thrombosis is recurrent, lifelong anticoagulation is usually recommended.
- LMWH is still the preferred agent for treatment of cancer-related VTE
- Patients with APS should be anticoagulated for life
  — Treat nonpregnant patients with APS with warfarin to maintain an INR of 2.0 to 3.0
  — Patients who have recurrent thrombotic events at this level of anticoagulation may require higher doses of warfarin aiming for INRs > 3.0, but bleeding risk increases substantially
  — Pregnant women (or women of childbearing age) with APS are anticoagulated with subcutaneous heparin and low-dose aspirin (81 mg orally daily because of the teratogenic effects of warfarin)
  — In women with APS and recurrent pregnancy loss, unfractionated heparin and low-dose aspirin can reduce risk of spontaneous abortion
  — After the first trimester, heparin is generally continued through pregnancy and the early postpartum period for thromboprophylaxis
  — Although LMWH has also been used for this indication, it is not clear that it has the same beneficial effect on reducing the risk of recurrent abortion as unfractionated heparin

Therapeutic Procedures

- Inferior vena cava filters may be placed in patients with lower extremity DVT with temporary contraindication to anticoagulation; however, if not removed promptly these filters become a nidus for thrombosis

8. Outcomes

Complications

- DVT
- PE
- Paradoxical embolism with patent foramen ovale
- Renal vein thrombosis
- Recurrent abortion

Prevention

- Anticoagulation and mechanical devices (intermittent pneumatic compression devices, venous foot pumps, graduated compression stockings) may prevent recurrent thrombosis

9. When to Refer and When to Admit

When to Refer

- Patients with recurrent thrombosis may need to be referred to a hematologist

When to Admit

- Any patient with thromboembolism that is unstable or requires expedited workup

SUGGESTED REFERENCES

Agnelli G et al; AMPLIFY Investigators. Oral apixaban for the treatment of acute venous thromboembolism. *N Engl J Med*. 2013 Aug 29;369(9):799–808. [PMID: 23808982]

Barbar S et al. A risk assessment model for the identification of hospitalized medical patients at risk for venous thromboembolism: the Padua Prediction Score. *J Thromb Haemost*. 2010 Nov;8(11):2450–2457. [PMID: 20738765]

Brighton TA et al. ASPIRE Investigators. Low-dose aspirin for preventing recurrent venous thromboembolism. *N Engl J Med*. 2012 Nov 22;367(21):1979–1987. [PMID: 23121403]

Castellucci LA et al. Clinical and safety outcomes associated with treatment of acute venous thromboembolism: a systematic review and meta-analysis. *JAMA*. 2014 Sep 17;312(11):1122–1135. [PMID: 25226478]

Erkens PM et al. Does the Pulmonary Embolism Severity Index accurately identify low risk patients eligible for outpatient treatment? *Thromb Res*. 2012 Jun;129(6):710–714. [PMID: 21906787]

Falck-Ytter Y et al. Prevention of VTE in orthopedic surgery patients: Antithrombotic Therapy and Prevention of Thrombosis, 9th ed: American College of Chest Physicians Evidence-Based Clinical Practice Guidelines. *Chest*. 2012 Feb;141(2 Suppl):e278S–e325S. [PMID: 22315265]

Gould MK et al. Prevention of VTE in nonorthopedic surgical patients: Antithrombotic Therapy and Prevention of Thrombosis, 9th ed: American College of Chest Physicians Evidence-Based Clinical Practice Guidelines. *Chest*. 2012 Feb;141(2 Suppl):e227S–e277S. Erratum in: *Chest*. 2012 May;141(5):1369. [PMID: 22315263]

Heidbuchel H et al. European Heart Rhythm Association Practical Guide on the use of new oral anticoagulants in patients with non-valvular atrial fibrillation. *Europace*. 2013 May;15(5):625–651. [PMID: 23625942]

Jiménez D et al. Simplification of the Pulmonary Embolism Severity Index for prognostication in patients with acute symptomatic pulmonary embolism. *Arch Intern Med*. 2010;170(15):1383–1389. [PMID: 20696966]

Kaatz S et al. Reversal of target-specific oral anticoagulants. *J Thromb Thrombolysis*. 2013 Aug;36(2):195–202. [PMID: 23657589]

Kahn SR et al. Prevention of VTE in nonsurgical patients: Antithrombotic Therapy and Prevention of Thrombosis, 9th ed: American College of Chest Physicians Evidence-Based Clinical Practice Guidelines. *Chest*. 2012 Feb;141(2 suppl):e195S–e226S. [PMID: 2231526]

Kearon C et al. Antithrombotic therapy for VTE disease: Antithrombotic Therapy and Prevention of Thrombosis, 9th ed: American College of Chest Physicians Evidence-Based Clinical Practice Guidelines. *Chest*. 2012 Feb;141(2 suppl):e419S–e494S. [PMID: 22315268]

Kearon C et al. Duration of anticoagulant therapy for deep vein thrombosis and pulmonary embolism. *Blood*. 2014 Mar 20;123(12):1794–1801. [PMID: 24497538]

Neumann I et al. Oral direct Factor Xa inhibitors versus low-molecular-weight heparin to prevent venous thromboembolism in patients undergoing total hip or knee replacement: a systematic review and meta-analysis. *Ann Intern Med*. 2012 May 15;156(10):710–719. [PMID: 22412038]

Qaseem A et al. Venous thromboembolism prophylaxis in hospitalized patients: a clinical practice guideline from the American College of Physicians. *Ann Intern Med*. 2011 Nov 1;155(9):625–632. [PMID: 22041951]

Scherz N et al. Prospective, multicenter validation of prediction scores for major bleeding in elderly patients with venous thromboembolism. *J Thromb Haemost*. 2013 Mar;11(3):435–443. [PMID: 23279158]

24

Iron Deficiency Anemia

A 65-year-old previously well man presents to the clinic with the complaint of fatigue of 3 months' duration. Questioning reveals diffuse weakness and feeling winded when walking uphill or climbing more than one flight of stairs. All of his symptoms have slowly worsened over time. Except for light-headedness, the review of systems is negative. The patient has no significant medical history, social history, or family history. On physical examination, he appears somewhat pale, with normal vital signs except for a resting pulse of 118 bpm. The physical examination is otherwise unremarkable except for his rectal examination, which reveals brown, guaiac-positive stool (consistent with occult blood in the stool). A complete blood count (CBC) reveals a microcytic anemia with low mean corpuscular volume (MCV).

LEARNING OBJECTIVES

▶ Know the underlying diseases that may cause iron deficiency anemia
▶ Learn the clinical manifestations and objective findings of iron deficiency anemia
▶ Know the differential diagnosis of iron deficiency anemia
▶ Learn the treatment for iron deficiency anemia

QUESTIONS

1. What are the salient features of this patient's problem?
2. How do you think through his problem?
3. What are the key features, including essentials of diagnosis, general considerations, and demographics, of iron deficiency anemia?
4. What are the symptoms and signs of iron deficiency anemia?
5. What is the differential diagnosis of iron deficiency anemia?
6. What are laboratory findings in iron deficiency anemia?
7. What are the treatments for iron deficiency anemia?
8. What is the outcome, including follow-up, of iron deficiency anemia?
9. When should patients with iron deficiency anemia be referred to a specialist?

ANSWERS

1. Salient Features

Fatigue, weakness, and dyspnea of insidious onset; pale on physical examination; guaiac-positive stool; and microcytic anemia

2. How to Think Through

Several of this patient's symptoms and signs—fatigue, dyspnea, lightheadedness, weakness, tachycardia—might suggest cardiac and pulmonary etiologies to your differential diagnosis. *But do not forget anemia!* Once you establish that the patient is anemic, look at the reticulocyte count. Hyperproliferative anemia indicates either hemolysis or active bleeding. Hypoproliferative anemia, which is more common, often indicates a deficiency state. Anemia is further assessed by looking at the MCV.

Is the reticulocyte count low or high in iron deficiency anemia? (Low.) What happens to the MCV? (Low.) What are other possible causes of this patient's microcytic anemia? In iron deficiency anemia, what is the pattern of abnormalities in the serum iron studies—ferritin, iron, transferrin (total iron-binding capacity), and % saturation? What features will you likely find on the peripheral smear in this iron-deficient patient? How can the platelet count provide a clue?

Whenever you determine that the etiology of anemia is iron deficiency, you MUST investigate its cause. Conceptualize the possible causes by tracing the path from dietary intake, to absorption, to bioavailability, to possible blood loss. What are the potential pathologies at each stage? For example, where is iron absorbed and what might disrupt this absorption? While the gastrointestinal (GI) tract is the most common source of blood loss, also be sure to consider other sources of blood loss (eg, uterine, urinary, pulmonary).

3. Key Features

Essentials of Diagnosis
- Iron deficiency is present if serum ferritin is < 12 µg/L or < 30 µg/L if also anemic
- Caused by bleeding in adults unless proved otherwise
- Response to iron therapy

General Considerations
- Most common cause of anemia worldwide
- Causes
  — Blood loss (GI, menstrual, repeated blood donation)
  — Dietary iron-deficiency
  — Decreased absorption of iron
  — Increased requirements (pregnancy, lactation)
  — Celiac disease (gluten enteropathy)
  — Hemoglobinuria
  — Iron sequestration (pulmonary hemosiderosis)
- Women with heavy menstrual losses may require more iron than can readily be absorbed; thus, they often become iron deficient
- Pregnancy and lactation also increase requirement for iron, necessitating medicinal iron supplementation
- Long-term aspirin use may cause GI blood loss even without documented structural lesion
- Search for a source of GI bleeding if other sites of blood loss (menorrhagia, other uterine bleeding, and repeated blood donations) are excluded

Demographics
- More common in women as a result of menstrual losses

4. Symptoms and Signs

- Symptoms of anemia (eg, easy fatigability, dyspnea, tachycardia, palpitations, and tachypnea on exertion)
- Skin and mucosal changes (eg, smooth tongue, brittle nails, spooning of nails [koilonychia], and cheilosis) in severe iron deficiency
- Dysphagia resulting from esophageal webs (Plummer–Vinson syndrome) may occur in severe iron deficiency
- Pica (ie, craving for specific foods [eg, ice chips, lettuce] often not rich in iron) is frequent

5. Differential Diagnosis

- Microcytic anemia resulting from other causes
  — Thalassemia
  — Anemia of chronic disease
  — Sideroblastic anemia
  — Lead poisoning

6. Laboratory Findings

Laboratory Tests

- Diagnosis can be made by
  — Laboratory confirmation of an iron-deficient state
  — Evaluation of response to a therapeutic trial of iron replacement
- The reticulocyte count is low or inappropriately normal
- A ferritin value < 12 µg/L is a highly reliable indicator of depletion of iron stores
- However, because serum ferritin levels may rise in response to inflammation or other stimuli, a normal ferritin level does not exclude a diagnosis of iron deficiency
- A ferritin level of < 30 µg/L almost always indicates iron deficiency in anyone who is anemic
- As iron deficiency progresses, serum iron values decline to < 30 µg/dL and transferrin levels rise to compensate, leading to transferrin saturations of $< 15\%$
- As deficiency progresses, anisocytosis (variation in red blood cell [RBC] size) and poikilocytosis (variation in RBC shape) develop
- Abnormal peripheral blood smear: markedly hypochromic cells, target cells, hypochromic pencil-shaped or cigar-shaped cells, and occasionally small numbers of nucleated RBCs in severe iron deficiency; platelet count is commonly increased, but it usually remains $< 800,000/\mu L$
- Bone marrow biopsy for evaluation of iron stores
  — Rarely performed
  — If done, shows the absence of iron in erythroid progenitor cells by Prussian blue staining
- As the MCV falls (ie, microcytosis), the blood smear shows hypochromic microcytic cells
- Low hepcidin level in isolated iron deficiency anemia; however, this is not yet a clinically available test

7. Treatments

Medications

- Ferrous sulfate, 325 mg orally three times daily
  — Taken on an empty stomach, it provides 180 mg of iron daily, of which up to 10 mg is absorbed
  — Treatment of choice
  — Nausea and constipation limit patient compliance
  — Extended-release ferrous sulfate with mucoprotease is the best tolerated oral preparation
- Compliance improved by introducing the medicine slowly in gradually escalating doses
- Taking ferrous sulfate with food reduces side effects and but also its absorption

- Continue iron therapy for 3 to 6 months after restoration of normal hematologic values to replenish iron stores
- Failure of response to iron therapy
  — Usually due to medication noncompliance
  — Pure iron deficiency might prove refractory to oral iron replacement. Refractoriness is defined as a hemoglobin increment of < 1 g/dL (10 g/L) after 4 to 6 weeks of 100 mg/d of elemental oral iron.
  — The differential diagnosis of refractory cases includes malabsorption from autoimmune gastritis, *Helicobacter pylori* gastric infection, and celiac disease; ongoing GI blood loss; hereditary iron-refractory iron deficiency; or incorrect diagnosis (anemia of chronic disease, thalassemia).
- Indications for parenteral iron
  — Intolerance of oral iron such as GI disease (usually inflammatory bowel disease) precluding use of oral iron
  — Refractoriness to oral iron
  — Continued blood loss that cannot be corrected
- Improvements in the formulation of parenteral iron preparations have greatly reduced the risks and increased the ease of its administration
  — Iron dextran is safe and can be given in < 5 min, but the maximum dose is 200 mg
  — Iron oxide coated with polyglucose sorbitol carboxymethylether can be given in doses up to 510 mg by intravenous bolus over 20 seconds, with no test dose required
  — Total body iron ranges between 2 and 4 g: ~50 mg/kg in men and 35 mg/kg in women
  — The iron deficit is calculated by determining the decrement in RBC mass from normal recognizing there is 1 mg of iron in each milliliter of RBCs
- For patients with end-stage chronic kidney disease, ferric pyrophosphate citrate (Triferic) can be added to the dialysate to replace the 5 to 7 mg of iron lost at each hemodialysis.

Therapeutic Procedures
- Treat underlying cause of the iron deficiency such as the source of GI bleeding

8. Outcome

Follow-Up
- Recheck complete blood cell count to observe for response to iron replacement by return of hematocrit to halfway toward normal within 3 weeks and fully to baseline after 2 months
- Iron supplementation during pregnancy and lactation: included in prenatal vitamins

9. When to Refer
- No response to iron therapy
- If suspected diagnosis is not confirmed

SUGGESTED REFERENCES

Cancelo-Hildago MJ et al. Tolerability of different oral iron supplements: a systematic review. *Curr Med Res Opin*. 2013 Apr;29(4):291–303. [PMID: 23252877]

Donker AE et al. Practice guidelines for the diagnosis and management of microcytic anemias due to genetic disorders of iron metabolism or heme synthesis. *Blood*. 2014 Jun 19;123(25):3873–3886. [PMID: 24665134]

Hershko C et al. How I treat unexplained refractory iron deficiency anemia. *Blood*. 2014 Jan 16;123(3):326–333. [PMID: 24215034]

Kautz L et al. Molecular liaisons between erythropoiesis and iron metabolism. *Blood*. 2014 Jul 24;124(4):479–482. [PMID: 24876565]

Larson DS et al. Update on intravenous iron choices. *Curr Opin Nephrol Hypertens*. 2014 Mar;23(2): 186–191. [PMID: 24401789]

25

Deep Venous Thrombosis and Thromboembolism

A 57-year-old man undergoes total knee replacement for severe degenerative joint disease. Four days after surgery, he develops acute onset of shortness of breath and right-sided pleuritic chest pain. His family history is remarkable in that his father died after a pulmonary embolism (PE). The patient is now in moderate respiratory distress with a respiratory rate 28/min, heart rate 120 bpm, and blood pressure 110/70 mm Hg. Oxygen saturation is 90% on room air. Lung examination is normal. Cardiac examination reveals tachycardia but is otherwise unremarkable. The right lower extremity is postsurgical, healing well, with 2+ pitting edema, calf tenderness, erythema, and warmth; the left leg is normal.

LEARNING OBJECTIVES

▶ Learn the clinical manifestations and objective findings of deep venous thrombosis (DVT) and thromboembolism

▶ Understand the factors that predispose to DVT and thromboembolism and how those factors relate to risk of recurrence

▶ Know the differential diagnosis of DVT and thromboembolism

▶ Learn the initial and subsequent treatment regimens for DVT and thromboembolism

▶ Understand how to prevent DVT and thromboembolism in hospitalized patients

QUESTIONS

1. What are the salient features of this patient's problem?

2. How do you think through his problem?

3. What are the key features, including essentials of diagnosis and general considerations, of DVT and thromboembolism?

4. What are the symptoms and signs of DVT and thromboembolism?

5. What is the differential diagnosis of DVT and thromboembolism?

6. What are laboratory, imaging, and procedural findings in DVT and thromboembolism?

7. What are the treatments for DVT and thromboembolism?

8. What are the outcomes, including complications, prevention, and prognosis, of DVT and thromboembolism?

9. When should patients with DVT and thromboembolism be referred to a specialist or admitted to the hospital?

ANSWERS

1. Salient Features

Recent orthopedic surgery; acute shortness of breath, pleuritic chest pain, tachycardia, and tachypnea suggesting PE; family history of thrombosis; lower extremity with edema, tenderness, erythema, and warmth

2. How to Think Through

Given the postsurgical context, acute symptoms, and vital sign abnormalities, PE is likely, and anticoagulation therapy should be started immediately. Computed tomography (CT)-angiography can be performed when the patient is stable. Whether to use thrombolytic therapy is the key management question in this case. Thrombolysis is known to improve outcomes in massive PE but is controversial in submassive PE. The patient has tachycardia, but is not frankly hypotensive at this point. What study would help with this decision? (Echocardiography to characterize the degree of right heart strain.)

When a reversible risk factor for DVT or PE is identified, such as immobility, cancer, recent surgery, or injury to a blood vessel wall, the event is said to be "provoked," an evaluation for thrombophilia is often not performed, and anticoagulation is prescribed for 3 to 6 months. When a DVT or PE is unprovoked, the risk of recurrence is as high as 7% to 10% per year, and lifelong anticoagulation is typically indicated. This case presents a circumstance in which evaluation for a hypercoagulable state will be needed to guide duration of anticoagulation: while his recent orthopedic surgery is a major reversible risk factor, he also has a family history of PE, suggesting a possible inherited thrombophilia. The evaluation should be delayed for 3 months, since factors such as protein C and S are consumed during the acute PE.

3. Key Features

Essentials of Diagnosis
- Predisposition to venous thrombosis
- Pain, swelling, and redness below the level of the thrombus
- Presence of thromboembolic disease such as PE

General Considerations
- DVT and PE are two manifestations of the same disease
- DVT is the most common source of PE
- DVT may be in the upper or lower extremity, though most commonly in the legs
- Deep venous thrombi confined to the calf rarely embolize; however, 20% of calf thrombi propagate proximally to the popliteal and iliofemoral veins
- Fifty to sixty percent of patients with proximal DVT will have pulmonary emboli; half of these pulmonary emboli are asymptomatic
- Fifty to seventy percent of patients with symptomatic PE will have lower extremity DVT
- Risk factors include venous stasis, injury to the vessel wall, and hypercoagulability
- Venous stasis causes
  — Immobility, eg, bed rest, obesity, or stroke
  — Hyperviscosity, eg, polycythemia
  — Increased central venous pressures, eg, low cardiac output, pregnancy
- Hypercoagulability causes
  — Oral contraceptives
  — Hormone replacement therapy
  — Malignancy
  — Surgery
  — Inherited hypercoagulable state
- Vessel injury includes surgery or placement of foreign material such as central venous catheters

4. Symptoms and Signs

- Pain, swelling, and redness below the level of the thrombus
- Usually unilateral
- Normal arterial pressures and perfusion in the distal extremity
- Homan sign: pain in the calf with dorsiflexion of the ankle (limited sensitivity)
- DVT may be detectable as a palpable cord in the calf
- DVT may be associated with symptoms and signs of PE, eg, dyspnea, chest pain, tachycardia, and tachypnea

5. Differential Diagnosis

- Muscular strain
- Baker cyst
- Achilles tendon rupture
- Cellulitis
- Superficial thrombophlebitis
- Lymphatic obstruction (eg, from pelvic tumor)
- Reflex sympathetic dystrophy
- Tumor or fibrosis obstructing venous flow
- May–Thurner syndrome (left iliac vein compressed by right common iliac artery)

6. Laboratory, Imaging, and Procedural Findings

Laboratory Tests

- A negative D-dimer (dimerized plasmin fragment D) can rule out DVT in patients with low pretest probability
- Patients may need further laboratory tests for inherited hypercoagulable disorders. The evaluation should be delayed for 3 months because factors such as protein C and S are consumed during the acute PE.

Imaging Studies

- Ultrasonography (USG) with Doppler is diagnostic of DVT and is the preferred study
- MRI may also be diagnostic though more expensive; it may be useful in nonextremity thrombosis
- Helical CT scan or ventilation–perfusion scanning is used for patients with symptoms of PE

Diagnostic Procedures

- Venography is the gold standard test for DVT, but it is invasive, expensive, and rarely used
- Impedance plethysmography, which relies on changes in electrical impedance between patent and obstructed veins, is comparable to USG in accuracy

7. Treatments

Medications

- Anticoagulant therapy is the cornerstone of medical therapy
- LMWHs are more effective than unfractionated heparin in the immediate treatment of DVT and PE and are preferred because of predictable pharmacokinetics.
- Fondaparinux (a factor Xa inhibitor) may be used for immediate treatment and shows no increase in bleeding risk. Its lack of reversibility, long half-life, and primarily kidney clearance are limitations to its use.
- After initial therapy with either LMWH or fondaparinux, oral anticoagulation is started with a vitamin K antagonist (eg, warfarin) with dose adjustment based on a target INR value of 2.0 to 3.0
- The target-specific oral anticoagulants rivaroxaban and apixaban are approved as monotherapy immediately following diagnosis and eliminate the need for parenteral therapy. Dabigatran requires 5 to 10 days of parenteral anticoagulation followed by transition to this oral agent. All three are approved and noninferior to LMWH and warfarin with

Table 25-1. Initial anticoagulation for VTE[a].

Anticoagulant	Dose/Frequency	DVT, Lower Extremity	DVT, Upper Extremity	PE	VTE, With Concomitant Severe Renal Impairment[b]	VTE, Cancer-Related	Comment
Unfractionated heparin							
Unfractionated heparin	80 units/kg intravenous bolus then continuous intravenous infusion of 18 units/kg/h	×	×	×	×		Bolus may be omitted if risk of bleeding is perceived to be elevated. Maximum bolus, 10,000 units. Requires aPTT monitoring. Most patients: begin warfarin at time of initiation of heparin
	330 units/kg subcutaneously × 1 then 250 units/kg subcutaneously every 12 h	×					Fixed-dose; no aPTT monitoring required
LMWH and fondaparinux							
Enoxaparin[c]	1 mg/kg subcutaneously every 12 h	×	×	×			Most patients: begin warfarin at time of initiation of LMWH
Dalteparin[c]	200 units/kg subcutaneously once daily for first month, then 150 units/kg/d	×	×	×		×	Cancer: administer LMWH for ≥ 3–6 mo; reduce dose to 150 units/kg after first month of treatment
Fondaparinux	5–10 mg subcutaneously once daily (see Comment)	×	×	×			Use 7.5 mg for body weight 50–100 kg, 10 mg for body weight > 100 kg
Target-specific oral anticoagulants							
Rivaroxaban	15 mg orally twice daily with food for first 21 d, then 20 mg orally daily with food						Contraindicated if CrCl < 30 mL/min
Apixaban	10 mg orally twice daily for first 7 d then 5 mg twice daily						Contraindicated if CrCl < 25 mL/min
Dabigatran	5–10 d of parenteral anticoagulation then 150 mg twice daily						Contraindicated if CrCl < 30 mL/min

DVT, deep venous thrombosis; LMWH, low-molecular-weight heparin; PE, pulmonary embolism; VTE, venous thromboembolic disease (includes DVT and PE).

Note: An "×" denotes appropriate use of the anticoagulant.

[a]Obtain baseline hemoglobin, platelet count, aPTT, PT/INR, creatinine, urinalysis, and stool occult blood test prior to initiation of anticoagulation. *Anticoagulation is contraindicated in the setting of active bleeding.*

[b]Defined as creatinine clearance < 30 mL/min.

[c]Body weight < 50 kg: reduce dose and monitor anti-Xa levels.

respect to prevention of recurrent VTE; both rivaroxaban and apixaban boast a lower bleeding risk. These agents have a predictable dose effect, few drug–drug interactions, and freedom from laboratory monitoring
- LMWH is still the preferred agent for treatment of cancer-related VTE
- Duration of treatment for provoked DVT (eg, that occurs in the presence of a major and reversible risk factor such as surgery) is a minimum of 3 months; lifelong anticoagulation should be considered in patients with unprovoked DVTs (Tables 25-1 and 25-2)

Surgery
- Surgical thrombectomy is an option, especially in large iliofemoral thromboses

Therapeutic Procedures
- Inferior vena cava (IVC) filters may be used in patients with documented DVT and an absolute contraindication for anticoagulation to reduce the risk of PE
- Retrievable IVC filter is preferred as the filter increases the risk of further thrombosis with long-term placement

Table 25-2. Duration of treatment of VTE.

Scenario	Suggested Duration of Therapy	Comments
Major transient risk factor (eg, major surgery, major trauma, and major hospitalization)	At least 3 mo	VTE prophylaxis upon future exposure to transient risk factors
Minor transient risk factor (eg, exposure to exogenous estrogens/progestins, pregnancy, and airline travel lasting > 6 h)	At least 3 mo	VTE prophylaxis upon future exposure to transient risk factors
Cancer-related	≥ 3–6 mo or as long as cancer active, whichever is longer	LMWH recommended for initial treatment (see Table 25-1)
Unprovoked thrombosis	At least 3 mo, consider indefinite if bleeding risk allows	May individually risk-stratify for recurrence with follow-up ultrasound, D-dimer, clinical risk score, and clinical presentation
Recurrent unprovoked	Indefinite	
Underlying significant thrombophilia (eg, antiphospholipid antibody syndrome, antithrombin deficiency, protein C deficiency, protein S deficiency, ≥ 2 concomitant thrombophilic conditions)	Indefinite	To avoid false positives, consider delaying investigation for laboratory thrombophilia until 3 mo after event

LMWH, low-molecular-weight heparin; VTE, venous thromboembolic disease.

- Graduated compression stockings may provide symptomatic relief from swelling but have failed to show a decrease in the likelihood of post-thrombotic syndrome (swelling, pain, and skin ulceration) and are contraindicated in patients with peripheral arterial disease.
- Directed thrombolytic therapies may be used for large thromboses with high-risk, massive PE (hemodynamic instability). Thrombolytic therapy has been used in selected patients with intermediate-risk, submassive PE (without hemodynamic instability but with evidence of right ventricular compromise and myocardial injury). A "safe dose" of tPA (≤ 50% of the standard dose [100 mg]) shows similar efficacy and a better safety profile in small trials

8. Outcomes
Complications
- PE
- Paradoxical embolism with patent foramen ovale

Prevention
- Prophylactic therapy is effective and underused in hospitalized patients, in which thromboembolic disease is common (Tables 25-3 and 25-4)

Prognosis
- Prognosis and recurrence is based on clinical scenario in which disease occurred
- Provoked disease recurrence is 3%; unprovoked disease recurs 8% of the time; patients with cancer have > 20% recurrence rates
- Death from thromboemboli is uncommon, occurring in < 3%

9. When to Refer and When to Admit
When to Refer
- Large iliofemoral venous thromboembolism (VTE), IVC thrombosis, portal vein thrombosis, or Budd–Chiari syndrome
- Passive PE
- Need for IVC filter placement

Table 25-3. Pharmacologic prophylaxis of VTE in selected clinical scenarios[a].

Anticoagulant	Dose	Frequency	Clinical Scenario	Comment
Enoxaparin	40 mg	Once daily	Most medical inpatients and critical care patients	—
			Surgical patients (moderate risk for VTE)	Consider continuing for 4 wk total duration for cancer surgery and high-risk medical patients
			Abdominal/pelvic cancer surgery	
		Twice daily	Bariatric surgery	Higher doses may be required
	30 mg	Twice daily	Orthopedic surgery[b]	Give for at least 10 d. For THR, TKA, or HFS, consider continuing up to 1 mo after surgery in high-risk patients
			Major trauma	Not applicable to patients with isolated lower extremity trauma
			Acute spinal cord injury	—
Dalteparin	2500 units	Once daily	Most medical inpatients	—
			Abdominal surgery (moderate risk for VTE)	Give for 5–10 d
	5000 units	Once daily	Orthopedic surgery[b]	First dose = 2500 units. Give for at least 10 d. For THR, TKA, or HFS, consider continuing up to 1 mo after surgery in high-risk patients
			Abdominal surgery (higher risk for VTE)	Give for 5–10 d
			Medical inpatients	—
Fondaparinux	2.5 mg	Once daily	Orthopedic surgery[b]	Give for at least 10 d. For THR, TKA, or HFS, consider continuing up to 1 mo after surgery in high-risk patients
Rivaroxaban	10 mg	Once daily	Orthopedic surgery—total hip and total knee replacement	Give for 12 d following total knee replacement; give for 35 d following total hip replacement
Apixaban	2.5 mg orally	Twice daily	following hip or knee replacement surgery	Give for 12 d following total knee replacement; give for 35 d following total hip replacement
Unfractionated heparin	5000 units	Three times daily	Higher VTE risk with low bleeding risk	Includes gynecologic surgery for malignancy and urologic surgery, medical patients with multiple risk factors for VTE
	5000 units	Twice daily	Hospitalized patients at intermediate risk for VTE	Includes gynecologic surgery (moderate risk)
			Patients with epidural catheters	LMWHs usually avoided due to risk of spinal hematoma
			Patients with severe renal insufficiency[c]	LMWHs contraindicated
Warfarin	Variable	Once daily	Orthopedic surgery[b]	Titrate to goal INR = 2.5. Give for at least 10 d. For high-risk patients undergoing THR, TKA, or HFS, consider continuing up to 1 mo after surgery

HFS, hip fracture surgery; LMWH, low-molecular-weight heparin; THR, total hip replacement; TKA, total knee arthroplasty; VTE, venous thromboembolic disease.

[a]All regimens administered subcutaneously, except for warfarin.

[b]Includes TKA, THR, and HFS.

[c]Defined as creatinine clearance < 30 mL/min.

When to Admit

- Documented or suspected PE that is not considered low risk
- DVT with poorly controlled pain, high bleeding risk, or contraindications to LMWH
- Large iliofemoral DVT
- Acute DVT with absolute contraindication to anticoagulation for IVC filter placement

Table 25-4. Contraindications to VTE prophylaxis for medical or surgical hospital inpatients at high risk for VTE.

Absolute contraindications
Acute hemorrhage from wounds or drains or lesions
Intracranial hemorrhage within prior 24 h
Heparin-induced thrombocytopenia (HIT) considering using fondaparinux
Severe trauma to head or spinal cord or extremities
Epidural anesthesia/spinal block within 12 h of initiation of anticoagulation (concurrent use of an epidural catheter and LMWH thromboprophylaxis should require approval by service who performed the epidural or spinal procedure, eg, anesthesia/pain service)
Currently receiving warfarin or heparin or LMWH or direct thrombin inhibitor for other indications

Relative contraindications
Coagulopathy (INR > 1.5)
Intracranial lesion or neoplasm
Severe thrombocytopenia (platelet count < 50 000/μL)
Intracranial hemorrhage within past 6 mo
Gastrointestinal or genitourinary hemorrhage within past 6 mo

INR, international normalized ratio; LMWH, low-molecular-weight heparin; VTE, venous thromboembolism.
Adapted from Guidelines used at the VA Medical Center, San Francisco, CA.

SUGGESTED REFERENCES

American College of Emergency Physicians Clinical Policies Subcommittee on Critical Issues in the Evaluation and Management of Adult Patients Presenting to the Emergency Department With Suspected Pulmonary Embolism, Fesmire FM et al. Critical issues in the evaluation and management of adult patients presenting to the emergency department with suspected pulmonary embolism. *Ann Emerg Med.* 2011 Jun;57(6):628–652.e75. [PMID: 21621092]

Burns SK et al. Diagnostic imaging and risk stratification of patients with acute pulmonary embolism. *Cardiol Rev.* 2012 Jan–Feb;20(1):15–24. [PMID: 22143281]

Goldhaber SZ et al. Pulmonary embolism and deep vein thrombosis. *Lancet.* 2012 May 12;379(9828):1835–1846. [PMID: 22494827]

Hunt JM et al. Clinical review of pulmonary embolism: diagnosis, prognosis, and treatment. *Med Clin North Am.* 2011 Nov;95(6):1203–1222. [PMID: 22032435]

Jaff MR et al. American Heart Association Council on Cardiopulmonary, Critical Care, Perioperative and Resuscitation; American Heart Association Council on Peripheral Vascular Disease; American Heart Association Council on Arteriosclerosis, Thrombosis and Vascular Biology. Management of massive and submassive pulmonary embolism, iliofemoral deep vein thrombosis, and chronic thromboembolic pulmonary hypertension: a scientific statement from the American Heart Association. *Circulation.* 2011 Apr 26;123(16):1788–1830. [PMID: 21422387]

Kearon C et al. Antithrombotic therapy for VTE disease: Antithrombotic Therapy and Prevention of Thrombosis, 9th ed: American College of Chest Physicians Evidence-Based Clinical Practice Guideline. *Chest.* 2012 Feb;141(2 suppl):e419S–e494S. [PMID: 22315268]

Lucassen W et al. Clinical decision rules for excluding pulmonary embolism: a meta-analysis. *Ann Intern Med.* 2011 Oct 4;155(7):448–460. [PMID: 21969343]

Merrigan JM et al. JAMA patient page. Pulmonary embolism. *JAMA.* 2013 Feb 6;309(5):504. [PMID: 23385279]

Moores LK et al. Current approach to the diagnosis of acute nonmassive pulmonary embolism. *Chest.* 2011 Aug;140(2):509–518. [PMID: 21813530]

Singh B et al. Diagnostic accuracy of pulmonary embolism rule-out criteria: a systematic review and meta-analysis. *Ann Emerg Med.* 2012 Jun;59(6):517–520. [PMID: 22177109]

Tapson VF. Treatment of pulmonary embolism: anticoagulation, thrombolytic therapy, and complications of therapy. *Crit Care Clin.* 2011 Oct;27(4):825–839. [PMID: 22082516]

Vitamin B$_{12}$ Deficiency Anemia

26

A 58-year-old woman presents to the emergency department with complaints of progressive fatigue and weakness for the past 6 months. She is short of breath after walking several blocks. On review of systems, she mentions mild diarrhea. She has noted intermittent numbness and tingling of her lower extremities and a loss of balance while walking. She denies other neurologic or cardiac symptoms and has no history of black or bloody stools or other blood loss. On physical examination she is tachycardic to 110 bpm; other vital signs are within normal limits. Head and neck examination is notable for pale conjunctivas and a beefy red tongue with loss of papillae. Cardiac examination shows a rapid regular rhythm with a grade 2/6 systolic murmur at the left sternal border. Lung, abdominal, and rectal examination findings are normal. Neurologic examination reveals decreased sensation to position and vibration in the lower extremities. Laboratory testing shows a low hematocrit level.

LEARNING OBJECTIVES

▶ Learn the clinical manifestations and objective findings of vitamin B$_{12}$ deficiency
▶ Understand the factors that predispose to vitamin B$_{12}$ deficiency
▶ Know the differential diagnosis of vitamin B$_{12}$ deficiency
▶ Learn the treatments for vitamin B$_{12}$ deficiency
▶ Understand how to prevent vitamin B$_{12}$ deficiency

QUESTIONS

1. What are the salient features of this patient's problem?
2. How do you think through her problem?
3. What are the key features, including essentials of diagnosis and general considerations, of vitamin B$_{12}$ deficiency?
4. What are the symptoms and signs of vitamin B$_{12}$ deficiency?
5. What is the differential diagnosis of vitamin B$_{12}$ deficiency?
6. What are laboratory and procedural findings in vitamin B$_{12}$ deficiency?
7. What are the treatments for vitamin B$_{12}$ deficiency?

8. What are the outcomes, including follow-up, complications, and prognosis, of vitamin B_{12} deficiency?

ANSWERS

1. Salient Features

Fatigue, weakness, and dyspnea of insidious onset; neurologic symptoms including peripheral neuropathy and ataxia; tachycardia and paleness with anemia; glossitis; posterior column neurologic findings on examination

2. How to Think Through

Here, the combination of two clinical presentations should raise the possibility of vitamin B_{12} deficiency: anemia plus neurological symptoms. While peripheral neuropathy is the most common neurologic manifestation, what other neurological symptoms can result from advanced B_{12} deficiency? Regarding the anemia, in what range does the typical mean corpuscular volume (MCV) fall in B_{12} deficiency; are there exceptions? What are the other common causes of macrocytic anemia? Specifically, what other metabolic derangements? Medication effects? Toxic ingestions? What are the findings on a peripheral blood smear in B_{12} deficiency? What would the reticulocyte count be? Can this patient's symptoms of fatigue, weakness, and dyspnea be caused by her anemia? In this patient, what would be the most common cause of B_{12} deficiency? How would you diagnose it? What might be some other possible causes? Surgical? Infectious? Inflammatory? Dietary?

3. Key Features

Essentials of Diagnosis
- Macrocytic anemia
- Megaloblastic peripheral blood smear (macro-ovalocytes and hypersegmented neutrophils)
- Low serum vitamin B_{12} level

General Considerations
- All vitamin B_{12} is absorbed from the diet (foods of animal origin)
- After ingestion, vitamin B_{12} binds to intrinsic factor, a protein secreted by gastric parietal cells
- Vitamin B_{12}–intrinsic factor complex is absorbed in the terminal ileum by cells with specific receptors for the complex; it is then transported through the plasma and stored in the liver
- Liver stores are of such magnitude that it takes at least 3 years for vitamin B_{12} deficiency to develop after vitamin B_{12} absorption ceases
- Causes of vitamin B_{12} deficiency
  — Decreased intrinsic factor production: pernicious anemia (most common cause), gastrectomy
  — Dietary deficiency (rare but seen in vegans)
  — Competition for B_{12} in gut: blind loop syndrome, fish tapeworm (rare)
  — Decreased ileal B_{12} absorption: surgical resection, Crohn disease
  — Pancreatic insufficiency
  — *Helicobacter pylori* infection
  — Transcobalamin II deficiency (rare)
- Pernicious anemia is associated with atrophic gastritis and other autoimmune diseases, eg, immunoglobulin A (IgA) deficiency, polyglandular endocrine failure syndromes

4. Symptoms and Signs
- Causes a moderate to severe anemia of slow onset such that patients may have few symptoms relative to their degree of anemia

- Pallor and mild icterus or sallow complexion
- Glossitis and vague gastrointestinal disturbances (eg, anorexia, diarrhea)
- Neurologic manifestations
  — Peripheral neuropathy usually occurs first
  — Then, subacute combined degeneration of the spinal cord affecting posterior columns may develop, causing difficulty with position and vibration sensation and balance
  — In advanced cases, dementia and other neuropsychiatric changes may occur
  — Neurologic manifestations occasionally precede hematologic changes; patients with suspicious neurologic symptoms and signs should be evaluated for vitamin B$_{12}$ deficiency despite normal mean cell volume (MCV) and absence of anemia

5. Differential Diagnosis

- Folic acid deficiency (another cause of megaloblastic anemia)
- Myelodysplastic syndrome (another cause of macrocytic anemia with abnormal morphology)
- Other causes of peripheral neuropathy, ataxia, or dementia

6. Laboratory and Procedural Findings

Laboratory Tests

- Normal vitamin B$_{12}$ level is > 210 pg/mL
- Serum vitamin B$_{12}$ levels in overt deficiency: < 170 pg/mL
- Serum vitamin B$_{12}$ levels in symptomatic patients: < 100 pg/mL
- The diagnosis is best confirmed by an elevated level of serum methylmalonic acid (> 1000 nmol/L) or serum homocysteine (> 16.2 mmol/L)
- The anemia of vitamin B$_{12}$ deficiency is typically moderate to severe with the MCV quite elevated (110–140 fL); however, MCV may be normal
- Peripheral blood smear is megaloblastic, defined as red blood cells that appear as macro-ovalocytes (although other shape changes are usually present) and neutrophils that are hypersegmented (6 [or greater]-lobed neutrophils or mean neutrophil lobe counts > 4)
- Reticulocyte count is reduced
- In severe cases, white blood cell count and platelet count are reduced
- Serum lactate dehydrogenase (LDH) is elevated and indirect bilirubin modestly increased

Diagnostic Procedures

- Bone marrow morphology is characteristic
  — Marked erythroid hyperplasia
  — Megaloblastic changes in erythroid series
  — Giant bands and metamyelocytes in myeloid series

7. Treatments

Medications

- Intramuscular or subcutaneous injections of 100 μg of vitamin B$_{12}$ are adequate for each dose
- Replacement is usually given daily for the first week, weekly for the first month, and then monthly for life
- Oral or sublingual methylcobalamin (1 mg/d) may be used instead of parenteral therapy once initial correction of the deficiency has occurred
- Oral or sublingual replacement is effective, even in pernicious anemia, since approximately 1% of the dose is absorbed in the intestine via passive diffusion in the absence of active transport
- Vitamin B$_{12}$ replacement must be continued indefinitely and serum vitamin B$_{12}$ levels must be monitored to ensure adequate replacement

- Simultaneous folic acid replacement (1 mg daily) is recommended for the first several months of vitamin B_{12} replacement
- Red blood cell transfusions are rarely needed despite the severity of anemia, but when given, diuretics are also recommended to avoid heart failure

8. Outcomes

Follow-Up

- Pernicious anemia is a lifelong disorder; if patients discontinue monthly therapy, the vitamin deficiency will recur
- Brisk reticulocytosis occurs 5 to 7 days after therapy, and the hematologic picture normalizes in 2 months
- Follow serum vitamin B_{12} level

Complications

- Nervous system complications include a complex neurologic syndrome (eg, altered cerebral function and dementia)
- Hypokalemia may complicate the first several days of parenteral vitamin B_{12} therapy in pernicious anemia, particularly if anemia is severe

Prognosis

- Patients with pernicious anemia respond to parenteral vitamin B_{12} therapy with immediate improvement in sense of well-being
- Nervous system manifestations are reversible if they are of relatively short duration (< 6 months) but may be permanent if treatment is not initiated promptly

SUGGESTED REFERENCES

Bunn HF. Vitamin B_{12} and pernicious anemia—the dawn of molecular medicine. *N Engl J Med.* 2014 Feb 20;370(8):773–776. [PMID: 24552327]

Oberley MJ et al. Laboratory testing for cobalamin deficiency in megaloblastic anemia. *Am J Hematol.* 2013 Jun;88(6):522–526. [PMID: 23423840]

Stabler SP. Clinical practice. Vitamin B_{12} deficiency. *N Engl J Med.* 2013 Jan 10;368(2):149–160. [PMID: 23301732]

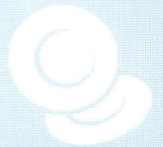

Gastrointestinal/Liver/Pancreas Disorders

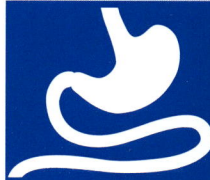

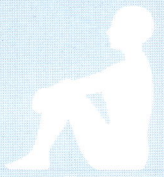

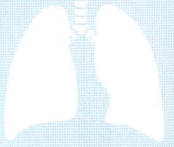

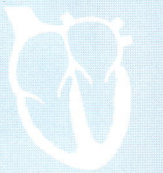

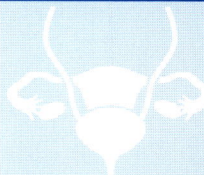

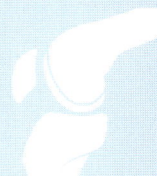

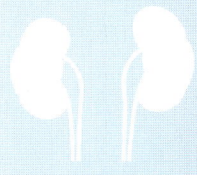

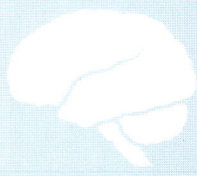

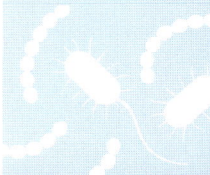

27

Acute Cholecystitis

A 52-year-old man presents to the emergency room with right upper quadrant (RUQ) abdominal pain for 8 hours. He states that it is steady and unrelenting, and began about 1 hour after he ate a hamburger with French fries. Since the pain began, he has experienced episodic nausea and he vomited once. On physical examination, he is febrile and extremely tender to palpation in the RUQ of the abdomen, with a positive Murphy sign on inspiration. The white blood cell (WBC) count is 19,000/μL (19 × 10^9/L). An abdominal ultrasound reveals a thickened gallbladder with multiple gallstones and pericholecystic fluid.

LEARNING OBJECTIVES

▶ Learn the clinical manifestations and objective findings of cholecystitis
▶ Understand the factors that predispose to both gallstone and acalculous cholecystitis
▶ Know the differential diagnosis of cholecystitis
▶ Learn the medical and surgical treatment for cholecystitis, and which patients can avoid surgery

QUESTIONS

1. What are the salient features of this patient's problem?
2. How do you think through his problem?
3. What are the key features, including essentials of diagnosis and general considerations, of cholecystitis?
4. What are the symptoms and signs of cholecystitis?
5. What is the differential diagnosis of cholecystitis?
6. What are laboratory and imaging findings in cholecystitis?
7. What are the treatments for cholecystitis?
8. What are the outcomes, including follow-up, complications, and prognosis, of cholecystitis?
9. When should patients with cholecystitis be admitted to the hospital?

ANSWERS

1. Salient Features

RUQ abdominal pain; onset after fatty meal; nausea and vomiting; fever and elevated WBC count; positive Murphy sign; thickened gallbladder and pericholecystic fluid on abdominal ultrasound

2. How to Think Through

Based solely on the history and physical examination in this case (before the ultrasound), what causes of RUQ pain are important to consider in the differential diagnosis? (Acute cholecystitis, acute pancreatitis, acute hepatitis, intra-abdominal abscess, right lower lobe pneumonia, and cardiac ischemia.) Could this be biliary colic? (The duration and unrelenting nature of the pain, along with the fever, indicate true inflammation rather than the transient obstruction of biliary colic.) How would the presence of jaundice change your assessment? (Cholangitis, hepatitis, and hemolysis would rise on the differential diagnosis.) Would the presence of gallstones alone on ultrasound be sufficient to make the diagnosis of cholecystitis? (No. Cholelithiasis is common. The diagnosis of cholecystitis is a clinical one based on findings from the history, examination, WBC, and ultrasound. Gallbladder wall edema on ultrasound strongly suggests cholecystitis.)

What are the initial steps in his management? (Intravenous fluids, analgesia, and surgical consultation.) Are antibiotics indicated? (Yes, given the fever and leukocytosis. About 40% of patients have positive biliary cultures, especially with *Escherichia coli*. This patient would almost certainly receive empiric antibiotics.) When should surgery be performed? (Immediate cholecystectomy improves outcomes, and would be optimal in this case. However, medical comorbidities or acute shock confer high surgical risk and may necessitate delay in surgery.) How are high-risk patients managed? (Often with percutaneous cholecystostomy and antibiotics, with subsequent cholecystectomy.)

3. Key Features

Essentials of Diagnosis
- Steady, severe pain and tenderness in the abdominal RUQ or epigastrium
- Nausea and vomiting
- Fever and leukocytosis

General Considerations
- Associated with gallstones in over 90% of cases
- Occurs when a stone becomes impacted in the cystic duct and inflammation develops behind the obstruction
- Acalculous cholecystitis should be considered when
  — Unexplained fever or RUQ pain occurs within 2 to 4 weeks of major surgery
  — A critically ill patient has had no oral intake for a prolonged period
- Acute cholecystitis may be caused by infectious agents (eg, cytomegalovirus, crypto-sporidiosis, or microsporidiosis) in patients with AIDS or by vasculitis (eg, polyarteritis nodosa, Henoch–Schönlein purpura)

4. Symptoms and Signs
- The acute attack is often precipitated by a large or fatty meal
- Relatively sudden, severe, and steady pain that is localized to the abdominal RUQ or epigastrium and that may gradually subside over a period of 12 to 18 hours
- Vomiting occurs in about 75% of patients and affords variable relief in 50%

- RUQ abdominal tenderness
  — Almost always present
  — Usually associated with muscle guarding and rebound pain
- A palpable gallbladder is present in about 15% of cases
- Jaundice
  — Present in about 25% of cases
  — When persistent or severe, suggests the possibility of choledocholithiasis
- Fever is usually present

5. Differential Diagnosis

- Perforated peptic ulcer
- Acute pancreatitis
- Appendicitis
- Perforated colonic carcinoma or diverticulum of hepatic flexure
- Acute hepatitis or liver abscess
- Pneumonia with pleurisy on right side
- Myocardial infarction
- Radicular pain in T6–T10 dermatome, eg, preeruptive zoster

6. Laboratory and Imaging Findings

Laboratory Tests

- The WBC count is usually high (12,000–15,000/µL [12–15 × 10⁹/L])
- Total serum bilirubin values of 1 to 4 mg/dL (17.1–68.4 µmol/L) may be seen even in the absence of common bile duct obstruction
- Serum aminotransferase and alkaline phosphatase levels are often elevated—the former as high as 300 units/mL, or even higher when associated with ascending cholangitis
- Serum amylase may also be moderately elevated

Imaging Studies

- Plain films of the abdomen may show radiopaque gallstones in 15% of cases
- ^{99m}Tc hepatobiliary imaging (using iminodiacetic acid compounds) (HIDA scan)
  — Useful in demonstrating an obstructed cystic duct, which is the cause of acute cholecystitis in most patients
  — This test is reliable if the bilirubin is under 5 mg/dL (85.5 µmol/L) (98% sensitivity and 81% specificity for acute cholecystitis)
- RUQ abdominal ultrasound
  — May show gallstones
  — However, it is not sensitive for acute cholecystitis (67% sensitivity, 82% specificity)
- CT may show complications of acute cholecystitis, such as gallbladder perforation or gangrene

7. Treatments

Medications

- Cholecystitis will usually subside on a conservative regimen (withholding of oral feedings, intravenous alimentation, analgesics, and antibiotics, eg, cefoperazone 1 to 2 g intravenously every 12 hours)
- Meperidine or morphine may be given for pain

Surgery

- Cholecystectomy (generally laparoscopic) should be performed within 24 hours after admission to the hospital for acute cholecystitis because of the high risk of recurrent attacks (up to 10% by 1 month and over 30% by 1 year)
- Compared with delayed surgery, surgery within 24 hours is associated with a reduced risk of major bile duct injury and death

- Surgical treatment of chronic cholecystitis is the same as for acute cholecystitis
  — If indicated, cholangiography can be performed during laparoscopic cholecystectomy
  — Choledocholithiasis can also be excluded by either preoperative or postoperative endoscopic retrograde or magnetic resonance cholangiopancreatography

Therapeutic Procedures
- In high-risk patients, the following may postpone or even avoid the need for surgery
  — Ultrasound-guided aspiration of the gallbladder
  — Percutaneous cholecystostomy
  — Endoscopic insertion of a stent or nasobiliary drain into the gallbladder
- Cholecystectomy is mandatory when there is evidence of gangrene or perforation

8. Outcomes

Follow-Up
- If treating nonsurgically, watch the patient (especially if diabetic or elderly) for
  — Recurrent symptoms of cholecystitis
  — Evidence of gangrene of the gallbladder
  — Cholangitis

Complications
Gangrene of the Gallbladder
- After 24 to 48 hours, the following suggests severe inflammation and possible gangrene of the gallbladder
  — Continuation or progression of RUQ abdominal pain
  — Tenderness
  — Muscle guarding
  — Fever
  — Leukocytosis
- Necrosis may develop without specific signs in the obese, diabetic, elderly, or immuno-suppressed patient
- May lead to gallbladder perforation, usually with formation of a pericholecystic abscess, and rarely to generalized peritonitis
- Other serious acute complications include emphysematous cholecystitis (secondary infection with a gas-forming organism) and empyema

Chronic Cholecystitis
- Chronic cholecystitis results from repeated episodes of acute cholecystitis or chronic irritation of the gallbladder wall by stones
- Calculi are usually present

Other Complications
- Gallbladder villi may undergo polypoid enlargement due to cholesterol deposition ("strawberry gallbladder," cholesterolosis) (4%–5%)
- Marked adenomatous hyperplasia of the gallbladder resembles a myoma (adenomyomatosis)
- Hydrops of the gallbladder results when acute cholecystitis subsides but cystic duct obstruction persists, producing distention of the gallbladder with a clear mucoid fluid
- A stone in the neck of the gallbladder may compress the common bile duct and cause jaundice (Mirizzi syndrome)
- Cholelithiasis with chronic cholecystitis may be associated with
  — Acute exacerbations of gallbladder inflammation
  — Bile duct stone
  — Fistulization to the bowel
  — Pancreatitis
  — Carcinoma of the gallbladder (rarely)

- Calcified (porcelain) gallbladder may have a high association with gallbladder carcinoma (particularly when the calcification is mucosal rather than intramural) and appears to be an indication for cholecystectomy

Prognosis
- The mortality rate of cholecystectomy is < 0.2%
- Hepatobiliary tract surgery in the elderly has a higher mortality rate
- Mortality rate is also higher in patients who have diabetes mellitus
- A successful surgical procedure is generally followed by complete resolution of symptoms

9. When to Admit
- All patients with acute cholecystitis should be hospitalized

SUGGESTED REFERENCES

de Mestral C et al. Comparative operative outcomes of early and delayed cholecystectomy for acute cholecystitis: a population-based propensity score analysis. *Ann Surg.* 2014 Jan;259(1):10–15. [PMID: 23979286]

Gutt CN et al. Acute cholecystitis: early versus delayed cholecystectomy, a multicenter randomized trial (ACDC study, NCT00447304). *Ann Surg.* 2013 Sep;258(3):385–393. [PMID: 24022431]

Hasan MK et al. Endoscopic management of acute cholecystitis. *Gastrointest Endosc Clin N Am.* 2013 Apr;23(2):453–459. [PMID: 23540969]

Karamanos E et al. Effect of diabetes on outcomes in patients undergoing emergent cholecystectomy for acute cholecystitis. *World J Surg.* 2013 Oct;37(10):2257–2264. [PMID: 23677561]

Pitt HA. Patient value is superior with early surgery for acute cholecystitis. *Ann Surg.* 2014 Jan;259(1):16–17. [PMID: 24326747]

Cirrhosis

28

A 63-year-old man with a long history of alcoholism presents to his new primary care clinician with a 6-month history of increasing abdominal girth. He has also noted easy bruising and worsening fatigue. He denies any history of gastrointestinal (GI) bleeding. He says he drinks three or four cocktails at night but is trying to cut down. Physical examination reveals a cachectic man who appears older than his stated age. Blood pressure is 108/70 mm Hg. His scleras are anicteric. His neck veins are flat, and chest examination demonstrates gynecomastia and multiple spider angiomas. Abdominal examination is significant for a protuberant abdomen with a detectable fluid wave, shifting dullness, and an enlarged spleen. The liver edge is difficult to appreciate. He has trace pitting pedal edema. Laboratory evaluation shows anemia, mild thrombocytopenia, and an elevated prothrombin time. An abdominal ultrasound shows splenomegaly, significant ascites, and a shrunken, heterogeneous liver consistent with cirrhosis.

LEARNING OBJECTIVES

▶ Learn the clinical manifestations and objective findings of cirrhosis
▶ Understand the factors that predispose to cirrhosis
▶ Know the differential diagnosis of cirrhosis
▶ Learn what laboratory and diagnostic imaging findings are typical of cirrhosis
▶ Learn the treatments for cirrhosis
▶ Understand the complications and prognosis of cirrhosis

QUESTIONS

1. What are the salient features of this patient's problem?

2. How do you think through his problem?

3. What are the key features, including essentials of diagnosis, general considerations, and demographics, of cirrhosis?

4. What are the symptoms and signs of cirrhosis?

5. What is the differential diagnosis of cirrhosis?

6. What are laboratory, imaging, and procedural findings in cirrhosis?

7. What are the treatments for cirrhosis?

8. What are the outcomes, including complications and prognosis, of cirrhosis?

9. When should patients with cirrhosis be referred to a specialist or admitted to the hospital?

ANSWERS

1. Salient Features

Chronic alcoholism; ascites, coagulopathy, and thrombocytopenia; peripheral edema, gynecomastia, spider angiomas, and splenomegaly; ultrasound demonstrating a shrunken liver

2. How to Think Through

Portal hypertension, inadequate protein synthesis, and inadequate clearance of circulating estrogens explain most of this patient's symptoms and signs. Which elements are due to portal hypertension? (Ascites, lower extremity edema, splenomegaly, and thrombocytopenia due to splenic sequestration.) What other complications of portal hypertension is he at risk for? (Infection, eg, bacterial peritonitis, hepatocellular carcinoma [HCC], hepatorenal syndrome, and encephalopathy.) How would you determine if he has encephalopathy? What would you expect his liver enzymes to show? His liver biopsy? Besides chronic heavy alcohol intake (his major risk factor), what are other major risk factors for cirrhosis? How would you test for each?

Is his cirrhosis currently compensated or decompensated? How should his ascites be treated? (Sodium restriction; a loop diuretic and aldosterone receptor blocker; large volume paracentesis.) What data are needed to establish his prognosis? (Serum creatinine, albumin, and bilirubin; imaging to evaluate for HCC, endoscopy, and esophageal varices.) What scoring systems can help establish disease severity? Is he a candidate for liver transplantation? (Not while actively drinking alcohol.)

3. Key Features

Essentials of Diagnosis

- End result of injury that leads to both fibrosis and regenerating nodules
- May be reversible if cause is removed
- Clinical features result from hepatic cell dysfunction, portosystemic shunting, and portal hypertension

General Considerations

- The most common histologic classification of cirrhosis is micronodular, macronodular, and mixed
- Each form may be seen at different stages of the disease
- Risk factors
  — Chronic viral hepatitis
  — Alcoholism
  — Drug toxicity
  — Autoimmune and metabolic liver diseases
  — Miscellaneous disorders
- Many patients have more than one risk factor (eg, chronic hepatitis and alcoholism)
- Three clinical stages
  — Compensated
  — Compensated with varices
  — Decompensated (ascites, variceal bleeding, encephalopathy, or jaundice)

Micronodular cirrhosis
- Regenerating nodules are < 1 mm
- Typical of alcoholic liver disease (Laennec cirrhosis)

Macronodular cirrhosis
- Characterized by larger nodules, up to several centimeters in diameter, that may contain central veins
- Corresponds to postnecrotic (posthepatitic) cirrhosis; may follow episodes of massive necrosis and stromal collapse

Demographics
- Twelfth leading cause of death in the United States
- Mexican Americans and African Americans have a higher frequency of cirrhosis than whites because of a higher rate of risk factors
- Celiac disease appears to be associated with an increased risk of cirrhosis

4. Symptoms and Signs
- Can be asymptomatic for long periods
- Symptoms are usually insidious in onset, but may be abrupt
- Fatigue, disturbed sleep, muscle cramps, anorexia, and weight loss are common
- Nausea and occasional vomiting
- Reduced muscle strength and exercise capacity
- Jaundice—usually not an initial sign—is mild at its onset, then increases in severity
- Abdominal pain can result from hepatic enlargement and stretching of Glisson capsule or from ascites
- Hematemesis is the presenting symptom in 15% to 25% of cases
- Fever
  — May be a presenting symptom in up to 35%
  — Usually reflects associated alcoholic hepatitis, spontaneous bacterial peritonitis, or intercurrent infection
- Amenorrhea in women
- Erectile dysfunction, loss of libido, sterility, and gynecomastia in men
- In 70% of cases, the liver is enlarged and firm with a sharp or nodular edge; the left lobe may predominate
- Splenomegaly occurs in 35% to 50%
- Ascites, pleural effusions, peripheral edema, and ecchymoses are late findings
- Relative adrenal insufficiency appears common in advanced cirrhosis, even in absence of sepsis

Encephalopathy
- Characterized by
  — Day–night reversal
  — Asterixis
  — Tremor
  — Dysarthria
  — Delirium
  — Drowsiness
  — Coma
- Occurs late except when precipitated by an acute hepatic insult or an episode of GI bleeding or infection

Skin
- Spider telangiectasias on the upper half of the body
- Palmar erythema, Dupuytren contractures
- Glossitis and cheilosis from vitamin deficiencies
- Dilated superficial veins of the abdomen and thorax that fill from below when compressed

5. Differential Diagnosis

- Chronic viral hepatitis
- Alcoholism
- Nonalcoholic fatty liver disease
- Metabolic, eg, hemochromatosis, α_1-antiprotease deficiency, Wilson disease, Celiac disease (gluten enteropathy)
- Primary biliary cirrhosis
- Secondary biliary cirrhosis (chronic obstruction due to stone, stricture, and neoplasm)
- Cryptogenic cirrhosis
- Heart failure or constrictive pericarditis
- Hereditary hemorrhagic telangiectasia

6. Laboratory, Imaging, and Procedural Findings

Laboratory Tests

- Laboratory abnormalities are either absent or minimal in early or compensated cirrhosis
- Anemia
  — Usually macrocytic, from suppression of erythropoiesis by alcohol, folate deficiency, hypersplenism, hemolysis, and blood loss from the GI tract
- White blood cell count
  — May be low, reflecting hypersplenism
  — May be high, suggesting infection
- Thrombocytopenia is secondary to
  — Marrow suppression by alcohol
  — Sepsis
  — Folate deficiency
  — Splenic sequestration
- Hypoalbuminemia and prolongation of the prothrombin time decreased synthetic function
- Modest elevations of serum aspartate aminotransferase (AST) and alkaline phosphatase and progressive elevation of serum bilirubin
- γ-Globulin is increased and may be very high in autoimmune hepatitis
- Vitamin D deficiency has been reported in 91% of patients with cirrhosis
- Patients with alcoholic cirrhosis may have elevated serum cardiac troponin I and brain natriuretic peptide levels
- Combinations of tests (eg, AST and platelet count) are under study for predicting cirrhosis in patients with chronic liver diseases such as chronic hepatitis C

Imaging Studies

- Ultrasonography
  — Can assess liver size and consistency and detect ascites or hepatic nodules, including small hepatocellular carcinomas
  — May establish patency of the splenic, portal, and hepatic veins together with Doppler studies
- Hepatic nodules can be characterized by contrast-enhanced computed tomography (CT) or magnetic resonance imaging (MRI)
- Nodules suspicious for malignancy may be biopsied under ultrasound or CT guidance

Diagnostic Procedures

- Esophagogastroduodenoscopy confirms the presence of varices and detects specific causes of bleeding
- Liver biopsy confirms cirrhosis, HCC
- Paracentesis and ascitic fluid analysis to rule out spontaneous bacterial peritonitis
- Wedged hepatic vein pressure measurement may establish the presence and cause of portal hypertension

7. Treatments

Medications

Ascites and Edema

- Restrict sodium intake to 400 to 800 mg/d
- Restrict fluid intake (800–1000 mL/d) for hyponatremia (sodium < 125 mEq/L)
- Ascites may rapidly decrease on bed rest and dietary sodium restriction alone
- Use spironolactone (usually with furosemide) if there is no response to salt restriction
  — The initial dose of spironolactone is 100 mg daily orally
  — May be increased by 100 mg every 3 to 5 days (up to a maximal conventional daily dose of 400 mg/d, though higher doses have been used) until diuresis is achieved, typically preceded by a rise in the urinary sodium concentration
  — Monitor for hyperkalemia
- Substitute amiloride, 5 to 10 mg daily orally, if painful gynecomastia develops from spironolactone
- Diuresis can be augmented with the addition of furosemide, 40 to 160 mg daily orally. Monitor blood pressure, urinary output, mental status, and serum electrolytes, especially potassium

Anemia

- Iron deficiency anemia: ferrous sulfate, 0.3 g enteric-coated tablets, 3 times daily orally after meals
- Macrocytic anemia associated with alcoholism: folic acid, 1 mg/d once daily orally
- Packed red blood cell transfusions may be necessary in GI bleeding to replace blood loss

Hemorrhagic Tendency

- Treat severe hypoprothrombinemia with vitamin K (eg, phytonadione, 5 mg once daily orally or subcutaneously)
- If this treatment is ineffective, use large volumes of fresh frozen plasma. Because the effect is transient, plasma infusions are indicated only for active bleeding or before an invasive procedure
- Use of recombinant factor VII may be an alternative
- Hepatic encephalopathy
- Lactulose or polyethylene glycol 3350-electrolyte solution
- Rifaximin

Surgery

- Liver transplantation is indicated in selected cases of irreversible, progressive liver disease
- Absolute contraindications include
  — Malignancy (except small hepatocellular carcinomas in a cirrhotic liver)
  — Sepsis
  — Advanced cardiopulmonary disease (except hepatopulmonary syndrome)

Therapeutic Procedures

- Most important is abstinence from alcohol
- Diet
  — Should have adequate calories (25–35 kcal/kg/d) in compensated cirrhosis and 35 to 45 kcal/kg/d in those with malnutrition
  — Protein should include 1.0 to 1.5 g/kg/d in compensated cirrhosis and 1.5 g/kg/d in those with malnutrition
  — For hepatic encephalopathy, protein intake should be reduced to 60 to 80 g/d
- Vitamin supplementation is desirable
- Patients should receive following vaccines
  — Hepatitis A virus (HAV), hepatitis B virus (HBV)
  — Pneumococcal
  — Influenza (yearly)

- The goal of weight loss with ascites without associated peripheral edema should not exceed 0.5 to 0.7 kg/d
- Large-volume paracentesis (> 5 L) is effective in patients with
  — Massive ascites and consequent respiratory compromise
  — Ascites refractory to diuretics
  — Intolerable diuretic side effects
- Transjugular intrahepatic portosystemic shunt (TIPS)
  — In refractory ascites, reduces ascites recurrence and the risk of hepatorenal syndrome.
  — Preferred to peritoneovenous shunts because of the high rate of complications from the latter
  — Increases the risk of hepatic encephalopathy compared with repeated large-volume paracentesis

8. Outcomes

Complications
- Upper GI tract bleeding may occur from
  — Varices
  — Portal hypertensive gastropathy
  — Gastroduodenal ulcer
- Portal vein thrombosis, which also causes varices
- Hepatorenal syndrome occurs in up to 10% of patients with advanced cirrhosis
- Spontaneous bacterial peritonitis; performance of diagnostic paracentesis in patients with new ascites and hospitalization can reduce mortality in cirrhosis
- Liver failure may be precipitated by alcoholism, surgery, and infection
- The risk of carcinoma of the liver is increased greatly in patients with cirrhosis
- Hepatic Kupffer cell (reticuloendothelial) dysfunction and decreased opsonic activity lead to an increased risk of systemic infection
- Osteoporosis

Prognosis
- Prognostic scoring systems for cirrhosis include the Child–Turcotte–Pugh score (Table 28-1) and the Model for End-Stage Liver Disease (MELD) score

Table 28-1. Child–Turcotte–Pugh and model for end-stage liver disease (MELD) scoring systems for staging cirrhosis.

Child–Turcotte–Pugh Scoring System			
Numerical Score			
Parameter	**1**	**2**	**3**
Ascites	None	Slight	Moderate to severe
Encephalopathy	None	Slight to moderate	Moderate to severe
Bilirubin, mg/dL (µmol/L)	< 2.0 (34.2)	2–3 (34.2–51.3)	> 3.0 (51.3)
Albumin, mg/dL (g/L)	> 3.5 (35)	2.8–3.5 (28–35)	< 2.8 (28)
Prothrombin time, seconds increased	1–3	4–6	> 6.0
Total Numerical Score and Corresponding Child Class			
		Score	**Class**
		5–6	A
		7–9	B
		10–15	C

MELD Scoring System

$$MELD = 11.2 \log_e (INR) + 3.78 \log_e (bilirubin [mg/dL]) + 9.57 \log_e (creatinine [mg/dL]) + 6.43 \quad (range\ 6{-}40).$$

INR, international normalized ratio.

- MELD is used to determine priorities for liver transplantation
- In patients with a low MELD score (< 21), a low serum sodium concentration (< 130 mEq/L), an elevated hepatic venous pressure gradient, and persistent ascites predict a high mortality rate
- Only 50% of patients with severe hepatic dysfunction (serum albumin < 3 mg/dL, bilirubin > 3 mg/dL, ascites, encephalopathy, cachexia, and upper GI bleeding) survive 6 months
- The risk of death is associated with
  — Muscle wasting
  — Age ≥ 65 years
  — Mean arterial pressure < 82 mm Hg
  — Chronic kidney disease
  — Cognitive dysfunction
  — Ventilatory insufficiency
  — Prothrombin time ≥ 16 seconds
  — Delayed and suboptimal treatment of sepsis
  — Secondary infections
- Liver transplantation has markedly improved survival, particularly for patients referred early for evaluation

9. When to Refer and When to Admit

When to Refer
- For liver biopsy
- Before the MELD score is ≥ 14
- For upper endoscopy to screen for gastroesophageal varices

When to Admit
- GI bleeding
- Stage 3 to 4 hepatic encephalopathy
- Worsening kidney function
- Severe hyponatremia
- Serious infection
- Profound hypoxia
- Palliative care for end-stage liver disease

SUGGESTED REFERENCES

Fagundes C et al. A modified acute kidney injury classification for diagnosis and risk stratification of impairment of kidney function in cirrhosis. *J Hepatol.* 2013 Sep;59(3):474–481. [PMID: 23669284]

Ge PS et al. The changing role of beta-blocker therapy in patients with cirrhosis. *J Hepatol.* 2014 Mar;60(3):643–653. [PMID: 24076364]

Kimer N et al. Systematic review with meta-analysis: the effects of rifaximin in hepatic encephalopathy. *Aliment Pharmacol Ther.* 2014 Jul;40(2):123-132. [PMID: 24849268]

Kim JJ et al. Delayed paracentesis is associated with increased in-hospital mortality in patients with spontaneous bacterial peritonitis. *Am J Gastroenterol.* 2014 Sep;109(9):1436–1442. [PMID: 25091061]

Machicao VI et al. Pulmonary complications in chronic liver disease. *Hepatology.* 2014 Apr;59(4):1627–1637. [PMID: 24089295]

Mandorfer M et al. Nonselective beta blockers increase risk for hepatorenal syndrome and death in patients with cirrhosis and spontaneous bacterial peritonitis. *Gastroenterology.* 2014 Jun;146(7):1680–1690. [PMID: 24631577]

Martin P et al. Evaluation for liver transplantation in adults: 2013 practice guideline by the American Association for the Study of Liver Diseases and the American Society of Transplantation. *Hepatology.* 2014 Mar;59(3):1144–1165. [PMID: 24716201]

Mullen KD et al. Rifaximin is safe and well tolerated for long-term maintenance of remission from overt hepatic encephalopathy. *Clin Gastroenterol Hepatol.* 2014 Aug;12(8):1390–1397. [PMID: 24365449]

Orman ES et al. Paracentesis is associated with reduced mortality in patients hospitalized with cirrhosis and ascites. *Clin Gastroenterol Hepatol.* 2014 Mar;12(3):496–503. [PMID: 23978348]

Poonja Z et al. Patients with cirrhosis and denied liver transplants rarely receive adequate palliative care or appropriate management. *Clin Gastroenterol Hepatol.* 2014 Apr;12(4):692–698. [PMID: 23978345]

Rahimi RS et al. Lactulose vs polyethylene glycol 3350-electrolyte solution for treatment of overt hepatic encephalopathy: the HELP randomized clinical trial. *JAMA Intern Med.* 2014 Nov 1;174(11):1727–1733. [PMID: 25243839]

Runyon BA et al. Introduction to the revised American Association for the Study of Liver Diseases Practice Guideline management of adult patients with ascites due to cirrhosis 2012. *Hepatology.* 2013 Apr;57(4):1651–1653. [PMID: 23463403]

Salerno F et al. Albumin infusion improves outcomes of patients with spontaneous bacterial peritonitis: a meta-analysis of randomized trials. *Clin Gastroenterol Hepatol.* 2013 Feb;11(2):123–130. [PMID: 23178229]

Singal AK et al. Prevalence and in-hospital mortality trends of infections among patients with cirrhosis: a nationwide study of hospitalised patients in the United States. *Aliment Pharmacol Ther.* 2014 Jul;40(1):105–112. [PMID: 24832591]

Tsochatzis EA et al. Liver cirrhosis. *Lancet.* 2014 May 17;383(9930):1749–1761. [PMID: 24480518]

Vilstrup H et al. Hepatic encephalopathy in chronic liver disease: 2014 Practice Guideline by the American Association for the Study of Liver Diseases and the European Association for the Study of the Liver. *Hepatology.* 2014 Aug;60(2):715–735. [PMID: 25042402]

Colorectal Cancer

29

A 54-year-old man presents to the clinic for a routine checkup. He is well, with no physical complaints. The history is remarkable only for a father with colon cancer at age 55. Physical examination is normal. Cancer screening is discussed, and the patient is sent home with fecal occult blood testing supplies. The fecal occult blood test results are positive. Subsequent colonoscopy reveals a villous adenoma as well as a 2-cm carcinoma.

LEARNING OBJECTIVES

▶ Learn about recommended screening tests for colorectal cancer
▶ Learn the clinical manifestations and objective findings of colorectal cancer
▶ Understand the factors that predispose to colorectal cancer
▶ Know the differential diagnosis of colorectal cancer
▶ Learn the treatment for colorectal cancer
▶ Know how to prevent colorectal cancer

QUESTIONS

1. What are the salient features of this patient's situation?

2. How do you think through his problem?

3. What are the key features, including essentials of diagnosis, general considerations, and demographics, of colorectal cancer?

4. What are the symptoms and signs of colorectal cancer?

5. What is the differential diagnosis of colorectal cancer?

6. What are laboratory, imaging, and procedural findings in colorectal cancer?

7. What are the treatments for colorectal cancer?

8. What are the outcomes, including follow-up, prognosis, and prevention, of colorectal cancer?

9. When should patients with colorectal cancer be referred to a specialist or admitted to the hospital?

ANSWERS

1. Salient Features

Family history of colon cancer at similar age; routine screening after age 50 years; fecal occult blood test positive; and subsequent colonoscopy with both an adenoma and a carcinoma

2. How to Think Through

What are the recommended colon cancer screening modalities? When does screening start for a patient with no family history of polyposis or colon cancer? (At age 50 years.) When should screening have begun for the patient in this case? (10 years earlier than the age at which his father was diagnosed.) What pathological characteristics of polyps found on colonoscopy are considered high risk for progression to cancer? (Tubular adenoma, villous adenoma, serrated polyp, and, less commonly, hyperplastic polyp.) In addition to family history, what are the other known risk factors for colon cancer? (Inflammatory bowel disease; diets low in fiber, high in red meat and fat; black > white race.)

How does right-sided colon cancer present? How does left-sided colon cancer present?

What is the next step for this patient? (Computed tomography [CT] scan of the chest, abdomen, and pelvis for preoperative staging.) For which stages of colon cancer is chemotherapy a recommended part of the treatment?

3. Key Features

Essentials of Diagnosis

- Personal or family history of adenomatous polyps or colorectal cancer are important risk factors
- Symptoms or signs depend on tumor location
- Proximal colon cancer—fecal occult blood, anemia
- Distal colon cancer—change in bowel habits, hematochezia
- Diagnosis established with colonoscopy

General Considerations

- Colon cancers are usually adenocarcinomas
- About 50% occur distal to the splenic flexure (descending rectosigmoid) within reach of detection by flexible sigmoidoscopy
- Most colorectal cancers arise from malignant transformation of an adenomatous polyp (tubular, tubulovillous, or villous adenoma), serrated polyp (traditional serrated adenoma, or sessile serrated adenoma), or less commonly, hyperplastic polyp
- Up to 5% of colorectal cancers are caused by inherited autosomal dominant germline mutations resulting in polyposis syndromes or hereditary nonpolyposis colorectal cancer
- Risk factors
  — Age
  — History of colorectal cancer or adenomatous polyps
  — Family history of colorectal cancer
  — Inflammatory bowel disease (ulcerative colitis and Crohn colitis)
  — Diets rich in fats and red meat
  — Race (higher risk in blacks than in whites)

Demographics

- Second leading cause of death due to malignancy in the United States
- Colorectal cancer will develop in ~6% of Americans and 40% of those will die of the disease
- In 2014, there were an estimated 96,830 new cases of colon cancer and 40,000 new cases of rectal cancer in the United States, with combined estimated 50,310 deaths

4. Symptoms and Signs

- Adenocarcinomas grow slowly and may be asymptomatic
- Right-sided colon cancers cause
  — Iron deficiency anemia
  — Fatigue
  — Weakness from chronic blood loss
- Left-sided colon cancers cause
  — Obstructive symptoms
  — Colicky abdominal pain
  — Change in bowel habits
  — Constipation alternating with loose stools
  — Stool streaked with blood
- Rectal cancers cause
  — Rectal tenesmus
  — Urgency
  — Recurrent hematochezia
- Weight loss is uncommon unless cancer is metastatic
- Physical examination usually normal, except in advanced disease: mass may be palpable in the abdomen
- Hepatomegaly suggests metastatic spread

5. Differential Diagnosis

- Diverticulosis or diverticulitis
- Hemorrhoids
- Adenomatous polyps
- Ischemic colitis
- Inflammatory bowel disease
- Irritable bowel syndrome
- Infectious colitis
- Iron deficiency from another cause

6. Laboratory, Imaging, and Procedural Findings

Laboratory Tests

- Complete blood cell count may reveal iron deficiency anemia
- Elevated liver tests, particularly the alkaline phosphatase, are suggestive of metastatic disease
- Fecal occult blood tests are positive
- Carcinoembryonic antigen (CEA) level should normalize after complete surgical resection; persistently elevated levels suggest the presence of persistent disease and warrant further evaluation

Imaging Studies

- Barium enema or CT colonography ("virtual colonoscopy") for initial diagnosis, if colonoscopy not available
- Chest, abdominal, and pelvic CT scan for preoperative staging
- Pelvic magnetic resonance imaging (MRI) and endorectal ultrasonography may guide operative management of rectal cancer

Diagnostic Procedures

- Colonoscopy is the diagnostic procedure of choice because it visualizes the whole colon and permits biopsy of lesions
- Staging by the TNM (tumor, node, metastasis) system correlates with the patient's long-term survival; it is used to determine which patients should receive adjuvant therapy

7. Treatments

Medications

Stage II Disease

- Adjuvant chemotherapy is beneficial for persons at high risk for recurrence

Stage III Disease

- Postoperative adjuvant chemotherapy
  — Significantly increases disease-free survival as well as overall survival by up to 30%
  — Recommended for all fit patients
- FOLFOX (oxaliplatin, fluorouracil, and leucovorin) is the preferred adjuvant therapy for most patients with Stage III disease
- The addition of a biologic agent (bevacizumab or cetuximab) to FOLFOX does not improve outcomes in the adjuvant setting

Stage IV (Metastatic) Disease

- FOLFOX or FOLFIRI (addition of irinotecan to fluorouracil and leucovorin)
  — Preferred first-line regimens
  — Median survival is improved (15–20 months)
- Patients progressing with one regimen may respond to the alternative regimen, prolonging mean survival to > 20 months
- Aflibercept, a novel antiangiogenic agent, is FDA-approved for use in second-line colorectal cancer in combination with FOLFIRI
- Biological agents (bevacizumab, cetuximab, panitumumab, and ramucirumab,) demonstrate further improvement in response rates in stage IV disease
- Regorafenib, a multitargeted kinase inhibitor, is FDA-approved for patients with metastatic, refractory colorectal cancer after progression on standard regimens

Surgery

- Resection of the primary colonic or rectal cancer
- Regional lymph node removal to assist in staging
- For rectal carcinoma, in selected patients, transanal excision
- For all other patients with rectal cancer, low anterior resection with a colorectal anastomosis or an abdominoperineal resection with a colostomy
- For unresectable rectal cancer, diverting colostomy, radiation therapy, laser fulguration, or placement of an expandable wire stent
- For metastatic disease, resection of isolated liver or lung metastases

Therapeutic Procedures

- Local ablative techniques (cryosurgery, embolization) for unresectable hepatic metastases
- Following surgical resection with total mesorectal excision, adjuvant 5-FU–based therapy (generally with the FOLFOX regimen, extrapolating from its benefit in patients with similarly staged colon cancers) is recommended for a total of approximately 6 months of perioperative therapy including any neoadjuvant chemoradiation

8. Outcomes

Follow-Up

- After resection surgery, patients should be evaluated every 3 to 6 months for 2 years and then every 6 months for a total of 5 years with
  — History
  — Physical examination
  — Fecal occult blood testing
  — Liver tests
  — Serum CEA level
- A rise in CEA level that had normalized initially after surgery is suggestive of cancer recurrence

- Obtain colonoscopy
  — Twelve months after surgical resection for persons who had complete preoperative colonoscopy
  — Three to six months postoperatively for persons who did not have complete preoperative colonoscopy
  — If negative, then repeat every 3 to 5 years thereafter
- Change in the patient's clinical picture, abnormal liver tests, or a rising CEA level warrant chest radiography and abdominal CT

Prognosis

- Colorectal cancer mortality has decreased by approximately 35% between 1990 and 2007, possibly due to improved screening and treatment modalities
- Five-year survival rates
  — Stage I—90% to 100%, even with no adjuvant therapy
  — Stage II (node-negative disease)—80%
  — Stage III (node-positive disease)—30% to 50%
- Long-term survival rates
  — Stage I— > 90%
  — Stage II— > 70% to 85%
  — Stage III with fewer than 4 positive lymph nodes—67%
  — Stage III with > 4 positive lymph nodes—33%
  — Stage IV—5% to 7%
- For each stage, rectal cancers have a worse prognosis

Prevention

- Screening for colorectal neoplasms should be offered to every patient age > 50 years (Table 29-1)
- Chemoprevention
  — Prolonged regular use of aspirin and other nonsteroidal anti-inflammatory drugs may decrease the risk of colorectal neoplasia
  — However, routine use as chemoprevention agents is not recommended currently
- Prospective studies have not shown a reduction in colon cancer or recurrence of adenomatous polyps with diets that are low in fat or high in fiber, fruits or vegetables or with calcium, folate, β-carotene, or vitamins A, C, D, or E supplements

Table 29-1. Recommendations for colorectal cancer screening.

Average-Risk Individuals ≥ 50 y old[a]
Annual fecal occult blood testing using higher sensitivity tests (Hemoccult SENSA)
Annual fecal immunochemical test (FIT)
Fecal DNA test (interval uncertain)
Flexible sigmoidoscopy every 5 y
Colonoscopy every 10 y
CT colonography every 5 y
Individuals With a Family History of a First-Degree Member With Colorectal Neoplasia[b]
Single first-degree relative with colorectal cancer diagnosed at age ≥ 60 y: Begin screening at age 40. Screening guidelines same as average-risk individual; however, preferred method is colonoscopy every 10 y
Single first-degree relative with colorectal cancer or advanced adenoma diagnosed at age < 60 y, or two first-degree relatives: Begin screening at age 40 or at age 10 y younger than age at diagnosis of the youngest affected-relative, whichever is first in time. Recommended screening: colonoscopy every 5 y

[a]Joint Guideline from the American Cancer Society, the US Multi-Society Task Force on Colorectal Cancer, and the American College of Radiology. *Gastroenterology*. 2008;134(5):1570.

[b]American College of Gastroenterology. Guidelines for colorectal cancer screening. *Am J Gastroenterol*. 2009; 104(3):739.

9. When to Refer and When to Admit

When to Refer

- Patients with symptoms (change in bowel habits, hematochezia), signs (mass on abdominal examination or digital rectal examination), or laboratory tests (iron deficiency anemia) suggestive of colorectal neoplasia should be referred for colonoscopy
- Patients with suspected colorectal cancer or adenomatous polyps of any size should be referred for colonoscopy
- Virtually all patients with proven colorectal cancer should be referred to a surgeon for resection. Patients with clinical stage T3 and/or node-positive rectal tumors also should be referred to an oncologist preoperatively for neoadjuvant therapy
- Patients with stage III or IV disease should be referred to an oncologist

When to Admit

- Patients with complications of colorectal cancer (obstruction, acute bleeding) requiring urgent evaluation and intervention
- Patients with severe complications of chemotherapy
- Patients with advanced metastatic disease requiring palliative care

SUGGESTED REFERENCES

Bennouna J et al; ML18147 Study Investigators. Continuation of bevacizumab after first progression in metastatic colorectal cancer (ML18147): a randomised phase 3 trial. *Lancet Oncol.* 2013 Jan;14(1):29–37. [PMID: 23168366]

Bokemeyer C et al. Addition of cetuximab to chemotherapy as first-line treatment for *KRAS* wild-type metastatic colorectal cancer: pooled analysis of the CRYSTAL and OPUS randomised clinical trials. *Eur J Cancer.* 2012 Jul;48(10):1466–1475. [PMID: 22446022]

Brenner H et al. Protection from colorectal cancer after colonoscopy: a population-based, case-control study. *Ann Intern Med.* 2011 Jan 4;154(1):22–30. [PMID: 21200035]

Grothey A et al; CORRECT Study Group. Regorafenib monotherapy for previously treated metastatic colorectal cancer (CORRECT): an international, multicentre, randomised, placebo-controlled, phase 3 trial. *Lancet.* 2013 Jan 26;381(9863):303–312. [PMID: 23177514]

Imperiale TF et al. Multitarget stool DNA testing for colorectal-cancer screening. *N Engl J Med.* 2014 Jul 10;371(2):187–188. [PMID: 25006736]

Kahi CJ et al. Screening and surveillance for colorectal cancer: state of the art. *Gastrointest Endosc.* 2013 Mar;77(3):335–350. [PMID: 23410695]

Lee JK et al. Accuracy of fecal immunochemical tests for colorectal cancer: systematic review and meta-analysis. *Ann Intern Med.* 2014 Feb 4;160(3):171. [PMID: 24658694]

Limketkai BN et al. The cutting edge of serrated polyps: a practical guide to approaching and managing serrated colon polyps. *Gastrointest Endosc.* 2013 Mar;77(3):360–375. [PMID: 23410696]

Nishihara R et al. Long-term colorectal-cancer incidence and mortality after lower endoscopy. *N Engl J Med.* 2013 Sep 19;369(12):1095–1105. [PMID: 24047059]

Quintero E et al; COLONPREV Study Investigators. Colonoscopy versus fecal immunochemical testing in colorectal-cancer screening. *N Engl J Med.* 2012 Feb 23;366(8):697–706. [PMID: 22356323]

Sauer R et al. Preoperative versus postoperative chemoradiotherapy for locally advanced rectal cancer: results of the German CAO/ARO/AIO-94 randomized phase III trial after a median follow-up of 11 years. *J Clin Oncol.* 2012 Jun 1;30(16):1926–1933. [PMID: 22529255]

Shaukat A et al. Long-term mortality after screening for colorectal cancer. *N Engl J Med.* 2013 Sep 19;369(12):1106–1114. [PMID: 24047060]

Siegel R et al. Cancer statistics, 2014. *CA Cancer J Clin.* 2015 Jan–Feb;65(1):5–29. [PMID: 25559415]

Singh S et al. Prevalence, risk factors, and outcomes of interval colorectal cancers: a systematic review and meta-analysis. *Am J Gastroenterol.* 2014 Sep;109(9):1375–1389. [PMID: 24957158]

Van Cutsem E et al. Addition of aflibercept to fluorouracil, leucovorin, and irinotecan improves survival in a phase III randomized trial in patients with metastatic colorectal cancer previously treated with an oxaliplatin-based regimen. *J Clin Oncol.* 2012 Oct 1;30(28):3499–3506. [PMID: 22949147]

Yang DX et al. Estimating the magnitude of colorectal cancers prevented during the era of screening: 1976 to 2009. *Cancer.* 2014 Sep 15;120(18):2893–2901. [PMID: 24894740]

Crohn Disease

30

A 28-year-old woman arrives in the urgent care clinic complaining of cramping abdominal pain. She states she has had the pain intermittently over the past 5 months, accompanied by diarrhea. During this time period she has lost 16 pounds and has had significant malaise. On physical examination, she has a diffusely tender abdomen, worst in the right lower quadrant (RLQ), without signs of rebound or guarding. Complete blood count (CBC) reveals anemia and serum testing shows vitamin B_{12} deficiency. Her stool sample is sent for culture, ova, and parasites, all of which are negative. She is referred for colonoscopy.

LEARNING OBJECTIVES

▶ Learn the clinical manifestations and objective findings of Crohn disease and its complications

▶ Understand the natural history of Crohn disease

▶ Know the differential diagnosis of Crohn disease

▶ Learn the treatments for chronic manifestations and acute exacerbations of Crohn disease

▶ Know the indications for surgery in Crohn disease

QUESTIONS

1. What are the salient features of this patient's problem?

2. How do you think through her problem?

3. What are the key features, including essentials of diagnosis and general considerations, of Crohn disease?

4. What are the symptoms and signs of Crohn disease?

5. What is the differential diagnosis of Crohn disease?

6. What are laboratory, imaging, and procedural findings in Crohn disease?

7. What are the treatments for Crohn disease?

8. What are the outcomes, including complications, prognosis, and prevention, of Crohn disease?

9. When should patients with Crohn disease be referred to a specialist or admitted to the hospital?

ANSWERS

1. Salient Features

Chronic cramping abdominal pain and diarrhea; weight loss; malaise; anemia (presumably from poor vitamin B_{12} absorption in the terminal ileum); and negative stool culture and ova and parasite testing

2. How to Think Through

Diarrhea, a common symptom, requires a framework for clinical reasoning to determine its cause. The time course of this patient's presentation places it in the category of chronic diarrhea. From there, what are the common pathologic categories to frame your differential diagnosis? (Infectious, inflammatory, functional, malabsorption, and medication side effects. Less common causes, such as neuroendocrine tumors and vasculitis, may be considered, but can be explored after the common causes.) What characteristics make inflammatory bowel disease (IBD) likely in this patient? (Chronic abdominal pain; weight loss; and low serum vitamin B_{12} level, indicating likely involvement of the terminal ileum. Ulcerative colitis commonly causes hematochezia, and Crohn disease causes heme-positive stools without gross blood. Her anemia may be caused by anemia of chronic disease, iron deficiency from gastrointestinal blood loss, or vitamin B_{12} deficiency.) Is fecal leukocyte testing useful in diagnosis of IBD? (No. Test specificity is poor due to the presence of fecal leukocytes in infectious diarrhea.) What extra-intestinal symptoms and signs would increase your suspicion for IBD? (Fever, uveitis, arthritis, oral ulcers, and erythema nodosum. See below.) What is her colonoscopy likely to show, and how do the gross and pathologic colonoscopic findings differ between Crohn disease and ulcerative colitis? What are the most serious complications of Crohn disease? (Fistulae, intra-abdominal abscesses, and intestinal obstruction.) What are the common steroid-sparing agents in the treatment of Crohn disease? (Azathioprine; mercaptopurine; methotrexate; infliximab, adalimumab, and certolizumab; vedolizumab.)

3. Key Features

Essentials of Diagnosis

- Insidious onset
- Intermittent bouts of low-grade fever, diarrhea, and RLQ pain
- RLQ mass and tenderness
- Perianal disease with abscess, fistulas
- Radiographic or endoscopic evidence of ulceration, stricturing, or fistulas of the small intestine or colon

General Considerations

- Crohn disease is a transmural process
- Crohn disease may involve
  — Small bowel only, most commonly the terminal ileum (ileitis), in ~33% of cases
  — Small bowel and colon, most often the terminal ileum and adjacent proximal ascending colon (ileocolitis), in ~50%
  — Colon alone in 20%
- Chronic illness with exacerbations and remissions
- One-third of patients have associated perianal disease (fistulas, fissures, abscesses)
- Fewer than 5% of patients have symptomatic involvement of the upper intestinal tract
- Smokers are at increased risk
- Treatment is directed both toward symptomatic improvement and controlling the disease process

4. Symptoms and Signs

- Abdominal pain
- Liquid bowel movements
- Abdominal tenderness or abdominal mass

Chronic Inflammatory Disease
- Malaise, loss of energy
- Diarrhea, nonbloody, intermittent
- Cramping or steady RLQ or periumbilical pain
- Focal RLQ tenderness,
- Palpable, tender mass in the lower abdomen

Intestinal Obstruction
- Postprandial bloating, cramping pains, and loud borborygmi
- Narrowing of the small bowel may occur as a result of inflammation, spasm, or fibrotic stenosis

Fistulization With or Without Infection
- Sinus tracts and fistulas can result in intra-abdominal or retroperitoneal abscesses manifested by fevers, chills, a tender abdominal mass, and leukocytosis
- Fistulas between the small intestine and colon commonly are asymptomatic but can result in diarrhea, weight loss, bacterial overgrowth, and malnutrition
- Fistulization can cause bladder or vagina recurrent infections
- Cutaneous fistulas
- Perianal disease
  — Skin tags
  — Anal fissures
  — Perianal abscesses
  — Fistulas

Extraintestinal Manifestations
- Arthralgias, arthritis
- Iritis or uveitis
- Pyoderma gangrenosum
- Erythema nodosum
- Oral aphthous lesions
- Gallstones
- Nephrolithiasis

5. Differential Diagnosis
- Ulcerative colitis
- Irritable bowel syndrome
- Appendicitis
- *Yersinia enterocolitica* enteritis
- Mesenteric adenitis
- Intestinal lymphoma
- Segmental colitis due to ischemic colitis, tuberculosis, amebiasis, and *Chlamydia*
- Diverticulitis with abscess
- Nonsteroidal anti-inflammatory drug-induced colitis
- Perianal fistula due to other cause

6. Laboratory, Imaging, and Procedural Findings

Laboratory Tests
- Obtain CBC, erythrocyte sedimentation rate (ESR), or C-reactive protein, serum albumin
- Anemia of chronic inflammation, blood loss, iron deficiency, or vitamin B_{12} malabsorption
- Leukocytosis with abscesses
- Elevated ESR or C-reactive protein
- Send stool for culture (routine pathogens), ova and parasites, leukocytes, fat, and *Clostridium difficile* toxin

Imaging Studies
- Barium upper gastrointestinal series with small bowel follow-through
- Computed tomography (CT) enterography
- Capsuled (video) imaging of small intestine

Diagnostic Procedures
- Colonoscopy
- Biopsy of intestine reveals granulomas in 25%

7. Treatments

Medications

Symptomatic Treatment of Diarrhea
- Antidiarrheal agents
  — Loperamide (2 to 4 mg), diphenoxylate with atropine (one tablet), or tincture of opium (5 to 15 drops) four times daily as needed
  — Should not be used in patients with active severe colitis
- Broad-spectrum antibiotics if bacterial overgrowth
- Cholestyramine 2 to 4 g, colestipol 5 g, or colesevelam 625 mg one to two times daily before meals to bind the malabsorbed bile salts

Treatment of Exacerbations
- Early introduction of biologic therapy should be strongly considered in patients with risk factors for aggressive disease, including young age, perianal disease, stricturing disease, or need for corticosteroids
- 5-Aminosalicylic acid agents
  — Mesalamine (Asacol 2.4 to 4.8 g/d orally; Pentasa 4 g/d orally) has long been used as initial therapy for the treatment of mild to moderately active colonic and ileocolonic Crohn disease
  — Current treatment guidelines recommend against use of these agents for Crohn disease
- Antibiotics may reduce inflammation through alteration of gut flora, reduce bacterial overgrowth, or treat microperforations
  — Metronidazole, 10 mg/kg/d for 6 to 12 weeks
  — Ciprofloxacin, 500 mg twice daily orally for 6 to 12 weeks
  — Rifaximin, 400 mg three times daily, for 6 to 12 weeks
- Ileal-release preparation of topically active compound budesonide, 9 mg once daily orally for 8 to 16 weeks, induces remission in 50% to 70% of patients with mild-to-moderate Crohn disease involving the terminal ileum or ascending colon
  — After initial treatment, budesonide is tapered over 2 to 4 weeks in 3 mg increments
  — Low-dose budesonide (6 mg/d) may be used for up to 1 year to maintain remission
  — Budesonide is superior to mesalamine but somewhat less effective than prednisone
- Corticosteroids
  — Prednisone, 40 to 60 mg/d for 2 to 3 weeks
  — Taper by 5 mg/wk until dosage is 20 mg/d, then by 2.5 mg/wk or every other week for acute episodes of moderate-to-severe disease
- Immunomodulatory drugs
  — Mercaptopurine and azathioprine are more commonly used than methotrexate in the United States
  — Methotrexate (25 mg subcutaneously weekly for 12 weeks, followed by 12.5 to 15 mg once weekly) is used in patients who are unresponsive to, or intolerant of, mercaptopurine or azathioprine
  — Because oral absorption may be erratic, parenteral administration of methotrexate is preferred
  — These agents do not appear to be effective at inducing remission, thus guidelines recommend against using thiopurine monotherapy to induce remission

- Anti-TNF therapies: infliximab, adalimumab, and certolizumab are used to induce and maintain remission in moderate to severe Crohn disease as well as to treat extraintestinal manifestations (except optic neuritis)
  — Induction therapy
    › Infliximab: three-dose regimen of 5 mg/kg at 0, 2, and 6 weeks
    › Adalimumab: 160 mg at week 0 and 80 mg at week 2
    › Certolizumab: 400 mg at weeks 0, 2, and 4
  — Maintenance therapy
    › Infliximab: 5 mg/kg infusion every 8 weeks
    › Adalimumab: 40 mg subcutaneous infection every 2 weeks
    › Certolizumab: 400 mg subcutaneous injection every 4 weeks
- Anti-integrins
  — Due to the recognized risk of reactivation of JC virus and the development of progressive multifocal encephalopathy (PML) and the advent of more gut-specific anti-integrins, natalizumab has little use in inflammatory bowel disease
  — Vedolizumab is primarily used in patients with moderate to severe Crohn disease in whom anti-TNF therapy has failed or is not tolerated
- Vedolizumab: 300 mg intravenously at weeks 0 and 2 OR 300 mg intravenously every 8 weeks

Surgery
- At least one surgical procedure required by > 50% of patients
- Indications for surgery
  — Intractability to medical therapy
  — Intra-abdominal abscess
  — Massive bleeding
  — Obstruction with fibrous stricture
- Incision and drainage for abscess
- Surgical resection of the stenotic area or stricturoplasty in small bowel obstruction

Therapeutic Procedures
- Percutaneous drainage for abscess
- Nasogastric suction and intravenous fluids for small bowel obstruction
- Well-balanced diet
- Avoid lactose-containing foods since lactose intolerance is common
- Fiber supplementation for patients with colonic involvement
- Low-roughage diet for patients with obstructive symptoms
- Low-fat diet for patients with fat malabsorption
- Vitamin B_{12} 100 µg intramuscularly every month if prior terminal ileal resection
- Total parenteral nutrition
  — Used short term in patients with active disease and progressive weight loss or in malnourished patients awaiting surgery
  — Used long term in subset of patients with extensive intestinal resections resulting in short bowel syndrome with malnutrition

8. Outcomes
Complications
- Abscess
- Small bowel obstruction
- Fistulas
- Perianal disease
- Carcinoma
- Hemorrhage (unusual)
- Malabsorption

Prognosis

- With proper medical and surgical treatment, most patients are able to cope with this chronic disease and its complications
- Few patients die of Crohn disease

Prevention

- Annual colonoscopy screening to detect dysplasia or cancer recommended for patients with a history of ≥ 8 years of Crohn colitis

9. When to Refer and When to Admit

When to Refer

- For expertise in endoscopic procedures or capsule endoscopy
- Any patient requiring hospitalization for follow-up
- Patients with moderate-to-severe disease for whom therapy with immunomodulators or biologic agents is being considered
- When surgery may be necessary
- For annual colonoscopy after ≥ 8 years of Crohn colitis

When to Admit

- An intestinal obstruction is suspected
- An intra-abdominal or perirectal abscess is suspected
- A serious infectious complication is suspected, especially in patients who are immuno-compromised due to concomitant use of corticosteroids, immunomodulators, antitumor necrosis factor, or anti-integrin agents
- Patients with severe symptoms of diarrhea, dehydration, weight loss, or abdominal pain
- Patients with severe or persisting symptoms despite treatment with corticosteroids

SUGGESTED REFERENCES

Cheifetz AS. Management of active Crohn disease. *JAMA*. 2013 May 22;309(20):2150–2158. [PMID: 23695484]

Cho SM et al. Postoperative management of Crohn disease. *Med Clin North Am*. 2010 Jan;94(1):179–188. [PMID: 19944804]

Colombel JF et al; SONIC Study Group. Infliximab, azathioprine, or combination therapy for Crohn's disease. *N Engl J Med*. 2010 Apr 15;362(15):1383–1395. [PMID: 20393175]

Cosnes J et al; Groupe d'Etude Thérapeutique des Affections Inflammatoires du Tube Digestif (GETAID). Early administration of azathioprine vs conventional management of Crohn's Disease: a randomized controlled trial. *Gastroenterology*. 2013 Oct;145(4):758–765.e2. [PMID: 23644079]

D'Haens GR et al. The London Position Statement of the World Congress of Gastroenterology on Biological Therapy for IBD with the European Crohn's and Colitis Organization: when to start, when to stop, which drug to choose, and how to predict response? *Am J Gastroenterol*. 2011 Feb;106(2):199–212. [PMID: 21045814]

Ford AC et al. Efficacy of 5-aminosalicylates in Crohn's disease: systematic review and meta-analysis. *Am J Gastroenterol*. 2011 Apr;106(4):617–629. [PMID: 21407190]

Ford AC et al. Efficacy of biologic therapies in inflammatory bowel disease: systematic review and meta-analysis. *Am J Gastroenterol*. Apr; 2011;106(4):644–659. [PMID: 21407183]

Panés J et al; AZTEC Study Group. Early azathioprine therapy is no more effective than placebo for newly diagnosed Crohn's disease. *Gastroenterology*. 2013 Oct;145(4):766–774.e1. [PMID: 23770132]

Sandborn WJ et al; GEMINI 2 Study Group. Vedolizumab as induction and maintenance therapy for Crohn's disease. *N Engl J Med*. 2013 Aug 22;369(8):711–721. [PMID: 23964933]

Sands BE et al. Effects of vedolizumab induction therapy for patients with Crohn's disease in whom tumor necrosis factor antagonist treatment failed. *Gastroenterology*. 2014 Sep;147(3):618–627.e3. [PMID: 24859203]

Savarino E et al. Adalimumab is more effective than azathioprine and mesalamine at preventing post-operative recurrence of Crohn's disease: a randomized controlled trial. *Am J Gastroenterol*. 2013 Nov;108(11):1731–1742. [PMID: 24019080]

Terdiman JP et al. American Gastroenterological Association Institute guideline on the use of thio-purines, methotrexate, and anti-TNF-α biologic drugs for the induction and maintenance of remission in inflammatory Crohn's disease. *Gastroenterology*. 2013 Dec;145(6):1459–1463. [PMID: 24267474]

Diarrhea

31

A 62-year-old woman presents to her primary care clinician with complaints of 2 weeks of diarrhea, starting after a recent hospitalization for pneumonia. She describes the diarrhea as watery stool mixed with small amounts of blood, large in volume, and occurring 7 to 10 times per day. She was treated in the hospital with antibiotics for her pneumonia, and for this diarrheal episode received a recent course of a ciprofloxacin from an urgent care clinic without resolution. On physical examination, she has dry mucous membranes and a diffusely tender abdomen.

LEARNING OBJECTIVES

► Learn the historical factors, symptoms, and signs of diarrhea that help elucidate the cause of a patient's diarrhea
► Understand the factors that predispose to the development of rare causes of diarrhea
► Know the differential diagnosis of the different types of diarrhea
► Learn the medical treatments for diarrhea and in which patients antibiotics or antidiarrheals are contraindicated
► Know the warning signs that diarrhea requires further diagnostic testing

QUESTIONS

1. What are the salient features of this patient's problem?
2. How do you think through her problem?
3. What are the key features, including essentials of diagnosis, general considerations, and demographics, of diarrhea?
4. What are the symptoms and signs of diarrhea?
5. What is the differential diagnosis of acute, chronic, and traveler's diarrhea?
6. What are laboratory, imaging, and procedural findings in diarrhea?
7. What are the treatments for diarrhea?
8. What are the outcomes, including prevention, prognosis, and complications, of diarrhea?
9. When should patients with diarrhea be referred to a specialist or admitted to the hospital?

ANSWERS

1. Salient Features

Frequent stools; 2-week time course; recent hospitalization and antibiotic use; large-volume watery stool with blood; no resolution with ciprofloxacin; dehydration and abdominal tenderness

2. How to Think Through

Acute diarrhea is defined as occurring for less than 2 weeks. Given that this patient was recently hospitalized and received two courses of antibiotics, what are the most likely causes of her diarrhea? (Direct medication toxicity vs infectious diarrhea—specifically *Clostridium difficile* colitis or another hospital-acquired pathogen.) When following antibiotic exposure does diarrhea due to *C difficile* typically begin? (5–10 days, though the interval can be up to several weeks.) What are the next diagnostic steps? (Send stool *C difficile* toxin assay immediately. Stool culture for *Campylobacter*, *Shigella*, and *Salmonella* is reasonable. There are no risk factors for parasitic disease. A complete blood count, and serum electrolytes and creatinine should be sent.)

What is the next treatment step? (Due to the high prevalence of *C difficile*—up to 20% of hospitalized patients are carriers—and the potential severity of the complications, empiric antibiotic treatment for *C difficile* is appropriate. Her dry mucous membranes on examination suggest dehydration and, based on her vital signs and overall assessment, readmission to the hospital for supportive care should be strongly considered.)

What are the serious sequelae of *C difficile* colitis? (Fulminant colitis with systemic toxicity; toxic megacolon.) What clinical signs would prompt imaging and escalation of care? (High fever, severe pain, leukocytosis [WBC of 15,000/μL is typical for mild-to-moderate disease, 40,000/μL is more consistent with fulminant disease], and shock.)

3. Key Features

Essentials of Diagnosis
- Acute diarrhea has duration of < 2 weeks
- Chronic diarrhea is present for > 4 weeks
- Traveler's diarrhea is usually a benign, self-limited disease occurring about a week into travel
- Severity of any diarrhea ranges from mild and self-limited to severe and life-threatening
- Before embarking on extensive workup, common causes should be excluded, including medications, chronic infections, and irritable bowel syndrome
- Classification
  — Medications
  — Osmotic diarrhea
  — Secretory conditions
  — Inflammatory conditions
  — Malabsorption conditions
  — Motility disorders
  — Acute or chronic infections
  — Systemic disorders
- Prophylaxis for traveler's diarrhea is not recommended unless there is a comorbid disease (inflammatory bowel syndrome, HIV, and immunosuppressive medication)
- Single-dose therapy of a fluoroquinolone is usually effective for traveler's diarrhea if symptoms develop

General Considerations
- Acute diarrhea is most commonly caused by infectious agents, bacterial toxins (Table 31-1), or drugs
- Recent illnesses in family members suggest infectious diarrhea

Table 31-1. Acute bacterial diarrheas and "food poisoning."

Organism	Incubation Period	Vomiting	Diarrhea	Fever	Associated Foods	Diagnosis	Clinical Features and Treatment
Staphylococcus (preformed toxin)	1–8 h	+++	±	±	Staphylococci grow in meats, dairy, and bakery products and produce enterotoxin	Clinical. Food and stool can be tested for toxin	Abrupt onset, intense nausea and vomiting for up to 24 h, recovery in 24–48 h. Supportive care
Bacillus cereus (preformed toxin)	1–8 h	+++	±	−	Reheated fried rice causes vomiting or diarrhea	Clinical. Food and stool can be tested for toxin	Acute onset, severe nausea and vomiting lasting 24 h. Supportive care
B cereus (diarrheal toxin)	10–16 h	±	+++	−	Toxin in meats, stews, and gravy	Clinical. Food and stool can be tested for toxin	Abdominal cramps, watery diarrhea, and nausea lasting 24–48 h. Supportive care
Clostridium perfringens	8–16 h	±	+++	−	Clostridia grow in rewarmed meat and poultry dishes and produce an enterotoxin	Stools can be tested for enterotoxin or cultured	Abrupt onset of profuse diarrhea, abdominal cramps, nausea; vomiting occasionally. Recovery usual without treatment in 24–48 h. Supportive care; antibiotics not needed
Clostridium botulinum	12–72 h	±	−	−	Clostridia grow in anaerobic acidic environment, eg, canned foods, fermented fish, foods held warm for extended periods	Stool, serum, and food can be tested for toxin. Stool and food can be cultured	Diplopia, dysphagia, dysphonia, respiratory embarrassment. Treatment requires clear airway, ventilation, and intravenous polyvalent antitoxin. Symptoms can last for days to months
Clostridium difficile	Usually occurs after 7–10 d of antibiotics. Can occur after a single dose or several weeks after completion of antibiotics	−	+++	++	Associated with antimicrobial drugs; clindamycin and β-lactams most commonly implicated. Fluoroquinolones associated with hypervirulent strains	Stool tested for toxin	Abrupt onset of diarrhea that may be bloody; fever. Oral metronidazole for mild to moderate cases. Oral vancomycin for more severe disease
Enterohemorrhagic *Escherichia coli*, including Shiga toxin–producing *E coli* (STEC)	1–8 d	+	+++	−	Undercooked beef, especially hamburger; unpasteurized milk and juice; raw fruits and vegetables	Shiga-toxin producing *E coli* can be cultured on special medium. Other toxins can be detected in stool	Usually abrupt onset of diarrhea, often bloody; abdominal pain. In adults, it is usually self-limited to 5–10 d. In children, it is associated with hemolytic-uremic syndrome (HUS). Antibiotic therapy may increase risk of HUS. Plasma exchange may help patients with STEC-associated HUS
Enterotoxigenic *E coli* (ETEC)	1–3 d	±	+++	±	Water, food contaminated with feces	Stool culture. Special tests required to identify toxin-producing strains	Watery diarrhea and abdominal cramps, usually lasting 3–7 d. In travelers, fluoroquinolones shorten disease
Vibrio parahaemolyticus	2–48 h	+	+	±	Undercooked or raw seafood	Stool culture on special medium	Abrupt onset of watery diarrhea, abdominal cramps, nausea and vomiting. Recovery is usually complete in 2–5 d
Vibrio cholerae	24–72 h	+	+++	−	Contaminated water, fish, shellfish, street vendor food	Stool culture on special medium	Abrupt onset of liquid diarrhea in endemic area. Needs prompt intravenous or oral replacement of fluids and electrolytes. Tetracyclines and azithromycin shorten excretion of vibrios
Campylobacter jejuni	2–5 d	±	+++	+	Raw or undercooked poultry, unpasteurized milk, water	Stool culture on special medium	Fever, diarrhea that can be bloody, cramps. Usually self-limited in 2–10 d. Treat with azithromycin or fluoroquinolones for severe disease. May be associated with Guillain–Barré syndrome

(continued)

Table 31-1. Acute bacterial diarrheas and "food poisoning." (continued)

Organism	Incubation Period	Vomiting	Diarrhea	Fever	Associated Foods	Diagnosis	Clinical Features and Treatment
Shigella species (mild cases)	24–48 h	±	+	+	Food or water contaminated with human feces. Person-to-person spread	Routine stool culture	Abrupt onset of diarrhea, often with blood and pus in stools, cramps, tenesmus, and lethargy. Stool cultures are positive. Therapy depends on sensitivity testing, but the fluoroquinolones are most effective. Do not give opioids. Often mild and self-limited
Salmonella species	1–3 d	−	+ +	+	Eggs, poultry, unpasteurized milk, cheese, juices, raw fruits and vegetables	Routine stool culture	Gradual or abrupt onset of diarrhea and low-grade fever. No antimicrobials unless high risk or systemic dissemination is suspected, in which case give a fluoroquinolone. Prolonged carriage can occur
Yersinia enterocolitica	24–48 h	±	+	+	Undercooked pork, contaminated water, unpasteurized milk, tofu	Stool culture on special medium	Severe abdominal pain, (appendicitis-like symptoms) diarrhea, fever. Polyarthritis, erythema nodosum in children. If severe, give tetracycline or fluoroquinolone. Without treatment, self-limited in 1–3 wk
Rotavirus	1–3 d	+ +	+ + +	+	Fecally contaminated foods touched by infected food handlers	Immunoassay on stool	Acute onset, vomiting, watery diarrhea that lasts 4–8 d. Supportive care
Noroviruses and other caliciviruses	12–48 h	+ +	+ + +	+	Shellfish and fecally contaminated foods touched by infected food handlers	Clinical diagnosis with negative stool cultures. PCR available on stool	Nausea, vomiting (more common in children) diarrhea (more common in adults), fever, myalgias, abdominal cramps. Lasts 12–60 h. Supportive care

PCR, polymerase chain reaction.

- Community outbreaks (schools, nursing homes, and cruise ships) suggest viral etiology or common food source
- Ingestion of improperly stored or prepared food implicates toxin-secreting or invasive bacteria
- Exposure to unpurified water suggests *Giardia* or *Cryptosporidium*
- Large *Cyclospora* outbreaks have been traced to contaminated produce
- Recent travel abroad suggests "traveler's diarrhea"
- Antibiotic administration suggests *C difficile* colitis
- HIV infection or sexually transmitted diseases suggest AIDS-associated diarrhea
- Proctitis and rectal discharge suggest gonorrhea, syphilis, lymphogranuloma venereum (LGV), and herpes simplex
- Acute noninflammatory diarrhea
  — Fecal leukocytes and blood are absent
  — Diarrhea may be voluminous with periumbilical cramps, bloating, nausea, or vomiting
  — Usually arises from small bowel due to a toxin-producing bacterium or other agents (viruses, *Giardia*)
  — Prominent vomiting suggests viral enteritis or *Staphylococcus aureus* food poisoning
  — May cause dehydration, hypokalemia, and metabolic acidosis
- Acute inflammatory diarrhea
  — Fecal leukocytes are present; blood mixed with stool may also be present (dysentery)
  — Diarrhea usually arises from colon, is small volume (< 1 L/d), with left lower quadrant cramps, urgency, and tenesmus

- Usually caused by invasive organisms (shigellosis, salmonellosis, *Campylobacter*, or *Yersinia* infection, amebiasis, cytomegalovirus) or a toxin (*C difficile*, Shiga toxin–producing *Escherichia coli* (also called enterohemorrhagic *E coli*)
- Medications that can commonly cause diarrhea include
  — Cholinesterase inhibitors
  — Selective serotonin reuptake inhibitors
  — Angiotensin II–receptor blockers
  — Proton pump inhibitors
  — Nonsteroidal anti-inflammatory drugs
  — Metformin
  — Allopurinol
  — Orlistat
- Osmotic diarrheas resolve during fasting
- Secretory diarrhea is caused by increased intestinal secretion or decreased absorption with little change in stool output during fasting
- The major causes of malabsorption are small mucosal intestinal diseases, intestinal resections, lymphatic obstruction, small intestinal bacterial overgrowth, and pancreatic insufficiency
- Motility disorders are secondary to systemic disorders or surgery that lead to rapid transit or to stasis of intestinal contents with bacterial overgrowth, malabsorption
- Immunocompromised patients are susceptible to *Microsporidia, Cryptosporidium,* cytomegalovirus, *Isospora belli, Cyclospora,* and *Mycobacterium avium-intracellulare* complex (MAC) infections
- Chronic systemic conditions such as thyroid disease, diabetes mellitus, and collagen vascular disorders may cause diarrhea through alterations in motility or intestinal absorption
- Whenever a person travels from one country to another—particularly if the change involves a marked difference in climate, social conditions, or sanitation standards and facilities—diarrhea may develop within 2 to 10 days
- Bacteria cause 80% of cases of traveler's diarrhea, but contributory causes include
  — Unusual food and drink
  — Change in living habits
  — Occasional viral infections (adenoviruses or rotaviruses)
  — Change in bowel flora
- Traveler's diarrhea is a risk factor for development of irritable bowel syndrome

Demographics
- Lactase deficiency
  — Occurs in 75% of nonwhite adults and 25% of whites
  — May be acquired with viral gastroenteritis, medical illness, or gastrointestinal surgery

4. Symptoms and Signs
- Increased stool frequency or liquidity
- Rectal discharge suggests proctitis
- Physical examination may reveal abdominal tenderness, peritonitis
- When cause is invasive bacterial pathogens (eg, *Shigella, Campylobacter, Salmonella*), stools may be bloody and fever may be present
- When cause is enterotoxigenic *E coli*, stools are usually watery and fever usually is absent
- Osmotic diarrheas
  — Abdominal distention
  — Bloating
  — Flatulence due to increased colonic gas production
- Secretory diarrhea
  — High-volume (> 1 L/d) watery diarrhea
  — Dehydration
  — Electrolyte imbalance

- Inflammatory conditions
  — Abdominal pain
  — Fever
  — Weight loss
  — Hematochezia
- Malabsorption syndromes
  — Weight loss
  — Osmotic diarrhea
  — Steatorrhea
  — Nutritional deficiencies

5. Differential Diagnosis

Acute Diarrhea

- Infectious: noninflammatory (nonbloody)
  — Viruses: Norwalk virus, rotavirus, adenoviruses, astrovirus, and coronavirus
  — Preformed toxin (food poisoning): *S aureus*, *Bacillus cereus*, *Clostridium perfringens*
  — Toxin production: enterotoxigenic *E coli*, *Vibrio cholerae*, and *V parahaemolyticus*
  — Protozoa: *Giardia lamblia*, *Cryptosporidium*, *Cyclospora*, and *Isospora*
- Infectious: invasive or inflammatory
  — *Shigella*, *Salmonella*, *Campylobacter*, enteroinvasive *E coli*, Shiga toxin-producing *E coli*, *Yersinia enterocolitica*, *C difficile* (eg, pseudomembranous colitis), *Entamoeba histolytica*, *Neisseria gonorrhoeae*, and *Listeria monocytogenes*
- Associated with unprotected anal intercourse
  — *N gonorrhoeae*
  — Syphilis
  — LGV
  — Herpes simplex
- Noninfectious
  — Drug reaction, especially antibiotics
  — Ulcerative colitis, Crohn disease (inflammatory)
  — Ischemic colitis (inflammatory)
  — Fecal impaction (stool may leak around impaction)
  — Laxative abuse
  — Radiation colitis (inflammatory)
  — Emotional stress

Chronic Diarrhea

- Common
  — Irritable bowel syndrome
  — Parasites
  — Caffeine
  — Laxative abuse
- Osmotic
  — Lactase deficiency
  — Medications: antacids, lactulose, sorbitol, and olestra
  — Factitious: magnesium-containing antacids or laxatives
- Secretory
  — Hormonal: Zollinger–Ellison syndrome (gastrinoma), carcinoid, VIPoma, medullary thyroid carcinoma, and adrenal insufficiency
  — Laxative abuse: cascara, senna
  — Medications
- Inflammatory conditions
  — Inflammatory bowel disease
  — Microscopic colitis (lymphocytic or collagenous)

— Cancer with obstruction and pseudodiarrhea

— Radiation colitis

- Malabsorption
  — Small bowel: celiac disease (gluten enteropathy), Whipple disease, tropical sprue, eosinophilic gastroenteritis, small bowel resection, and Crohn disease
  — Lymphatic obstruction: lymphoma, carcinoid, tuberculosis, *M avium-intracellulare* complex (MAC) infection, Kaposi sarcoma, sarcoidosis, and retroperitoneal fibrosis
  — Pancreatic insufficiency: chronic pancreatitis, cystic fibrosis, and pancreatic cancer
  — Bacterial overgrowth, eg, diabetes mellitus
  — Reduced bile salts: ileal resection, Crohn disease, postcholecystectomy
- Motility disorders
  — Irritable bowel syndrome
  — Postsurgical: vagotomy, partial gastrectomy, blind loop with bacterial overgrowth
  — Systemic disease: diabetes mellitus, hyperthyroidism, and scleroderma
  — Caffeine or alcoholism
- Chronic infections
  — Parasites: giardiasis, amebiasis, and strongyloidiasis

Traveler's Diarrhea

- Most common
  — Enterotoxigenic *E coli*
  — *Shigella*
  — *Campylobacter*
- Less common
  — *Aeromonas*
  — *Salmonella*
  — Noncholera vibrios
  — *E histolytica*
  — *G lamblia*
  — Adenoviruses
  — Rotavirus
- Chronic watery diarrhea
  — *E histolytica*
  — *G lamblia*
  — Tropical sprue (rare)

6. Laboratory, Imaging, and Procedural Findings

Laboratory Tests

Acute Diarrhea

- Noninflammatory diarrhea
  — Ninety percent mild, self-limited, resolving within 5 days
  — Stool cultures positive in < 3%; therefore, initial symptomatic treatment given for mild symptoms
  — If diarrhea worsens or persists for > 7 to 10 days, send stools for leukocytes or lactoferrin, cultures, ova and parasites (3 samples), *Giardia* antigen
- Diarrhea that requires prompt evaluation
  — Inflammatory diarrhea: fever (> 38.5°C), WBC > 15,000/μL, bloody diarrhea, or severe abdominal pain
  — Passage of ≥ 6 unformed stools in 24 hours
  — Profuse watery diarrhea and dehydration
  — Frail older patients or nursing home residents
  — Immunocompromised patients (AIDS, posttransplantation)
  — Hospital-acquired diarrhea (onset following at least 3 days of hospitalization)

— Exposure to antibiotics

— Systemic illness

- Three stool examinations for ova and parasites to look for amebiasis should be obtained if diarrhea persists > 10 days, in those who engage in oral–anal sexual practices, and those with recent travel to amebiasis endemic areas
- Stool *C difficile* toxin assay if recent history of antibiotic exposure or hospitalization
- Rectal swab cultures for *Chlamydia*, *N gonorrhoeae*, and herpes simplex virus in sexually active patients with suspected proctitis

Chronic Diarrhea

- A complete blood cell count, serum electrolytes, liver biochemical tests, calcium, phosphorus, albumin, and thyroid-stimulating hormone; prothrombin time/INR, erythrocyte sedimentation rate, and C-reactive protein should be obtained in most patients
- Serologic testing for celiac disease (gluten enteropathy) with serum IgA tissue transglutaminase test may be recommended for most patients with chronic diarrhea and all patients with signs of malabsorption
- Stool studies for chronic diarrhea
  - Analyze stool sample for ova and parasites, electrolytes (to calculate osmotic gap), qualitative staining for fat (Sudan stain), occult blood, and leukocytes or lactoferrin
  - The presence of fecal leukocytes or lactoferrin may suggest inflammatory bowel disease
  - The presence of *Giardia* and *E histolytica* may be detected in wet mounts; however, fecal antigen detection tests are a more sensitive and specific detection method
  - *Cryptosporidium* and *Cyclospora* are found with modified acid-fast staining
  - An increased osmotic gap suggests an osmotic diarrhea or disorder of malabsorption
  - A positive fecal fat stain suggests a disorder of malabsorption
  - Twenty-four-hour stool collection for weight and quantitative fecal fat
    - Stool weight < 200 to 300 g/24 h excludes diarrhea and suggests a functional disorder such as irritable bowel syndrome
    - Stool weight > 200 g/24 h confirms diarrhea
    - Stool weight > 1000 to 1500 g/24 h suggests secretory diarrhea, including neuroendocrine tumors
    - Fecal fat > 10 g/24 h indicates a malabsorption syndrome
- If malabsorption is suspected
  - Obtain serum folate, B_{12}, iron, vitamin A and D levels, prothrombin time
  - Serologic tests for celiac disease: serum IgA tissue transglutaminase antibody
- If a secretory cause is suspected
  - Obtain serum VIP (for VIPoma), chromogranin A (carcinoid), calcitonin (medullary thyroid carcinoma), gastrin (Zollinger–Ellison syndrome), and glucagon (glucagonoma)
  - Obtain urine 5-hydroxyindoleacetic acid (for carcinoid)

Traveler's Diarrhea

- A stool culture is indicated for patients with fever and bloody diarrhea, but in most cases cultures are reserved for those who do not respond to antibiotics

Imaging Studies

- Abdominal computed tomography (CT) for suspected chronic pancreatitis, pancreatic cancer, and neuroendocrine tumors
- Small intestinal imaging with barium, CT, or magnetic resonance imaging (MRI) is helpful in the diagnosis of Crohn disease, small bowel lymphoma, carcinoid, and jejunal diverticula
- Somatostatin receptor scintigraphy in suspected neuroendocrine tumors

Diagnostic Procedures

- In > 90% of cases, acute diarrhea is mild and self-limited, and diagnostic investigation is unnecessary

- Prompt sigmoidoscopy for severe proctitis (tenesmus, discharge, and rectal pain) or for suspected *C difficile* colitis, ulcerative colitis, or ischemic colitis
- Sigmoidoscopy or colonoscopy with mucosal biopsy to diagnose inflammatory bowel disease and melanosis coli
- Upper endoscopy with small bowel biopsy to diagnose suspected celiac disease, Whipple disease, and AIDS-related *Cryptosporidium, Microsporidia*, and *M avium-intracellulare* complex (MAC) infection
- Breath hydrogen tests to diagnose bacterial overgrowth

7. Treatments

Medications

- Opioid agents help decrease the stool number and liquidity and control fecal urgency
- Antidiarrheal agents may be used safely in mild-to-moderate noninflammatory diarrhea
- Loperamide, 4 mg orally initially, followed by 2 mg after each loose stool (maximum: 16 mg/24 h)
- Bismuth subsalicylate (Pepto-Bismol), 2 tablets or 30 mL four times daily orally
- Diphenoxylate with atropine (anticholinergic) contraindicated in acute diarrhea because of the rare precipitation of toxic megacolon; 1 tablet three to four times daily in chronic diarrhea
- Codeine 15 to 60 mg every 4 hours orally; tincture of opium, 0.03 to 1.2 mL every 6 hours as needed, safe in most patients with chronic, intractable diarrhea
- Clonidine, 0.1 to 0.6 mg twice daily orally, or a clonidine patch, 0.1 to 0.2 mg/d, helpful in secretory diarrheas, diabetic diarrhea, and cryptosporidiosis
- Octreotide, 50 to 250 μg three times daily subcutaneously, for secretory diarrheas due to neuroendocrine tumors (VIPomas, carcinoid). A once monthly depot formulation of octreotide is available.
- Cholestyramine or colestipol (2–4 g once to three times daily) or colesevelam (625 mg, 1–3 tablets once or twice daily) in patients with bile salt-induced diarrhea secondary to intestinal resection or ileal disease
- Neither opioid nor antidiarrheal agents should be used in patients with bloody diarrhea, high fever, or systemic toxicity, and both agents should be discontinued in patients whose diarrhea is worsening despite therapy
- Empiric antibiotic treatment
  — Regimens include
    ◦ Fluoroquinolones (eg, ciprofloxacin 500 mg, ofloxacin 400 mg, or norfloxacin 400 mg, twice daily orally) for 5 to 7 days
    ◦ Trimethoprim–sulfamethoxazole, 160/800 mg twice daily orally, or doxycycline, 100 mg twice daily orally
  — Indications include
    ◦ Moderate-to-severe fever
    ◦ Tenesmus
    ◦ Bloody stools
    ◦ Presence of fecal leukocytes while the stool bacterial culture is incubating
    ◦ Immunocompromised patients
    ◦ Significant dehydration
- Specific antimicrobial treatment is recommended in
  — Shigellosis
  — Cholera
  — Extraintestinal salmonellosis
- Listeriosis
  — Traveler's diarrhea
  — *C difficile* infection
  — Giardiasis
  — Amebiasis

- Antibiotics not recommended in nontyphoid *Salmonella*, *Campylobacter*, *Aeromonas*, *Yersinia*, or Shiga toxin–producing *E coli* infection except in severe disease
- Oral rehydration solutions or salts to treat dehydration are available over the counter in the United States (Infalyte, Pedialyte, Gatorade, and others) and in many foreign countries
- Ciprofloxacin (750 mg), levofloxacin (500 mg), or ofloxacin (200 mg) cures most cases of traveler's diarrhea
- Azithromycin is drug of choice for traveler's diarrhea in pregnant women and for cases due to invasive bacteria or resistant to fluoroquinolones

Therapeutic Procedures
- Diet
  — Adequate oral fluids containing carbohydrates and electrolytes
  — Avoidance of high-fiber foods, fats, milk products, caffeine, and alcohol
  — Frequent feedings of tea; "flat" carbonated beverages; and soft, easily digested foods (eg, soups, crackers, bananas, applesauce, rice, and toast)
- Rehydration
  — Oral electrolyte solutions (eg, Infalyte, Pedialyte, Gatorade)
  — Intravenous fluids (lactated Ringer injection) for severe dehydration
- Consider discontinuing medications that could be causing chronic diarrhea

8. Outcomes

Prevention
- When traveling, eat only "peeled, packaged, and piping hot" foods; recommend avoidance of fresh foods and water sources in developing countries, where infectious diarrheal illnesses are endemic
- Traveler's prophylaxis is recommended for
  — Patients with significant underlying disease (inflammatory bowel disease, AIDS, diabetes, heart disease in the elderly, and conditions requiring immunosuppressive medications)
  — Patients whose full activity status during the trip is so essential that even short periods of diarrhea would be unacceptable
- Prophylaxis is started upon entry into the destination country and is continued for 1 or 2 days after leaving
- For stays of > 3 weeks, prophylaxis is not recommended because of the cost and increased toxicity
- Numerous antimicrobial regimens for once-daily oral prophylaxis of traveler's diarrhea are effective, such as
  — Norfloxacin, 400 mg
  — Ciprofloxacin, 500 mg
  — Rifaximin, 200 mg
- Bismuth subsalicylate for traveler's diarrhea prevention
  — Effective, but rarely used
  — Turns the tongue and the stools black
  — Can interfere with doxycycline absorption, which may be needed for malaria prophylaxis
- Because not all travelers will have diarrhea and because most episodes are brief and self-limited, an alternative approach currently recommended is to provide the traveler with a supply of antimicrobials to be taken if significant diarrhea occurs during the trip

Prognosis
- Cause is identifiable and treatable in almost all patients
- Most traveler's diarrhea is short-lived and resolves without specific therapy

Complications
- Dehydration
- Electrolyte abnormalities
- Malabsorption: weight loss, vitamin deficiencies

9. When to Refer and When to Admit

When to Refer
- Cases refractory to treatment
- Persistent infection
- Immunocompromised patient

When to Admit
- Severe dehydration for intravenous fluids, especially if vomiting or unable to maintain sufficient oral fluid intake
- Organ failure
- Bloody diarrhea that is severe or worsening in order to distinguish infectious versus noninfectious cause
- Severe abdominal pain, worrisome for toxic colitis, inflammatory bowel disease, intestinal ischemia, or surgical abdomen
- Signs of severe infection or sepsis (fever > 39.5°C, leukocytosis, and rash)
- Hemodynamically unstable
- Severe or worsening diarrhea in patients who are > 70 years old or immunocompromised
- Secretory diarrhea with dehydration
- Signs of hemolytic-uremic syndrome (acute kidney injury, thrombocytopenia, hemolytic anemia)

SUGGESTED REFERENCES

Buchholz U et al. German outbreak of *Escherichia coli* O104:H4 associated with sprouts. *N Engl J Med.* 2011 Nov 10;365(19):1763–1770. [PMID: 22029753]

DuPont HL. Acute infectious diarrhea in immunocompetent adults. *N Engl J Med.* 2014 Apr 17;370(16):1532–1540. [PMID: 24738670]

Li Z et al. Treatment of chronic diarrhea. *Best Pract Res Clin Gastroenterol.* 2012 Oct;26(5):677–687. [PMID: 23384811]

Money ME et al. Review: management of postprandial diarrhea syndrome. *Am J Med.* 2012 Jun;125(6):538–544. [PMID: 22624684]

Schiller LR. Definitions, pathophysiology, and evaluation of chronic diarrhoea. *Best Pract Res Clin Gastroenterol.* 2012 Oct;26(5):551–562. [PMID: 23384801]

32 Lower Gastrointestinal Bleeding

A 53-year-old man comes to the emergency room with a 3-hour history of bright red blood per rectum. The man states that he had been feeling well until 3 hours before when he had the sudden urge to defecate and passed a large amount of bright red blood that seemed to fill the toilet bowl. After the initial episode, he has passed similar amounts of blood mixed with maroon stool four more times. He is feeling light-headed, but denies abdominal pain, nausea, vomiting, hematemesis, or melena. He endorses having had a similar but less severe episode some years ago, which resolved quickly without treatment. His past medical history includes diverticulosis coli, diagnosed on a prior computed tomography (CT) scan. On physical examination, his heart rate is 130 bpm.

LEARNING OBJECTIVES

► Learn the clinical manifestations and objective findings that characterize the different types of lower gastrointestinal (GI) bleeding
► Understand how to distinguish upper tract from lower tract GI bleeding
► Know the differential diagnosis of lower GI bleeding
► Understand the strategies for determining the source of lower GI bleeding
► Learn about the treatments for lower GI bleeding

QUESTIONS

1. What are the salient features of this patient's problem?
2. How do you think through his problem?
3. What are the key features, including essentials of diagnosis, general considerations, and demographics, of lower GI bleeding?
4. What are the symptoms and signs of lower GI bleeding?
5. What is the differential diagnosis of lower GI bleeding?
6. What are laboratory, imaging, and procedural findings in lower GI bleeding?
7. What are the treatments for lower GI bleeding?
8. What are the outcomes, including complications and prognosis, of lower GI bleeding?
9. When should patients with lower GI bleeding be admitted to the hospital?

ANSWERS

1. Salient Features

Hematochezia (recurrent episodes); no melena; painless; history of diverticulosis coli and prior episode of self-limited bleeding; symptoms and signs of volume depletion (light-headedness, tachycardia)

2. How to Think Through

GI bleeding is common and rapid initial triage is essential. What single feature in the case indicates the need for urgent management, and what is your first priority? (The heart rate of 130 bpm indicates hypovolemia; rapid intravenous [IV] access is needed.) Would a normal hematocrit (Hct) reassure you that a hemorrhage is insignificant? (No. The Hct in acute blood loss is often normal.) Are lower GI sources of blood loss more or less common than upper GI sources? Do they generally present higher or lower risk of death? (Lower GI sources are less common and generally less morbid.) What features make a lower GI source more likely in this case? (Bright red blood, history of diverticulosis coli.) What are the common causes of lower GI bleeding and which of these fit with the data in this case? Would you assess risk factors for upper GI bleeding as well? (Yes. A brisk upper GI bleed may appear as red blood per rectum.) If hematochezia continues, with persistent tachycardia despite transfusions, what are further diagnostic and treatment options? (Rapid purge colonoscopy; and angiography and embolization by interventional radiology.) Is intervention typically needed in lower GI bleeding? (No, the majority of lower GI bleeds stop spontaneously. Supportive care and subsequent colonoscopy are the more common course.)

3. Key Features

Essentials of Diagnosis

- Hematochezia is usually present
- Ten percent of cases of hematochezia are due to an upper GI source
- Stable patients can be evaluated by colonoscopy
- Massive active bleeding calls for evaluation with sigmoidoscopy, upper endoscopy, nuclear bleeding scan, or angiography

General Considerations

- Lower GI bleeding is defined as that arising below the ligament of Treitz, ie, (nonduodenal) small intestine or colon; up to 95% of cases arise in the colon
- Lower tract bleeding
  - Thirty-three percent less common than upper tract bleeding
  - Tends to have a more benign course
  - Is less likely to present with shock or orthostasis (< 20% of cases) or to require transfusions (< 40%)
- Spontaneous cessation occurs in > 85%; hospital mortality is < 4%
- Most common causes in patients age < 50 years include
  - Infectious colitis
  - Anorectal disease
  - Inflammatory bowel disease (ulcerative colitis or Crohn disease)
- Most common causes in patients age > 50 years include
  - Diverticulosis coli (50% of cases)
  - Angioectasias (4%)
  - Neoplasms (polyps or carcinoma) (7%)
  - Ischemia
  - Radiation-induced proctitis
  - Solitary rectal ulcer
  - Nonsteroidal anti-inflammatory drug (NSAID)-induced ulcers

— Small bowel diverticula
— Colonic varices
- In 20% of cases, no source of bleeding can be identified
- Diverticular bleeding
  — Acute, painless, large-volume maroon or bright red hematochezia occurs in 3% to 5% of patients with diverticulosis coli, often associated with the use of NSAIDs
  — Bleeding more commonly originates on the right side, though diverticula are more prevalent on the left side
  — More than 95% require < 4 units of blood transfusion
  — Bleeding subsides spontaneously in 80% but may recur in up to 25% of patients
- Angioectasias
  — Painless bleeding, ranging from occult blood loss to melena or hematochezia
  — Bleeding most commonly originates in the cecum and ascending colon
  — Causes: congenital; hereditary hemorrhagic telangiectasia (HHT); autoimmune disorders, typically scleroderma
- Neoplasms: benign polyps and colorectal carcinoma cause chronic occult blood loss or intermittent anorectal hematochezia
- Anorectal disease
  — Small amounts of bright red blood noted on the toilet paper, blood streaking of the stool, or blood dripping into the toilet bowl
  — Clinically significant blood loss can sometimes occur
- Ischemic colitis
  — Hematochezia or bloody diarrhea associated with mild cramps
  — In most cases, bleeding is mild and self-limited

Demographics
- Diverticular bleeding is more common in patients > 50 years
- Angioectasia bleeding is more common in patients > 70 years and with chronic kidney disease (CKD)
- Ischemic colitis is most commonly seen
  — In older patients due to atherosclerotic disease—postoperatively after ileoaortic or abdominal aortic aneurysm surgery
  — In younger patients due to vasculitis, coagulation disorders, estrogen therapy, and long-distance running

4. Symptoms and Signs
- Brown stools mixed or streaked with blood suggest rectosigmoid or anal source
- Painless large-volume bleeding suggests diverticular bleeding
- Maroon stools suggest a right colon or small intestine source
- Black stools (melena) suggest a source proximal to the ligament of Treitz, but dark maroon stools arising from small intestine or right colon may be misinterpreted as "melena"
- Bright red blood per rectum occurs uncommonly with upper tract bleeding and almost always in the setting of massive hemorrhage with shock
- Bloody diarrhea associated with cramping abdominal pain, urgency, or tenesmus suggests inflammatory bowel disease (especially ulcerative colitis), infectious colitis, or ischemic colitis

5. Differential Diagnosis
- Diverticulosis coli
- Angioectasias, eg, idiopathic arteriovenous malformations, CREST (calcinosis, Raynaud syndrome, esophageal dysmotility, sclerodactyly, and telangiectasia) syndrome, and hereditary hemorrhagic telangiectasias
- Colonic polyps
- Colorectal cancer

- Inflammatory bowel disease (ulcerative colitis or Crohn disease)
- Hemorrhoids
- Anal fissure
- Ischemic colitis
- Infectious colitis
- Radiation colitis or proctitis
- Nonsteroidal anti-inflammatory drug-induced ulcers of small bowel or right colon

6. Laboratory, Imaging, and Procedural Findings

Laboratory Tests
- Complete blood cell count, platelet count, prothrombin time and international normalized ratio (INR)
- Serum creatinine, blood urea nitrogen
- Type and cross-match for transfusion

Imaging Studies
- Nuclear technetium-labeled red blood cell scan may be helpful in patients with significant active bleeding (bright red or maroon stools at the time of the scan)
  — Because most bleeding is slow or intermittent, less than half of nuclear studies are diagnostic
  — Scintigraphy is mainly used to see if bleeding is ongoing in order to proceed with angiography
  — Less than half of patients with a positive nuclear study have positive angiography
- Selective mesenteric angiography is used in patients with massive bleeding or positive technetium scans
- Nuclear scan or angiography may allow more limited surgical resection

Diagnostic Procedures
- Nasogastric tube aspiration or upper endoscopy in massive hematochezia to exclude upper GI tract source
- Anoscopy
- Colonoscopy in patients in whom bleeding has ceased or in patients with moderate active bleeding immediately after rapid purge with 4 to 10 L polyethylene glycol solution to clear the colon (rapid purge colonoscopy) or in whom no bleeding is detected on scintigraphy
- Small intestine push enteroscopy or video capsule imaging in patients with unexplained recurrent hemorrhage of obscure origin, suspected as originating from the small intestine

7. Treatments

Surgery
- Surgery is indicated in patients with ongoing bleeding that requires > 6 units of blood transfusion within 24 hours or > 10 total units in whom endoscopic or angiographic therapy failed
- Limited resection of the bleeding segment of small intestine or colon, if possible, which may be guided by nuclear scan or angiography
- Total abdominal colectomy with ileorectal anastomosis, if a bleeding site cannot be precisely identified in cases of ongoing hemorrhage

Therapeutic Procedures
- Excellent vascular access with (usually) two 18-gauge (or larger) peripheral IV lines
- Volume repletion with IV fluids
- Close monitoring of blood counts and coagulation panel with transfusion support as needed
- Therapeutic colonoscopy: high-risk lesions (eg, diverticulum with active bleeding or a visible vessel, or an angioectasia) can be treated endoscopically with saline or epinephrine injection, cautery (bipolar or heater probe), or application of metallic clips or bands
- Angiography with selective embolization achieves immediate hemostasis in > 95% of patients when a bleeding lesion is identified

8. Outcomes

Complications

- Major complications from intra-arterial embolization (mainly ischemic colitis) occur in 5%; rebleeding occurs in up to 25%

Prognosis

- Twenty-five percent of patients with diverticular hemorrhage have recurrent bleeding

9. When to Admit

- All patients with significant hematochezia or hemodynamic instability

SUGGESTED REFERENCES

Allen TW et al. Nuclear medicine tests for acute gastrointestinal conditions. *Semin Nucl Med.* 2013 Mar;43(2):88–101. [PMID: 23414825]

ASGE Standards of Practice Committee; Pasha SF et al. The role of endoscopy in the patient with lower GI bleeding. *Gastrointest Endosc.* 2014 Jun;79(6):875–885. [PMID: 24703084]

Kaltenbach T et al. Colonoscopy with clipping is useful in the diagnosis and treatment of diverticular bleeding. *Clin Gastroenterol Hepatol.* 2012 Feb;10(2):131–137. [PMID: 22056302]

Navaneethan U et al. Timing of colonoscopy and outcomes in patients with lower GI bleeding: a nationwide population-based study. *Gastrointest Endosc.* 2014 Feb;79(2):297–306. [PMID: 24060518]

Strate LL et al. Use of aspirin or nonsteroidal anti-inflammatory drugs increases risk for diverticulitis and diverticular bleeding. *Gastroenterology.* 2011 May;140(5):1427–1433. [PMID: 21320500]

Upper Gastrointestinal Bleeding

33

A 74-year-old man with severe osteoarthritis presents to the emergency room reporting two episodes of melena (black stools) without hematochezia (bright red blood in the stools) or hematemesis (bloody vomitus). He takes 600 mg of ibuprofen three times a day to control his arthritis pain. He denies alcoholism. On examination, his blood pressure (BP) is 150/70 mm Hg and his resting pulse is 96/min. His epigastrium is minimally tender to palpation. Rectal examination reveals black tarry stool in the vault, which is grossly positive for occult blood. Endoscopy demonstrates a 3-cm gastric ulcer. *Helicobacter pylori* is identified on biopsies of the ulcer site.

LEARNING OBJECTIVES

▶ Learn the clinical manifestations and objective findings of upper gastrointestinal (UGI) bleeding

▶ Understand the factors that predispose to UGI bleeding

▶ Know the differential diagnosis of UGI bleeding

▶ Learn the treatment for UGI bleeding

▶ Understand how to prevent UGI bleeding

QUESTIONS

1. What are the salient features of this patient's problem?

2. How do you think through his problem?

3. What are the key features, including essentials of diagnosis, general considerations, and demographics, of UGI bleeding?

4. What are the symptoms and signs of UGI bleeding?

5. What is the differential diagnosis of UGI bleeding?

6. What are laboratory and procedural findings in UGI bleeding?

7. What are the treatments for UGI bleeding?

8. What is the outcome, including prognosis, of UGI bleeding?

9. When should patients with UGI bleeding be referred to a specialist or admitted to the hospital?

ANSWERS

1. Salient Features

Melena; nonsteroidal anti-inflammatory drug (NSAID) use; mild tachycardia from anemia; tender epigastrium, occult blood positive; endoscopy showing gastric ulcer; biopsy positive for *H pylori*

2. How to Think Through

UGI bleeding is a common clinical problem and rapid initial triage is essential. As soon as melena is confirmed by physical examination, you must determine if the patient is hemodynamically stable. What is the most sensitive marker of a hemodynamically significant hemorrhage? (An elevated heart rate.)

What are key factors in determining if an urgent upper endoscopy is indicated? (Evidence of hemodynamic instability; ongoing bleeding.) How could you assess ongoing hemorrhage? (Nasogastric lavage.) Does hematochezia rule out the UGI tract as a bleeding source? (No. A brisk UGI bleed may appear as red blood.) Would a normal hematocrit reassure you that a hemorrhage is insignificant? (No.) What is the first priority if you suspect a significant GI bleed? (Intravenous [IV] access.)

What are important risk factors to consider for UGI bleeding? (Alcoholism and other risk factors for cirrhosis, NSAID use, retching [Mallory–Weiss tear], *H pylori* risk factors, and symptoms suggesting gastric cancer.) What raises the likelihood of *H pylori*? (Patients born in an endemic country; older age.) How is *H pylori* treated?

3. Key Features

Essentials of Diagnosis

- Hematemesis (bright red blood or "coffee grounds")
- Melena in most cases; hematochezia in massive UGI bleeding
- Use volume (hemodynamic) status to determine severity of blood loss; hematocrit is a poor early indicator of blood loss
- Endoscopy is diagnostic and may be therapeutic

General Considerations

- Most common presentation is hematemesis or melena; severe hematochezia in 10% of cases
- Hematemesis is either bright red blood or brown "coffee grounds" material
- Melena develops after as little as 50 to 100 mL of blood loss
- Hematochezia requires > 1000 mL of blood loss
- UGI bleeding is self-limited in 80% of cases; urgent medical therapy and endoscopic evaluation are required in the remainder
- Bleeding > 48 hours prior to presentation carries a low risk of recurrent bleeding
- Peptic ulcers account for ~40% of cases
- Portal hypertension bleeding (10%–20% of cases) occurs from varices (most commonly esophageal)
- Mallory–Weiss tears are lacerations of the gastroesophageal junction (5% to 10% of cases)
- Vascular anomalies account for 7% of cases
  - Angioectasias
    - Most common
    - 1–10 mm distorted, aberrant submucosal vessels
    - Have bright red stellate appearance
    - Occur throughout GI tract but most commonly in right colon
  - Telangiectasias
    - Small cherry red lesions
    - Occur sporadically

— Dieulafoy lesion
  ◦ Aberrant, large caliber submucosal artery
  ◦ Most common in proximal stomach and causes recurrent, intermittent bleeding
- Gastric neoplasms (1% of cases)
- Erosive gastritis (< 5% of cases) due to NSAIDs, alcohol, or severe medical or surgical illness (stress-related mucosal disease)

Demographics
- 250,000 hospitalizations a year in the United States

4. Symptoms and Signs

- Signs of chronic liver disease implicate bleeding due to portal hypertension, but a different lesion is identified in 25% of patients with cirrhosis
- Dyspepsia, NSAID use, or history of previous peptic ulcer suggests peptic ulcer disease
- Heavy alcohol ingestion or retching suggests a Mallory–Weiss tear

5. Differential Diagnosis

- Hemoptysis
- Peptic ulcer disease
- Esophageal or gastric varices
- Erosive gastritis, eg, NSAIDs, alcohol, and stress
- Mallory–Weiss tear
- Portal hypertensive gastropathy
- Angioectasias (angiodysplasias), eg, idiopathic arteriovenous malformation, CREST (calcinosis, Raynaud syndrome, esophageal dysmotility, sclerodactyly, and telangiectasia) syndrome, hereditary hemorrhagic telangiectasias
- Gastric cancer
- Rare causes
  — Erosive esophagitis
  — Duodenal varices
  — Aortoenteric fistula
  — Dieulafoy lesion (aberrant gastric submucosal artery)
  — Hemobilia (from hepatic tumor, angioma, and penetrating trauma)
  — Pancreatic cancer
  — Hemosuccus pancreaticus (pancreatic pseudoaneurysm)

6. Laboratory and Procedural Findings

Laboratory Tests
- Complete blood cell count
- Platelet count
- Prothrombin time (PT) and international normalized ratio (INR)
- Serum creatinine
- Liver enzymes
- Blood typing and screening or cross-matching
- Hematocrit is not a reliable indicator of the severity of acute bleeding

Diagnostic Procedures
- Assess volume (hemodynamic) status
  — Systolic BP
  — Heart rate
  — Postural hypotension
- Upper endoscopy after the patient is hemodynamically stable
  — To identify the source of bleeding
  — To determine the risk of rebleeding and guide triage

— To render endoscopic therapy such as cautery or injection of a sclerosant or epinephrine or application of a rubber band or metallic clips
— To biopsy ulcers for *H pylori*

7. Treatments

Medications
- Intravenous proton pump inhibitor (eg, esomeprazole or pantoprazole 80-mg bolus, followed by 8 mg/h continuous infusion for 72 hours) reduces risk of rebleeding in patients with peptic ulcers with high-risk features (active bleeding, visible vessel, or adherent clot) after endoscopic treatment
- Oral proton pump inhibitors (omeprazole, esomeprazole, or pantoprazole 40 mg, lansoprazole or dexlansoprazole 30–60 mg, once or twice daily are sufficient for lesions at low-risk for rebleeding (esophagitis, gastritis, clean-based ulcers, and Mallory–Weiss tears)
- Octreotide, 100-µg bolus, followed by 50 to 100 µg/h, for bleeding related to portal hypertension
- In countries where it is available (not in United States), terlipressin may be preferred to octreotide to treat bleeding related to portal hypertension

Therapeutic Procedures
- Insert two 18-gauge or larger intravenous lines
- In patients without hemodynamic compromise or overt active bleeding, aggressive fluid repletion can be delayed until extent of bleeding clarified
- Patients with hemodynamic compromise should be given 0.9% saline or lactated Ringer injection and cross-matched for 2 to 4 units of packed red blood cells (RBC)
- Nasogastric tube placed for aspiration
- Blood replacement to maintain a hemoglobin of 7 to 9 g/dL
- In the absence of continued bleeding, the hematocrit should rise 4% for each unit of transfused packed red cells
- Transfuse blood in patients with massive active bleeding regardless of the hematocrit
- Transfuse platelets if platelet count < 50,000/µL or if impaired platelet function due to aspirin or clopidogrel use
- Uremic patients with active bleeding should be given three doses of desmopressin (DDAVP), 0.3 µg/kg intravenously at 12-hour intervals
- Fresh frozen plasma should be given for actively bleeding patients with a coagulopathy and an INR > 1.8
- However, endoscopy may be performed safely if the INR is < 2.5
- In massive bleeding, 1 unit of fresh frozen plasma should be given for each 5 units of packed RBC transfused
- Intra-arterial embolization in patients who are poor operative risks and with persistent bleeding from ulcers, angiomas, or Mallory–Weiss tears in whom endoscopic therapy has failed
- Transvenous intrahepatic portosystemic shunts (TIPS) to decompress the portal venous system and control acute variceal bleeding are indicated in patients in whom endoscopic modalities have failed

8. Outcome

Prognosis
- Mortality rate is 4% to 10%, and even higher in patients older than age 60, though rates have been declining steadily; often mortality is from complications of underlying diseases
- Hemorrhage from peptic ulcers has an overall mortality rate of 6%
- Portal hypertension has a hospital mortality rate of 15%; mortality rate of 60% to 80% at 1 to 4 years

9. When to Refer and When to Admit

When to Refer

- Refer to gastroenterologist for endoscopy
- Refer to surgeon for uncontrollable, life-threatening hemorrhage

When to Admit

- Very low-risk patients who meet following criteria do not require hospital admission and can be evaluated as outpatients
  - No serious comorbid medical illnesses or advanced liver disease and normal hemodynamic status
  - No evidence of overt bleeding (hematemesis or melena) within 48 hours
  - Negative nasogastric lavage
  - Normal laboratory tests
- Low-to-moderate-risk patients are admitted to hospital
  - Upper endoscopy after appropriate stabilization and further treatment
  - Based on findings, may then be discharged and monitored as outpatients
- High-risk patients with any of the following require intensive care unit (ICU) admission
  - Active bleeding manifested by hematemesis or bright red blood on nasogastric aspirate
  - Shock
  - Persistent hemodynamic derangement despite fluid resuscitation
  - Serious comorbid medical illness
  - Evidence of advanced liver disease

SUGGESTED REFERENCES

Almadi MA et al. Antiplatelet and anticoagulant therapy in patients with gastrointestinal bleeding: an 86-year-old woman with peptic ulcer disease. *JAMA.* 2011 Dec 7;306(21):2367–2374. [PMID: 22045703]

Greenspoon J et al; International Consensus Upper Gastrointestinal Bleeding Conference Group. Management of patients with nonvariceal upper gastrointestinal bleeding. *Clin Gastroenterol Hepatol.* 2012 Mar;10(3):234–239. [PMID: 21820395]

Lau JY et al. Challenges in the management of acute peptic ulcer bleeding. *Lancet.* 2013 Jun 8;381(9882):2033–2043. [PMID: 23746903]

Marmo R et al; PNED 1 and PNED 2 Investigators. Predicting mortality in patients with in-hospital nonvariceal upper GI bleeding: a prospective, multicenter database study. *Gastrointest Endosc.* 2014 May;79(5):741–749. [PMID: 24219820]

Srygley FD et al. Does this patient have a severe upper gastrointestinal bleed? *JAMA.* 2012 Mar 14;307(10):1072–1079. [PMID: 22416103]

Villanueva C et al. Transfusion for acute upper gastrointestinal bleeding. *N Engl J Med.* 2013 Apr 4;368(1):11–21. [PMID: 23550677]

34

Viral Hepatitis

A 27-year-old woman presents to her primary care clinician complaining of nausea and vomiting. She returned 1 week ago from an international trip to South America where she ate at local restaurants and food carts. On physical examination, her skin is jaundiced, her abdomen is tender to palpation in the right upper quadrant (RUQ), and there is mild hepatomegaly. Serum bilirubin and aminotransferases are elevated. Anti-hepatitis A virus (HAV) IgM is positive.

LEARNING OBJECTIVES

► Learn the clinical manifestations and objective findings of viral hepatitis
► Understand the factors that predispose to the contraction of each type of viral hepatitis
► Know the differential diagnosis of viral hepatitis
► Learn the treatment for acute viral hepatitis
► Know the possible complications of viral hepatitis

QUESTIONS

1. What are the salient features of this patient's problem?
2. How do you think through her problem?
3. What are the key features, including essentials of diagnosis, general considerations, and demographics, of viral hepatitis?
4. What are the symptoms and signs of viral hepatitis?
5. What is the differential diagnosis of viral hepatitis?
6. What are laboratory and procedural findings in viral hepatitis?
7. What are the treatments for viral hepatitis A, B, and C?
8. What are the outcomes, including complications, prognosis, and prevention, of viral hepatitis?
9. When should patients with viral hepatitis be referred to a specialist or admitted to the hospital?

ANSWERS

1. Salient Features

Nausea, vomiting; recent travel with possibly unsanitary food exposure; jaundice; tender abdomen; hepatomegaly; elevated serum bilirubin and aminotransferase tests; positive antibody to hepatitis A (anti-HAV) IgM antibody

2. How to Think Through

Acute nausea and vomiting in a returning traveler can be due to infectious gastroenteritis, but their overlap with jaundice places viral hepatitis high in the differential diagnosis. What risk factors for hepatitis in general should be assessed? (Acetaminophen use, alcoholism, toxin [eg, *Amanita* mushroom consumption], unprotected sexual risk behaviors, injection drug use, recent tattoos, or blood transfusion.) The duration of travel and of her symptoms should be elicited. The incubation period of the hepatitis viruses varies, and this can help narrow the differential diagnosis. All of them can cause the acute symptoms seen in this patient. What viral hepatitis serologies are detectable during the acute illness and would be most informative here? (Anti-HAV IgM; HBV surface antigen and anti-HBc IgM; anti-HCV and, if a high suspicion, assay for HCV RNA.) If all these study results are negative, what other infectious causes of hepatitis should be considered? (Mononucleosis [Epstein–Barr virus (EBV)], cytomegalovirus (CMV), leptospirosis, brucellosis, yellow fever, Middle East respiratory syndrome, Ebola virus, influenza.) Would a serum alanine aminotransferase level > 1000 IU/dL, or a bilirubin level > 8 mg/dL suggest that the diagnosis of viral hepatitis may be incorrect? (No. This degree of elevation is common.) How should she be managed? (Supportive care, intravenous [IV] hydration and glucose if needed, avoidance of alcohol and hepatotoxic medications.) What is the likelihood of her developing fulminant hepatic failure? (Very rare in hepatitis A, unless underlying HCV or cirrhosis.) Hand washing by the patient and care providers is important.

3. Key Features

Essentials of Diagnosis

Acute hepatitis A, B, C

- Prodrome of anorexia, nausea, vomiting, malaise, aversion to smoking
- Fever, enlarged and tender liver, jaundice
- Markedly elevated aminotransferases
- Normal to low white blood cell (WBC) count
- Hepatitis C is often asymptomatic; source of hepatitis C infection is unknown in many

Chronic hepatitis A, B, and C

- Patients with acute hepatitis A almost always recover, do not develop chronic hepatitis
- Chronic hepatitis B and C are defined as a continuing inflammatory reaction of the liver after > 3 to 6 months
- Chronic hepatitis B is characterized by persistent detection of serum hepatitis B surface antigen (HBsAg)
- This is most often accompanied by persistently elevated aminotransferase levels
- Chronic hepatitis C is also characterized by persistent detection of serum antibody to hepatitis C virus (HCV) and persistently abnormal serum aminotransferase levels

General Considerations

Acute hepatitis A

- Transmission of HAV is by the fecal–oral route; the incubation period averages 30 days
- HAV is excreted in feces for up to 2 weeks before the clinical illness and rarely persists in feces after the first week of illness (there is no chronic carrier state)

Acute hepatitis B

- HBV contains an inner core protein (hepatitis B core antigen, HBcAg) and outer surface coat (hepatitis B surface antigen, HBsAg)
- The incubation period for hepatitis B is 6 weeks to 6 months (average 3 months) and the onset of HBV is more insidious and the aminotransferase levels higher on average than in HAV infection
- Eight genotypes of HBV (A–H) have been identified
- Four phases of HBV infection are recognized
  — Immune tolerant phase
  — Immune clearance phase

— Inactive HBsAg carrier state
— Reactivated chronic hepatitis B phase

- Early in the course, hepatitis Be antigen (HBeAg) and hepatitis B virus (HBV) DNA are present in serum
  — HBeAg is indicative of active viral replications and necroinflammatory activity in the liver
  — These persons are at risk for progression to cirrhosis and for hepatocellular carcinoma
  — Low-level IgM anti-HBc is also present in about 70%
- Clinical and biochemical improvement may coincide with
  — Disappearance of HBeAg and HBV DNA from serum
  — Appearance of anti-HBe
  — Integration of the HBV genome into the host genome in infected hepatocytes
- If cirrhosis has not yet developed, such persons are at a lower risk for cirrhosis and hepatocellular carcinoma

Acute hepatitis C

- The HCV is a single-stranded RNA virus (Hepacivirus) with properties similar to those of flavivirus
- Six major genotypes of HCV have been identified
- Coinfection with HCV is found in at least 30% of persons infected with HIV, and HIV leads to more rapid progression of chronic hepatitis C to cirrhosis
- Anti-HCV is not protective; in patients with acute or chronic hepatitis, its presence in serum generally signifies that HCV is the cause

Chronic hepatitis B, C

- Chronic hepatitis B and C can be characterized on the basis of liver biopsy findings
  — The grade of portal, periportal, and lobular inflammation (minimal, mild, moderate, or severe)
  — The stage of fibrosis (none, mild, moderate, severe, cirrhosis)
- HCV may be the most common etiology of chronic hepatitis
- HCV coinfection is found in 30% of persons infected with HIV
- Anti-HCV is not protective; in chronic hepatitis its presence in serum signifies that HCV is the cause

Demographics
Hepatitis A

- HAV spread is favored by crowding and poor sanitation, with outbreaks often resulting from contaminated water or food, though outbreaks among injection drug users have been reported
- Since introduction of HAV vaccine in the United States in 1995, the incidence rate of HAV infection has declined from 14 to 1.3 per 100,000 population

Hepatitis B

- Chronic hepatitis B afflicts 400 million people worldwide and 2.2 million (predominantly men) in the United States
- Incidence of HBV has decreased from 8.5 to 1.5 cases per 100,000 population since the 1990s
- HBV is usually transmitted by infected blood or blood products and by sexual contact
- HBV is present in saliva, semen, and vaginal secretions
- HBsAg-positive mothers may transmit HBV to the newborn at the time of delivery ("vertical transmission")
- The risk of chronic HBV infection in the infant approaches 90% if the mother is HBeAg positive
- HBV is prevalent in men who have sex with men and injection drug users, but most cases result from heterosexual transmission
- About 7% of HIV-infected persons are coinfected with HBV
- Groups at risk for HBV infection include

— Patients and staff at hemodialysis centers
— Physicians, dentists, and nurses
— Personnel working in clinical and pathology laboratories and blood banks
• The risk of HBV infection from a blood transfusion is < 1 in 60,000 units transfused in the United States

Hepatitis C

• Chronic hepatitis C develops in up to 85% of patients with acute hepatitis C
• There are about 2.3 million HCV carriers in the United States as of 2013, down from 3.2 million in 2001 (184 million worldwide) and another 1.3 million previously exposed persons who have cleared the virus
• In the past, HCV caused over 90% of cases of posttransfusion hepatitis, yet only 4% of cases of hepatitis C were attributable to blood transfusions
• Over 50% of HCV cases are transmitted by injection drug use
• Body piercing, tattoos, and hemodialysis may be risk factors for HCV infection
• The risk of sexual and maternal–neonatal transmission of HCV is low and may be greatest in those with high circulating levels of HCV RNA
— Multiple sexual partners may increase the risk of HCV infection
— Transmission via breast-feeding has not been documented
• Hospital-acquired transmission of HCV may occur between patients on a liver unit or via
— Multidose vials of saline
— Reuse of disposable syringes
— Contamination of shared saline, radiopharmaceutical, and sclerosant vials

4. Symptoms and Signs

Acute hepatitis A, B, and C

• Onset may be abrupt or insidious
• Malaise, myalgia, arthralgia, easy fatigability, upper respiratory symptoms, and anorexia
• A distaste for smoking, paralleling anorexia, may occur early
• Nausea and vomiting are frequent, and diarrhea or constipation may occur
• Defervescence and a fall in pulse rate often coincide with the onset of jaundice
• Abdominal pain
— Usually mild and constant in the RUQ or epigastrium
— Often aggravated by jarring or exertion
— Rarely severe enough to simulate cholecystitis
• Jaundice
— Never develops in many patients
— Occurs after 5 to 10 days but may appear at the same time as the initial symptoms
— With its onset, prodromal symptoms often worsen, followed by progressive clinical improvement
— Stools may be acholic (clay-colored)
• Hepatomegaly—rarely marked—is present in over 50% of cases. Liver tenderness is usually present
• Splenomegaly occurs in 15% of patients
• Soft, enlarged lymph nodes—especially in the cervical or epitrochlear areas—may occur
• The acute illness usually subsides over 2 to 3 weeks

Hepatitis A

• Clinical, biochemical, and serologic recovery from hepatitis A may be followed by one or two relapses, but recovery is the rule; however, a protracted course has been reported to be associated with HLA *DRB1*1301*

Hepatitis B

• In 5% to 10% of cases of hepatitis B, the course may be more protracted, but < 1% will have a fulminant course
• Hepatitis B may become chronic

- Chronic hepatitis B is clinically indistinguishable from chronic hepatitis due to other causes
- Immune clearance phase
  — HBeAg and HBV DNA are present in serum, indicative of active viral replication
  — Serum aminotransferase levels are normal, with little necroinflammation in the liver
  — This phase is common in infants and young children whose immature immune system fails to mount an immune response to HBV
- Inactive HBsAg carrier state
  — Patients have entered this phase when biochemical improvement follows immune clearance and cirrhosis has not yet developed
  — Patients in this phase are at a low risk for cirrhosis and hepatocellular carcinoma
  — Patients with persistently normal serum aminotransferase levels infrequently have histologically significant liver disease
- Reactivated chronic hepatitis B phase
  — Risk factors for reactivation include male sex and HBV genotype C, advanced age, alcohol use, cigarette smoking, and coinfection with HCV or HDV
  — In patients with either HBeAg-positive or HBeAg-negative chronic hepatitis B, the risk of cirrhosis and of hepatocellular carcinoma correlates with the serum HBV DNA level
  — HIV coinfection is also associated with an increased frequency of cirrhosis when the CD4 count is low

Hepatitis C
- The incubation period of HCV averages 6 to 7 weeks
- Clinical illness in HCV is
  — Often mild
  — Usually asymptomatic
  — Characterized by waxing and waning aminotransferase elevations and a high rate (> 80%) of chronic hepatitis
- In patients with the HCV CC genotype
  — Spontaneous clearance of HCV following acute infection is more common (64%)
  — Jaundice is more likely to develop during the course of acute hepatitis C

5. Differential Diagnosis
- Viruses: hepatitis A, B, C, D (delta agent, always in presence of B), E, infectious mononucleosis, cytomegalovirus (CMV), Epstein–Barr virus (EBV), herpes simplex virus (HSV), parvovirus B19, yellow fever, Middle East respiratory syndrome, Ebola virus, influenza; hepatitis G rarely, if ever, causes frank hepatitis
- CMV, EBV, and HSV are found particularly in immunocompromised persons
- Other infections: leptospirosis, secondary syphilis, brucellosis, Q fever
- Alcoholic hepatitis and nonalcoholic steatohepatitis
- Drugs and toxins (predictable): acetaminophen, *Amanita* mushrooms, tetracycline, valproic acid
- Drugs and toxins (idiosyncratic): isoniazid, nonsteroidal anti-inflammatory drugs, statins, azole antifungals, halothane, ecstasy, kava
- Vascular: right-sided HF, shock liver, portal vein thrombosis, Budd–Chiari syndrome
- Metabolic: Wilson disease, hemochromatosis, acute fatty liver of pregnancy, Reye syndrome
- Autoimmune hepatitis
- α1-Antiprotease (α1-antitrypsin) deficiency
- Lymphoma or metastatic cancer
- TT virus (TTV)
  — Found in up to 7.5% of blood donors
  — Readily transmitted by blood transfusions
  — However, an association between this virus and liver disease has not been established

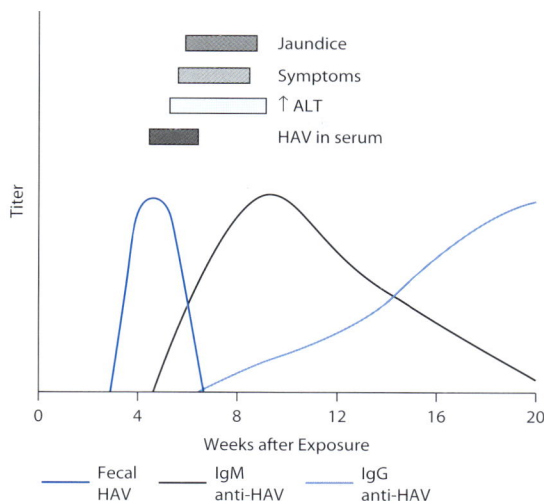

Figure 34-1. The typical course of acute type A hepatitis. (ALT, alanine aminotransferase; anti-HAV, antibody to hepatitis A virus; HAV, hepatitis A virus.) (Reproduced with permission from Koff RS. Acute viral hepatitis. In: Friedman LS, Keeffe EB, eds. *Handbook of Liver Disease*, 3rd ed. Philadelphia: Saunders Elsevier; 2012.)

- A related virus known as SEN-V has been found in 2% of US blood donors
  — Is transmitted by transfusion
  — May account for some cases of transfusion-associated non-ABCDE hepatitis

6. Laboratory Findings

Laboratory Tests

Hepatitis A

- Anti-HAV appears early in the course of the illness
- See Figure 34-1
- Both IgM and IgG anti-HAV are detectable in serum soon after the onset
- Peak titers of IgM anti-HAV occur during the first week of clinical disease and disappear within 3 to 6 months
- Detection of IgM anti-HAV is an excellent test for diagnosing acute hepatitis A (but is not recommended for evaluation of asymptomatic patients with persistent aminotransferase elevations)
- Titers of IgG anti-HAV peak after 1 month of the disease and may persist for years
- IgG anti-HAV indicates previous exposure to HAV, noninfectivity, and immunity. In the United States, about 30% of the population have serologic evidence of previous infection
- The WBC count is normal to low, especially in the preicteric phase. Large atypical lymphocytes may occasionally be seen
- Mild proteinuria is common, and bilirubinuria often precedes the appearance of jaundice
- Strikingly elevated aspartate or alanine aminotransferases occur early, followed by elevations of bilirubin and alkaline phosphatase; in a small number of patients, the latter persist after aminotransferase levels have normalized
- Cholestasis is occasionally marked

Hepatitis B

- Antibodies to hepatitis B appear early in the course of the illness (Table 34-1)
- See Figure 34-2

HBsAg

- Appears before biochemical evidence of liver disease, and persists throughout the clinical illness
- After the acute illness, it may be associated with chronic hepatitis

Table 34–1. Common serologic patterns in hepatitis B virus infection and their interpretation.

HBsAg	Anti-HBs	Anti-HBc	HBeAg	Anti-HBe	Interpretation
+	–	IgM	+	–	Acute hepatitis B
+	–	IgG[a]	+	–	Chronic hepatitis B with active viral replication
+	–	IgG	–	+	Chronic hepatitis B generally with low viral replication
+	+	IgG	+ or –	+ or –	Chronic hepatitis B with heterotypic anti-HBs (about 10% of cases)
–	–	IgM	+ or –	–	Acute hepatitis B
–	+	IgG	–	+ or –	Recovery from hepatitis B (immunity)
–	+	–	–	–	Vaccination (immunity)
–	–	IgG	–	–	False-positive; less commonly, infection in remote past

[a]Low levels of IgM anti-HBc may also be detected.

Anti-HBs
- Appears after clearance of HBsAg and after successful vaccination against hepatitis B
- Signals recovery from HBV infection, noninfectivity, and immunity

Anti-HBc
- IgM anti-HBc appears shortly after HBsAg is detected. (HBcAg alone does not appear in serum)
  — Its presence in acute hepatitis indicates a diagnosis of acute hepatitis B
  — It fills the rare serologic gap when HBsAg has cleared but anti-HBs is not yet detectable
  — Can persist for 3 to 6 months or more and reappear during flares of chronic hepatitis B
- IgG anti-HBc also appears during acute hepatitis B but persists indefinitely
- In asymptomatic blood donors, an isolated anti-HBc with no other positive HBV serologic results may represent a falsely positive result or latent infection

HBeAg
- Found only in HBsAg-positive serum and indicates viral replication and infectivity
- Persistence beyond 3 months indicates an increased likelihood of chronic hepatitis B
- Its disappearance is often followed by the appearance of anti-HBe, generally signifying diminished viral replication and decreased infectivity

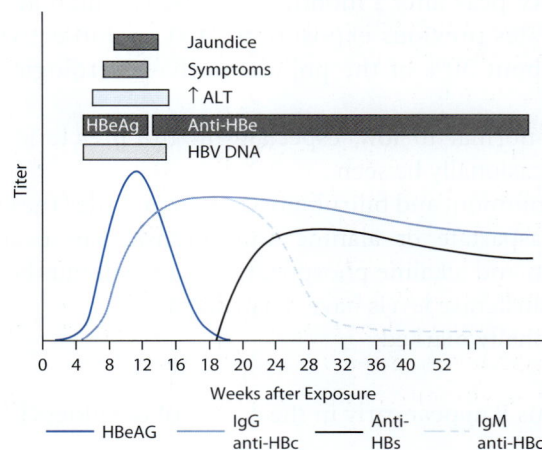

Figure 34-2. The typical course of acute type B hepatitis. (ALT, alanine aminotransferase; anti-HBc, antibody to hepatitis B core antigen; anti-HBe, antibody to HBeAg; anti-HBs, antibody to HBsAg; HBeAg, hepatitis Be antigen; HBsAg, hepatitis B surface antigen.) (Reproduced with permission from Koff RS. Acute viral hepatitis. In: Friedman LS, Keeffe EB, eds. *Handbook of Liver Disease*, 3rd ed. Philadelphia: Saunders Elsevier; 2012.)

HBV DNA

- Generally parallels the presence of HBeAg, though HBV DNA is a more sensitive and precise marker of viral replication and infectivity
- Very low levels of HBV DNA are detectable only by polymerase chain reaction (PCR)
  — May persist in serum after recovery from acute hepatitis B
  — However, HBV DNA is bound to IgG and is rarely infectious

Immune Tolerant Phase

- HBeAg and HBV DNA are present in serum, indicative of active viral replication
- When HBV infection is acquired in infancy or early childhood, serum aminotransferase levels often are normal and little necroinflammation is present in the liver

Immune Clearance Phase

- Aminotransferase levels are elevated

Inactive HBsAg Carrier State

- Disappearance of HBeAg and reduced HBV DNA levels ($< 10^5$ copies/mL, or $< 20,000$ international units/mL) in serum, appearance of anti-HBe, and integration of the HBV genome into the host genome in infected hepatocytes

Reactivated Chronic Hepatitis B Phase

- May result from infection by a precore mutant of HBV or spontaneous mutation of the precore or core promoter region of the HBV genome during the course of chronic hepatitis caused by wild-type HBV
- There is a rise in serum HBV DNA levels and possible progression to cirrhosis (at a rate of 8%–10% per year), particularly when additional mutations in the core gene of HBV are present
  — Elevated serum bilirubin level, low albumin level, and prolonged prothrombin time reflect advanced disease (severe inflammation or cirrhosis, or both)
  — Normal to low WBC count and large atypical lymphocytes
  — Mild proteinuria is common
  — Bilirubinuria often precedes the appearance of jaundice
  — Elevated aspartate or alanine aminotransferase occurs early, followed by elevations of bilirubin and alkaline phosphatase
  — Marked prolongation of prothrombin time in severe hepatitis correlates with increased mortality

Hepatitis C

- Serum anti-HCV by enzyme immunoassay (EIA) is present (Figure 34-3)
  — The immunoassay has moderate sensitivity (false negatives) for the diagnosis early in the course and in healthy blood donors and low specificity (false positives) in persons with elevated γ-globulin levels
  — In these situations, a diagnosis of hepatitis C may be confirmed by use of a polymerase chain reaction (PCR) assay for HCV RNA
  — Occasional persons are found to have anti-HCV in serum without HCV RNA in serum, suggesting recovery from HCV infection in the past
  — In pregnant patients, serum aminotransferase levels frequently normalize despite persistence of viremia, only to increase again after delivery
  — The WBC count is normal to low, especially in the preicteric phase
  — Large atypical lymphocytes may occasionally be seen
  — Mild proteinuria is common, and bilirubinuria often precedes the appearance of jaundice
  — Elevated aspartate or alanine aminotransferase levels occur early, followed by elevations of bilirubin and alkaline phosphatase; in a small number of patients, the latter persist after aminotransferase levels have normalized
  — In approximately 40% of cases of chronic hepatitis C, serum aminotransferase levels are persistently normal

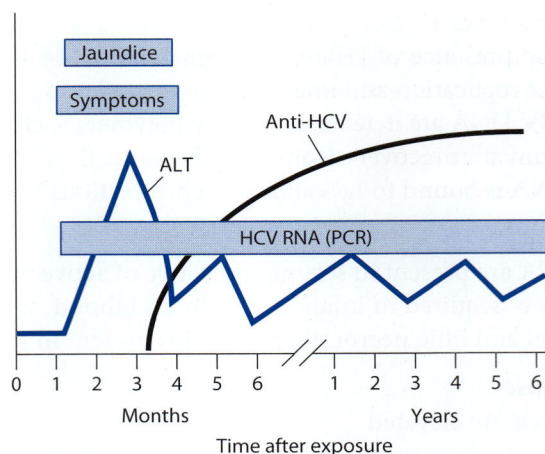

Figure 34-3. The typical course of acute and chronic hepatitis C. (ALT, alanine aminotransferase; anti-HCV, antibody to hepatitis C virus by enzyme immunoassay; HCV RNA [PCR], hepatitis C viral RNA by polymerase chain reaction.) (Reproduced with permission from Koff RS. Acute viral hepatitis. In: Friedman LS, Keeffe EB, eds. *Handbook of Liver Disease*, 3rd ed. Philadelphia: Saunders Elsevier; 2012.)

Diagnostic Procedures
• Liver biopsy may be indicated for diagnosis, staging, and predicting response to therapy
• Serum FibroSure testing or ultrasound elastography may be used to identify the absence of fibrosis or presence of cirrhosis in chronic hepatitis C

7. Treatments
Medications
Acute Hepatitis A, B, and C
• If nausea and vomiting are pronounced or if oral intake is substantially decreased, intravenous 10% glucose is indicated
• Small doses of oxazepam are safe, as metabolism is not hepatic; morphine sulfate is to be avoided

Acute Hepatitis B
• Antiviral therapy is generally unnecessary but it is usually prescribed in cases of fulminant hepatitis B as well as in spontaneous reactivation of chronic hepatitis B presenting as acute-on-chronic liver failure
• Corticosteroids produce no benefit

Chronic Hepatitis B
• Treated with antiviral agents in selected patients with active viral replication
  — HBeAg is present and HBV DNA elevated [$\geq 10^5$ copies/mL, or $\geq 20,000$ international units/mL] in serum
  — Elevated aminotransferase levels
• Entecavir
  — Dosage: 0.5 mg orally daily for patients not resistant to lamivudine and 1 mg orally daily for patients who are resistant to lamivudine
  — Entecavir resistance is rare unless a patient is already resistant to lamivudine
  — Histologic improvement is observed in 70% of treated patients and suppression of HBV DNA in serum occurs in nearly all treated patients
  — Entecavir has been reported to cause lactic acidosis when used in patients with decompensated cirrhosis
• Tenofovir
  — Dosage: 300 mg orally daily
  — Equally effective against HBV as entecavir; used as a first-line agent or when resistance to a nucleoside analog has developed

— Has a low rate of resistance when used as initial therapy

— Long-term use may lead to an elevated serum creatinine level and reduced serum phosphate level (Fanconi-like syndrome) that is reversible with discontinuation of the drug

— Classified as pregnancy category B; treatment is recommended starting in the third trimester when a mother's serum HBV DNA level is > 200,000 international units/mL to reduce levels at time of delivery

• Adefovir dipivoxil

— Dosage: 10 mg orally once daily for at least 1 year

— Has activity against wild-type and lamivudine-resistant HBV but is the least potent of the oral antiviral agents for HBV

— Adding the drug may be effective in patients who have become resistant to lamivudine

— A small number of patients achieve sustained suppression of HBV replication; long-term suppressive therapy is often required

— Resistance is less frequent than with lamivudine but is seen in up to 29% of patients treated for 5 years

— Patients with underlying kidney dysfunction are at risk for nephrotoxicity

• Telbivudine

— Dosage: 600 mg orally daily

— More potent than either lamivudine or adefovir

— Resistance to this drug may develop, however, particularly in patients who are resistant to lamivudine

— Elevated creatine kinase levels are common

— Classified as pregnancy category B; treatment is recommended starting in the third trimester when mother's serum HBV DNA level is > 200,000 international units/mL to reduce levels at time of delivery

• Lamivudine

— Dosage: 100 mg orally daily

— By the end of 1 year, however, 15%–30% of responders experience a relapse (and occasionally frank decompensation)

— The rate of resistance reaches 70% by 5 years of therapy; consequently, lamivudine is no longer considered first-line therapy in the United States but may be used in countries in which its relative low cost is a deciding factor

— Classified as pregnancy category C; safe to use in pregnant women with HIV; treatment is recommended starting in the third trimester when a mother's serum HBV DNA level is > 200,000 international units/mL to reduce levels at time of delivery

• Peginterferon alfa-2a

— Dosage: 180 μg subcutaneously once weekly for 48 weeks

— Leads to sustained normalization of aminotransferase levels, disappearance of HBeAg and HBV DNA from serum, appearance of anti-HBe, and improved survival in up to 40% of treated patients

— Response is most likely in patients with a low baseline HBV DNA level and high aminotransferase levels and is more likely in those infected with HBV genotype A than with other genotypes (especially genotype D) and who have certain favorable polymorphisms of the *IL28B* gene

— Most complete responders eventually clear HBsAg and develop anti-HBs in serum, and are thus cured

— Relapses are uncommon in complete responders who seroconvert from HBeAg to anti-HBe

— Patients with HBeAg-negative chronic hepatitis B have a response rate of 60% after 48 weeks of therapy but the response may not be durable

— Response to interferon is poor in patients with HIV coinfection

Chronic Hepatitis C

- The introduction of direct-acting and host-targeting antiviral agents has revolutionized the treatment of HCV; now regimens are often all-oral and peginterferon is often not needed (Table 34-2)
- HCV genotype 1 has become easy to cure with oral direct-acting agents, with expected sustained virologic response rates above 90%, and virtually all HCV genotype 2 infection is curable with all-oral regimens
- Newer therapies are very effective, but costly and insurance coverage may be a barrier to treatment

Table 34-2. Direct-acting antiviral agents for HCV infection.

Agent	Genotype(s)	Dose[b]	Comment
NS3/4A Protease Inhibitors			
Boceprevir	1	800 mg orally three times daily	Used in combination with pegylated interferon and ribavirin; no longer recommended
Telaprevir	1	1125 mg orally twice daily	Used in combination with pegylated interferon and ribavirin; no longer recommended
Simeprevir	1 and 4	150 mg orally once daily	Used in combination with pegylated interferon and ribavirin or with sofosbuvir
Paritaprevir	1 and 4	150 mg orally once daily	Used in combination with ombitasvir and dasabuvir; ritonavir (100 mg) boosted[c]; for genotype 1b with cirrhosis and genotype 1a, used with ribavirin
Asunaprevir[a]	1 and 4	200 mg orally twice daily	Used in combination with daclatasvir or with daclatasvir and beclabuvir
Grazoprevir[a]	1, 2, 4–6	100 mg orally once daily	Used in combination with elbasvir
NS5A Inhibitors			
Daclatasvir[a]	1–6	60 mg orally once daily	Used in combination with sofosbuvir (genotypes 1–6) or with pegylated interferon and ribavirin (genotype 4) or with asunaprevir (with or without beclabuvir; under study)
Ledipasvir	1, 3, and 4	90 mg orally once daily	Used in combination with sofosbuvir[d]
Ombitasvir[a]	1 and 4	25 mg orally once daily	Used in combination with paritaprevir (ritonavir boosted) and dasabuvir with or without ribavirin as per paritaprevir above
Elbasvir[a]	1–6	50 mg orally once daily	Used in combination with grazoprevir
GS-5816[a]	1–6	100 mg orally once daily	Used in combination with sofosbuvir
NS5B Nucleos(t)ide Polymerase Inhibitor			
Sofosbuvir	1–6	400 mg orally once daily	Used in combination with pegylated interferon and ribavirin (all genotypes) or with ribavirin alone (genotypes 2 and 3) or with simeprevir (genotypes 1 and 4) or with daclatasvir (all genotypes) or with ledipasvir (genotypes 1, 3, and 4) or with GS-5861 (under study)
NS5B Non-nucleos(t)ide Polymerase Inhibitors			
Dasabuvir	1 and 4	250 mg orally twice daily	Used in combination with paritaprevir (ritonavir boosted) and ombitasvir with or without ribavirin as per paritaprevir above
Beclabuvir[a]	1	75 mg orally twice daily	Used in combination with daclatasvir and asunaprevir

[a]Agent has not been approved by the FDA as of early 2015; additional drugs are under study.

[b]The preferred regimen and duration of treatment may vary depending on HCV genotype, presence or absence of cirrhosis, or nonresponse to prior therapy for HCV infection.

[c]Marketed as Viekira Pak (AbbVie).

[d]Marketed as Harvoni (Gilead Sciences).

- Treatment of HCV genotype 3 infection, particularly in association with cirrhosis, remains a challenge
- Two peginterferon formulations are available
  — Peginterferon alfa-2b, with a 12-kDa polyethylene glycol (PEG), in a dose of 1.5 µg/kg weekly subcutaneously
  — Peginterferon alfa-2a, with a 40-kDa PEG, in a dose of 180 µg once per week for 48 weeks subcutaneously
- When ribavirin is used with peginterferon alfa-2b
  — Dose of ribavirin is based on the patient's weight
  — May range from 800 to 1400 mg daily in two divided doses
- When ribavirin is used with peginterferon alfa-2a
  — Dose of ribavirin is again based on the patient's weight
  — Dose is 1000 mg for patients weighing < 75 kg and 1200 mg for those > 75 kg)
- When peginterferon alfa plus ribavirin therapy is undertaken, obtain a CBC at weeks 1, 2, and 4 after therapy is started and monthly thereafter; monitor patients on ribavirin for hemolysis
- Peginterferon alfa with ribavirin may be effective treatment for cryoglobulinemia associated with chronic hepatitis C
- Coinfection of HCV and HIV may benefit from treatment of HCV
- Treatment with peginterferon alfa plus ribavirin is costly, has side effects (flu-like symptoms) that are almost universal, and serious toxicity can include psychiatric symptoms, thyroid dysfunction, bone marrow suppression, and retinopathy (especially in patients with hypertension)
- Contraindications for interferon therapy include pregnancy and breast-feeding, decompensated cirrhosis, prior solid organ transplants (except liver), profound cytopenias, severe psychiatric disorders, autoimmune diseases, inability to self-administer subcutaneous injections
- Ribavirin should be avoided in persons over age 65 and in patients for whom hemolysis could pose a risk of angina or stroke
- Rash, itching, headache, cough, and shortness of breath also occur with ribavirin; lactic acidosis is a concern if also taking highly active antiretroviral therapy for HIV

Therapeutic Procedures
- Activity is modified according to symptoms; bed rest is not necessary except for marked symptoms
- Dietary management in acute viral hepatitis consists of palatable meals as tolerated, without overfeeding; breakfast is usually best tolerated; in late stage chronic hepatitis B or C, sodium or protein restriction is undertaken if needed for fluid overload or encephalopathy
- Strenuous physical exertion, alcohol, and hepatotoxic agents should be avoided

8. Outcomes
Complications
Hepatitis A
- Fulminant hepatitis A is uncommon; its frequency is increased when hepatitis A occurs in a patient with chronic hepatitis C

Hepatitis B
- Acute hepatitis B can lead to chronic infection and fulminant liver failure (particularly if the patient is coinfected with the delta agent, hepatitis D)
- Chronic hepatitis B may be complicated by
  — Cirrhosis and liver failure
  — Hepatocellular carcinoma
  — Extrahepatic manifestations include polyarteritis nodosa, membranous glomerulonephritis

- The 5-year mortality rate for chronic hepatitis B
  — 0% to 2% in those without cirrhosis
  — 14% to 20% in those with compensated cirrhosis
  — 70% to 86% in those with decompensated cirrhosis
- The risk of cirrhosis and hepatocellular carcinoma correlates with serum HBV DNA levels, and a focus of therapy is to suppress HBV DNA levels below 300 copies/mL (60 international units/mL)
- There is some evidence that HBV genotype C is associated with a higher risk of cirrhosis and hepatocellular carcinoma than other genotypes
- Antiviral treatment improves the prognosis in responders

Hepatitis C
- Hepatitis C associated diseases
  — Mixed cryoglobulinemia and membranoproliferative glomerulonephritis
  — Possibly lichen planus, autoimmune thyroiditis, lymphocytic sialadenitis, idiopathic pulmonary fibrosis, porphyria cutanea tarda, monoclonal gammopathy, and non-Hodgkin lymphoma

Prognosis
Hepatitis A
- Generally, clinical recovery in hepatitis A is complete in 9 weeks
- Hepatitis A does not cause chronic liver disease, though it may persist for up to 1 year, and clinical and biochemical relapses may occur before full recovery
- The mortality rate is < 0.6% for hepatitis A

Hepatitis B
- Mortality rate for acute hepatitis B is 0.1% to 1% but is higher with superimposed hepatitis D
- The risk of fulminant hepatitis is < 1%, with a 60% mortality rate
- Following acute hepatitis B
  — HBV infection persists in 1% to 2% of immunocompetent persons
  — Risk is higher in immunocompromised persons
- Chronic hepatitis B, particularly when HBV infection is acquired early in life and viral replication persists
  — Confers a substantial risk of cirrhosis and hepatocellular carcinoma (up to 25%–40%)
  — Men are at greater risk than women
- Universal vaccination of neonates in countries endemic for HBV reduces the incidence of hepatocellular carcinoma

Hepatitis C
- In most patients, clinical recovery is complete in 3 to 6 months
- Liver function returns to normal in chronic hepatitis C infection, though aminotransferase elevations persist in most patients in whom chronic hepatitis C ensues
- The mortality rate of hepatitis C is < 1%, but the rate is higher in older people
- Fulminant hepatitis C is rare in the United States
- Chronic hepatitis develops in as many as 80% of all persons with acute hepatitis C, which in many cases progresses very slowly
- Cirrhosis develops in up to 20% to 30% of those with chronic hepatitis C; the risk is higher in men, in those who drink > 50 g of alcohol daily, and possibly in those who acquire HCV infection after age 40, as well as in patients coinfected with both HCV and HBV or with HCV and HIV
- Immunosuppressed persons (hypogammaglobulinemia, HIV infection with a low CD4 count, or organ transplant recipients receiving immunosuppressants) progress more rapidly to cirrhosis than immunocompetent persons
- Patients with cirrhosis are at risk for hepatocellular carcinoma at a rate of 3% to 5% per year
  — Patients with HCV genotype 1b at higher risk than those with other genotypes

Prevention

Acute Hepatitis A, B, and C

- Strict isolation is not necessary, but hand washing after bowel movements is required
- Thorough hand washing by anyone who may contact contaminated utensils, bedding, or clothing is essential
- Testing of donated blood for A, B, and C virus
  — For example, testing for HCV has helped reduce the risk of transfusion-associated hepatitis C from 1 in 10 to about 1 in 2 million units

Hepatitis A

Immune Globulin

- Give to all close (eg, household) personal contacts and consider giving it to persons who consume food prepared by an infected food handler
- The recommended dose, 0.02 mL/kg intramuscularly, is protective if administered during incubation

Vaccination

- Two effective inactivated hepatitis A vaccines are available in the United States and recommended for
  — Persons living in or traveling to endemic areas (including military personnel)
  — Patients with chronic liver disease on diagnosis
  — Persons with clotting-factor disorders who are treated with concentrates
  — Men who have sex with men
  — Animal handlers
  — Illicit drug users
  — Sewage workers
  — Food handlers
  — Close personal contacts of international adoptees
  — Children and caregivers in day care centers and institutions
- HAV vaccine is effective in the prevention of secondary spread to household contacts of primary cases
- The recommended dose for adults
  — A volume of 1 mL (1440 ELISA units) of Havrix (GlaxoSmithKline) or 1 mL (50 units) of Vaqta (Merck) intramuscularly
  — Follow with a booster dose at 6 to 18 months
- A combined hepatitis A and B vaccine (Twinrix, GlaxoSmithKline) is available

Hepatitis B

- Strict isolation of patients is not necessary but thorough hand washing by anyone who may contact contaminated utensils, bedding, or clothing is essential
- Screening of donated blood for HBsAg and anti-HBc has reduced the risk of transfusion-associated hepatitis markedly
- Test pregnant women for HBsAg
- Cesarean delivery, in combination with immunoprophylaxis of the neonate, reduces the risk of perinatal transmission when the mother's serum HBV DNA level is $\geq$ 200,000 international units/mL
- Counsel patients with HBV to practice safe sex
- Vaccinate against HAV (after prescreening for prior immunity) in those with chronic hepatitis B

Hepatitis B Immune Globulin (HBIG)

- May be protective, or may attenuate the severity of illness, if given within 7 days after exposure (dose is 0.06 mL/kg body weight) followed by HBV vaccine
- Use this approach after exposure to HBsAg-contaminated material via mucous membranes or breaks in the skin, after sexual contact, and for infants born to HBsAg-positive mothers (in combination with the vaccine series)

Vaccination

- The current vaccines are recombinant-derived
- Centers for Disease Control and Prevention (CDC) recommends universal vaccination of infants and children and all at-risk adults
- Over 90% of recipients mount protective antibody to hepatitis B
- Give 10 to 20 μg (depending on the formulation), repeated again at 1 and 6 months, but alternative schedules are approved, including accelerated schedules of 0, 1, 2, and 12 months
- Check postimmunization anti-HBs titers if need to document seroconversion
- Protection appears to be excellent—at least for 20 years—even if the titer of anti-HBs wanes
- Booster reimmunization is not routinely recommended but is advised for immunocompromised persons in whom anti-HBs titers fall below 10 milli-international units/mL
- For vaccine nonresponders, three additional vaccine doses may elicit seroprotective anti-HBs levels in 30% to 50%

Hepatitis C

- Strict isolation of patients is not necessary, but hand washing by patients after bowel movements is required
- Thorough hand washing by anyone who may contact contaminated utensils, bedding, or clothing is essential
- Testing blood for HCV has helped reduce the risk of transfusion-associated hepatitis C
- Screening of persons born between 1945 and 1965 ("baby boomers") for HCV infection is now recommended by the CDC and the United States Preventive Services Task Force and could identify over 900,000 new cases

9. When to Refer and When to Admit

When to Refer

- For liver biopsy
- For antiviral therapy

When to Admit

- The patient is unable to maintain hydration
- Suspected impending fulminant hepatic failure (eg, hepatic encephalopathy, INR prolongation > 1.6)

SUGGESTED REFERENCES

Afdhal N et al; ION-1 Investigators. Ledipasvir and sofosbuvir for untreated HCV genotype 1 infection. *N Engl J Med.* 2014 May 15;370(20):1889–1898. [PMID: 24725239]

Chien YC et al. Incomplete hepatitis B immunization, maternal carrier status, and increased risk of liver diseases: a 20-year cohort study of 3.8 million vaccinees. *Hepatology.* 2014 Jul;60(1):125–132. [PMID: 24497203]

Chou R et al. Screening for hepatitis B virus infection in adolescents and adults: a systematic review to update the U.S. Preventive Services Task Force recommendation. *Ann Intern Med.* 2014 Jul 1;161(1):31–45. [PMID: 24861032]

Collier MG et al; Hepatitis A Outbreak Investigation Team. Outbreak of hepatitis A in the USA associated with frozen pomegranate arils imported from Turkey: an epidemiological case study. *Lancet Infect Dis.* 2014 Oct;14(10):976–981. [PMID: 25195178]

Kabiri M et al. The changing burden of hepatitis C virus infection in the US: model-based predictions. *Ann Intern Med.* 2014 Aug 5;161(3):170–180. [PMID: 25089861]

LeFevre ML et al. Screening for hepatitis B virus infection in nonpregnant adolescents and adults: U.S. Preventive Services Task Force recommendation statement. *Ann Intern Med.* 2014 Jul 1;161(1):58–66. [PMID: 24863637]

Lo Re V 3rd et al. Hepatic decompensation in antiretroviral-treated patients co-infected with HIV and hepatitis C virus compared with hepatitis C virus-monoinfected patients: a cohort study. *Ann Intern Med.* 2014 Mar 18;160(6):369–379. [PMID: 24723077]

Trépo C et al. Hepatitis B virus infection. *Lancet.* 2014 Dec 6;384(9959):2053–2063. [PMID: 24954675]

Wenzel JJ et al. Hepatitis A as a foodborne infection. *Lancet Infect Dis.* 2014 Oct;14(10):907–908. [PMID: 25195177]

Acute Pancreatitis

A 58-year-old woman presents to the emergency department with a 2-day history of fever, anorexia, nausea, and abdominal pain. She was seen 2 months ago for an episode of right upper quadrant abdominal pain, at which time ultrasound imaging demonstrated multiple gallstones without evidence of gallbladder wall edema. Today, serum amylase and lipase levels are both markedly elevated and she is admitted to the hospital. On day 3 of her hospital course, the clinician is called urgently to evaluate the patient for hypotension, increased shortness of breath, and ensuing respiratory failure. She requires endotracheal intubation and mechanical ventilation. A chest radiograph and severe hypoxia support the diagnosis of acute respiratory distress syndrome (ARDS).

LEARNING OBJECTIVES

► Learn the clinical manifestations and objective findings of acute pancreatitis
► Understand the causes of and factors that predispose to acute pancreatitis
► Know the differential diagnosis of acute pancreatitis
► Learn the medical treatment for acute pancreatitis and the indications for surgical intervention
► Know how to use Ranson criteria to assess the prognosis in acute pancreatitis

QUESTIONS

1. What are the salient features of this patient's problem?

2. How do you think through her problem?

3. What are the key features, including essentials of diagnosis and general considerations, of acute pancreatitis?

4. What are the symptoms and signs of acute pancreatitis?

5. What is the differential diagnosis of acute pancreatitis?

6. What are laboratory, imaging, and procedural findings in acute pancreatitis?

7. What are the treatments for acute pancreatitis?

8. What are the outcomes, including follow-up, complications, and prognosis, of acute pancreatitis?

9. When should patients with acute pancreatitis be admitted to the hospital?

ANSWERS

1. Salient Features

Fever; anorexia, nausea, abdominal pain; history of gallstones; elevated lipase and amylase; associated ARDS

2. How to Think Through

Undifferentiated abdominal pain is a common clinical challenge. In this case, elevated serum amylase and lipase levels point to a diagnosis of acute pancreatitis. What are the leading causes of acute pancreatitis? (Alcoholism, gallstones, hypertriglyceridemia, medication side effect, pancreatic duct stricture or obstruction, pancreatic or other malignancy, or compressive adenopathy.) Even without the history provided in this case, cholelithiasis would be the most likely cause, given her age and sex. Nevertheless, alcoholism should be assessed. What were the important elements of her treatment on admission? (Supportive care including IV hydration, nothing by mouth, and pain control.)

The major challenge is to identify the 15% to 25% of cases that will progress to severe, necrotizing pancreatitis. Predictive models, such as the Ranson criteria, are employed, though they have low specificity. Should the patient receive an imaging study when her condition deteriorates? (Yes. Imaging may be omitted at presentation if the diagnosis is relatively clear. Worsening clinical status, however, is an indication for computed tomography [CT] scan or magnetic resonance cholangiopancreatography [MRCP], both of which can distinguish necrosis from edema.)

Does development of shock and ARDS in this case indicate necrosis and/or infection? (Necrosis is likely, and cytokine-mediated systemic inflammatory response syndrome can precipitate these complications, even in the absence of infection.) What are the treatment options for severe pancreatitis? (Opioids; calcium gluconate for tetany; fresh frozen plasma for coagulopathy with bleeding; vasopressor medications for shock; nutritional support; broad-spectrum antibiotics and debridement for infection.)

3. Key Features

Essentials of Diagnosis

- Abrupt onset of deep epigastric pain, often with radiation to the back
- Nausea, vomiting, sweating, weakness, fever
- Abdominal tenderness and distention
- Leukocytosis, elevated serum amylase, elevated serum lipase
- History of previous episodes, often related to alcohol intake

General Considerations

- Most often due to passed gallstone, usually ≤ 5 mm in diameter, or heavy alcohol intake
- Rarely, may be the initial manifestation of a pancreatic or ampullary neoplasm
- Pathogenesis may include edema or obstruction of the ampulla of Vater, bile reflux into pancreatic ducts, and direct injury of the pancreatic acinar cells

4. Symptoms and Signs

- There may be a history of alcohol intake or a heavy meal immediately preceding the attack, or a history of milder similar episodes or biliary pain in the past
- One classification of the severity of acute pancreatitis has been proposed, as follows
  - Mild: absence of organ failure and pancreatic or peripancreatic necrosis or fluid collections or systemic complications
  - Moderate: presence of sterile (peri)pancreatic necrosis and/or transient (< 48 hours) organ failure (using the Sequential Organ Failure Assessment [SOFA] score) or local or systemic complications, or both
  - Severe: presence of infected (peri)pancreatic necrosis or persistent (≥ 48 hours) organ failure

- Pain
  - Severe, steady, boring epigastric pain, generally abrupt in onset. Usually radiates into the back but may radiate to the right or left
  - Often made worse by walking and lying and better by sitting and leaning forward
- The upper abdomen is tender, most often without guarding, rigidity, or rebound
- There may be distention and absent bowel sounds from paralytic ileus
- Nausea and vomiting
- Weakness, sweating, and anxiety in severe attacks
- Fever of 38.4°C to 39.0°C, tachycardia, hypotension (even true shock), pallor, and cool clammy skin are present in severe cases
- Mild jaundice is common
- Occasionally, an upper abdominal mass may be palpated
- Acute kidney injury (usually prerenal) may occur early in the course

5. Differential Diagnosis

- Acute cholecystitis
- Acutely perforated duodenal ulcer
- Acute intestinal obstruction
- Leaking aortic aneurysm
- Renal colic and acute mesenteric ischemia

6. Laboratory, Imaging, and Procedural Findings

Laboratory Tests

- Serum amylase and lipase increase, usually > 3 times normal, within 24 hours in 90% of cases; lipase remains elevated longer than amylase for more accurate diagnosis
- Leukocytosis (10,000–30,000/μL [10–30 × 10^9/L]), proteinuria, granular casts, glycosuria (10%–20% of cases), hyperglycemia, and elevated serum bilirubin may be present
- Blood urea nitrogen (BUN) and alkaline phosphatase may be elevated and coagulation tests abnormal
- An elevated serum creatinine level (> 1.8 mg/dL [> 159.1 μmol/L]) at 48 hours is associated with the development of pancreatic necrosis
- A serum alanine aminotransferase level of > 150 units/L (3 mkat/L) suggests biliary pancreatitis
- Hypocalcemia correlates with severity of disease. Serum calcium levels < 7 mg/dL (1.75 mmol/L) (when serum albumin is normal) are associated with tetany
- Early hemoconcentration, hematocrit value > 44%, predicts pancreatic necrosis
- An elevated C-reactive protein concentration (> 15 mg/dL [150 mg/L]) after 48 hours suggests severe disease
- The fluid amylase content is high in ascites or left pleural effusions

Imaging Studies

- Plain abdominal radiographs may show
  - Gallstones (if calcified)
  - A "sentinel loop" (a segment of air-filled left upper quadrant small intestine)
  - A "colon cutoff sign" (a gas-filled segment of transverse colon abruptly ending at the inflamed pancreas)
  - Focal linear atelectasis of the lower lobe of the lungs with or without pleural effusion
- Ultrasonography may identify gallstones but is otherwise often unhelpful for diagnosis
- CT scan
  - Can demonstrate an enlarged pancreas and pseudocysts
  - Can differentiate pancreatitis from other possible intra-abdominal catastrophes
  - Can provide initial assessment of prognosis (Table 35-1)
- Dynamic intravenous (IV) contrast-enhanced CT
  - Of particular value after the first 3 days of severe disease to identify necrotizing pancreatitis and assess prognosis

Table 35-1. Severity index for acute pancreatitis.

CT Grade	Points	Pancreatic Necrosis	Additional Points	Severity Index[a]	Mortality Rate[b]
A Normal pancreas	0	0%	0	0	0%
B Pancreatic enlargement	1	0%	0	1	0%
C Pancreatic inflammation and/or peripancreatic fat	2	< 30%	2	4	< 3%
D Single acute peripancreatic fluid collection	3	30–50%	4	7	6%
E Two or more acute peripancreatic fluid collections or retroperitoneal air	4	> 50%	6	10	> 17%

[a]Severity index = CT Grade Points + Additional Points.

[b]Based on the severity index.

Adapted with permission from Balthazar EJ. Acute pancreatitis: assessment of severity with clinical and CT evaluation. *Radiology.* 2002;223(3):603–613.

— Avoid IV contrast when the serum creatinine level is > 1.5 mg/dL (132.6 μmol/L); order MRI instead
• Endoscopic ultrasonography (EUS) is useful for occult biliary disease (eg, small stones, sludge)

Diagnostic Procedures
• ECG may show ST–T wave changes
• CT-guided needle aspiration of necrotizing pancreatitis may diagnose infection
• Endoscopic retrograde cholangiopancreatography (ERCP) is generally not indicated unless there is associated cholangitis or jaundice
• However, aspiration of bile for crystal analysis may confirm microlithiasis

7. Treatments
Medications
• Treat pain with meperidine up to 100 to 150 mg every 3 to 4 hours intramuscularly as needed for pain
• Keep NPO (nothing by mouth) and administer IV fluids until patient is pain-free and has bowel sounds
• Then begin clear liquids and gradually advance to a low-fat diet, guided by the patient's tolerance and by absence of pain
• For mild pancreatitis
  — Early fluid resuscitation (one-third of the total 72-hour fluid volume administered within 24 hours of presentation, 250–500 mL/h initially) may reduce the frequency of systemic inflammatory response syndrome and organ failure
  — Lactated Ringer solution may be preferable to normal saline
  — However, overly aggressive fluid resuscitation may lead to morbidity as well
• For severe pancreatitis, large quantities of IV fluids are needed to maintain intravascular volume
  — Risk factors for high levels of fluid sequestration include younger age, alcoholism as cause, higher hematocrit value, higher serum glucose, and systemic inflammatory response syndrome in the first 48 hours of hospital admission
• Give calcium gluconate IV for hypocalcemia with tetany
• Infusions of fresh frozen plasma or serum albumin may be needed for coagulopathy or hypoalbuminemia
• If shock persists after adequate volume replacement (including packed red cells), vasopressors may be required
• Enteral nutrition via a nasogastric or nasojejunal tube is preferable to parenteral nutrition in patients who will otherwise be without oral nutrition for at least 7–10 days

but it may not be tolerated in some patients with an ileus. Enteral nutrition does not reduce the rates of infection and death compared with the introduction of an oral diet after 72 hours
- Parenteral nutrition (including lipids) should be considered in patients who have severe pancreatitis and an ileus
- Imipenem (500 mg every 8 hours IV), ciprofloxacin (750 mg twice daily IV) combined with metronidazole (500 mg three times daily IV or orally or three times daily), or cefuroxime (1.5 g three times daily IV, then 250 mg twice daily orally) given for 14 days for sterile pancreatic necrosis may reduce the risk of pancreatic infection
- The role of IV somatostatin is uncertain, but octreotide is not beneficial

Surgery
- For mild pancreatitis with cholelithiasis, cholecystectomy, or cholecystostomy may be justified
- Infected pancreatic necrosis is an absolute indication for debridement
- Biliary sphincterotomy
  — Used to treat recurrent acute pancreatitis attributable to sphincter of Oddi dysfunction
  — As effective as combined biliary and pancreatic sphincterotomy in reducing frequency of recurrent acute pancreatitis
  — However, treated patients may still develop chronic pancreatitis
- Necrosectomy may improve survival in necrotizing pancreatitis and prevent clinical deterioration with multiorgan failure or lack of resolution by 4 weeks

Therapeutic Procedures
- The pancreatic rest program includes
  — Nothing by mouth
  — Bed rest
  — Nasogastric suction for moderately severe pain, vomiting, or abdominal distention
- ERCP with endoscopic sphincterotomy and stone extraction is indicated when severe pancreatitis results from choledocholithiasis, particularly if jaundice (serum total bilirubin > 5 mg/dL [85.5 μmol/L]) or cholangitis is present

8. Outcomes

Follow-Up
- Monitor severely ill patients closely
  — White blood cell count
  — Hematocrit
  — Serum electrolytes
  — Serum calcium
  — Serum creatinine
  — BUN
  — Serum aspartate aminotransferase and lactate dehydrogenase (LDH)
  — Arterial blood gases
- Cultures of blood, urine, sputum, and pleural effusion (if present) and needle aspirations of pancreatic necrosis (with CT guidance) should be obtained
- Following recovery from acute biliary pancreatitis, laparoscopic cholecystectomy is generally performed, although endoscopic sphincterotomy alone may be done

Complications
- Acute tubular necrosis
- Necrotizing pancreatitis and infected pancreatic necrosis
- ARDS; cardiac dysfunction may be superimposed
- Pancreatic abscess may develop after ≥ 6 weeks; it requires prompt percutaneous or surgical drainage
- Treat pancreatic infections with imipenem, 500 mg every 8 hours IV

Table 35-2. Ranson criteria for assessing the severity of acute pancreatitis.

Three or More of the Following Predict a Severe Course Complicated by Pancreatic Necrosis With a Sensitivity of 60%–80%	
Age > 55 y	
White blood cell count > $16 \times 10^3/\mu L$ ($16 \times 10^9/L$)	
Blood glucose > 200 mg/dL (11 mmol/L)	
Serum lactic dehydrogenase > 350 units/L (7 mkat/L)	
Aspartate aminotransferase > 250 units/L (5 mkat/L)	
Development of the Following in the First 48 h Indicates a Worsening Prognosis	
Hematocrit drop of > 10 percentage points	
Blood urea nitrogen rise > 5 mg/dL (1.8 mmol/L)	
Arterial P_{O_2} of < 60 mm Hg (7.8 kPa)	
Serum calcium of < 8 mg/dL (0.2 mmol/L)	
Base deficit > 4 mEq/L	
Estimated fluid sequestration of > 6 L	

Mortality Rates Correlate With the Number of Criteria Present[a]

Number of Criteria	Mortality Rate
0–2	1%
3–4	16%
5–6	40%
7–8	100%

[a]An APACHE II score ≥ 8 also correlates with mortality.

- Pseudocysts < 6 cm in diameter often resolve spontaneously
  — They are multiple in 14% of cases
  — They may become secondarily infected and need drainage
  — Drainage may also help persisting pain or pancreatitis
  — Erosion into a blood vessel can result in a major hemorrhage into the cyst
- Pancreatic ascites may occur after recovery from acute pancreatitis even in absence of frank abdominal pain. Marked elevations in the ascitic fluid protein (> 3 mg/dL) and amylase (> 1000 units/L) levels are typical
- Portosplenomesenteric venous thrombosis frequently develops in patients with necrotizing acute pancreatitis but rarely leads to complications
- Chronic pancreatitis develops in about 10% of cases
- Permanent diabetes mellitus and exocrine pancreatic insufficiency occur uncommonly after a single acute episode
- The risk of chronic pancreatitis following an episode of acute alcoholic pancreatitis is 13% in 10 years and 16% in 20 years, and the risk of diabetes mellitus is increased more than twofold over 5 years

Prognosis
- Use of Ranson criteria helps assess disease severity (Table 35-2)
- When three or more of the Ranson criteria are present on admission, a severe course complicated by pancreatic necrosis can be predicted with a sensitivity of 60% to 80%. Mortality rates correlate with the number of criteria

9. When to Admit
- Nearly all patients with severe pancreatitis

SUGGESTED REFERENCES

Acevedo-Piedra NG et al. Validation of the determinant-based classification and revision of the Atlanta classification systems for acute pancreatitis. *Clin Gastroenterol Hepatol.* 2014 Feb;12(2):311–316. [PMID: 23958561]

Alsamarrai A et al. Factors that affect risk for pancreatic disease in the general population: a systematic review and meta-analysis of prospective cohort studies. *Clin Gastroenterol Hepatol.* 2014 Oct;12(10):1635–1644. [PMID: 24509242]

de-Madaria E et al. Early factors associated with fluid sequestration and outcomes of patients with acute pancreatitis. *Clin Gastroenterol Hepatol.* 2014 Jun;12(6):997–1002. [PMID: 24183957]

Fogel EL et al. ERCP for gallstone pancreatitis. *N Engl J Med.* 2014 Jan 9;370(2):150–157. [PMID: 24401052]

Freeman ML (editor). Effective endoscopic management of pancreatic diseases. *Gastrointest Endosc Clin N Am* [entire issue]. 2013 Oct;23(4):735–934. [PMID: 24079799]

Johnson CD et al. Acute pancreatitis. *BMJ.* 2014 Aug 12;349:g4859. [PMID: 25116169]

Mouli VP et al. Efficacy of conservative treatment, without necrosectomy, for infected pancreatic necrosis: a systematic review and meta-analysis. *Gastroenterology.* 2013 Feb;144(2):333–340. [PMID: 23063972]

Nawaz H et al. Revised Atlanta and determinant-based classification: application in a prospective cohort of acute pancreatitis patients. *Am J Gastroenterol.* 2013 Dec;108(12):1911–1917. [PMID: 24126632]

Tenner S et al. American College of Gastroenterology guideline: management of acute pancreatitis. *Am J Gastroenterol.* 2013 Sep;108(9):1400–1416. [PMID: 23896955]

Trikudanathan G et al. Endoscopic interventions for necrotizing pancreatitis. *Am J Gastroenterol.* 2014 Jul;109(7):969–981. [PMID: 24957157]

Vipperla K et al. Risk of and factors associated with readmission after a sentinel attack of acute pancreatitis. *Clin Gastroenterol Hepatol.* 2014 Nov;12(11):1911–1919. [PMID: 24815327]

Working Group IAP/APA Acute Pancreatitis Guidelines. IAP/APA evidence-based guidelines for the management of acute pancreatitis. *Pancreatology.* 2013 Jul–Aug;13(4 suppl 2):e1–e15. [PMID: 24054878]

Wu BU et al. Clinical management of patients with acute pancreatitis. *Gastroenterology.* 2013 Jun;144(6):1272–1281. [PMID: 23622137]

36

Chronic Pancreatitis

A 52-year-old man with a 20-year history of alcoholism presents to his primary care clinician complaining of recurrent episodes of epigastric and left upper quadrant (LUQ) abdominal pain. Over the past month, the pain has become almost continuous, and he has requested morphine for better pain control. He also notes that recently his stool has been bulky and foul smelling. He has a history of alcoholism-related acute pancreatitis. Examination reveals a 10-pound weight loss over the past 6 months. He has some mild muscle guarding over the epigastrium with tenderness to palpation. Bowel sounds are somewhat decreased. Serum amylase and lipase are mildly elevated. A plain film of the abdomen demonstrates pancreatic calcifications.

LEARNING OBJECTIVES

► Learn the clinical manifestations and objective findings of chronic pancreatitis
► Understand the risk factors for the development of chronic pancreatitis
► Know the differential diagnosis of chronic pancreatitis
► Understand the options for diagnosing chronic pancreatitis, and which tests may be normal despite the presence of the disease
► Learn the effective medical and surgical treatments for chronic pancreatitis

QUESTIONS

1. What are the salient features of this patient's problem?
2. How do you think through his problem?
3. What are the key features, including essentials of diagnosis, general considerations, and demographics, of chronic pancreatitis?
4. What are the symptoms and signs of chronic pancreatitis?
5. What is the differential diagnosis of chronic pancreatitis?
6. What are laboratory, imaging, and procedural findings in chronic pancreatitis?
7. What are the treatments for chronic pancreatitis?
8. What are the outcomes, including complications, prognosis, and prevention, of chronic pancreatitis?
9. When should patients with chronic pancreatitis be referred to a specialist or admitted to the hospital?

ANSWERS

1. Salient Features

Long-standing alcoholism and repeated acute pancreatitis episodes; chronic epigastric abdominal pain; bulky and foul smelling stool (steatorrhea) representing pancreatic insufficiency; tender epigastrium on examination; elevated serum amylase and lipase; pancreatic calcifications

2. How to Think Through

Epigastric pain has a broad differential diagnosis, and malabsorptive symptoms develop at an advanced stage of chronic pancreatitis. These features highlight the importance of history gathering—the pattern and timing of the pain, alcoholism, prior acute episodes of abdominal pain, nausea, and anorexia—and careful physical examination. If the serum amylase and lipase were normal, could the patient have a diagnosis of chronic pancreatitis? (Yes, this is common. While these enzymes are often mildly elevated in chronic pancreatitis, their sensitivity and utility is far greater in the diagnosis of acute pancreatitis.) How could you confirm your diagnosis? (With the history and physical examination provided in this case, confirmation of steatorrhea alone would be sufficient to make the diagnosis. Calcification of the pancreas on X-ray provides sufficient confirmation as well. Computed tomography [CT] scan, magnetic resonance cholangiopancreatography [MRCP], and endoscopic retrograde cholangiopancreatography [ERCP] are available if needed.) Should his endocrine function be assessed? (Yes. Such patients can develop impaired glucose tolerance and, eventually, diabetes mellitus.) What lifestyle modification will improve his symptoms? (Abstinence from alcohol; small meals; low fat diet.) What medications should be considered? (Pancreatic enzymes.) Are there procedural interventions that might help his symptoms? (ERCP with stenting of the pancreatic duct, sphincterotomy; celiac plexus nerve block.) What complications might arise for this patient? (Opioid addiction; diabetes; pancreatic pseudocyst, abscess, or cancer; bile duct stricture; cholestasis; malnutrition; peptic ulcer.)

3. Key Features

Essentials of Diagnosis
- Epigastric pain
- Steatorrhea
- Weight loss
- Abnormal pancreatic imaging
- A mnemonic for predisposing factors is TIGAR-O
  — Toxic-metabolic
  — Idiopathic
  — Genetic
  — Autoimmune
  — Recurrent and severe acute pancreatitis
  — Obstructive

General Considerations
- Occurs most often with alcoholism (45% to 80% of all cases)
- Risk of chronic pancreatitis increases with duration and amount of alcohol consumed, but it develops in only 5% to 10% of heavy drinkers
- Tobacco smoking is a risk factor for idiopathic chronic pancreatitis and may accelerate progression of alcoholic chronic pancreatitis
- Pancreatitis develops in about 2% of patients with hyperparathyroidism
- In tropical Africa and Asia, tropical pancreatitis, related in part to malnutrition, is most common cause of chronic pancreatitis
- A stricture, stone, or tumor obstructing the pancreas can lead to obstructive chronic pancreatitis

- Autoimmune pancreatitis is associated with hypergammaglobulinemia and is responsive to corticosteroids
  — Type 1 autoimmune pancreatitis is characterized by lymphoplasmacytic sclerosing pancreatitis on biopsy, associated bile duct strictures, retroperitoneal fibrosis, renal and salivary gland lesions, and a high rate of relapse after treatment
  — Type 2 autoimmune pancreatitis is characterized by idiopathic duct centric pancreatitis on biopsy, lack of systemic IgG4 involvement, and lack of relapse after treatment
  — Affected persons are at increased risk for various cancers
- Between 10% and 30% of cases are idiopathic
- The pathogenesis of chronic pancreatitis may be explained by the SAPE (sentinel acute pancreatitis event) hypothesis; a first episode of acute pancreatitis initiates an inflammatory process that results in injury fibrosis

Demographics
- Genetic factors may predispose to chronic pancreatitis in some cases. —For example, mutations of the cystic fibrosis transmembrane conductance regulator (*CFTR*) gene, the pancreatic secretory trypsin inhibitor gene (*PSTI*, serine protease inhibitor, *SPINK 1*), and possibly the gene for uridine 5′-diphosphate-glucuronosyltransferase

4. Symptoms and Signs
- Persistent or recurrent episodes of epigastric and LUQ pain with referral to the upper left lumbar region are typical
- Anorexia, nausea, vomiting, constipation, flatulence, and weight loss are common
- During attacks tenderness over the pancreas, mild muscle guarding, and ileus may be noted
- Attacks may last only a few hours or as long as 2 weeks; pain may eventually be almost continuous
- Steatorrhea (as indicated by bulky, foul, fatty stools) may occur late in the course

5. Differential Diagnosis
- Cholelithiasis
- Diabetes mellitus
- Malabsorption due to other causes
- Intractable duodenal ulcer
- Pancreatic cancer
- Irritable bowel syndrome

6. Laboratory, Imaging, and Procedural Findings

Laboratory Tests
- Serum amylase and lipase may be elevated during acute attacks; normal values do not exclude the diagnosis
- Serum alkaline phosphatase and bilirubin may be elevated owing to compression of the bile duct
- Glycosuria may be present
- Excess fecal fat may be demonstrated in the stool
- Pancreatic insufficiency
  — May be confirmed by response to therapy with pancreatic enzyme supplements or a secretin stimulation test if available (which has a high negative predictive value for early chronic pancreatitis)
  — May be diagnosed by detection of decreased fecal chymotrypsin or elastase levels (if test available), though the tests lack sensitivity and specificity
- Vitamin B_{12} malabsorption is detectable in about 40% of patients, but clinical deficiency of vitamin B_{12} and fat-soluble vitamins is rare
- Accurate genetic tests are available for the major trypsinogen gene mutations

- Elevated IgG4 levels, antinuclear antibody (ANA), and antibodies to lactoferrin and carbonic anhydrase II are often seen in cases of autoimmune pancreatitis
- Elevated antibodies to peptide A1P1-7 and to ubiquitin-protein ligase E3 component n-recognin 2 have been reported in a high percentage of patients with autoimmune pancreatitis but also in some patients with pancreatic cancer

Imaging Studies
- Plain radiographs show calcifications due to pancreatolithiasis in 30% of patients
- CT may show calcifications not seen on plain radiographs as well as ductal dilatation and heterogeneity or atrophy of the gland
- MRCP (including secretin-enhanced MRCP) and endoscopic ultrasonography (with pancreatic tissue sampling) are less-invasive diagnostic tools than ERCP
- In autoimmune chronic pancreatitis, imaging shows diffuse enlargement of the pancreas, peripheral rim hypoattenuation, and irregular narrowing of the main pancreatic duct

Diagnostic Procedures
- ERCP
  — Most sensitive study for chronic pancreatitis
  — May show dilated ducts, intraductal stones, strictures, or pseudocysts
  — However, results may be normal in patients with so-called minimal change pancreatitis
  — Endoscopic ultrasonographic ("Rosemont") criteria
    ◦ Hyperechoic foci with shadowing indicative of calculi in the main pancreatic duct and lobularity with honeycombing of the pancreatic parenchyma

7. Treatments

Medications
- Steatorrhea
  — Treat with pancreatic supplements (Table 36-1), total dose of 40,000 units of lipase
  — Tablets should be taken at the start of, during, and at the end of a meal
  — Doses of 90,000 units or more of lipase per meal may be required in some cases
  — Concurrent administration of H_2-receptor antagonists (eg, ranitidine, 150 mg twice daily orally), or a proton-pump inhibitor (eg, omeprazole, 20 to 60 mg daily orally), or sodium bicarbonate, 650 mg before and after meals orally, may further decrease steatorrhea
- In selected cases of alcoholic pancreatitis and in cystic fibrosis, enteric-coated microencapsulated preparations may help
- However, in cystic fibrosis, high-dose pancreatic enzyme therapy has been associated with strictures of the ascending colon
- Pain secondary to idiopathic chronic pancreatitis may be alleviated by the use of pancreatic enzymes (not enteric-coated) or octreotide, 200 μg three times daily subcutaneously
- Associated diabetes should be treated
- Autoimmune pancreatitis is treated with prednisone 40 mg per day orally for 1 to 2 months, followed by a taper of 5 mg every 2 to 4 weeks

Surgery
- Correctable coexistent biliary tract disease should be treated surgically
- Surgery may be indicated to drain persistent pseudocysts, treat other complications, or relieve pain
- When the pancreatic duct is diffusely dilated, anastomosis between the duct after it is split longitudinally and a defunctionalized limb of jejunum (modified Puestow procedure), in some cases combined with local resection of the head of the pancreas (Beger or Frey procedure), is associated with relief of pain in 80% of cases
- In advanced cases, subtotal or total pancreatectomy may be considered a last resort but has variable efficacy and is associated with high rates of pancreatic insufficiency and diabetes

Table 36-1. FDA-approved pancreatic enzyme (pancrelipase) preparations.

Product	Enzyme Content/Unit Dose, USP units		
	Lipase	Amylase	Protease
Immediate Release Capsule			
Nonenteric-coated			
Viokace 10,440	10,440	39,150	39,150
Viokace 20,880	20,880	78,300	78,300
Delayed Release Capsules			
Enteric-coated minimicrospheres			
Creon 3000	3000	15,000	9500
Creon 6000	6000	30,000	19,000
Creon 12,000	12,000	60,000	38,000
Creon 24,000	24,000	120,000	76,000
Creon 36,000	36,000	180,000	114,000
Enteric-coated minitablets			
Ultresa 13,800	13,800	27,600	27,600
Ultresa 20,700	20,700	46,000	41,400
Ultresa 23,000	23,000	46,000	41,400
Enteric-coated beads			
Zenpep 3000	3000	16,000	10,000
Zenpep 5000	5000	27,000	17,000
Zenpep 10,000	10,000	55,000	34,000
Zenpep 15,000	15,000	82,000	51,000
Zenpep 20,000	20,000	109,000	68,000
Zenpep 25,000	25,000	136,000	85,000
Enteric-coated microtablets			
Pancreaze 4200	4200	17,500	10,000
Pancreaze 10,500	10,500	43,750	25,000
Pancreaze 16,800	16,800	70,000	40,000
Pancreaze 21,000	21,000	61,000	37,000
Bicarbonate-buffered enteric-coated microspheres			
Pertyze 8000	8000	30,250	28,750
Pertyze 16,000	16,000	60,500	57,500

FDA, US Food and Drug Administration; USP, US Pharmacopeia.

- Endoscopic or surgical (including laparoscopic) drainage is indicated for symptomatic pseudocysts and those over 6 cm in diameter

Therapeutic Procedures
- A low-fat diet should be prescribed
- Alcohol is forbidden because it frequently precipitates attacks
- Opioids should be avoided if possible
- When obstruction of the duodenal end of the pancreatic duct can be demonstrated by ERCP, dilation of the duct, placement of a stent in the duct, pancreatic duct stone lithotripsy, or resection of the tail of the pancreas with implantation of the distal end of the duct by pancreaticojejunostomy may be performed
- Pancreatic ascites or pancreaticopleural fistulas due to a disrupted pancreatic duct can be treated with endoscopic placement of a stent across the duct

- Fragmentation of pancreatic duct stones by lithotripsy and endoscopic removal of stones from the duct, pancreatic sphincterotomy, or pseudocyst drainage may relieve pain in selected patients
- Endoscopic therapy is successful in about 50% of cases
- Surgery is successful in about 50% of patients who do not respond to endoscopic therapy
- For patients with chronic pain and nondilated ducts, a percutaneous celiac plexus nerve block may be considered under either CT or endoscopic ultrasound guidance, with pain relief (often short-lived) in approximately 50% of patients

8. Outcomes

Complications

- Opioid addiction is common
- Brittle diabetes mellitus, pancreatic pseudocyst or abscess, cholestatic liver enzymes with or without jaundice, bile duct stricture, malnutrition related to steatorrhea, and peptic ulcer
- Pancreatic cancer develops in 4% of patients after 20 years; the risk may relate to tobacco use and alcoholism

Prognosis

- Chronic pancreatitis often leads to disability and reduced life expectancy; pancreatic cancer is the main cause of death
- In many cases, it is a self-perpetuating disease characterized by chronic pain or recurrent episodes of acute pancreatitis and ultimately by pancreatic exocrine or endocrine insufficiency
- After many years, chronic pain may resolve spontaneously or as a result of surgery tailored to the cause of pain
- Diabetes mellitus develops in over 80% of adults within 25 years after the clinical onset of chronic pancreatitis
- Prognosis is best with recurrent acute pancreatitis caused by a remediable condition such as cholelithiasis, choledocholithiasis, stenosis of the sphincter of Oddi, or hyperparathyroidism
- In alcoholic pancreatitis, pain relief is most likely when a dilated pancreatic duct can be decompressed

Prevention

- Abstinence from alcohol
- Medical management of the hyperlipidemia frequently associated with pancreatitis may prevent recurrent attacks

9. When to Refer and When to Admit

When to Refer

- All patients should be referred for diagnostic procedures (eg, ERCP) and therapeutic procedures (eg, lithotripsy, sphincterotomy, pseudocyst drainage, celiac plexus block)

When to Admit

- Severe pain
- New jaundice
- New fever

SUGGESTED REFERENCES

Bang UC et al. Mortality, cancer, and comorbidities associated with chronic pancreatitis: a Danish nationwide matched-cohort study. *Gastroenterology*. 2014 Apr;146(4):989–994. [PMID: 24389306]

Duggan SN et al. High prevalence of osteoporosis in patients with chronic pancreatitis: a systematic review and meta-analysis. *Clin Gastroenterol Hepatol*. 2014 Feb;12(2):219–228. [PMID: 23856359]

Forsmark CE. Management of chronic pancreatitis. *Gastroenterology*. 2013 Jun;144(6):1282–1291. [PMID: 23622138]

Fritz S et al. Diagnosis and treatment of autoimmune pancreatitis types 1 and 2. *Br J Surg*. 2014 Sep;101(10):1257–1265. [PMID: 25047016]

Issa Y et al. Treatment options for chronic pancreatitis. *Nat Rev Gastroenterol Hepatol*. 2014 Sep;11(9):556–564. [PMID: 24912390]

Kamisawa T et al. Recent advances in autoimmune pancreatitis: type 1 and type 2. *Gut*. 2013 Sep;62(9):1373–1380. [PMID: 23749606]

Trang T et al. Pancreatic enzyme replacement therapy for pancreatic exocrine insufficiency in the 21(st) century. *World J Gastroenterol*. 2014 Sep 7;20(33):11467–11485. [PMID: 25206255]

Ulcerative Colitis

37

A 43-year-old man presents to the urgent care clinic with bloody diarrhea. He states that he has had 5 to 6 stools per day for the past 7 days, associated with crampy abdominal pain and a feeling of incomplete emptying of his bowels. He has had similar episodes in the past, though this one is particularly severe. Physical examination shows tender abdomen and blood on digital rectal examination. His blood hemoglobin is 8.3 g/dL. Sigmoidoscopy reveals a friable colonic mucosa and biopsies show inflammation confined to the mucosal surface.

LEARNING OBJECTIVES

▶ Learn the clinical manifestations and objective findings of ulcerative colitis (UC)
▶ Understand the extraintestinal manifestations of UC
▶ Know the differential diagnosis of UC
▶ Learn the treatment for UC by disease severity, and the indications for surgery
▶ Understand how to prevent colon cancer in patients with UC

QUESTIONS

1. What are the salient features of this patient's problem?
2. How do you think through his problem?
3. What are the key features, including essentials of diagnosis, general considerations, and demographics of UC?
4. What are the symptoms and signs of UC?
5. What is the differential diagnosis of UC?
6. What are laboratory, imaging, and procedural findings in UC?
7. What are the treatments for UC?
8. What are the outcomes, including complications, prognosis, and prevention, of UC?
9. When should patients with UC be referred to a specialist or admitted to the hospital?

ANSWERS

1. Salient Features

Bloody diarrhea; abdominal pain and tenesmus; episodic nature with exacerbations; abdominal tenderness; blood on rectal examination; anemia; inflammation of the mucosal surface that is not transmural

2. How to Think Through

How should the clinical problem in this case be framed in order to construct a differential diagnosis? (Bloody diarrhea, or simply lower gastrointestinal bleeding.) What is the differential diagnosis? (Infectious colitis due to *Escherichia coli* O157:H7, *Shigella*, *Campylobacter*, and *Salmonella* species; inflammatory bowel disease [IBD]; ischemic colitis; colon cancer; and diverticulosis.) While the friable mucosa in ischemic colitis can resemble IBD, this patient is young for that diagnosis and no atherosclerotic risk factors are mentioned. Colon cancer does not fit the tempo of his presentation. Diverticular bleeding is usually painless. What medical history helps distinguish between IBD from infection? (His prior similar episodes favor the diagnosis of IBD.)

What extraintestinal signs and symptoms, if present, would increase your suspicion for IBD? (Fever; uveitis; arthritis or ankylosing spondylitis; erythema nodosum or pyoderma gangrenosum; sclerosing cholangitis; thromboembolism.)

What studies should be obtained? (A complete blood count [CBC] to assess for anemia [present in this case]; serum electrolytes and creatinine given the frequent diarrhea; a stool culture to exclude infection. Ova and parasite testing is low yield without a risk factor such as travel to an endemic region, or men who have sex with men. Fecal leukocyte testing is not useful due to poor specificity. Sigmoidoscopy, as in this case, is diagnostic. It is easier and safer than pancolonoscopy in the setting of acute colitis.) How should his IBD be treated? (Treatment depends on the severity: for mild-to-moderate disease, 5-aminosalicylic acid [ASA] derivatives [eg, mesalamine, balsalazide, sulfasalazine] rectally or orally, corticosteroids [delayed-release budesonide] orally; for moderate-to-severe disease with inadequate response to agents listed above, corticosteroids [eg, prednisone orally; methylprednisolone or hydrocortisone intravenously; hydrocortisone enemas], infliximab, adalimumab, golimumab, or vedolizumab; for severe or refractory disease: corticosteroids [methylprednisolone intravenously] or cyclosporine or infliximab; for toxic megacolon: add broad-spectrum antibiotics to infliximab or cyclosporine.)

3. Key Features

Essentials of Diagnosis
- Bloody diarrhea
- Lower abdominal cramps and fecal urgency
- Anemia, low serum albumin
- Negative stool cultures
- Sigmoidoscopy is key to diagnosis

General Considerations
- UC is an idiopathic inflammatory condition that involves the mucosal surface of the colon, resulting in diffuse friability and erosions with bleeding
- One-third of patients have disease confined to the rectosigmoid region (proctosigmoiditis); one-third have disease that extends to the splenic flexure (left-sided colitis); and one-third have disease that extends more proximally (extensive colitis)
- In patients with distal colitis, the disease progresses with time to more extensive involvement in 25% to 50%
- Most affected patients experience periods of symptomatic flare-ups and remissions

Demographics
- More common in nonsmokers and former smokers, severity may worsen in patients who stop smoking
- Appendectomy before age 20 reduces risk

4. Symptoms and Signs

- Bloody diarrhea
- Cramps, abdominal pain

- Fecal urgency and tenesmus
- Tenderness, evidence of peritoneal inflammation
- Bright red blood on digital rectal examination

Mild Disease
- Diarrhea infrequent
- Rectal bleeding and mucus intermittent
- Left lower quadrant cramps, relieved by defecation
- No significant abdominal tenderness

Moderate Disease
- Diarrhea more severe with frequent bleeding
- Abdominal pain and tenderness (but not severe)
- Mild fever, anemia, and hypoalbuminemia

Severe Disease
- More than 6 bloody bowel movements per day
- Signs of hypovolemia and impaired nutrition
- Abdominal pain and tenderness

Fulminant Disease
- Rapid progression of symptoms and signs of severe toxicity (hypovolemia, hemorrhage requiring transfusion, and abdominal distention with tenderness) over 1 to 2 weeks

Toxic Megacolon
- Colonic dilation of > 6 cm on radiographs with signs of toxicity, occurring in < 2%, heightens risk of perforation

Extracolonic Manifestations
- Occur in 50% of cases
- Oral ulcers
- Erythema nodosum, pyoderma gangrenosum
- Episcleritis or uveitis
- Spondylitis or sacroiliitis
- Thromboembolic events
- Oligoarticular or polyarticular nondeforming arthritis
- Sclerosing cholangitis

5. Differential Diagnosis
- Infectious colitis
  - *Salmonella*
  - *Shigella*
  - *Campylobacter*
  - Amebiasis
  - *C difficile*
  - Enteroinvasive *E coli*
- Ischemic colitis
- Crohn disease
- Diverticular disease
- Colon cancer
- Antibiotic-associated diarrhea or pseudomembranous colitis
- Infectious proctitis: gonorrhea, chlamydia, herpes, syphilis
- Radiation colitis or proctitis
- Cytomegalovirus colitis in immunocompromised persons

6. Laboratory, Imaging, and Procedural Findings

Laboratory Tests

- The degree of abnormality of the hemoglobin, sedimentation rate, and serum albumin reflects disease severity
- Stools for bacterial (including *C difficile*) culture, ova and parasites

Imaging Studies

- Abdominal radiographs
- Barium enema is of little usefulness and may precipitate toxic megacolon

Diagnostic Procedures

- Sigmoidoscopy establishes diagnosis
- Colonoscopy should not be performed in patients with fulminant disease because of the risk of perforation
- However, after improvement, colonoscopy is recommended to determine extent of disease

7. Treatments

Medications

Mild-to-Moderate Colitis

- Oral 5-ASA agents (mesalamine, balsalazide, sulfasalazine)
  - Best for treating disease extending above the sigmoid colon; symptomatic improvement seen in 50% to 75% of patients
  - Mesalamine
    - Optimal dose of mesalamine for inducing remission of mild disease is 2.4 g/d and of moderate disease is 2.4 to 4.8 g/d
    - Most patients improve within 3 to 6 weeks, although some require 2 to 3 months
  - Sulfasalazine
    - Comparable in efficacy to mesalamine
    - Commonly used as first-line agent because of its low cost but is associated with greater side effects
    - To minimize side effects, dosing is started at 500 mg twice daily and increased gradually over 1 to 2 weeks to 2 g twice daily
    - Total doses of 5 to 6 g/d may have greater efficacy but are poorly tolerated
- Folic acid, 1 mg once daily orally, should be given to all patients taking sulfasalazine
- Corticosteroid therapy to patients who do not improve after 2 to 3 weeks
  - Delayed-release budesonide (Uceris) 9 mg once daily
  - Has shown modest benefit in mild to moderate colitis, achieving remission in 17.5% after 8 weeks compared with 12.5 % with placebo
  - Because of its low incidence of steroid-associated side effects, it may be considered in patients with mild colitis for whom systemic corticosteroids are deemed high risk
- Antidiarrheal agents (eg, loperamide, 2 mg orally, or diphenoxylate with atropine, 1 tablet up to 4 times daily)
  - Should not be given in the acute phase of illness
  - However, they are particularly useful at nighttime and when taken prophylactically when patients may not have access to toilet facilities

Distal Colitis

- Mesalamine rectal suppositories 1000 mg per rectum once daily for proctitis or mesalamine rectal suspension, 4 g per rectum at bedtime for proctosigmoiditis, for 3 to 12 weeks; 75% of patients improve
- Hydrocortisone suppository or foam for proctitis and hydrocortisone enema (80–100 mg) for proctosigmoiditis; less effective

Moderate-to-Severe Colitis

- Corticosteroid therapy improves 50% to 75%
  - Prednisone 40 to 60 mg once daily orally for 1 to 2 weeks; then taper by 5 to 10 mg/wk
  - Severe disease: methylprednisolone, 48 to 64 mg intravenously, or hydrocortisone 300 mg intravenously, in 4 divided doses or by continuous infusion
  - Hydrocortisone enemas, 100 mg twice daily
- Infliximab, 5 mg/kg intravenously, given at 0, 2, and 6 weeks for patients with inadequate response to corticosteroids or mesalamine; clinical response in 65% and remission in 35%
- Adalimumab, 160 mg subcutaneously at 0 weeks; 80 mg at 2 weeks; then 40 mg every other week
  - After 8 weeks, clinical response was reported in 52% and remission in 17%
  - Although the response and remission rates appear lower with adalimumab than infliximab, differences in study design and patient populations limit comparisons
- Golimumab, 200 mg subcutaneously once, followed by 100 mg subcutaneously monthly, is an alternative
- Vedolizumab, 300 mg intravenously at weeks 0 and 2, or 300 mg intravenously every 8 weeks, is primarily used in patients with moderate to severe ulcerative colitis in whom other therapies have failed or are not tolerated

Severe Colitis

- Cyclosporine, 4 mg/kg/d intravenously, improves 60% to 75% of patients with severe colitis who did not improve after 7 to 10 days of intravenous corticosteroids (methylprednisolone)
- Infliximab, 5 mg/kg intravenously, for patients with inadequate response to 4 to 7 days of intravenous corticosteroids (methylprednisolone)

Fulminant Colitis and Toxic Megacolon

- Broad-spectrum antibiotics targeting anaerobes and gram-negative bacteria
- Intravenous corticosteroids, cyclosporine, or infliximab, as discussed above

Maintenance Therapy

- Long-term oral maintenance therapy with sulfasalazine, 1.0 to 1.5 g twice daily, or mesalamine, 1.6 to 2.4 g once daily have been shown to reduce relapse rates to < 35%
- For distal colitis: oral mesalamine, balsalazide, or sulfasalazine reduce the relapse rate from 80% to 90% to < 20% within 1 year
- Immunomodulators: 6-mercaptopurine 1.0 to 1.5 mg/kg or azathioprine 2.0 to 2.5 mg/kg of benefit in 60% of patients with severe or refractory disease, allowing tapering of corticosteroids and maintenance of remission
- Infliximab 5 mg/kg intravenously every 8 weeks for moderate-to-severe disease; up to half of patients maintain clinical response at 1 year

Refractory Disease

- Mercaptopurine or azathioprine

Surgery

- Total proctocolectomy with ileostomy (standard ileostomy, continent ileostomy, or ileoanal anastomosis) required in 25% of patients
- Indications for surgery include
  - Patients with severe disease (eg, severe hemorrhage) who do not improve at 7 to 10 days
  - Patients with fulminant disease who do not improve after 48 to 72 hours of corticosteroid, infliximab, or cyclosporine therapy
  - Unresponsive toxic megacolon or perforation
  - Refractory disease requiring long-term corticosteroids to control symptoms
  - Dysplasia or carcinoma on surveillance colonoscopic biopsies

Therapeutic Procedures

Mild-to-Moderate Colitis
- Regular diet
- Limit intake of caffeine and gas-producing vegetables

Severe Colitis
- Discontinue all oral intake
- Avoid opioid and anticholinergic agents
- Restore circulating volume with fluids and blood
- Correct electrolyte abnormalities

Fulminant Colitis and Toxic Megacolon
- Nasogastric suction, roll patients from side to side on the abdomen
- Serial examinations and abdominal radiographs to look for worsening dilation

8. Outcomes

Complications
- Toxic megacolon
- Colon cancer
- Venous thromboembolism

Prognosis
- Lifelong disease characterized by exacerbations and remissions
- In most patients, disease is readily controlled by medical therapy without need for surgery
- Majority never require hospitalization
- Surgery results in complete cure of the disease

Prevention
- Colon cancer occurs in ~0.5% to 1.0% per year of patients who have had colitis for > 10 years
- Colonoscopy with multiple random mucosal biopsies recommended every 1 to 2 years in patients with extensive colitis, beginning 8 to 10 years after diagnosis; chromoendoscopy with methylene blue or indigo carmine enhances detection of subtle mucosal lesions
- Folic acid, 1 mg once daily orally, decreases risk of colon cancer
- Venous thromboembolism prophylaxis for all hospitalized patients

9. When to Refer and When to Admit

When to Refer
- Colonoscopy: for evaluation of activity and extent of active disease and for surveillance for neoplasia in patients with quiescent disease for > 8 to 10 years
- When hospitalization is required
- When surgical colectomy is indicated

When to Admit
- Patients with severe disease manifested by frequent bloody stools, anemia, weight loss, and fever
- Patients with fulminant disease manifested by rapid progression of symptoms, worsening abdominal pain, distention, high fever, tachycardia
- Patients with moderate-to-severe symptoms that do not respond to oral corticosteroids and require a trial of bowel rest and intravenous corticosteroids

SUGGESTED REFERENCES

Bitton A et al; Canadian Association of Gastroenterology Severe Ulcerative Colitis Consensus Group. Treatment of hospitalized adult patients with severe ulcerative colitis: Toronto consensus statements. *Am J Gastroenterol.* 2012 Feb;107(2):179–194. [PMID: 22108451]

Danese S et al. Biological agents for moderately to severely active ulcerative colitis: a systematic review and network meta-analysis. *Ann Intern Med*. 2014 May 20;160(10):704–711. [PMID: 24842416]

Feagan BG et al; GEMINI 1 Study Group. Vedolizumab as induction and maintenance therapy for ulcerative colitis. *N Engl J Med*. 2013 Aug 22;369(8):699–710. [PMID: 23964932]

Kornbluth A et al. Ulcerative colitis practice guidelines in adults: American College of Gastroenterology, Practice Parameters Committee. *Am J Gastroenterol*. 2010 Mar;105(3):501–523. [PMID: 20068560]

Marshall JK et al. Rectal 5-aminosalicylic acid for maintenance of remission in ulcerative colitis. *Cochrane Database Syst Rev*. 2012 Nov 14;11:CD004118. [PMID: 23152224]

Ordás I et al. Ulcerative colitis. *Lancet*. 2012 Nov 3;380(9853):1606–1619. [PMID: 22914296]

Gynecologic/Urologic Disorders

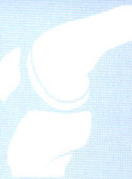

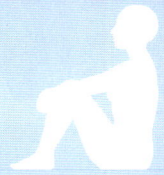
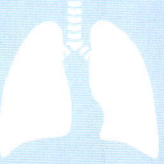
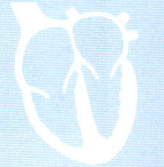
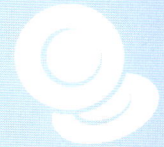
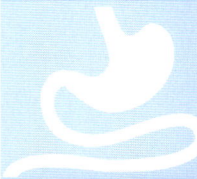
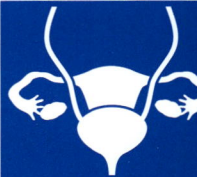
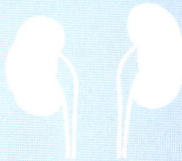
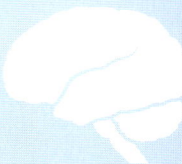

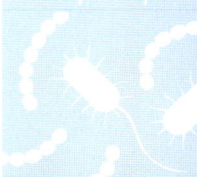

38

Breast Cancer

A 53-year-old nulliparous woman presents to her clinician for evaluation of a painless breast lump that she first noted a few months ago. She came for evaluation when she noticed bloody discharge from the ipsilateral nipple. She takes no medications, and her family history is remarkable for her mother and sister having breast cancer. On physical examination, there is a firm 2-cm mass with poorly defined margins in the left breast, and firm left axillary lymph nodes.

LEARNING OBJECTIVES

► Learn the common and uncommon clinical manifestations and objective findings of breast cancer and how they differ by stage
► Understand the risk factors for the development of breast cancer
► Know the differential diagnosis of breast cancer including both benign and malignant disorders
► Learn the surgical and chemotherapy treatments for both localized and metastatic breast cancer

QUESTIONS

1. What are the salient features of this patient's problem?
2. How do you think through her problem?
3. What are the key features, including essentials of diagnosis, general considerations, and demographics, of breast cancer?
4. What are the symptoms and signs of breast cancer?
5. What is the differential diagnosis of breast cancer?
6. What are laboratory, imaging, and procedural findings in breast cancer?
7. What are the treatments for breast cancer?
8. What are the outcomes, including follow-up, complications, prognosis, and prevention, of breast cancer?
9. When should patients with breast cancer be referred to a specialist or admitted to the hospital?

ANSWERS

1. Salient Features

Nulliparous woman; painless and firm breast lump; nipple discharge; family history of breast cancer in first-degree relatives; ipsilateral firm axillary lymphadenopathy

2. How to Think Through

Breast cancer is the second most common cause of cancer death in women, and is a major source of morbidity. This woman's presentation is highly concerning for breast cancer and prompt evaluation is essential. This patient is nulliparous with a strong family history. What other factors increase a woman's risk for breast cancer? (Total duration of menses, ie, early menarche and late menopause; alcoholism, high dietary fat, and lack of exercise; high breast density on mammography.) If the physical examination is accurate, this patient's presentation is concerning for invasive breast cancer, stage IIIa or greater, as defined by T2 (2 cm mass), N2 (ipsilateral matted axillary lymph nodes), with no comment on possible distant metastasis. Fortunately, < 10% of women present with metastatic disease.

How should she be evaluated? (Bilateral mammography and ultrasound of breast and axilla; core needle biopsy of the mass is preferred over fine-needle biopsy.) What special studies should be conducted on the biopsy tissue? (Assays for hormone receptors and human epidermal growth factor receptor 2 expression, both of which guide treatment and prognosis.) Computed tomography (CT) scan, possibly with positron emission tomography (PET) scan, is needed to detect metastases.

Treatment will depend on histology, tumor markers, metastatic disease, and comorbidities, but may include surgery, chemotherapy, radiation, and hormonal therapy. Should the patient or her family members undergo genetic testing for *BRCA1* mutations? (A family history of breast cancer is common, due to its prevalence. While only 10% of breast cancers are associated with inherited genetic mutations, referral to genetic counseling is important in this circumstance because two first-degree relatives had it.)

3. Key Features

Essentials of Diagnosis

- Early findings
  — Single, nontender, firm-to-hard mass with ill-defined margins
  — Mammographic abnormalities
  — No palpable mass
- Later findings
  — Skin or nipple retraction
  — Axillary lymphadenopathy
  — Breast enlargement, redness, edema, pain
  — Fixation of mass to skin or chest wall

General Considerations

- Next to skin cancer, it is the most common cancer in women
- Second most common cause of cancer death in women
- About 231,840 new cases and about 40,290 deaths from breast cancer in US women estimated for 2015

Demographics

- Risk of breast cancer rises rapidly until early 60s, peaks in 70s and then declines
- More common in whites

- Risk is doubled in those who have one first-degree relative (mother, daughter, or sister) diagnosed with breast cancer; risk is tripled in those with two first-degree relatives diagnosed with breast cancer
- Risk is further increased if disease in affected family member has bilateral breast cancer or is diagnosed before menopause
- Nulliparous women and women whose first full-term pregnancy occurred after the age of 30 have an elevated risk
- Slight increased risk if menarche at age < 12 or natural menopause at age > 55
- Combined oral contraceptive pills may increase the risk of breast cancer
- Alcoholism, high dietary intake of fat, and lack of exercise may also increase breast cancer risk
- Increased incidence in fibrocystic disease with
  — Proliferative changes
  — Papillomatosis
  — Increased breast density on mammogram
  — Atypical epithelial hyperplasia
- Contralateral cancer develops in women with prior breast cancer at a rate of 1% to 2% per year
- Increased risk if history of uterine cancer
- Estimated 85% lifetime risk in women with *BRCA1* gene mutations
- Increased risk with *BRCA2*, ataxia-telangiectasia, and *p53* gene mutations

4. Symptoms and Signs

- Presenting complaint is a lump (usually painless) in 70%
- Less frequently
  — Breast pain
  — Nipple discharge
  — Erosion, retraction, enlargement, or itching of the nipple
  — Redness, generalized hardness, enlargement, or shrinking of the breast
  — Axillary mass or swelling of the arm (rare)
- With metastatic disease, back or bone pain, jaundice, or weight loss
- Physical examination is done with patient sitting arms at sides and then overhead, and supine with arm abducted
- Findings include
  — Nontender, firm or hard mass with poorly delineated margins
  — Skin or nipple retraction or dimpling
  — Breast asymmetry
  — Erosions of nipple epithelium
  — Watery, serous, or bloody discharge
- Metastatic disease suggested by
  — Firm or hard axillary nodes > 1 cm
  — Axillary nodes that are matted or fixed to skin or deep structures indicate advanced disease (at least stage III)
- Advanced stage (stage III or IV) cancer suggested by ipsilateral supraclavicular or infraclavicular nodes

5. Differential Diagnosis

- Fibrocystic condition of breast
- Fibroadenoma
- Intraductal papilloma
- Lipoma
- Fat necrosis

6. Laboratory, Imaging, and Procedural Findings

Laboratory Tests
- Alkaline phosphatase is increased in liver or bone metastases
- Serum calcium is elevated in advanced disease
- Carcinoembryonic antigen (CEA) and CA 15-3 or CA 27-29 are tumor markers, but are not recommended for diagnosis of early lesions nor for routine surveillance for recurrence after a breast cancer diagnosis

Imaging Studies
- Mammography
  — Full-field digital mammography provides an easier method to maintain and review mammograms and may improve image quality, but it has not been proven to improve overall cancer detection and is less economical
  — Full-field digital mammography may offer screening benefits to younger women (< 50 years of age) and to women with dense breasts versus plain film mammography
  — Computer-assisted detection may increase the sensitivity of mammography, but it has not been shown to improve mortality rates
- Tomosynthesis
  — Creates tomographic "slices" of the breast volume with a single acquisition
  — May improve the sensitivity of mammogram especially in patients with dense breast tissue
- Breast ultrasound may differentiate cystic from solid masses
- Magnetic resonance imaging (MRI) and ultrasound may be useful in women at high risk for breast cancer but not for general population
- Chest imaging with CT or radiographs may be done to evaluate for pulmonary metastases
- Abdominal imaging with CT or ultrasound may be done to evaluate for liver metastases
- Bone scan may show bony metastases in symptomatic patients
- PET scanning alone or combined with CT may also be used for detecting soft tissue or visceral metastases in patients with symptoms or signs of metastatic disease

Diagnostic Procedures
- Fine-needle aspiration (FNA) or core biopsy
- Open biopsy under local anesthesia if needle biopsy inconclusive
- Computerized stereotactic or ultrasound guided core needle biopsies for nonpalpable lesions found on mammogram
- TNM staging (I–IV) (Table 38-1)
- Cytologic examination of breast nipple discharge may be helpful on rare occasions

7. Treatments

Medications

Potentially Curable Disease
- Adjuvant chemotherapy improves survival
- CMF (cyclophosphamide, methotrexate, fluorouracil)
- AC (adriamycin [doxorubicin], cyclophosphamide) with taxanes (docetaxel or paclitaxel)
- Tamoxifen or aromatase inhibitors in hormone receptor-positive patients
  — Young women with high-risk ER-positive cancers have fewer relapses with the aromatase inhibitor, exemestane, plus ovarian suppression compared to tamoxifen plus ovarian suppression

Metastatic Disease
- Treatment options are outlined in Table 38-2
- For hormone receptor-positive postmenopausal patients
  — Tamoxifen (20 mg orally once daily)
  — Aromatase inhibitors (eg, anastrozole 1 mg orally once daily)

Table 38-1. TNM staging for breast cancer.

Primary Tumor (T)		
Primary Tumor (T)		
Definitions for classifying the primary tumor (T) are the same for clinical and for pathologic classification. If the measurement is made by physical examination, the examiner will use the major headings (T1, T2, or T3). If other measurements, such as mammographic or pathologic measurements, are used, the subsets of T1 can be used. Tumors should be measured to the nearest 0.1 cm increment		
TX	Primary tumor cannot be assessed	
T0	No evidence of primary tumor	
Tis	Carcinoma in situ	
Tis (DCIS)	Ductal carcinoma in situ	
Tis (LCIS)	Lobular carcinoma in situ	
Tis (Paget)	Paget disease of the nipple with no tumor	
Note: Paget disease associated with a tumor is classified according to the size of the tumor		
T1	Tumor ≤ 2 cm in greatest dimension	
T1mic	Microinvasion ≤ 0.1 cm in greatest dimension	
T1a	Tumor > 0.1 cm but not > 0.5 cm in greatest dimension	
T1b	Tumor > 0.5 cm but not > 1 cm in greatest dimension	
T1c	Tumor > 1 cm but not > 2 cm in greatest dimension	
T2	Tumor > 2 cm but not > 5 cm in greatest dimension	
T3	Tumor > 5 cm in greatest dimension	
T4	Tumor of any size with direct extension to (a) chest wall or (b) skin, only as described below	
T4a	Extension to chest wall, not including pectoralis muscle	
T4b	Edema (including peau d'orange or ulceration of the skin of the breast, or satellite skin nodules confined to the same breast)	
T4c	Both T4a and T4b	
T4d	Inflammatory carcinoma	
Regional Lymph Nodes (N)		
Clinical		
NX	Regional lymph nodes cannot be assessed (eg, previously removed)	
N0	No regional lymph node metastasis	
N1	Metastasis in movable ipsilateral axillary lymph node(s)	
N2	Metastases in ipsilateral axillary lymph nodes fixed or matted, or in clinically apparent[a] ipsilateral internal mammary nodes in the *absence* of clinically evident axillary lymph node metastasis	
pN2	Metastasis in four to nine axillary lymph nodes, or in clinically apparent[a] internal mammary lymph nodes in the *absence* of axillary lymph node metastasis	
pN2a	Metastasis in four to nine axillary lymph nodes (at least one tumor deposit > 2.0 mm)	

N2a	Metastasis in ipsilateral axillary lymph nodes fixed to one another (matted) or to other structures	
N2b	Metastasis only in clinically apparent[a] ipsilateral internal mammary nodes and in the *absence* of clinically evident axillary lymph node metastasis	
N3	Metastasis in ipsilateral infraclavicular lymph node(s) with or without axillary lymph node involvement, or in clinically apparent[a] ipsilateral internal mammary lymph node(s) and in the *presence* of clinically evident axillary lymph node metastasis; or metastasis in ipsilateral supraclavicular lymph node(s) with or without axillary or internal mammary lymph node involvement	
N3a	Metastasis in ipsilateral infraclavicular lymph node(s)	
N3b	Metastasis in ipsilateral internal mammary lymph node(s) and axillary lymph node(s)	
N3c	Metastasis in ipsilateral supraclavicular lymph node(s)	
Regional Lymph Nodes (pN)[b]		
pNX	Regional lymph nodes cannot be assessed (eg, previously removed, or not removed for pathologic study)	
pN0	No regional lymph node metastasis histologically, no additional examination for isolated tumor cells	
Note: Isolated tumor cells (ITC) are defined as single tumor cells or small cell clusters not > 0.2 mm, usually detected only by immunohistochemical (IHC) or molecular methods but which may be verified on hematoxylin and eosin stains. ITCs do not usually show evidence of malignant activity, eg, proliferation or stromal reaction		
pN0(i⁻)	No regional lymph node metastasis histologically, negative IHC	
pN0(i⁺)	No regional lymph node metastasis histologically, positive IHC, no IHC cluster > 0.2 mm	
pN0(mol⁻)	No regional lymph node metastasis histologically, negative molecular findings (RT-PCR)	
pN0(mol⁺)	No regional lymph node metastasis histologically, positive molecular findings (RT-PCR)	
pN1	Metastasis in one to three axillary lymph nodes, and/or in internal mammary nodes with microscopic disease detected by sentinel lymph node dissection but not clinically apparent[c]	
pN1mi	Micrometastasis (> 0.2 mm, none > 2.0 mm)	
pN1a	Metastasis in one to three axillary lymph nodes	
pN1b	Metastasis in internal mammary nodes with microscopic disease detected by sentinel lymph node dissection but not clinically apparent[c]	
pN1c	Metastasis in one to three axillary lymph nodes and in internal mammary lymph nodes with microscopic disease detected by sentinel lymph node dissection but not clinically apparent[c]. (If associated with greater than three positive axillary lymph nodes, the internal mammary nodes are classified as pN3b to reflect increased tumor burden)	
Distant Metastasis (M)		
MX	Distant metastasis cannot be assessed	
M0	No distant metastasis	
M1	Distant metastasis	

(continued)

Table 38-1. TNM staging for breast cancer. (continued)

		Stage Grouping		
pN2b	Metastasis in clinically apparent[a] internal mammary lymph nodes in the *absence* of axillary lymph node metastasis	**Stage 0** Tis	N0	M0
		Stage I T1[d]	N0	M0
pN3	Metastasis in 10 or more axillary lymph nodes, or in infraclavicular lymph nodes, or in clinically apparent[a] ipsilateral internal mammary lymph nodes in the *presence* of one or more positive axillary lymph nodes; or in > 3 axillary lymph nodes with clinically negative microscopic metastasis in internal mammary lymph nodes; or in ipsilateral supraclavicular lymph nodes	**Stage IIA** T0	N1	M0
		T1[d]	N1	M0
		T2	N0	M0
		Stage IIB T2	N1	M0
		T3	N0	M0
		Stage IIIA T0	N2	M0
		T1[d]	N2	M0
		T2	N2	M0
		T3	N1	M0
		T3	N2	M0
pN3a	Metastasis in 10 or more axillary lymph nodes (at least one tumor deposit > 2.0 mm), or metastasis to the infraclavicular lymph nodes	**Stage IIIB** T4	N0	M0
		T4	N1	M0
		T4	N2	M0
pN3b	Metastasis in clinically apparent[a] ipsilateral internal mammary lymph nodes in the *presence* of one or more positive axillary lymph nodes; or in > 3 axillary lymph nodes and in internal mammary lymph nodes with microscopic disease detected by sentinel lymph node dissection but not clinically apparent[c]	**Stage IIIC** Any T	N3	M0
		Stage IV Any T	Any N	M1
pN3c	Metastasis in ipsilateral supraclavicular lymph nodes	*Note:* Stage designation may be changed if postsurgical imaging studies reveal the presence of distant metastases, provided that the studies are carried out within 4 months of diagnosis in the absence of disease progression and provided that the patient has not received neoadjuvant therapy		

RT-PCR, reverse transcriptase/polymerase chain reaction.

[a]*Clinically apparent* is defined as detected by imaging studies (excluding lymphoscintigraphy) or by clinical examination or grossly visible pathologically.

[b]Classification is based on axillary lymph node dissection with or without sentinel lymph node dissection. Classification based solely on sentinel lymph node dissection without subsequent axillary lymph node dissection is designated (sn) for "sentinel node," eg, pN0(i+)(sn).

[c]*Not clinically apparent* is defined as not detected by imaging studies (excluding lymphoscintigraphy) or by clinical examination.

[d]T1 includes T1mic.

Reproduced, with permission, of the American Joint Committee on Cancer (AJCC), Chicago, Illinois, *AJCC Cancer Staging Manual*, 7th ed. New York: Springer-Science and Business Media LLC; 2010, www.springer.com.

Table 38-2. Agents commonly used for hormonal management of metastatic breast cancer.

Drug	Action	Dose, Route, Frequency	Major Side Effects
Tamoxifen citrate (Nolvadex)	SERM	20 mg orally daily	Hot flushes, uterine bleeding, thrombophlebitis, rash
Fulvestrant (Faslodex)	Steroidal estrogen receptor antagonist	500 mg intramuscularly day 1, 15, 29 and then monthly	Gastrointestinal upset, headache, back pain, hot flushes, pharyngitis
Toremifene citrate (Fareston)	SERM	40 mg orally daily	Hot flushes, sweating, nausea, vaginal discharge, dry eyes, dizziness
Diethylstilbestrol (DES)	Estrogen	5 mg orally three times daily	Fluid retention, uterine bleeding, thrombophlebitis, nausea
Goserelin (Zoladex)	Synthetic luteinizing hormone releasing analogue	3.6 mg subcutaneously monthly	Arthralgias, blood pressure changes, hot flushes, headaches, vaginal dryness
Megestrol acetate (Megace)	Progestin	40 mg orally four times daily	Fluid retention
Letrozole (Femara)	AI	2.5 mg orally daily	Hot flushes, arthralgia/arthritis, myalgia, bone loss
Anastrozole (Arimidex)	AI	1 mg orally daily	Hot flushes, skin rashes, nausea and vomiting, bone loss
Exemestane (Aromasin)	AI	25 mg orally daily	Hot flushes, increased arthralgia/arthritis, myalgia, bone loss

AI, aromatase inhibitor; SERM, selective estrogen receptor modulator.

— Bisphosphonates have shown a 35% to 40% relative reduction in the risk of cancer recurrence for hormone receptor-positive nonmetastatic breast cancer in two studies
- For patients who initially respond to tamoxifen, but then relapse, consider aromatase inhibitors
- For metastatic disease, chemotherapy should be considered
  — If visceral metastases (especially brain or lung lymphangitic)
  — If hormonal treatment is unsuccessful or disease progresses after initial response to hormonal manipulation
  — If tumor is estrogen receptor negative
- Pamidronate, zoledronic acid and denosumab (all given monthly) are Food and Drug Administration (FDA)-approved for metastatic cancer involving the bones
- AC achieves response rate of ~85%
- Combinations of cyclophosphamide, vincristine, methotrexate, fluorouracil, and taxanes achieve response rates of up to 60% to 70%
- Paclitaxel achieves response rate of 30% to 50%
- Trastuzumab, a monoclonal antibody that binds to *HER-2/neu* receptors on the cancer cell, is highly effective in *HER-2/neu*-expressive cancers
- Lapatinib
  — In combination with capecitabine is FDA-approved for the treatment of trastuzumab-resistant *HER-2/neu*-positive metastatic breast cancer
  — In combination with trastuzumab has been shown to be more effective than lapatinib alone for trastuzumab-resistant metastatic breast cancer
- Pertuzumab
  — A monoclonal antibody that targets the extracellular domain of *HER-2* receptors at a different epitope than targeted by trastuzumab and that inhibits dimerization of the receptor
  — A phase III placebo-controlled randomized study (CLEOPATRA) showed that patients treated with the combination of pertuzumab, trastuzumab, and docetaxel had a significantly longer progression-free survival time compared with those treated with docetaxel and trastuzumab alone
  — Longer follow-up revealed a significant overall survival benefit associated with pertuzumab as well
- Neoadjuvant chemotherapy plus dual *HER-2*-targeted therapy with trastuzumab and pertuzumab
  — Standard care option for patients with nonmetastatic *HER-2*-positive breast cancer
  — Prevents dimerization of *HER-2* with *HER-3*
  — Has been shown to be synergistic in combination with trastuzumab
- High-dose chemotherapy and autologous bone marrow or stem cell transplantation produce no improvement in survival over conventional chemotherapy

Surgery
- Surgery indicated for stage I and II cancers
- Disease-free survival rates are similar with partial mastectomy plus axillary dissection followed by radiation therapy and with modified radical mastectomy (total mastectomy plus axillary dissection)
- Relative contraindications to breast-conserving therapy
  — Large size and multifocal tumors
  — Clinically detectable multifocality
  — Fixation to the chest wall
  — Involvement of the nipple or overlying skin
  — Concomitant scleroderma
  — Prior therapeutic radiation to the ipsilateral breast or chest wall
- Axillary dissection generally indicated in women with invasive cancer

Table 38-3. Approximate survival (%) of patients with breast cancer by TNM stage.

TNM Stage	Five Years	Ten Years
0	95	90
I	85	70
IIA	70	50
IIB	60	40
IIIA	55	30
IIIB	30	20
IV	5–10	2
All	65	30

- Sentinel node biopsy is an alternative to axillary dissection in selected patients with invasive cancer
- If sentinel node biopsy reveals no evidence of axillary metastases, it is highly likely that the remaining lymph nodes are free of disease and axillary dissection may be omitted

Therapeutic Procedures
- Radiotherapy after partial mastectomy
  — Improves local control
  — Five to seven weeks of five daily fractions to a total dose of 5000 to 6000 cGy
  — May also improve survival after total mastectomy

8. Outcomes

Follow-Up
- Examine patient every 6 months for the first 2 years after diagnosis; thereafter, annually

Complications
- Pleural effusion occurs in almost half of patients with metastatic breast cancer
- Local recurrence occurs in 8%
- Significant edema of the arm occurs in about 10% to 30%; more commonly if radiotherapy to axilla after surgery

Prognosis
- Stage of breast cancer is the most reliable indicator of prognosis (Table 38-3)
- Clinical cure rate of localized invasive breast cancer treated with most accepted methods of therapy is 75% to > 90%
- When axillary lymph nodes are involved, the survival rate drops to 50% to 70% at 5 years and 25% to 40% at 10 years
- Estrogen and progesterone receptor-positive primary tumors have a more favorable course
- Tumors with marked aneuploidy have a poor prognosis
- Table 38-4 lists prognostic factors in node-negative breast cancer

Prevention
- American Cancer Society no longer recommends monthly breast self-examination; however, women should recognize and report any breast changes to their clinician
- Clinical examination every 3 years in women age 20 to 39, annually in women starting at age 40
- American Cancer Society recommends annual mammography beginning at age 40
- Mammography every 1 to 2 years in women age 50 to 69
- For women at high risk for developing breast cancer
  — Tamoxifen yields a 50% reduction in breast cancer if taken for 5 years
  — Raloxifene also prevents invasive breast cancer in high-risk population

Table 38-4. Prognostic factors in node-negative breast cancer.

Prognostic Factors	Increased Recurrence	Decreased Recurrence
Size	T3, T2	T1, T0
Hormone receptors	Negative	Positive
DNA flow cytometry	Aneuploid	Diploid
Histologic grade	High	Low
Tumor labeling index	< 3%	> 3%
S phase fraction	> 5%	< 5%
Lymphatic or vascular invasion	Present	Absent
Cathepsin D	High	Low
HER-2/neu oncogene	High	Low
Epidermal growth factor receptor	High	Low

9. When to Refer and When to Admit

When to Refer

- Women with exceptional family histories should be referred for genetic counseling and testing

When to Admit

- For definitive therapy by lumpectomy, axillary node dissection or sentinel node biopsy, or mastectomy after diagnosis by FNA or core needle biopsy
- For complications of metastatic disease

SUGGESTED REFERENCES

Baselga J et al; CLEOPATRA Study Group. Pertuzumab plus trastuzumab plus docetaxel for metastatic breast cancer. *N Engl J Med.* 2012 Jan 12;366(2):109–119. [PMID: 22149875]

Bleyer A et al. Effect of three decades of screening mammography on breast-cancer incidence. *N Engl J Med.* 2012 Nov 22;367(21):1998–2005. [PMID: 23171096]

Cuzick J et al. SERM Chemoprevention of Breast Cancer Overview Group. Selective oestrogen receptor modulators in prevention of breast cancer: an updated meta-analysis of individual participant data. *Lancet.* 2013 May 25;381(9880):1827–1834. [PMID: 23639488]

Cuzick J et al; IBIS-II investigators. Anastrozole for prevention of breast cancer in high-risk postmenopausal women (IBIS-II): an international, double-blind, randomised placebo-controlled trial. *Lancet.* 2014 Mar 22;383(9922):1041–1048. [PMID: 24333009]

Davies C et al; Adjuvant Tamoxifen: Longer Against Shorter (ATLAS) Collaborative Group. Long-term effects of continuing adjuvant tamoxifen to 10 years versus stopping at 5 years after diagnosis of oestrogen receptor-positive breast cancer: ATLAS, a randomised trial. *Lancet.* 2013 Mar 9;381(9869): 805–816. Erratum in: *Lancet.* 2013 Mar 9;381(9869):804. [PMID: 23219286]

Dengel LT et al. Axillary dissection can be avoided in the majority of clinically node-negative patients undergoing breast-conserving therapy. *Ann Surg Oncol.* 2014 Jan;21(1):22–27. [PMID: 23975314]

DeSantis CE et al. Cancer treatment and survivorship statistics, 2014. *CA Cancer J Clin.* 2014 Jul–Aug;64(4):252–271. [PMID: 24890451]

Giuliano AE et al. Association of occult metastases in sentinel lymph nodes and bone marrow with survival among women with early-stage invasive breast cancer. *JAMA.* 2011 Jul 27;306(4)385–393. [PMID: 21791687]

Giuliano AE et al. Axillary dissection vs no axillary dissection in women with invasive breast cancer and sentinel node metastasis: a randomized clinical trial. *JAMA.* 2011 Feb 9; 305(6):569–575. [PMID: 21304082]

Goldhirsch A et al; Herceptin Adjuvant (HERA) Trial Study Team. 2 years versus 1 year of adjuvant trastuzumab for HER2-positive breast cancer (HERA): an open-label, randomised controlled trial. *Lancet.* 2013 Sep 21;382(9897):1021–1028. [PMID: 23871490]

Goss PE et al; CTG MAP.3 Study Investigators. Exemestane for breast-cancer prevention in postmenopausal women. *N Engl J Med.* 2011 Jun 23;364(25):2381–2391. [PMID: 21639806]

Haviland JS et al. The UK Standardisation of Breast Radiotherapy (START) trials of radiotherapy hypofractionation for treatment of early breast cancer: 10-year follow-up results of two randomised controlled trials. *Lancet Oncol.* 2013 Oct;14(11):1086–1094. [PMID: 24055415]

Hendrick RE et al. United States Preventive Services Task Force screening mammography recommendations: science ignored. *AJR Am J Roentgenol*. 2011 Feb;196(2):W112–W116. [PMID: 21257850]

Independent UK Panel on Breast Cancer Screening. The benefits and harms of breast cancer screening: an independent review. *Lancet*. 2012 Nov 17;380(9855):1778–1786. [PMID: 23117178]

Jagsi R et al. Progress and controversies: radiation therapy for invasive breast cancer. *CA Cancer J Clin*. 2014 Mar–Apr;64(2):135–152. [PMID: 24357525]

Kümmel S et al. Surgical treatment of primary breast cancer in the neoadjuvant setting. *Br J Surg*. 2014 Jul;101(8):912–924. [PMID: 24838656]

Manson JE et al. Menopausal hormone therapy and health outcomes during the intervention and extended poststopping phases of the Women's Health Initiative randomized trials. *JAMA*. 2013 Oct 2;310(13):1353–1368. [PMID: 24084921]

Miller AB et al. Twenty five year follow-up for breast cancer incidence and mortality of the Canadian National Breast Screening Study: randomised screening trial. *BMJ*. 2014 Feb 11;348:g366. [PMID: 24519768]

National Comprehensive Cancer Network. NCCN Guidelines: Breast Cancer. http://www.nccn.org/professionals/physician_gls/f_guidelines.asp

Nelson HD et al. Risk assessment, genetic counseling, and genetic testing for BRCA-related cancer in women: a systematic review to update the U.S. Preventive Services Task Force recommendation. *Ann Intern Med*. 2014 Feb 18;160(4):255–266. [PMID: 24366442]

Nelson HD et al. Use of medications to reduce risk for primary breast cancer: a systematic review for the U.S. Preventive Services Task Force. *Ann Intern Med*. 2013 Apr 16;158(8):604–614. [PMID: 23588749]

Pace LE et al. A systematic assessment of benefits and risks to guide breast cancer screening decisions. *JAMA*. 2014 Apr 2;311(13):1327–1335. [PMID: 24691608]

Piccart M et al. Everolimus plus exemestane for hormone-receptor-positive, human epidermal growth factor receptor-2-negative advanced breast cancer: overall survival results from BOLERO-2. *Ann Oncol*. 2014 Dec;25(12):2357–2362. [PMID: 25231953]

Pivot X et al; PHARE trial investigators. 6 months versus 12 months of adjuvant trastuzumab for patients with HER2-positive early breast cancer (PHARE): a randomised phase 3 trial. *Lancet Oncol*. 2013 Jul;14(8):741–748. [PMID: 23764181]

Rakha EA. Pitfalls in outcome prediction of breast cancer. *J Clin Pathol*. 2013 Jun;66(6):458–464. [PMID: 23618694]

Roberston JF et al. Fulvestrant 500 mg versus anastrozole 1 mg for the first-line treatment of advanced breast cancer: follow-up analysis from the randomized 'FIRST' study. *Breast Cancer Res Treat*. 2012 Nov;136(2):503–511. [PMID: 23065000]

Schwartz MD et al. Long-term outcomes of BRCA1/BRCA2 testing: risk reduction and surveillance. *Cancer*. 2012 Jan 15;118(2):510–517. [PMID: 21717445]

Siegel R et al. Cancer statistics, 2015. *CA Cancer J Clin*. 2015 Jan–Feb;65(1):5–29.

Valachis A et al. Adjuvant therapy with zoledronic acid in patients with breast cancer: a systematic review and meta-analysis. *Oncologist*. 2013;18(4):353–361. [PMID: 23404816]

Verma S et al. EMILIA Study Group. Trastuzumab emtansine for HER2-positive advanced breast cancer. *N Engl J Med*. 2012 Nov 8;367(19):1783–1791. [PMID: 23020162]

Veronesi U et al. Intraoperative radiotherapy versus external radiotherapy for early breast cancer (ELIOT): a randomised controlled equivalence trial. *Lancet Oncol*. 2013 Dec;14(13):1269–1277. [PMID: 24225155]

von Minckwitz G et al. Neoadjuvant carboplatin in patients with triple-negative and HER2-positive early breast cancer (GeparSixto; GBG 66): a randomised phase 2 trial. *Lancet Oncol*. 2014 Jun;15(7):747–756. [PMID: 2479424]

Walter LC et al. Screening mammography in older women: a review. *JAMA*. 2014 Apr 2;311(13):1336–1347. [PMID: 24691609]

Warner E. Clinical practice. Breast-cancer screening. *N Engl J Med*. 2011 Sep 15;365(11):1025–1032. [PMID: 21916640]

39 Benign Prostatic Hyperplasia

A 68-year-old man presents to the primary care clinician with a complaint of urinary frequency. The patient has noted increased urinary urgency and frequency for approximately 1 year, which has progressively worsened. He now seems to have to urinate "all the time," including four times each night, and often feels like he has not completely emptied his bladder. In addition, in the last month he often has postvoid dribbling. The family history is negative for malignancy. On examination, he appears healthy. His prostate is diffusely enlarged without focal nodule or tenderness.

LEARNING OBJECTIVES

▶ Learn the clinical manifestations and objective findings of benign prostatic hyperplasia (BPH)
▶ Understand how to score the severity of BPH
▶ Know the differential diagnosis of BPH
▶ Learn the medical and surgical treatment for BPH, including the types of surgery and their complications

QUESTIONS

1. What are the salient features of this patient's problem?
2. How do you think through his problem?
3. What are the key features, including essentials of diagnosis, general considerations, etiology, and demographics, of BPH?
4. What are the symptoms and signs of BPH?
5. What is the differential diagnosis of BPH?
6. What are the procedural findings in BPH?
7. What are the treatments for BPH?
8. What is the outcome, specifically follow-up, of BPH?
9. When should patients with BPH be referred to a specialist?

ANSWERS

1. Salient Features

Older man; progressive urinary frequency and urgency; poor bladder emptying; nocturia; postvoid dribbling; prostate enlargement without nodules

2. How to Think Through

Progressive lower urinary tract symptoms are so common in older men that clinicians must maintain a broad differential before reaching a diagnosis of BPH. In addition to BPH, what other processes could account for this patient's symptoms? (Urinary tract infection [UTI], prostatitis, polyuria due to metabolic disturbance such as diabetes mellitus or insipidus, neurogenic bladder, urethral stricture, anticholinergic and sympathomimetic medications, or bladder or prostate cancer.) Is BPH a risk factor for prostate cancer? (Since both are common, analysis of data is complicated, but evidence suggests that it is not.)

How should this patient be evaluated? (Thorough review of systems [including constitutional symptoms and bone pain suggesting cancer]; family history; abdominal examination; prostatic digital rectal examination [DRE]; neurologic examination; and urinalysis [to detect infection or blood]. If there is concern for urinary retention, obtain a postvoid ultrasound of the bladder for residual urinary volume and serum creatinine.)

How should he be treated? (α-Blockers are the first-line therapy; 5α-reductase inhibitors are adjunctive agents, taking several months for maximal effect and being minimally effective without concurrent α-blocker. The phosphodiesterase-5 inhibitor tadalafil shows improvement between 2 and 4 weeks after treatment initiation. Surgical intervention, such as transurethral resection of the prostate [TURP], is considered for refractory symptoms, urinary retention, recurrent UTI, obstructive nephropathy.)

3. Key Features

Essentials of Diagnosis
- Obstructive or irritative voiding symptoms
- May have enlarged prostate on rectal examination
- Absence of UTI, neurologic disorder, urethral stricture disease, prostatic or bladder malignancy

General Considerations
- Smooth, firm, elastic enlargement of the prostate

Etiology
- Multifactorial
- Endocrine: dihydrotestosterone
- Aging

Demographics
- The most common benign tumor in men
- Incidence is age related
- Prevalence
  — ~20% in men aged 41 to 50
  — ~50% in men aged 51 to 60
  — > 90% in men aged ≥ 80
- Symptoms are also age related
  — At age 55, ~25% of men report obstructive voiding symptoms
  — At age 75 years, 50% of men report a decrease in the force and caliber of the urinary stream

4. Symptoms and Signs
- Can be divided into obstructive and irritative complaints
- Obstructive symptoms
  — Hesitancy
  — Decreased force and caliber of stream
  — Sensation of incomplete bladder emptying
  — Double voiding (urinating a second time within 2 hours)

Table 39-1. American Urological Association symptom index for benign prostatic hyperplasia[a].

Questions to Be Answered	Not at All	Less Than One Time in Five	Less Than Half the Time	About Half the Time	More Than Half the Time	Almost Always
1. Over the past month, how often have you had a sensation of not emptying your bladder completely after you finish urinating?	0	1	2	3	4	5
2. Over the past month, how often have you had to urinate again < 2 h after you finished urinating?	0	1	2	3	4	5
3. Over the past month, how often have you found you stopped and started again several times when you urinated?	0	1	2	3	4	5
4. Over the past month, how often have you found it difficult to postpone urination?	0	1	2	3	4	5
5. Over the past month, how often have you had a weak urinary stream?	0	1	2	3	4	5
6. Over the past month, how often have you had to push or strain to begin urination?	0	1	2	3	4	5
7. Over the past month, how many times did you most typically get up to urinate from the time you went to bed at night until the time you got up in the morning?	0	1	2	3	4	5

[a]Sum of seven circled numbers equals the symptom score.

Reproduced, with permission, from Barry MJ et al. The American Urological Association symptom index for benign prostatic hyperplasia. *J Urol*. 1992;148(5):1549–1557.

- — Straining to urinate
- — Postvoid dribbling
- Irritative symptoms
  - — Urgency
  - — Frequency
  - — Nocturia
- American Urological Association (AUA) Symptom Index (Table 39-1) should be calculated for all patients starting therapy
- Seven questions quantitate the severity of obstructive or irritative complaints on a scale of 0 to 5. Thus, the score can range from 0 to 35

5. Differential Diagnosis

- Prostate cancer
- UTI
- Neurogenic bladder
- Urethral stricture

6. Procedural Findings

Diagnostic Procedures

- History to exclude other possible causes of symptoms
- Physical examination, DRE, and a focused neurologic examination
- DRE: note size and consistency of the prostate
- Examine lower abdomen for a distended bladder
- If possibility of cancer, further evaluation is needed by serum prostate-specific antigen (PSA), transrectal ultrasound, and biopsy
- As included in the Choosing Wisely (ABIM Foundation) initiative, neither creatinine nor imaging should be routinely ordered for patients with benign prostatic hyperplasia

7. Treatments

Medications

- α-Blockers
  - Prazosin, 1 mg orally each night at bedtime for 3 nights, increasing to 1 mg twice daily orally and then titrating up to 5 mg twice daily orally if necessary
  - Terazosin, 1 mg once daily orally for 3 days, increasing to 2 mg once daily orally for 11 days, then 5 to 10 mg once daily if necessary
  - Doxazosin, 1 mg once daily orally for 7 days, increasing to 2 mg once daily orally for 7 days, then 4 to 8 mg once daily orally if necessary
  - Tamsulosin, 0.4 mg once daily orally after meal, increased to 0.8 mg once daily orally if necessary
    - ᵒ Caution: Patients who receive tamsulosin within 14 days before cataract surgery have an increased risk of developing the intraoperative complication of floppy iris syndrome and postoperative ophthalmic complications
  - Alfuzosin, 10 mg once daily orally; no dose titration needed
- 5α-reductase inhibitors
  - Finasteride, 5 mg once daily orally; 6 months of therapy required for maximum effects on prostate size (20% reduction) and symptomatic improvement
  - Dutasteride, 0.5 mg once daily orally
- Phosphodiesterase-5 inhibitor
  - Tadalafil is approved by the FDA to treat the signs and symptoms of benign prostatic hyperplasia
  - Also approved for use in men with both urinary symptoms and erectile dysfunction
- Saw palmetto is of no benefit
- Combination therapy
  - α-Blocker and 5α-reductase inhibitor (eg, long-term combination therapy with doxazosin and finasteride)
    - ᵒ Safe and reduces risk of overall clinical progression of BPH significantly more than either drug alone
    - ᵒ Reduces the long-term risk of acute urinary retention and the need for invasive therapy
    - ᵒ Entails the risks of additional side effects and the cost of two medications

Surgery

- Indications
  - Refractory urinary retention (failing at least one attempt at catheter removal)
  - Large bladder diverticula
  - Recurrent UTI
  - Recurrent gross hematuria
  - Bladder stones
  - Kidney failure
- TURP: operative complications
  - Bleeding
  - Urethral stricture or bladder neck contracture
  - Perforation of the prostate capsule with extravasation
  - Transurethral resection syndrome: hypervolemic, hyponatremic state resulting from the absorption of the hypotonic irrigating solution
- TURP: postoperative complications
  - Retrograde ejaculation (75%)
  - Erectile dysfunction (5%–10%)
  - Urinary incontinence (< 1%)
- Transurethral incision of the prostate
  - Removes the zone of the prostate around the urethra leaving the peripheral portion of the prostate and prostate capsule
  - Lower rate of retrograde ejaculation reported (25%)

- Consider open simple prostatectomy when
  — Prostate is too large to remove endoscopically (> 100 g)
  — Concomitant bladder diverticulum
  — Bladder stone is present
  — Dorsal lithotomy positioning is not possible
- Minimally invasive approaches
  — Transurethral laser-induced prostatectomy under transrectal ultrasound guidance
  — Visually directed laser techniques under cystoscopic control
  — Interstitial laser therapy usually under cystoscopic control
  — Advantages of laser surgery include
    ◦ Outpatient surgery
    ◦ Minimal blood loss
    ◦ Rare occurrence of transurethral resection syndrome
    ◦ Ability to treat patients while they are receiving anticoagulation therapy
  — Disadvantages of laser surgery include
    ◦ Lack of tissue for pathologic examination
    ◦ Longer postoperative catheterization time
    ◦ More frequent irritative voiding complaints
    ◦ Expense of laser fibers and generators
  — Transurethral needle ablation of the prostate has similar improvement outcomes to TURP
  — Transurethral electrovaporization and potassium titanyl phosphate laser photo-vaporization of the prostate
  — Hyperthermia—microwave thermotherapy
  — Implant to open prostatic urethra
    ◦ The implant retracts the enlarged lobes of the prostate in symptomatic men ≥ 50 years with an enlarged prostate
    ◦ Evidence suggests that the technique improves symptoms and voiding flow while having minimal impact on ejaculation
- See Table 39-2

Therapeutic Procedures
- With watchful waiting, ~10% progress to urinary retention, and half demonstrate marked improvement or resolution of symptoms

Table 39-2. Summary of benign prostatic hyperplasia treatment outcomes.[a]

Outcome	TUIP	Open Surgery	TURP	Watchful Waiting	α-Blockers	Finasteride[b]
Chance for improvement[a]	78%–83%	94%–99.8%	75%–96%	31%–55%	59%–86%	54%–78%
Degree of symptom improvement (% reduction in symptom score)	73%	79%	85%	Unknown	51%	31%
Morbidity and complications[a]	2.2%–33.3%	7%–42.7%	5.2%–30.7%	1%–5%	2.9%–43.3%	13.6%–8.8%
Death within 30–90 days[a]	0.2%–1.5%	1%–4.6%	0.5%–3.3%	0.8%	0.8%	0.8%
Total incontinence[a]	0.1%–1.1%	0.3%–0.7%	0.7%–1.4%	2%	2%	2%
Need for operative treatment for surgical complications[a]	1.3%–2.7%	0.6%–14.1%	0.7%–10.1%	0	0	0
Erectile dysfunction[a]	3.9%–24.5%	4.7%–39.2%	3.3%–34.8%	3%	3%	2.5%–5.3%
Retrograde ejaculation	6%–55%	36%–95%	25%–99%	0	4%–11%	0
Loss of work in days	7–21	21–28	7–21	1	3.5	1.5
Hospital stay in days	1–3	5–10	3–5	0	0	0

[a]90% confidence interval.

[b]Most of the data reviewed for finasteride are derived from three trials that have required an enlarged prostate for entry. The chance of improvement in men with symptoms yet minimally enlarged prostates may be much less, as noted from the VA Cooperative Trial.

TUIP, transurethral incision of the prostate; TURP, transurethral resection of the prostate.

8. Outcome

Follow-Up
- Follow AUA Symptom Index for BPH (Table 39-1)

9. When to Refer
- Progression to urinary retention
- Patient dissatisfaction with medical therapy

SUGGESTED REFERENCES

Juliao AA et al. American Urological Association and European Association of Urology guidelines in the management of benign prostatic hypertrophy: revisited. *Curr Opin Urol.* 2012 Jan;22(1):34–39. [PMID: 22123290]

McNicholas TA et al. Minimally invasive prostatic urethral lift: surgical technique and multinational experience. *Eur Urol.* 2013 Aug;64(2):292–299. [PMID: 23357348]

McVary KT et al. Update on AUA guideline on the management of benign prostatic hyperplasia. *J Urol.* 2011 May;185(5):1793–1803. [PMID: 21420124]

Toren P et al. Effect of dutasteride on clinical progression of benign prostatic hyperplasia in asymptomatic men with enlarged prostate: a post hoc analysis of the REDUCE study. *BMJ.* 2013 Apr 15;346:f2109. [PMID: 23587564]

40

Dysmenorrhea

A 24-year-old woman presents to the clinic complaining of painful menses. She states that for the last several years she has had cramping pain in the days preceding her menses as well as during her menses. In addition, she notes bloating, weight gain, and swelling of her hands and feet in the week before her menses. She has irritability and severe mood swings during that time; she cries easily and for no reason seems to become enraged at her family or boyfriend. On review of systems, she denies urinary symptoms, vaginal discharge, or gastrointestinal symptoms. She has no significant medical history. She has never been pregnant. She has never had a sexually transmitted disease. She is monogamous with her long-standing boyfriend and states that they always use condoms. She takes no medications. Her physical examination is unremarkable.

LEARNING OBJECTIVES

▶ Learn the clinical manifestations and objective findings of primary and secondary dysmenorrhea

▶ Understand the distinguishing features and demographics of primary and secondary dysmenorrhea

▶ Know the differential diagnosis of dysmenorrhea

▶ Learn the hormonal, nonhormonal, and surgical treatments for dysmenorrhea

QUESTIONS

1. What are the salient features of this patient's problem?

2. How do you think through her problem?

3. What are the key features, including essentials of diagnosis, general considerations, and demographics, of dysmenorrhea?

4. What are the symptoms and signs of dysmenorrhea?

5. What is the differential diagnosis of dysmenorrhea?

6. What are imaging and procedural findings in dysmenorrhea?

7. What are the treatments for dysmenorrhea?

8. When should patients with dysmenorrhea be referred to a specialist?

ANSWERS

1. Salient Features

Young woman; chronic painful menses that is cramping in character; bloating and weight gain with mood disturbance before menses; normal physical examination suggests primary dysmenorrhea

2. How to Think Through

Primary dysmenorrhea needs to be differentiated from secondary dysmenorrhea in this patient. Primary dysmenorrhea begins in adolescence. Symptoms begin 0 to 2 days prior to the onset of menses, and last up to 3 days; associated symptoms of nausea, back pain, fatigue, and headache are characteristic. Exclusion of secondary causes of menstrual pain often does not require additional testing, but careful assessment of risk factors, history, and pelvic examination is needed.

What history, not present in this case, would alert the clinician to possible secondary dysmenorrhea? (Onset after age 25, worsening of symptoms over time, unilateral pain, abnormal uterine bleeding.) Why is the low-risk sexual history important in this case? (Pelvic inflammatory disease is an important cause of secondary dysmenorrhea.) What are the other major secondary causes to consider? (Endometriosis is most common; adenomyosis.)

What is the natural history of primary dysmenorrhea and how should this patient be counseled? (Improvement over time is typical, often with marked improvement following parity.) What are the two major pharmacologic treatment strategies? (Hormonal contraception and nonsteroidal anti-inflammatory drugs [NSAIDs].) What nonpharmacologic treatments have the greatest evidentiary support? (Application of heat and physical activity.)

3. Key Features

Essentials of Diagnosis
- Primary dysmenorrhea is menstrual pain associated with menstrual cycles in the absence of pathologic findings
- Secondary dysmenorrhea is menstrual pain for which an organic cause exists, such as endometriosis or uterine fibroids

General Considerations
Primary Dysmenorrhea
- The pain usually begins within 1 to 2 years after the menarche and may become more severe with time
- The pain is produced by uterine vasoconstriction, anoxia, and sustained contractions mediated by prostaglandins

Demographics
Primary dysmenorrhea
- The frequency of cases increases up to age 20 and then decreases with age and markedly with parity
- Fifty percent to 75% of women are affected at some time, and 5% to 6% have incapacitating pain

Secondary Dysmenorrhea
- It usually begins well after menarche, sometimes even as late as the third or fourth decade of life

4. Symptoms and Signs

Primary Dysmenorrhea
- Pain is low, midline, wave-like, cramping pelvic pain often radiating to the back or inner thighs

- Cramps may last for 1 or more days and may be associated with nausea, diarrhea, headache, and flushing
- No pathologic findings on pelvic examination

Secondary Dysmenorrhea
- The history and physical examination commonly suggest endometriosis or fibroids
- Other causes may be pelvic inflammatory disease, submucous myoma, adenomyosis (presence of islands of endometrial tissue in the myometrium), intrauterine device (IUD) use, cervical stenosis with obstruction, or blind uterine horn (rare)

5. Differential Diagnosis

- Endometriosis
- Adenomyosis
- Pelvic inflammatory disease
- Uterine leiomyomas (fibroids)
- IUD
- Pelvic pain syndrome
- Endometrial polyp
- Cervicitis
- Cervical stenosis
- Cystitis
- Interstitial cystitis

6. Imaging and Procedural Findings

Imaging Studies
- Pelvic imaging is useful in detecting uterine fibroids or other anomalies
- MRI is the most reliable method to detect submucous myomas
- Ultrasound or, preferably, MRI is useful in identifying adenomyosis

Diagnostic Procedures
Secondary Dysmenorrhea
- Laparoscopy may be used to diagnose endometriosis or other pelvic abnormalities not visualized by imaging

7. Treatments

Medications
Primary Dysmenorrhea
- NSAIDs (ibuprofen, ketoprofen, mefenamic acid, naproxen) and cyclooxygenase-2 inhibitor (celecoxib) are generally helpful
- Drugs should be started 1 to 2 days before expected menses
- Symptoms can be suppressed and primary dysmenorrhea usually prevented by
  — Continuous use of oral contraceptives (to suppress menstruation completely)
  — Depot-medroxyprogesterone acetate
  — Levonorgestrel-containing IUD
- For women who do not want to use hormonal contraception, consider thiamine, 100 mg/d orally, or vitamin E, 200 units/d orally from 2 days prior to and for the first 3 days of menses

Secondary Dysmenorrhea
- Periodic use of analgesics, including the NSAIDs given for primary dysmenorrhea, may be beneficial
- Combined oral contraceptives can alleviate the symptoms of secondary dysmenorrhea, particularly in endometriosis
- Danazol and gonadotropin-releasing hormone agonists are also effective in the treatment of endometriosis

- Levonorgestrel-releasing intrauterine system, uterine artery embolization, or hormonal approaches to endometriosis are used to treat adenomyosis

Surgery

- If disability is marked or prolonged, laparoscopy or exploratory laparotomy is usually warranted
- Definitive surgery depends on the degree of disability and the findings at operation
- Hysterectomy is the treatment of choice for women with adenomyosis for whom child-bearing is not a consideration
- Uterine artery embolization done to remove or treat uterine fibroids; hysterectomy may be done if other treatments have not worked but is a last resort

Therapeutic Procedures

- Other modalities that may be helpful in primary dysmenorrhea include local heat and high-frequency transcutaneous electrical nerve stimulation
- Cervical stenosis may result from induced abortion, creating crampy pain at the time of expected menses with no blood flow; this is easily cured by passing a sound into the uterine cavity after administering a paracervical block

8. When to Refer

- Standard therapy fails to relieve pain
- Suspicion of pelvic pathology, such as endometriosis, leiomyomas, or adenomyosis

SUGGESTED REFERENCES

European Society of Human Reproduction and Embryology. Study finds convincing evidence that the combined oral contraceptive pill helps painful periods. 2012 Jan 18. http://www.eshre.eu/Press-Room/Press-releases/Press-releases--2012/Combined-oral-contraceptive-pill.aspx

Harel Z. Dysmenorrhea in adolescents and young adults: an update on pharmacological treatments and management strategies. *Expert Opin Pharmacother.* 2012 Oct;13(15):2157–2170. [PMID: 22984937]

Lindh I et al. The effect of combined oral contraceptives and age on dysmenorrhoea: an epidemiological study. *Hum Reprod.* 2012 Mar;27(3):676–682. [PMID: 22252090]

Osayande AS et al. Diagnosis and initial management of dysmenorrhea. *Am Fam Physician.* 2014 Mar 1;89(5):341–346. [PMID: 24695505]

41

Prostate Cancer

A 73-year-old African American man presents to a primary care clinician to establish care. He has not seen a doctor for some time, but low back pain and difficulty in initiating and maintaining a stream of urine have prompted his visit today. His family history is notable for his father having prostate cancer. On physical examination, he has tenderness to palpation over the lumbar spine, and his digital rectal examination (DRE) reveals a large focal hard prostate nodule. His laboratory testing reveals a serum PSA concentration of 21.3 ng/mL.

LEARNING OBJECTIVES

▶ Learn the clinical manifestations and objective findings of prostate cancer
▶ Understand the demographic and other risk factors that predispose to prostate cancer
▶ Know how to interpret PSA testing and how levels correlate with prostate cancer likelihood and disease progress
▶ Learn about the medical, surgical, and radiation treatments for prostate cancer
▶ Know the options available for prostate cancer screening

QUESTIONS

1. What are the salient features of this patient's problem?

2. How do you think through his problem?

3. What are the key features, including essentials of diagnosis, general considerations, and demographics, of prostate cancer?

4. What are the symptoms and signs of prostate cancer?

5. What is the differential diagnosis of prostate cancer?

6. What are laboratory, imaging, and procedural findings in prostate cancer?

7. What are the treatments for prostate cancer?

8. What are the outcomes, including follow-up, prognosis, and prevention of prostate cancer?

9. When should patients with prostate cancer be referred to a specialist?

ANSWERS

1. Salient Features

Older man; African American race; obstructive urinary symptoms; focal prostatic nodule; highly elevated PSA; low back pain and lumbar spine tenderness suggesting possible bony metastasis

2. How to Think Through

Prostate cancer detection is challenging. For every clinically important case of prostate cancer identified, routine PSA testing detects many cancers that will not progress to clinically significant disease. Prostate cancer, however, is a leading cause of cancer-related death among men.

What risk factors for prostate cancer are present in this patient? (Family history and African American heritage.) What is the most potentially alarming finding on physical examination in this case? (Lumbar tenderness suggesting metastatic disease.) What are the next diagnostic steps? (Transrectal ultrasound [TRUS] or MRI-guided biopsy of the prostate. Computed tomography [CT] of the abdomen and pelvis. Radionuclide bone scan.) Without the significant elevation in PSA, would a biopsy be warranted in this case? (Yes. Asymmetry or nodules on DRE should be evaluated histologically.) Does the high PSA value in this case increase the likelihood of extracapsular extension? (Yes. While PSA levels are challenging to interpret due to fluctuation and overlap with benign prostatic hyperplasia, a level > 10 ng/mL is a strong indication of extracapsular disease.) To what sites does prostate cancer metastasize? (Usually bone.) Are bony metastases in prostate cancer osteolytic or osteoblastic, and do they cause elevated serum alkaline phosphatase? (Osteoblastic. Yes, serum alkaline phosphatase and calcium may be elevated.) How is prostate cancer classified to guide treatment and prognosis? (The TNM staging system, incorporating the Gleason score for pathologic tumor grade, and the PSA value.)

3. Key Features

Essentials of Diagnosis
- Prostatic induration on DRE or elevated level of serum PSA
- Most often asymptomatic
- Rarely, systemic symptoms (weight loss, bone pain)

General Considerations
- Most common nondermatologic cancer detected in American men
- Second leading cause of cancer-related death in men
- In 2014 in the United States, an estimated 233,000 new cases of prostate cancer were diagnosed, and 29,480 deaths resulted
- At autopsy, > 40% of men aged > 50 years have prostate carcinoma, most often occult

Demographics
- Incidence increases with age: autopsy incidence ~30% of men aged 60 to 69 versus 67% in men aged 80 to 89 years
- Risk factors
  — Black race
  — Family history of prostate cancer
  — History of high dietary fat intake
- A 50-year-old American man has a lifetime risk of 40% for latent cancer, of 16% for clinically apparent cancer, and of 2.9% for death from prostate cancer
- Majority of prostate cancers are adenocarcinomas

4. Symptoms and Signs
- Focal nodules or areas of induration within the prostate on DRE
- Lymph node metastases
- Lower extremity lymphedema
- Back pain or pathologic fractures
- Obstructive voiding symptoms
- Rarely, signs of urinary retention (palpable bladder) or neurologic symptoms as a result of epidural metastases and cord compression

5. Differential Diagnosis

- Urinary obstruction, eg, urethral stricture, stone, bladder neck contracture
- Prostatitis
- Benign prostatic hyperplasia
- Prostatic stones
- Bladder cancer

6. Laboratory, Imaging, and Procedural Findings

Laboratory Tests

- Elevations in serum PSA (normal < 4 ng/mL)
- PSA correlates with the volume of both benign and malignant prostate tissue
- Between 18% and 30% of men with PSA 4.1 to 10.0 ng/mL have prostate cancer
- Age-specific PSA reference ranges exist
- Most organ-confined cancers have PSA levels < 10 ng/mL
- Advanced disease (seminal vesicle invasion, lymph node involvement, or occult distant metastases) have PSA levels > 40 ng/mL
- Elevations in blood urea nitrogen or serum creatinine in patients with urinary retention or those with ureteral obstruction due to locally or regionally advanced prostate cancers
- Elevations in serum alkaline phosphatase or calcium in patients with bony metastases
- Disseminated intravascular coagulation (DIC) in patients with advanced prostate cancers

Imaging Studies

- TRUS: most prostate cancers are hypoechoic
- Magnetic resonance imaging (MRI) of the prostate
- Positive predictive value for detection of both capsular penetration and seminal vesicle invasion is similar for both TRUS and MRI
- CT imaging can be useful in detecting regional lymphatic and intra-abdominal metastases
- Radionuclide bone scan for PSA level > 20 ng/mL for detecting bony metastases

Diagnostic Procedures

- TRUS-guided biopsy from the apex, mid portion, and base of the prostate
  — Done in men who have an abnormal DRE or an elevated PSA
  — Systematic rather than only lesion-directed biopsies are recommended
  — Extended pattern biopsies, including a total of at least 10 biopsies, are associated with improved cancer detection and risk stratification of newly diagnosed patients
- MRI-guided biopsy may improve not only overall cancer detection but discovery of clinically relevant disease

7. Treatments

Medications (by Target)

- Adrenal
  — Ketoconazole, 400 mg three times daily orally (adrenal insufficiency, nausea, rash, and ataxia)
  — Aminoglutethimide, 250 mg four times daily orally (adrenal insufficiency, nausea, rash, and ataxia)
  — Corticosteroids: prednisone, 20 to 40 mg once daily orally (gastrointestinal bleeding, fluid retention)
- Pituitary, hypothalamus
  — Diethylstilbestrol, 1 to 3 mg once daily orally (gynecomastia, hot flushes, thromboembolic disease, erectile dysfunction)
  — Luteinizing hormone-releasing hormone (LHRH) agonists, monthly or three-monthly depot injection (erectile dysfunction, hot flushes, gynecomastia, and rarely anemia)
- Prostate cell
  — Antiandrogens: flutamide, 250 mg three times daily orally, or bicalutamide, 50 mg once daily orally (no erectile dysfunction when used alone; nausea, diarrhea)

- Testis
  — Orchiectomy (gynecomastia, hot flushes, and impotence)
  — Ketoconazole for patients who have advanced prostate cancer with spinal cord compression, bilateral ureteral obstruction, or DIC
  — Complete androgen blockade by combining an antiandrogen with use of an LHRH agonist or orchiectomy
- Metastasis
  — Sipuleucel-T, an autologous cellular immunotherapy, is FDA-approved for metastatic hormone-refractory prostate cancer in asymptomatic or minimally symptomatic men
  — Denosumab, a RANK ligand inhibitor
    ◦ Approved for the prevention of skeletal-related events in patients with bone metastases from prostate cancer
    ◦ Appears to delay the development of these metastases
  — Chemotherapy: Docetaxel improves survival in men with hormone-refractory prostate cancer
  — Cabazitaxel, abiraterone, and enzalutamide
    ◦ Approved for advanced prostate cancer
    ◦ Improvements in survival have been shown in men having received prior docetaxel
    ◦ Abiraterone and enzalutamide are FDA-approved for use in the pre-chemotherapy metastatic setting
  — Radium-223 dichloride
    ◦ Approved for castration-resistant, symptomatic bone metastases
    ◦ Significant improvements reported in both overall survival and time to skeletal-related events (eg, fractures)

Therapeutic Procedures
- Patients need to be advised of all treatment options, including surveillance (watchful waiting), benefits, risks, and limitations
- For lower stage and grade cancers and those with lower serum PSA at diagnosis, consider surveillance (watchful waiting)
- For minimal capsular penetration, standard irradiation or surgery
- For locally extensive cancers, including seminal vesicle and bladder neck invasion, combination therapy (androgen deprivation combined with surgery or radiation, or both)
- For metastatic disease, androgen deprivation
- For localized disease
  — Optimal form of treatment controversial
  — Selected patients may be candidates for surveillance
  — Patients with an anticipated survival of > 10 years should be considered for radical prostatectomy or radiation therapy
- Radical prostatectomy
  — For stages T1 and T2 prostatic cancers, local recurrence is uncommon after radical prostatectomy
    ◦ Organ-confined cancers rarely recur
    ◦ Locally extensive cancers (capsular penetration, seminal vesicle invasion) have higher local (10%–25%) and distant (20%–50%) relapse rates
  — Adjuvant therapy (radiation for patients with positive surgical margins or androgen deprivation for lymph node metastases)
- Radiation therapy
  — Morbidity is limited; survival with localized cancers is 65% at 10 years
  — Newer techniques of radiation (implantation, conformal therapy using three-dimensional reconstruction of CT-based tumor volumes, heavy particle, charged particle, and heavy charged particle) improve local control rates
  — Brachytherapy is implantation of permanent or temporary radioactive sources (palladium, iodine, or iridium)

8. Outcomes

Follow-Up
• Surveillance alone may be appropriate for patients who are older and have very small and well-differentiated cancers

Prognosis
• Risk assessment tools can help predict the likelihood of success of surveillance or treatment by combining stage, grade, PSA level, and number and extent of positive prostate biopsies
  — Kattan nomogram predicts the likelihood that a patient will be disease-free by serum PSA at 5 years after radical prostatectomy or radiation therapy, depending on the tumor stage, grade, and PSA

Prevention
Screening for Prostate Cancer
• Screening tests currently available include DRE, serum PSA, TRUS
• Detection rates with DRE are low, varying from 1.5% to 7.0%
• TRUS has low specificity (and therefore high biopsy rate)

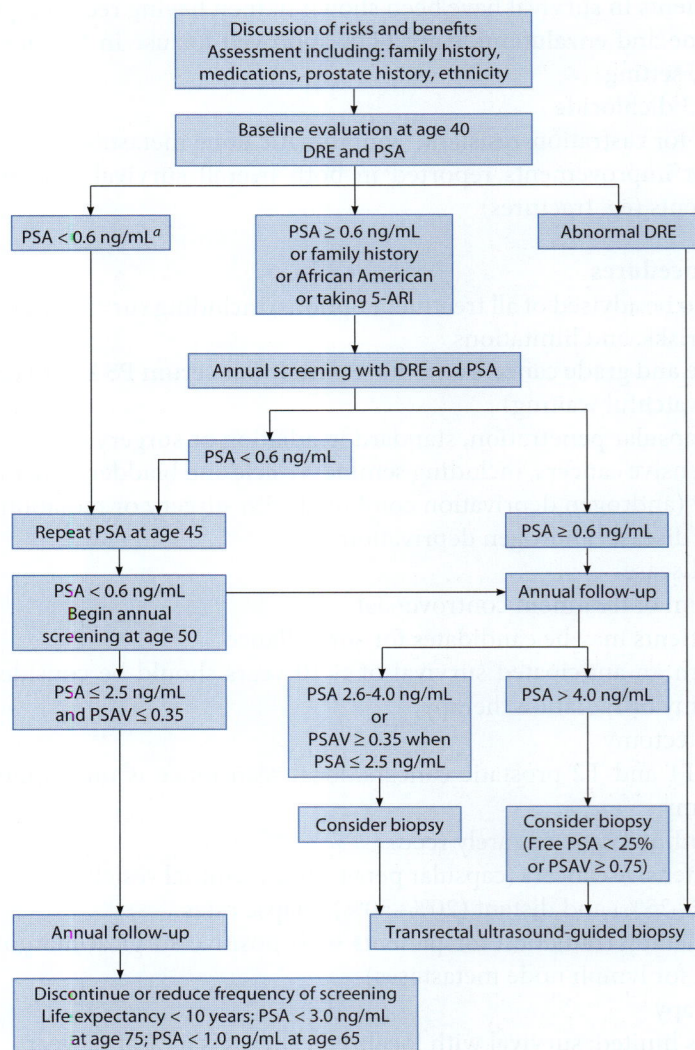

^aNCCN guidelines utilize PSA threshold of 1.0 ng/mL in men < 50 years, the 75th percentile range for this age group; the median PSA value for men 40–49 years is 0.6 ng/mL.

Figure 41-1. An algorithm for prostate cancer early detection. DRE, digital rectal examination; 5-ARI, 5α-reductase inhibitor; PSAV, PSA velocity (ng/mL/y) calculated on at least three consecutive values over at least an 18–24-month period. (Based on NCCN guidelines, data from the Baltimore Longitudinal Study on Aging, and Prostate Cancer Prevention Trial.)

- TRUS increases the detection rate very little when compared with the combined use of DRE and PSA testing
- To improve the performance of PSA as a screening test, alternative methods for its use have been developed
  - Establishment of age- and race-specific reference ranges
  - Measurement of free serum and protein-bound levels of PSA
  - Calculation of changes in PSA over time (PSA velocity)
- Traditional yearly screening may not be the most efficient approach, rather, earlier PSA testing at younger age may allow less frequent testing as well provide information regarding PSA velocity
- Studies from the Baltimore Longitudinal Study of Aging suggest that men with PSA above the age-based median when tested between 40 and 60 years are at significantly increased risk of subsequent cancer detection over 25 years
- Therefore, men with lower PSA ($\leq$ 0.6 ng/mL ages 40–50 and $\leq$ 0.71 ages 50–60) may require less-frequent PSA tests
- In addition, men with PSA velocity > 0.35 ng/mL per year measured 10–15 years before diagnosis had significantly worse cancer-specific survival compared with those with lower PSA velocity
- The National Comprehensive Cancer Network guidelines (http://www.nccn.org/professionals/physician_gls/f_guidelines.asp) for prostate cancer early detection incorporate many of these factors (Figure 41-1)
- The current European Association of Urology (EAU) recommend offering a baseline serum PSA to all men 40 to 45 years old and subsequently initiating a risk-adapted strategy

9. When to Refer

- Active surveillance may be appropriate in selected patients with very low-volume, low-grade prostate cancer.
- Localized disease may be managed by active surveillance, surgery, or radiation therapy.
- Locally extensive, regionally advanced, and metastatic disease often requires multimodal treatment strategies.

SUGGESTED REFERENCES

Beer TM et al; PREVAIL Investigators. Enzalutamide in metastatic prostate cancer before chemotherapy. N Engl J Med. 2014 Jul 31;371(5):424–433. [PMID: 24881730]

Bill-Axelson A et al. Radical prostatectomy or watchful waiting in early prostate cancer. N Engl J Med. 2014 Mar 6;370(10):932–942. [PMID: 24597866]

Ilic D et al. Screening for prostate cancer. Cochrane Database Syst Rev. 2013 Jan 31;1:CD004720. [PMID: 23440794]

Moyer VA. Screening for prostate cancer: U.S. Preventive Services Task Force recommendation statement. Ann Intern Med. 2012 Jul 17;157(2):120–134. [PMID: 22801674]

Niraula S et al. Treatment of prostate cancer with intermittent versus continuous androgen deprivation: a systematic review of randomized trials. J Clin Oncol. 2013 Jun 1;31(16):2029–2036. [PMID: 23630216]

Qaseem A et al. Screening for prostate cancer: a guidance statement from the Clinical Guidelines Committee of the American College of Physicians. Ann Intern Med. 2013 May 21;158(10):761–769. [PMID: 23567643]

Schröder FH et al; ERSPC Investigators. Prostate-cancer mortality at 11 years of follow-up. N Engl J Med. 2012 Mar 15;366(11):981–990. Erratum in: N Engl J Med. 2012 May 31;366(22):2137. [PMID: 22417251]

Thompson IM Jr et al. Long-term survival of participants in the prostate cancer prevention trial. N Engl J Med. 2013 Aug 15;369(7):603–610. [PMID: 23944298]

Wilt TJ et al; Prostate Cancer Intervention versus Observation Trial (PIVOT) Study Group. Radical prostatectomy versus observation for localized prostate cancer. N Engl J Med. 2012 Jul 19;367(3):203–213. Erratum in: N Engl J Med. 2012 Aug 9; 367(6):582. [PMID: 22808955]

Skin Disorders

Pulmonary/Ear, Nose, & Throat Disorders

Heart/Hypertension/Lipid Disorders

Hematologic Disorders

Gastrointestinal/Liver/Pancreas Disorders

Gynecologic/Urologic Disorders

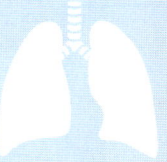

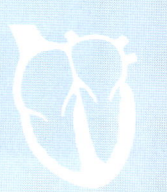

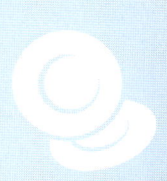

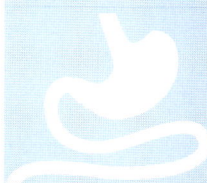

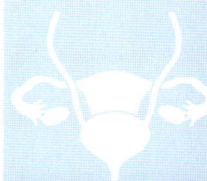

Musculoskeletal Disorders

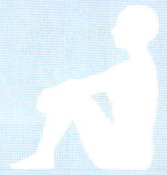

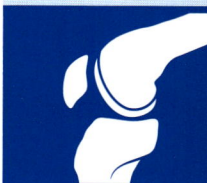

Kidney/Electrolyte Disorders

Nervous System/Psychiatric Disorders

Endocrine/Metabolic Disorders

Infectious Disorders

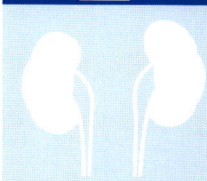

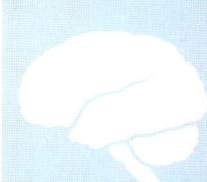

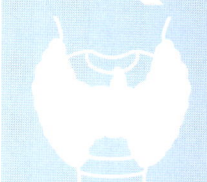

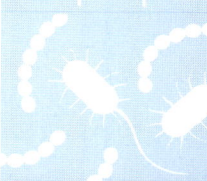

42

Low Back Pain

A 45-year-old man presents to urgent care clinic complaining of low back pain (LBP). He states that he was moving heavy boxes at work yesterday when he felt a sudden onset of LBP that radiated down his left buttock and left posterior thigh. His past medical history is unremarkable and he takes no medications. He denies any bowel or bladder incontinence. On physical examination, he has decreased sensation on the posterior left thigh, decreased strength on left ankle dorsiflexion, and an absent left ankle jerk deep tendon reflex. He has no saddle anesthesia and normal rectal tone. His straight leg raise test is positive, with pain reproduced on passive elevation of the right (contralateral) leg. After 4 weeks of conservative therapy, his symptoms resolve.

LEARNING OBJECTIVES

▶ Learn the clinical manifestations and objective findings of LBP and how to localize radicular symptoms
▶ Understand which patients with LBP need imaging
▶ Know the differential diagnosis of LBP
▶ Learn which medical and surgical treatments are effective for LBP
▶ Know the warning signs of cauda equina syndrome (CES)

QUESTIONS

1. What are the salient features of this patient's problem?
2. How do you think through his problem?
3. What are the key features, including essentials of diagnosis, general considerations, and demographics, of LBP?
4. What are the symptoms and signs of LBP?
5. What is the differential diagnosis of LBP?
6. What are imaging and procedural findings in LBP?
7. What are the treatments for LBP?
8. What is the outcome, including prognosis and complications, of LBP?
9. When should patients with LBP be referred to a specialist or admitted to the hospital?

ANSWERS

1. Salient Features

Acute onset of LBP; radiation down left buttock and posterior thigh with decreased sensation, decreased strength on ankle dorsiflexion, and loss of ankle jerk reflex consistent with L5-S1 radiculopathy; positive straight leg raise suggestive of disk herniation; no warning signs of CES

2. How to Think Through

Acute LBP is common in both primary care and emergency medicine settings. The challenge is to identify the high-risk patient who needs further urgent evaluation from the low-risk patient, who may be equally uncomfortable, but for whom a trial of conservative management is appropriate. Even with an apparent mechanical cause, such as in this case, key risk factors must be assessed. What are the major causes of high-risk back pain? (Infection, such as vertebral osteomyelitis or epidural abscess; metastatic cancer; rheumatologic spondylitis; CES; fracture.) This patient has no notable medical history, no history of cancer, corticosteroid use, or osteoporosis. What additional risk factor must be assessed? (Injection drug use.) What are the key "red flag" symptoms to elicit? (Fever, weight loss, nocturnal pain, change in bowel or bladder function, lower extremity or sphincter weakness.)

What is the most likely cause of this patient's pain, and can we localize the problem? (An L5-S1 radiculopathy, likely due to disk herniation. Less likely causes, given his age, include pyriformis syndrome, osteoarthritis [OA], and fracture.) What examination finding specifically supports the diagnosis of disk herniation? (Positive contralateral straight leg raise.)

Should he receive imaging? (No. He is very likely to improve with conservative management, including nonsteroidal anti-inflammatory drugs [NSAIDs], heat, and physical therapy, within 6 weeks.)

3. Key Features

Essentials of Diagnosis

- May be categorized by pain on flexion versus pain on extension
- Nerve root impingement is suspected when pain is leg-dominant rather than back-dominant
- Alarming ("red flag") symptoms or signs for serious spinal disease include unexplained weight loss, failure to improve with treatment, severe pain for more than 6 weeks, and night or rest pain
- The cauda equina syndrome often presents with bowel or bladder symptoms (or both) and is an emergency

General Considerations

- Cause is often multifactorial, although there are usually degenerative changes in the lumbar spine
- Alarming symptoms for back pain caused by cancer include
  — Unexplained weight loss
  — Failure to improve with treatment
  — Pain for > 6 weeks
  — Pain at night or rest
  — Age > 50 years
  — History of cancer
- Alarming symptoms for infection include
  — Fever
  — Rest pain
  — Recent infection (urinary tract infection, cellulitis, pneumonia)
  — History of immunocompromise or injection drug use

- The cauda equina syndrome is suggested by
  — Urinary retention or incontinence
  — Saddle anesthesia
  — Decreased anal sphincter tone or fecal incontinence
  — Bilateral lower extremity weakness
  — Progressive neurologic deficits
- Risk factors for back pain due to vertebral fracture include
  — Use of corticosteroids
  — Age > 70 years
  — History of osteoporosis
  — Recent severe trauma, presence of contusion or abrasion
  — Very severe focal pain
- Back pain may also be the presenting symptom in other serious medical problems including
  — Abdominal aortic aneurysm
  — Peptic ulcer disease
  — Kidney stones
  — Pancreatitis
- Annual prevalence is 15% to 45%
- Annual cost in the United States is over $50 billion

Demographics
- Most common cause of disability for patients under the age of 45
- Second most common cause for primary care visits

4. Symptoms and Signs

- Worsening with rest and improvement with activity is characteristic of seronegative spondyloarthropathies; degenerative disease usually improves with rest and is worse with activity
- Radiation down the buttock and below the knee, loss of reflexes, and a positive crossed straight-leg raise test result suggests nerve root irritation from a herniated disc

Physical Examination
- In the standing position
  — Observe the patient's posture
    ○ Commonly encountered spinal asymmetries include scoliosis, thoracic kyphosis, and lumbar hyperlordosis
  — Assess the active range of motion of the lumbar spine
  — Perform the one-leg standing extension test to assess for pain (the patient stands on one leg while extending the spine); a positive test can be caused by
    ○ Pars interarticularis fractures (spondylolysis or spondylolisthesis) or
    ○ Facet joint arthritis
- In the sitting position
  — Test motor strength, reflexes and sensation (Table 42-1)
  — Assess the major muscles in the lower extremities for weakness by eliciting a resisted isometric contraction for approximately 5 seconds
  — Compare the strength bilaterally to detect subtle muscle weakness
  — Similarly, check sensory testing to light touch in specific dermatomes for corresponding nerve root function
  — Finally, check the knee (femoral nerve L2–4), ankle (deep peroneal nerve L4–L5), and Babinski (sciatic nerve L5–S1) reflexes can be checked
- In the supine position
  — Evaluate the hip for range of motion, focusing on internal rotation
  — Perform the straight leg raise test; it puts traction and compression forces on the lower lumbar nerve roots (Table 42-1)

Table 42-1. Neurologic testing of lumbosacral nerve disorders.

Nerve Root	Motor	Reflex	Sensory Area
L1	Hip flexion	None	Groin
L2	Hip flexion	None	Thigh
L3	Extension of knee	Knee jerk	Knee
L4	Dorsiflexion of foot	Knee jerk	Medial calf
L5	Dorsiflexion of first toe	Babinski reflex	First dorsal web space between first and second toes
S1	Plantar flexion of foot, knee flexors, or hamstrings	Ankle jerk	Lateral foot
S2	Knee flexors or hamstrings	Knee flexor	Back of the thigh
S2-4	External anal sphincter	Anal reflex, rectal tone	Perianal area

- In the prone position
  — Carefully palpate each level of the spine and sacroiliac joints for tenderness
  — Perform a rectal examination if the cauda equina syndrome is suspected

5. Differential Diagnosis

- Muscular strain
- Herniated disk
- Lumbar spinal stenosis
- Compression fracture
- DJD
- Infectious diseases (eg, osteomyelitis, epidural abscess, subacute bacterial endocarditis)
- Neoplastic disease (vertebral metastases)
- Spondyloarthropathies, eg, ankylosing spondylitis
- Leaking abdominal aortic aneurysm
- Renal colic

6. Imaging and Procedural Findings

Imaging Studies

- The Agency for Healthcare Research and Quality guidelines for obtaining lumbar radiographs are summarized in Table 42-2
- Diagnostic imaging, including radiographs, is not typically recommended in the first 6 weeks unless alarming "red flag" symptoms suggesting infection, malignancy, or cauda equina syndrome are present
- If done, radiographs of the lumbar spine should include anteroposterior and lateral views
- Oblique views can be useful if the neural foramina or lesions need to be visualized
- MRI of the lumbosacral spine is the method of choice to evaluate symptoms not responding to conservative treatment or "red flags" for serious conditions

Diagnostic Procedures

- Electromyography or nerve conduction studies
  — May be useful in assessing patients with possible nerve root symptoms lasting longer than 6 weeks
  — Not usually necessary if the diagnosis of radiculopathy is clear

7. Treatments

Medications

- NSAIDs are effective in early treatment
- Muscle "relaxants" (diazepam, cyclobenzaprine, carisoprodol, methocarbamol)
  — Limited evidence that they provide short-term relief

Table 42-2. AHRQ criteria for lumbar radiographs in patients with acute low back pain.

Possible fracture
  Major trauma
  Minor trauma in patients > 50 years old
  Long-term corticosteroid use
  Osteoporosis
  > 70 years old

Possible tumor or infection
  > 50 years old
  < 20 years old
  History of cancer
  Constitutional symptoms
  Recent bacterial infection
  Injection drug use
  Immunosuppression
  Supine pain
  Nocturnal pain

AHRQ, Agency for Healthcare Research and Quality.

Reproduced, with permission, from Suarez-Almazor et al. Use of lumbar radiographs for the early diagnosis of low back pain. Proposed guidelines would increase utilization. *JAMA*. 1997;277:1782–1786.

— Best used if there is true muscle spasm that is painful
  — Should be used with care due to potential for addiction
• Opioids may be necessary to alleviate pain immediately
• Gabapentin, duloxetine, and nortriptyline may be helpful in treating more chronic neuropathic pain

Surgery
• Indications
  — Cauda equina syndrome
  — Ongoing morbidity with no response to > 6 months of conservative treatment
  — Cancer
  — Infection
  — Severe spinal deformity
• Surgery can improve pain but is unlikely to cure it

Therapeutic Procedures
• Nonpharmacologic treatments are key in the management of low back pain
• Education alone improves patient satisfaction with recovery and recurrence
• Physical therapy exercise programs can be tailored to the patient's symptoms and pathology
• Strengthening and stabilization exercises effectively reduce pain and functional limitation compared with usual care
• Improvements in posture, core stability strengthening, physical conditioning, and modifications of activities to decrease physical strain are keys for ongoing management
• Neither spinal manipulation nor traction have shown benefits, though the studies thus far are of low quality and small sample size
• Heat and cold treatments have no long-term benefits but may provide short-term symptom relief
• The efficacy of transcutaneous electrical nerve stimulation (TENS), back braces, physical agents, and acupuncture is unproven
• Epidural injections may provide improved pain reduction short term

8. Outcome

Prognosis
• Approximately 80% of episodes of low back pain resolve within 2 weeks and 90% resolve within 6 weeks

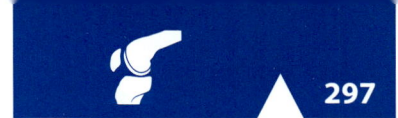

- Better prognosis when there is an anatomic lesion that can be corrected and when there are neurologic symptoms

Complications

- Depending on the surgery performed, possible complications include
  — Persistent pain
  — Surgical site pain, especially if bone grafting is needed
  — Infection
  — Neurologic damage
  — Nonunion
  — Cutaneous nerve damage
  — Implant failure
  — Deep venous thrombosis
  — Death

9. When to Refer and When to Admit

When to Refer

- Patients with cancer, infection, or severe spinal deformity
- Patients who have not responded to conservative treatment

When to Admit

- Neurologic signs indicative of the cauda equina syndrome
- Vertebral osteomyelitis

SUGGESTED REFERENCES

Downie A et al. Red flags to screen for malignancy and fracture in patients with low back pain: systematic review. *BMJ*. 2013 Dec 11;347:f7095. [PMID: 24335669]

Goodman DM et al. JAMA patient page. Low back pain. *JAMA*. 2013 Apr 24;309(16):1738. [PMID: 23613079]

Rubinstein SM et al. Spinal manipulative therapy for acute low back pain: an update of the Cochrane review. *Spine (Phila Pa 1976)*. 2013 Feb 1;38(3):E158–177. [PMID: 23169072]

43

Gout

A 58-year-old man with a long history of treated essential hypertension and mild chronic kidney disease presents to the urgent care clinic complaining of pain in the right knee. His primary care clinician saw him 1 week ago and added a thiazide diuretic to improve his blood pressure control. He had been feeling well until the night before the clinic visit, when he noted some redness and slight swelling of his knee. He went to sleep and was awakened early by significant swelling and pain. He was able to walk only with assistance. He has no history of knee trauma.

Physical examination confirmed the presence of a swollen right knee, which was erythematous and warm. Joint aspiration recovered copious dark yellow, cloudy synovial fluid. Microscopic analysis demonstrated 30,000 leukocytes/µL, a negative Gram stain, and many needle-like, negatively birefringent crystals.

LEARNING OBJECTIVES

▶ Learn the clinical manifestations and objective findings of gout
▶ Understand the factors that predispose to gout
▶ Know the differential diagnosis of gout—arthritis, podagra, and tophi
▶ Learn about treatments available for acute gout
▶ Understand how to prevent gout attacks

QUESTIONS

1. What are the salient features of this patient's problem?
2. How do you think through his problem?
3. What are the key features, including essentials of diagnosis and general considerations, of gout?
4. What are the symptoms and signs of gout?
5. What is the differential diagnosis of gout?
6. What are laboratory, imaging, and procedural findings in gout?
7. What are treatments available for gout?

8. What are the outcomes, including follow-up, complications, prognosis, and prevention, of gout?

9. When should patients with gout be referred to a specialist and admitted to the hospital?

ANSWERS

1. Salient Features

Chronic kidney disease; monoarticular joint pain; thiazide use; warm, red joint; synovial fluid with elevated WBC < 50 000/μL; negative Gram stain; negatively birefringent needle-shaped (urate) crystals

2. How to Think Through

A septic joint is the first consideration in any patient with monoarticular joint pain with evidence of inflammation (rubor [redness], dolor [pain], calor [warmth], and tumor [swelling])—ie, a true arthritis. The other two major etiologies of monoarticular arthritis are trauma and crystal-induced arthropathies. Does the patient fit the demographic predilections for gout? (Yes.) Is the joint in question one typically affected by gout? (Yes, most common are the great toe, mid-foot, and knee.) What is the tempo of the onset of pain in gout? (Rapid escalation.) What are the risk factors for gout? (Thiazides, myeloproliferative disorders, alcohol intake.) Can patients with gout have fever? (Yes.) How does synovial fluid analysis help? Where on the body might you find tophi? (Cartilage, external ears, hands, feet, olecranon, prepatellar pursue, tendons, and bone.) What might an x-ray show in gout? (Erosions.)

Joint aspiration is the priority in monoarticular arthritis, and is the right "next diagnostic step." Knowledge of the synovial fluid WBC ranges for inflammatory and septic joints is also essential for correct diagnosis. Gout is challenging in that it is the most likely noninfectious cause of a synovial fluid WBC > 50, 000/μL (although this patient's synovial fluid WBC was 30, 000/μL). However, while the joint aspirate Gram stain and culture help rule out infection, finding crystals establishes the diagnosis of gout definitively.

3. Key Features

Essentials of Diagnosis

- Acute onset, usually monoarticular, recurring attacks of arthritis, often involving the first metatarsophalangeal (MTP) joint
- Polyarticular involvement more common with long-standing disease
- Hyperuricemia in most; identification of urate crystals in joint fluid or tophi is diagnostic
- Dramatic therapeutic response to nonsteroidal anti-inflammatory drugs

General Considerations

- A metabolic disease of heterogeneous nature, often familial, associated with abnormal amounts of urates in the body and characterized early by a recurring acute arthritis, usually monoarticular, and later by chronic deforming arthritis
- Secondary gout is from acquired causes of hyperuricemia
  — Medication use (diuretics, low-dose aspirin, cyclosporine, and niacin)
  — Myeloproliferative disorders, multiple myeloma, hemoglobinopathies
  — Chronic kidney disease
  — Hypothyroidism, psoriasis, sarcoidosis, and lead poisoning
- Alcoholism promotes hyperuricemia by increasing urate production and decreasing the renal excretion of uric acid
- Hospitalized patients frequently suffer attacks of gout because of changes in diet (eg, inability to take oral feedings following abdominal surgery) or medications that lead to either rapid reductions or increases in the serum uric acid level

4. Symptoms and Signs

- Sudden onset of arthritis
  — Frequently nocturnal
  — Either without apparent precipitating cause or following rapid fluctuations in serum uric acid levels
  — The MTP joint of the great toe is the most susceptible joint ("podagra")
  — Other joints, especially those of the feet, ankles, and knees, are also commonly affected
  — May develop in periarticular soft tissues such as the arch of the foot
- As the attack progresses
  — The pain becomes intense
  — The involved joints are swollen and exquisitely tender
  — The overlying skin is tense, warm, and dusky red
  — Fever is common
- Tophi
  — May be found in cartilage, external ears, hands, feet, olecranon, prepatellar bursae, tendons, and bone
  — Usually seen only after several attacks of acute arthritis
- Asymptomatic periods of months or years commonly follow the initial attack
- After years of recurrent severe monoarthritis attacks, gout can evolve into a chronic, deforming polyarthritis of upper and lower extremities that mimics rheumatoid arthritis

5. Differential Diagnosis

- Arthritis: Cellulitis, septic arthritis, pseudogout, rheumatoid arthritis, reactive arthritis, osteoarthritis, chronic lead poisoning (saturnine gout), palindromic rheumatism
- Podagra: Trauma, cellulitis, sarcoidosis, pseudogout, psoriatic arthritis, bursitis of first MTP joint (inflamed bunion)
- Tophi: Rheumatoid nodules, erythema nodosum, coccidioidomycosis, endocarditis (Osler nodes), sarcoidosis, polyarteritis nodosa

6. Laboratory, Imaging, and Procedural Findings

Laboratory Tests

- During an acute flare, a single serum uric acid determination is normal in up to 25% of cases, and thus does not exclude gout
- However, serial measurements of serum uric acid detect hyperuricemia in 95% of patients

Imaging Studies

- Early in the disease, radiographs show no changes
- Later, punched-out erosions with an overhanging rim of cortical bone ("rat bite" erosions) develop. When these are adjacent to a soft tissue tophus, they are diagnostic of gout

Diagnostic Procedures

- Identification of sodium urate crystals in joint fluid or material aspirated from a tophus establishes the diagnosis
- The crystals, which may be extracellular or found within neutrophils, are needle-like and negatively birefringent when examined by polarized light microscopy

7. Treatments

Medications

Asymptomatic Hyperuricemia

- Should not be treated
- Uric acid-lowering drugs are not necessary until arthritis, renal calculi, or tophi become apparent

Acute Attack
- Treatment of the acute attack focuses on reducing inflammation, not lowering serum uric acid
- Nonsteroidal anti-inflammatory drugs are the treatment of choice
  - Naproxen 500 mg twice daily or indomethacin 25 to 50 mg every 8 hours
  - Should be continued until the symptoms have resolved (usually 5 to 10 days)
  - Contraindications include active peptic ulcer disease, impaired kidney function, and a history of allergic reaction to NSAIDs
- The pain of an acute attack may require opioids.
- Aspirin should be avoided since it aggravates hyperuricemia
- Oral colchicine is an appropriate treatment option for acute gout, provided the duration of the attack is <36 hours
  - For acute gout, administer orally as follows:
    › A loading dose of 1.2 mg followed by a dose of 0.6 mg 1 hour later
    › Then use prophylaxis dose (0.6 mg once or twice daily), beginning 12 hours later
  - For patients already taking prophylactic doses of colchicine who have an acute flare of gout
    › 1.2 mg followed by 0.6 mg 1 hour later provided they have not received this regimen within the preceding 14 days
    › If they have received regimen in preceding 14 days, NSAIDS or corticosteroids should be used
- Corticosteroids
  - May be given intravenously (eg, methylprednisolone, 40 mg/d tapered off over 7 days) or orally (eg, prednisone, 40 to 60 mg/d tapered off over 7 days)
  - May be given intra-articularly (eg, triamcinolone, 10 to 40 mg depending on the size of the joint) if the patient's gout is monarticular or oligoarticular
- Interleukin-1 inhibitor
  - Anakinra has efficacy for the management of acute gout
  - However, this drug has not been approved in the United States by the FDA for this indication

Surgery
- Surgical excision of large tophi rarely offers mechanical improvement in selected deformities

Therapeutic Procedures
- Corticosteroid injections for acute monoarticular disease
- Bed rest is important and should be continued for about 24 hours after the acute attack has subsided. Early ambulation may precipitate a recurrence
- Treat the acute arthritis first and hyperuricemia later, if at all. Sudden reduction of serum uric acid often precipitates further gouty arthritis

8. Outcomes
Follow-Up
- Maintain uric acid level within the normal range in nontophaceous gout
- Maintain serum uric acid below 6.0 mg/dL in tophaceous gout

Complications
- Chronic tophaceous arthritis can occur after repeated attacks of inadequately treated acute gout
- Uric acid kidney stones (5% to 10% of patients)
  - Hyperuricemia correlates highly with the likelihood of developing stones
  - The risk of stone formation reaches 50% with a serum uric acid level above 13 mg/dL
- Chronic urate nephropathy

- Although progressive renal failure occurs in a substantial percentage of patients with chronic gout, the etiologic role of hyperuricemia is controversial, because there are numerous confounding risk factors for renal failure

Prognosis

- Untreated, the acute attack may last from a few days to several weeks, but proper treatment quickly terminates the attack
- The intervals between acute attacks vary (up to years), but the asymptomatic periods often become shorter if the disease progresses

Prevention

- Potentially reversible causes of hyperuricemia
  — High-purine diet
  — Obesity
  — Frequent alcohol consumption
  — Use of certain medications (diuretics, niacin, low-dose aspirin)
- Colchicine, 0.6 mg once or twice daily orally
  — Can be used to prevent future attacks
  — Frequently prescribed to prevent attacks when probenecid, sulfinpyrazone, allopurinol, or febuxostat is being initiated
  — May be continued through an acute flare if patient already takes it in prophylactic doses
- Uricosuric drugs, xanthine oxidase inhibitors, and uricase can lower uric acid levels in patients with frequent episodes of arthritis, tophaceous deposits, or renal damage
  — Allopurinol
    ○ 300 mg/d orally is initial daily dose for patients with normal kidney function who are taking prophylactic colchicine
    ○ 100 mg/d orally is initial dose for patients not taking prophylactic colchicine
    ○ Maximum daily dose is 800 mg
    ○ Can be used in chronic kidney disease, but the dose must be reduced to decrease the chance of side effects
  — Probenecid
    ○ 0.5 g orally daily initially, with gradual increase to 1 to 2 g daily
    ○ Ineffective in patients with an estimated glomerular filtration rate (eGFR) of < 60 mL/min
  — Sulfinpyrazone
    ○ 50 to 100 mg orally twice daily initially, with gradual increase to 200 to 400 mg twice daily
    ○ Ineffective in patients with an eGFR of < 60 mL/min
  — Febuxostat
    ○ 40 mg/d orally is initial dose
    ○ Dose can be increased to 80 mg per day (maximum) if target serum uric acid is not reached within 2 weeks
    ○ Does not cause the hypersensitivity reactions seen with allopurinol
    ○ Can be given without dose adjustment to patients with mild-to-moderate renal disease
    ○ May increase liver function tests in 2% to 3% of patients
  — Pegloticase (recombinant uricase)
    ○ Must be administered intravenously (8 mg every 2 weeks)
    ○ Indicated for the rare patient with chronic tophaceous gout who is refractory to all other therapies
    ○ Converts uric acid to (readily excreted) allantoin
    ○ Carries a "Black Box Warning," which advises administering the drug only in health care settings and by health care professionals prepared to manage anaphylactic and other serious infusion reactions

9. When to Refer and When to Admit

When to Refer

• Refer to a rheumatologist if the patient has recurrent attacks despite treatment

When to Admit

• For suspected or proven superimposed septic arthritis

SUGGESTED REFERENCES

Becker MA et al. Long-term safety of pegloticase in chronic gout refractory to conventional treatment. *Ann Rheum Dis*. 2013 Sep 1;72(9):1469–1474. [PMID: 23144450]

Khanna D et al. 2012 American College of Rheumatology guidelines for management of gout. Part 1: systemic nonpharmacologic and pharmacologic therapeutic approaches to hyperuricemia. *Arthritis Care Res (Hoboken)*. 2012 Oct;64(10):1431–1446. [PMID: 23024028]

Khanna D et al. 2012 American College of Rheumatology guidelines for management of gout. Part 2: therapy and antiinflammatory prophylaxis of acute gouty arthritis. *Arthritis Care Res (Hoboken)*. 2012 Oct;64(10):1447–1461. [PMID: 23024029]

Neogi T. Clinical practice. Gout. *N Engl J Med*. 2011 Feb 3;364(5):443–452. [PMID: 21288096]

van Echteld I et al. Colchicine for acute gout. *Cochrane Database Syst Rev*. 2014 Aug 15;8:CD006190. [PMID: 25123076]

44

Knee Pain

A 41-year-old man presents to urgent care clinic complaining of right medial knee pain. He states that his pain began after he twisted his knee playing soccer 1 month ago. At the time, he had a significant amount of swelling and difficulty in bearing weight, both of which slowly resolved after 1 week of ice and rest. He did not seek medical attention at that time. Since then, he has had both pain and a frequent "locking" and "catching" of the joint when walking. On physical examination, he has tenderness to palpation at the medial joint line and a positive McMurray test. Magnetic resonance imaging (MRI) shows a tear of the medial meniscus.

LEARNING OBJECTIVES

▶ Learn the clinical manifestations and objective findings of the different causes for knee pain
▶ Understand the historical factors that suggest the etiology of knee pain
▶ Know the differential diagnosis of knee pain
▶ Learn the treatments for knee pain
▶ Learn which patients should see an orthopedist or rheumatologist

QUESTIONS

1. What are the salient features of this patient's problem?
2. How do you think through his problem?
3. What are the key features, including essentials of diagnosis and general considerations, of knee pain?
4. What are the symptoms and signs of knee pain?
5. What is the differential diagnosis of knee pain?
6. What are laboratory, imaging, and procedural findings in knee pain?
7. What are the treatments for knee pain?
8. What is the outcome, including prevention, of knee pain?
9. When should patients with knee pain be referred to a specialist or admitted to the hospital?

ANSWERS

1. Salient Features

Medial knee pain; trauma with twisting; immediate effusion; "locking" and "catching" sensation; positive McMurray test; MRI with meniscal tear

2. How to Think Through

When evaluating any acute arthritis, it is wise to begin with a mental checklist of systemic illnesses that manifest as acute arthritis. Otherwise, acute joint pain can be erroneously attributed to a traumatic mechanism as an explanation. If knee joint swelling and pain developed without clear-cut trauma, what study will likely provide the most important data? (Arthrocentesis.) Provided that this patient denies fevers or constitutional symptoms, and that the history supports trauma as the mechanism, the clinician's tasks are to identify the injured structure, weigh the utility of imaging, and assess the need for early intervention. Key historical data elicited in this case include the mechanism of injury, ability to bear weight following the injury, degree of swelling and pain, presence of "locking" and "catching." The exact location of the pain (best obtained by asking the patient to point with one finger) should also be assessed.

The tempo of swelling onset is not described here. When swelling develops rapidly after injury, hemarthrosis should be considered, possibly from an acute ligamentous tear. The symptoms of "catching" and "locking" described in this case strongly suggest what pathology? (A meniscal tear.) What knee joint structures should be evaluated on the physical examination? (anterior cruciate ligament [ACL], posterior cruciate ligament [PCL], medial collateral ligament [MCL], lateral collateral ligament [LCL], meniscus.) How is the meniscus assessed? (Two commonly performed tests load and stress the meniscus: McMurray test: flex/extend the knee with the patient supine while holding the ankle to internally/externally rotate the tibia; and Thessaly test: the patient twists left and right while standing on one leg with the knee bent 20 degrees.) What imaging modality is preferred if meniscus injury is suspected? (MRI.) What treatments are recommended? Symptomatic treatment aimed at the underlying cause may include anti-inflammatory medications, physical therapy (PT), bracing, ligamentous or meniscal repair.

3. Key Features

Essentials of Diagnosis

- Examination of range of motion, effusions, meniscus, and ligaments
- Evaluation of aspirated joint fluid if indicated

General Considerations

- The knee is stabilized by ligaments, limiting varus (LCL) and valgus (MCL) stresses as well as limiting anterior movement (ACL) and posterior movement (PCL)
- Bursa act to decrease friction of tendons and muscles
- The meniscal cartilage functions as a shock absorber during weight bearing
- Injuries may be caused from trauma, inflammation, infection, or degenerative changes
- Effusions can occur with intra-articular pathology such as osteoarthritis (OA) and meniscus or cruciate ligament tears
- Acute knee swelling (due to hemarthrosis) within 2 hours may indicate ligament injuries or patellar dislocation or fracture
- Runners may develop a variety of painful overuse syndromes of the knee, particularly those who overtrain or are not properly conditioned
  - Most of these conditions are forms of tendinitis or bursitis that can be diagnosed on examination
  - The most common conditions include
  - Anserine bursitis
  - Iliotibial band syndrome (ITBS)
  - Popliteal and patellar tendinitis
- Poor patellar tracking in the trochlear groove may also cause pain

4. Symptoms and Signs

- Location of knee symptoms is very helpful to diagnosis (Table 44-1)
- Evaluation should begin with general questions about duration and rapidity of symptom onset and the mechanism of injury or aggravating symptoms
- Overuse or degenerative problems can occur with stress or compression from sports, hobbies, or occupation
- A history of trauma as well as history of orthopedic problems requiring surgery should also be elicited
- Symptoms of infection (fever, recent bacterial infections, risk factors for sexually transmitted infections [such as *Neisseria gonorrhea*] or other bacterial infections [such as *Staphylococcus aureus*]) should always be evaluated
- Common symptomatic complaints
  - Presence of grinding, clicking, or popping with bending may be indicative of osteoarthritis or the patellofemoral syndrome
  - "Locking" or "catching" when walking suggests an internal derangement such as meniscal injury or a loose body in the knee
  - Intra-articular swelling of the knee or an effusion indicates an internal derangement or a synovial pathology. Large swelling may cause a popliteal (Baker) cyst. Acute swelling within minutes to hours suggests a hemarthrosis, most likely due to an anterior cruciate ligament injury, fracture or patellar dislocation, especially if trauma is involved
  - Lateral "snapping" with flexion and extension of the knee may indicate inflammation of the iliotibial band
  - Pain that is worsened with bending and walking downstairs suggests issues with the patellofemoral joint, such as chondromalacia of the patella or osteoarthritis
  - Pain that occurs when rising after prolonged sitting suggests a problem with tracking of the patella
- Swelling in the hollow or dimple around the patella and distention of the suprapatellar space may indicate knee joint effusion

Table 44-1. Location of common causes of knee pain.

Medial Knee Pain
Medial compartment osteoarthritis
Medial collateral ligament strain
Medial meniscal injury
Anserine bursitis (pain over the proximal medial tibial plateau)
Anterior Knee Pain
Patellofemoral syndrome (often bilateral)
Osteoarthritis
Prepatellar bursitis (associated with swelling anterior to the patella)
"Jumper's knee" (pain at the inferior pole of the patella)
Septic arthritis
Gout or other inflammatory disorder
Lateral Knee Pain
Lateral meniscal injury
Iliotibial band syndrome (pain superficially along the distal iliotibial band near lateral femoral condyle or lateral tibial insertion)
Lateral collateral ligament sprain
Posterior Knee Pain
Popliteal (Baker) cyst
Osteoarthritis
Meniscal tears
Hamstring or calf tendinopathy

- Specialized physical examination tests can help identify pathology (see Table 44-2)
  — Range of motion testing (Figure 44-2A)
  — Lachman test, anterior drawer test, and pivot shift test for ACL tear (Figures 44-2B, 44-2C, 44-2D)

Table 44-2. Knee examination, including specialized test maneuvers.

Maneuver	Description
Inspection	Examine for the alignment of the lower extremities (varus, valgus, knee recurvatum), ankle eversion and foot pronation, gait, SEADS
Palpation	Include important landmarks: patellofemoral joint, medial and lateral joint lines (especially posterior aspects), pes anserine bursa, distal iliotibial band and Gerdy tubercle (iliotibial band insertion)
A. Range of Motion Testing	Check range of motion actively (patient performs) and passively (clinician performs), especially with flexion and extension of the knee normally 0–10 degrees of extension and 120–150 degrees of flexion
Knee Strength Testing	Test resisted knee extension and knee flexion strength manually
Ligament Stress Tests	
B. Lachman test	Performed with the patient lying supine, and the knee flexed to 20–30 degrees. The examiner grasps the distal femur from the lateral side, and the proximal tibia with the other hand on the medial side. With the knee in neutral position, stabilize the femur, and pull the tibia anteriorly using a similar force to lifting a 10–15 pound weight. Excessive anterior translation of the tibia compared with the other side indicates injury to the anterior cruciate ligament
C. Anterior drawer	Performed with the patient lying supine and the knee flexed to 90 degrees. The clinician stabilizes the patient's foot by sitting on it and grasps the proximal tibia with both hands around the calf and pull anteriorly. A positive test finds anterior cruciate ligament laxity compared with the unaffected side
D. Pivot shift	Used to determine the amount of rotational laxity of the knee. The patient is examined while lying supine with the knee in full extension. It is then slowly flexed while applying internal rotation and a valgus stress. The clinician feels for a subluxation at 20–40 degrees of knee flexion. The patient must remain very relaxed to have a positive test

(continued)

Table 44-2. Knee examination, including specialized test maneuvers. (continued)

Maneuver	Description
E. Valgus stress Fix ankle	Performed with the patient supine. The clinician should stand on the outside of the patient's knee. With one hand, the clinician should hold the ankle while the other hand is supporting the leg at the level of the knee joint. A valgus stress is applied at the ankle to determine pain and laxity of the medial collateral ligament. The test should be performed at both 30 and 0 degrees of knee extension
F. Varus stress	The patient is again placed supine. For the right knee, the clinician should be standing on the right side of the patient. The left hand of the examiner should be holding the ankle while the right hand is supporting the lateral thigh. A varus stress is applied at the ankle to determine pain and laxity of the lateral collateral ligament. The test should be performed at both 30 and 0 degrees of knee flexion
The sag sign	The patient is placed supine and both hips and knees are flexed up to 90 degrees. Because of gravity, the posterior cruciate ligament-injured knee will have an obvious setoff at the anterior tibia, which is "sagging" posteriorly

(continued)

Table 44-2. Knee examination, including specialized test maneuvers. (continued)

Maneuver	Description
Posterior drawer	The patient is placed supine with the knee flexed at 90 degrees (see Anterior drawer figure above). In a normal knee, the anterior tibia should be positioned about 10 mm anterior to the femoral condyle. The clinician can grasp the proximal tibia with both hands and push the tibia posteriorly. The movement, indicating laxity and possible tear of the posterior cruciate ligament, is compared with the uninjured knee
Meniscal Signs	
McMurray test	Performed with the patient lying supine. The clinician flexes the knee until the patient reports pain. For this test to be valid, it must be flexed pain free beyond 90 degrees. The clinician externally rotates the patient's foot and then extends the knee while palpating the medial knee for "click" in the medial compartment of the knee or pain reproducing pain from a meniscus injury. To test the lateral meniscus, the same maneuver is repeated while rotating the foot internally (53% sensitivity and 59%–97% specificity)
G. Modified McMurray 	Performed with the hip flexed to 90 degrees. The knee is then flexed maximally with internally or externally rotation of the lower leg. The knee can then be rotated with the lower leg in internal or external rotation to capture the torn meniscus underneath the condyles. A positive test is pain over the joint line while the knee is being flexed and internally or externally rotated
H. Thessaly test 	Performed with the patient standing on one leg with knee slightly flexed. The patient is asked to twist the knee while standing on one leg. Pain can be elicited during twisting motion
Patellofemoral Joint Test	
Apprehension sign	Suggests instability of the patellofemoral joint and is positive when the patient becomes apprehensive when the knee is deviated laterally

SEADS, swelling; erythema, ecchymosis; atrophy, asymmetry; deformity; skin changes, scars, bruising.

— Valgus and varus stress tests for collateral ligament tears (Figures 44-2E, 44-2F)
— Posterior drawer test and "sag sign" for PCL tear
— McMurray test, modified McMurray test (Figure 44-2G), and Thessaly test (Figure 44-2H) for meniscal tear
— Apprehension sign for patellofemoral joint instability

5. Differential Diagnosis

• Meniscal injury
• Ligamentous tear or sprain
• OA
• Patellar dysfunction or misalignment
• Fracture of the patella or tibia
• Inflammatory arthritis
• Septic arthritis
• Ruptured popliteal (Baker) cyst
• Prepatellar or anserine bursitis

6. Laboratory, Imaging, and Procedural Findings

Laboratory Tests

• Complete blood count, uric acid level, and anticyclic citrullinated protein antibody testing may help identify infection, gout, or rheumatoid arthritis (RA) as the cause of an inflammatory arthritis
• Laboratory testing of aspirated joint fluid when indicated, can lead to a definitive diagnosis in most patients, eg, an acute hemarthrosis represents bloody swelling that usually occurs within the first 1 to 2 hours following trauma (see Tables 44-3 and 44-4)

Imaging Studies

• Plain weight-bearing radiographs may show degenerative changes or fractures
• MRI helps evaluate soft tissues, meniscus, and ligaments
• CT and ultrasound are sometimes useful

Diagnostic Procedures

• Physical examination includes palpating the relevant sites around the knee and special tests as noted above
• Arthrocentesis of joint fluid for laboratory diagnostic testing of effusions
• Note that overuse syndromes are not associated with joint effusions or synovitis

Table 44-3. Examination of joint fluid.

Measure	Normal	Group I (Noninflammatory)	Group II (Inflammatory)	Group III (Purulent)
Volume (mL) (knee)	< 3.5	Often > 3.5	Often > 3.5	Often > 3.5
Clarity	Transparent	Transparent	Translucent to opaque	Opaque
Color	Clear	Yellow	Yellow to opalescent	Yellow to green
WBC (per μL)	< 200	200–300	2000–75, 000[a]	> 100, 000[b]
Polymorphonuclear leukocytes	< 25%	< 25%	≥50%	≥75%
Culture	Negative	Negative	Negative	Usually positive[b]

WBC, white blood cell count.

[a]Gout, rheumatoid arthritis, and other inflammatory conditions occasionally have synovial fluid WBC counts > 75, 000/μL but rarely > 100, 000/μL.

[b]Most purulent effusions are due to septic arthritis. Septic arthritis, however, can present with group II synovial fluid, particularly if infection is caused by organisms of low virulence (eg, *Neisseria gonorrhoeae*) or if antibiotic therapy has been started.

Table 44-4. Differential diagnosis by joint fluid groups.

Group I (Noninflammatory) (< 2000 White Cells/µL)	Group II (Inflammatory) (2000–75, 000 White Cells/µL)	Group III (Purulent) (> 100, 000 White Cells/µL)	Hemorrhagic
Degenerative joint disease	Rheumatoid arthritis	Pyogenic bacterial infections	Hemophilia or other hemorrhagic diathesis
Trauma[a]	Acute crystal-induced synovitis (gout and pseudogout)		
Osteochondritis dissecans			Trauma with or without fracture
Osteochondromatosis	Reactive arthritis		Neuropathic arthropathy
Neuropathic arthropathy[a]	Ankylosing spondylitis		Pigmented villonodular synovitis
Subsiding or early inflammation	Rheumatic fever[b]		Synovioma
Hypertrophic osteoarthropathy[b]	Tuberculosis		Hemangioma and other benign neoplasms
Pigmented villonodular synovitis[a]			

[a]May be hemorrhagic.

[b]Noninflammatory or inflammatory group.

Reproduced, with permission, from Rodnan GP, ed. *Primer on the Rheumatic Diseases*, 7th ed. *JAMA*. 1973; 224(Suppl):662.

7. Treatments

Physical Therapy, Medications, and Surgery

- See treatment of specific disorders
  — Patellofemoral Pain
    ○ Conservative symptomatic management with ice, anti-inflammatory medications
    ○ Physical therapy (PT) targeted toward strengthening the posterolateral hip muscles which control rotation at the knee; brace or taping
    ○ Surgery is a last resort—lateral release or patellar realignment surgery
  — Meniscus Injury
    ○ In older patients with degenerative tears, treated conservatively with analgesics, PT
    ○ In younger patients with acute tears, arthroscopic meniscus debridement or repair
  — Posterior Cruciate Ligament (PCL) Injury
    ○ Unless there are associated neurovascular or other injuries (in up to one-third of cases), usually treated nonoperatively with knee brace locked in extension, crutches, gradual increase in range of motion
  — Collateral Ligament Injury
    ○ MCL injury, tears rarely require surgery—grades 1 to 2 tears: PT, weight bearing as tolerated; grade 2 tear: hinged knee brace; grade 3 tear: long leg brace, weight bearing only with brace locked in extension
    ○ LCL injury, tears—almost always require surgery, reconstruction
  — Anterior Cruciate Ligament (ACL) Injury
    ○ Arthroscopic surgical reconstruction using patellar or hamstring tendon (autograft) or cadaver graft (allograft)
    ○ In nonsurgical candidates, PT, ACL brace
  — Knee OA or RA
    ○ Acetaminophen; topical NSAIDs can be effective in the treatment of osteoarthritis and avoid many of the traditional NSAID complications in older patients
    ○ Viscosupplementation (hyaluronic acid) trial results are mixed, with possible small benefit and increased risk of serious adverse events

○ Platelet rich plasma injections contain high concentration of platelet-derived growth factors, which regulate some biological processes in tissue repair. The majority of trials showing improvement in pain have a high risk of bias.
○ Knee replacement surgery in patients with significant disability

Therapeutic Procedures
• In overuse syndromes, rest and abstention from causative physical activities for days to weeks are essential, with subsequent gentle stretching to prevent recurrence
• Joint aspiration (arthrocentesis) is often both diagnostic and therapeutic

8. Outcome

Prevention
• Stretching exercises to prevent OSs

9. When to Refer and When to Admit

When to Refer
• All patients with ACL tears
• Any ligamentous tear with joint instability
• Most meniscus injuries
• Severe OA or RA with disability that may benefit from knee replacement surgery
• Patients with persistent pain despite treatment

When to Admit
• Any patient with presumed septic arthritis

SUGGESTED REFERENCES

Altman RD. New guidelines for topical NSAIDs in the osteoarthritis treatment paradigm. *Curr Med Res Opin.* 2010 Dec;26(12):2871–2876. [PMID: 21070097]

Barrett AM et al. Anterior cruciate ligament graft failure: a comparison of graft type based on age and Tegner activity level. *Am J Sports Med.* 2011 Oct;39(10):2194–2198. [PMID: 21784999]

Collado H et al. Patellofemoral pain syndrome. *Clin Sports Med.* 2010 Jul;29(3):379–398. [PMID: 20610028]

Cram P et al. Total knee arthroplasty volume, utilization, and outcomes among Medicare beneficiaries, 1991–2010. *JAMA.* 2012 Sep 26;308(12):1227–1236. [PMID: 23011713]

Delincé P et al. Anterior cruciate ligament tears: conservative or surgical treatment? A critical review of the literature. *Knee Surg Sports Traumatol Arthrosc.* 2012 Jan;20(1):48–61. [PMID: 21773828]

Frobell RB et al. Treatment for acute anterior cruciate ligament tear: five year outcome of randomised trial. *BMJ.* 2013 Jan 24;346:f232. [PMID: 23349407]

Hammoud S et al. Outcomes of posterior cruciate ligament treatment: a review of the evidence. *Sports Med Arthrosc.* 2010 Dec;18(4):280–291. [PMID: 21079509]

Khayambashi K et al. Posterolateral hip muscle strengthening versus quadriceps strengthening for patellofemoral pain: a comparative control trial. *Arch Phys Med Rehabil.* 2014 May;95(5):900–907. [PMID: 24440362]

Laudy AB et al. Efficacy of platelet-rich plasma injections in osteoarthritis of the knee: a systematic review and meta-analysis. *Br J Sports Med.* 2014 Nov 21. [Epub ahead of print] [PMID: 25416198]

McDermott I. Meniscal tears, repairs and replacement: their relevance to osteoarthritis of the knee. *Br J Sports Med.* 2011 Apr;45(4):292–297. [PMID: 21297172]

Messier SP et al. Effects of intensive diet and exercise on knee joint loads, inflammation, and clinical outcomes among overweight and obese adults with knee osteoarthritis: the IDEA randomized clinical trial. *JAMA.* 2013 Sep 25;310(12):1263–1273. [PMID: 24065013]

Pacheco RJ et al. Posterolateral corner injuries of the knee: a serious injury commonly missed. *J Bone Joint Surg Br.* 2011 Feb;93(2):194–197. [PMID: 21282758]

Peeler J et al. Accuracy and reliability of anterior cruciate ligament clinical examination in a multidisciplinary sports medicine setting. *Clin J Sport Med.* 2010 Mar;20(2):80–85. [PMID: 20215888]

Sihvonen R et al; Finnish Degenerative Meniscal Lesion Study (FIDELITY) Group. Arthroscopic partial meniscectomy versus sham surgery for a degenerative meniscal tear. *N Engl J Med.* 2013 Dec 26;369(26):2515–2524. [PMID: 24369076]

van der Weegen W et al. No difference between intra-articular injection of hyaluronic acid and placebo for mild to moderate knee osteoarthritis: a randomized, controlled, double-blind trial. *J Arthroplasty.* 2014 Dec 13. [Epub ahead of print] [PMID: 25548079]

Rheumatoid Arthritis

45

A 47-year-old woman presents to the clinic with a 4-week history of fatigue, bilateral hand pain and stiffness, and hand and wrist joint swelling. About a month before presentation, she noticed that her hands were stiffer in the morning, but thought that it was due to too much typing. However, the stiffness has worsened, and she now needs about an hour each morning to "loosen up" her hands. As the day goes on, the stiffness improves, although it does not go away entirely. She has also noticed that her knuckles and wrists are swollen and feel somewhat warm. Physical examination reveals warm, erythematous wrists and metacarpal joints bilaterally. Hand x-ray films show periarticular demineralization and erosions, and blood test results are significant for mild anemia, elevated sedimentation rate, and positive rheumatoid factor (RF) and antibodies to cyclic citrullinated peptides (anti-CCP).

LEARNING OBJECTIVES

▶ Learn the clinical manifestations and objective findings of rheumatoid arthritis (RA)
▶ Know the differential diagnosis of RA
▶ Understand how to diagnose RA
▶ Know the extra-articular manifestations of RA
▶ Learn the treatment for RA
▶ Understand the long-term consequences of RA

QUESTIONS

1. What are the salient features of this patient's problem?
2. How do you think through her problem?
3. What are the key features, including essentials of diagnosis, general considerations, and demographics, of RA?
4. What are the symptoms and signs of RA?
5. What is the differential diagnosis of RA?
6. What are laboratory, imaging, and procedural findings in RA?

7. What treatments are available for RA?

8. What are the outcomes, including follow-up, complications, and prognosis, of RA?

9. When should patients with RA be referred to a specialist and when admitted to the hospital?

ANSWERS

1. Salient Features

Polyarticular joint pain and swelling; stiffness worse in the morning and lasting over 30 minutes; wrist and metacarpophalangeal (MCP) joint involvement; bilaterality of joint involvement; extra-articular features (fatigue and anemia); x-ray showing periarticular demineralization and erosions; elevated erythrocyte sedimentation rate (ESR) and RF; and anti-CCP antibodies

2. How to Think Through

Is this arthralgia (joint pain) or arthritis (joint inflammation)? What four things indicate joint inflammation? (Rubor [redness], dolor [pain], calor [warmth], and tumor [swelling].) How many joints are involved? (Mono- vs oligo- vs polyarthritis.) What is the pattern of joint involvement? (Small vs large vs both.) Which joints are involved? (Distal interphalangeal [DIP] vs proximal interphalangeal [PIP] vs MCP.) Is there morning stiffness for at least 30 minutes and prominent afternoon fatigue? Are there features of lupus (sicca symptoms, oral ulcers, malar rash, photosensitivity, chest pain, or Raynaud phenomenon)? Are there symptoms of psoriasis or inflammatory bowel disease? An ESR, while nonspecific, is useful marker of inflammation in subtle cases. A positive RF and characteristic erosions on hand films strengthen the case for RA, and positive anti-CCP antibodies are highly specific for the diagnosis. Would arthrocentesis help? If so, what might the synovial fluid show in this patient? (See Tables 45-1, 45-2, and 45-3.)

3. Key Features

Essentials of Diagnosis

- Usually insidious onset with morning stiffness and pain in affected joints
- Symmetric polyarthritis with predilection for small joints of the hands and feet; deformities common with progressive disease
- Radiographic findings
  — Juxta-articular osteoporosis
  — Joint erosions
  — Joint space narrowing
- RF and anti-CCP are present in 70% to 80%

Table 45-1. Diagnostic value of the joint pattern.

Characteristic	Status	Representative Disease
Inflammation	Present	Rheumatoid arthritis, systemic lupus erythematosus, gout
	Absent	Osteoarthritis
Number of involved joints	Monoarticular	Gout, trauma, septic arthritis, Lyme disease, osteoarthritis
	Oligoarticular (2–4 joints)	Reactive arthritis, psoriatic arthritis, inflammatory bowel disease
	Polyarticular (≥ 5 joints)	Rheumatoid arthritis, systemic lupus erythematosus
Site of joint involvement	Distal interphalangeal	Osteoarthritis, psoriatic arthritis (not rheumatoid arthritis)
	Metacarpophalangeal, wrists	Rheumatoid arthritis, systemic lupus erythematosus, calcium pyrophosphate deposition disease (not osteoarthritis)
	First metatarsal phalangeal	Gout, osteoarthritis

Table 45-2. Examination of joint fluid.

Measure	Normal	Group I (Noninflammatory)	Group II (Inflammatory)	Group III (Purulent)
Volume (mL) (knee)	< 3.5	Often > 3.5	Often > 3.5	Often > 3.5
Clarity	Transparent	Transparent	Translucent to opaque	Opaque
Color	Clear	Yellow	Yellow to opalescent	Yellow to green
WBC (per μL)	< 200	< 2000	2000–75, 000[a]	> 100, 000[b]
Polymorphonuclear leukocytes	< 25%	< 25%	≥ 50%	≥ 75%
Culture	Negative	Negative	Negative	Usually positive[b]

WBC, white blood cell count.

[a]Gout, rheumatoid arthritis, and other inflammatory conditions occasionally have synovial fluid WBC counts > 75, 000/μL but rarely > 100, 000/μL.

[b]Most purulent effusions are due to septic arthritis. Septic arthritis, however, can present with group II synovial fluid, particularly if infection is caused by organisms of low virulence (eg, *Neisseria gonorrhoeae*) or if antibiotic therapy has been started.

- Extra-articular manifestations
  — Subcutaneous nodules
  — Interstitial lung disease
  — Pleural effusion
  — Pericarditis
  — Splenomegaly with leukopenia
  — Vasculitis

General Considerations
- A chronic systemic inflammatory disease of unknown cause; major manifestation is synovitis of multiple joints
- The pathological findings in the joint include chronic synovitis with pannus formation
- The pannus erodes cartilage, bone, ligaments, and tendons

Demographics
- Female patients outnumber males almost 3:1
- Can begin at any age but peak onset is in fourth or fifth decade for women and sixth to eighth decades for men

Table 45-3. Differential diagnosis by joint fluid groups.

Group I (Noninflammatory) (< 2000 White Cells/μL)	Group II (Inflammatory) (2000–75, 000 White Cells/μL)	Group III (Purulent) (> 100, 000 White Cells/μL)	Hemorrhagic
Degenerative joint disease Trauma[a] Osteochondritis dissecans Osteochondromatosis Neuropathic arthropathy[a] Subsiding or early inflammation Hypertrophic osteoarthropathy[b] Pigmented villonodular synovitis[a]	Rheumatoid arthritis Acute crystal-induced synovitis (gout and pseudogout) Reactive arthritis Ankylosing spondylitis Rheumatic fever[b] Tuberculosis	Pyogenic bacterial infections	Hemophilia or other hemorrhagic diathesis Trauma with or without fracture Neuropathic arthropathy Pigmented villonodular synovitis Synovioma Hemangioma and other benign neoplasms

[a]May be hemorrhagic.

[b]Noninflammatory or inflammatory group.

Reproduced, with permission, from Rodnan GP, ed. *Primer on the Rheumatic Diseases*, 7th ed. *JAMA*. 1973; 224(suppl):662.

4. Symptoms and Signs

- Joint symptoms
  - Onset of articular signs of inflammation is usually insidious, with prodromal symptoms of vague periarticular pain or stiffness
  - Symmetric swelling of multiple joints with tenderness and pain is characteristic
  - Monoarticular disease is occasionally seen initially
  - Stiffness persisting for > 30 minutes (and usually many hours) is prominent in the morning
  - Stiffness may recur after daytime inactivity and be much more severe after strenuous activity
  - PIP joints of the fingers, MCP joints, wrists, knees, ankles, and MTP joints are most often involved
  - Synovial cysts and rupture of tendons may occur
  - Entrapment syndromes (eg, of the median nerve in the carpal tunnel of the wrist)
  - Neck can be affected but the other portions of the spine are usually spared and sacroiliac joints are not involved
  - In advanced disease, atlantoaxial (C1–C2) subluxation can lead to myelopathy
- Rheumatoid nodules
  - Present in about 20% of patients
  - Most commonly situated over bony prominences but also observed in the bursae and tendon sheaths
  - Occasionally seen in the lungs, the sclerae, and other tissues
  - Correlate with the presence of RF in serum ("seropositivity"), as do most other extra-articular manifestations
- Ocular symptoms
  - Dryness of the eyes, mouth, and other mucous membranes is found especially in advanced disease (see Sjögren syndrome)
  - Other manifestations include episcleritis, scleritis, and scleromalacia due to scleral nodules
- Other symptoms
  - Palmar erythema is common
  - Occasionally, a small vessel vasculitis develops and manifests as tiny hemorrhagic infarcts in the nail folds or finger pulps
  - Necrotizing arteritis is well reported but rare
  - Interstitial lung disease is not uncommon
  - Pericarditis and pleural disease, when present, are usually silent clinically

5. Differential Diagnosis

- Gout with tophi (mistaken for rheumatoid nodules)
- Systemic lupus erythematosus
- Parvovirus B19 infection
- Osteoarthritis or inflammatory osteoarthritis
- Polymyalgia rheumatica
- Hemochromatosis (MCP and wrist joints)
- Lyme disease
- Rheumatic fever
- Rubella arthritis
- Hepatitis B or C
- Palindromic rheumatism
- Hypertrophic pulmonary osteoarthropathy (paraneoplastic)
- Systemic vasculitis, especially
  - Polyarteritis nodosa
  - Mixed cryoglobulinemia
  - Antineutrophil cytoplasmic antibody-associated vasculitides

6. Laboratory, Imaging, and Procedural Findings

Laboratory Tests

- Anti-CCP antibodies and RF are present in 70% to 80% of patients with established RA
- RF has a sensitivity of only 50% in early disease
- Anti-CCP antibodies are the most specific blood test (specificity ~95%)
- Approximately 20% of patients have antinuclear antibodies
- ESR and levels of C-reactive protein are typically elevated in proportion to disease activity
- A moderate hypochromic normocytic anemia is common
- The white blood cell (WBC) count is normal or slightly elevated, but leukopenia may occur, often in the presence of splenomegaly (ie, Felty syndrome)
- The platelet count is often elevated, roughly in proportion to the severity of overall joint inflammation
- Joint fluid examination is valuable, reflecting abnormalities that are associated with varying degrees of inflammation (see Tables 45-1, 45-2, and 45-3)

Imaging Studies

- Radiographic changes are the most specific for RA
- However, radiographs are not sensitive in that most of those taken during the first 6 months are read as normal
- The earliest changes occur in the hands or feet and consist of soft tissue swelling and juxta-articular demineralization
- Later, diagnostic changes of uniform joint space narrowing and erosions develop

Diagnostic Procedures

- Arthrocentesis is needed to diagnose superimposed septic arthritis, which is a common complication of RA and should be considered whenever one joint is inflamed out of proportion to the rest

7. Treatments

Medications

- Nonsteroidal anti-inflammatory drugs (NSAIDs)
  - Provide some symptomatic relief but do not prevent erosions or alter disease progression
  - Not appropriate for monotherapy and should only be used in conjunction with disease-modifying antirheumatic drugs (DMARDs)
- Cyclooxygenase (COX)-2 inhibitor, celecoxib
  - Just as effective as NSAIDs
  - However, less likely to cause clinically significant upper gastrointestinal hemorrhage or ulceration
  - Long-term use, particularly without concomitant aspirin use, increases the risk of cardiovascular events
- DMARDs should be started as soon as the diagnosis is certain
- Methotrexate
  - Initial synthetic DMARD of choice
  - Is generally well tolerated and often produces a beneficial effect in 2 to 6 weeks
- Tumor necrosis factor (TNF) inhibitors work faster than methotrexate and may replace that drug as the remitting agent of first choice
  - Etanercept
    - A soluble recombinant TNF receptor: fragment crystallizable (Fc) fusion protein
    - Dosage: 50 mg subcutaneously once per week
  - Infliximab
    - A chimeric monoclonal antibody
    - Dosage: 3 to 10 mg/kg intravenously; infusions are repeated after 2, 6, 10, and 14 weeks and then are administered every 8 weeks

- Adalimumab
  - A human monoclonal antibody that binds to TNF
  - Dosage: 40 mg subcutaneously every other week
- Golimumab
  - A human anti-TNF monoclonal antibody
  - Dosage: 50 mg subcutaneously once monthly
- Certolizumab pegol
  - A PEGylated monoclonal antibody TNF inhibitor
  - Dosage: 200 to 400 mg subcutaneously every 2 to 4 weeks
- Cost is a consideration for TNF inhibitors (more than $10,000 per year)
- Hydroxychloroquine is useful for patients with mild disease
- Corticosteroids
  - Low doses (eg, oral prednisone 5–10 mg/d) produce a prompt anti-inflammatory effect and slow the rate of articular erosion
  - Intra-articular corticosteroids may be helpful if one or two joints are the chief source of difficulty
  - Intra-articular triamcinolone, 10–40 mg depending on the size of the joint to be injected, may be given for symptomatic relief but not more than four times a year
- Sulfasalazine
  - Second-line agent
  - Dosage: start at 0.5 g orally twice daily and then increase each week by 0.5 g until the patient improves or the daily dose reaches 3 g
- Leflunomide
  - A pyrimidine synthesis inhibitor
  - Dosage: start at 10 to 20 mg daily orally
  - Severe and fatal hepatotoxicity has been reported
  - Contraindicated in pregnancy
- Abatacept
  - A recombinant protein made by fusing a fragment of the Fc domain of human immunoglobulin G with the extracellular domain of a T-cell inhibitory receptor (CTLA4)
  - For moderate to severe RA
  - Dosing depends on body weight
  - For a 60 to 100 kg individual, dosage is 750 mg intravenously at weeks 0, 2, and 4, then every 4 weeks
- Rituximab
  - Can be effective for moderate to severe RA refractory to the combination of methotrexate and a TNF inhibitor
  - Dosage: 1000 mg intravenously every 2 weeks for two doses (after premedication with corticosteroids)
  - Fatal infusion reactions have been reported
- Tocilizumab
  - A monoclonal antibody that blocks the receptor for IL-6, an inflammatory cytokine involved in the pathogenesis of RA
  - For moderate-to-severe RA in combination with methotrexate or other nonbiologic DMARD for patients whose disease has been refractory to treatment with a TNF inhibitor
  - Increases the risk of opportunistic and other serious infections (patients should be screened and treated for latent tuberculosis prior to receiving the tocilizumab)
  - Tofacitinib
  - For use in severe rheumatoid arthritis that is refractory to methotrexate
  - Dosage: 5 mg orally twice daily
  - Can be used either as monotherapy or in combination with methotrexate or other nonbiologic DMARD

— Increases the risk of opportunistic and other serious infections (patients should be screened and treated for latent tuberculosis prior to receiving tofacitinib)
- DMARDs generally have greater efficacy in combination (the most common current combination is that of methotrexate with one of the TNF inhibitors)

Surgery
- Cases of advanced destruction from long-standing, severe, and erosive disease of hip, knee, shoulder, and MCP joints may benefit from joint replacement

Therapeutic Procedures
- Nonpharmacologic
  — Physical therapy
  — Occupational therapy
  — Joint rest
  — Exercise
  — Splinting
  — Heat and cold
  — Assist devices
  — Splints
- Intra-articular corticosteroids (triamcinolone, 10–40 mg) may be helpful if one or two joints are the primary source of difficulty

8. Outcomes

Follow-Up
- Frequent follow-up early after diagnosis to ensure appropriate patient education and response to treatment
- Patients taking DMARDs require monitoring of blood cell counts and hepatic and renal function every 6–8 weeks

Complications
- Joint destruction
- Joint deformities
  — Ulnar deviation of the fingers
  — Boutonnière deformity (hyperextension of the DIP joint with flexion of the PIP joint)
  — "Swan-neck" deformity (flexion of the DIP joint with extension of the PIP joint)
  — Valgus deformity of the knee
  — Volar subluxation of the MTP joints
- Septic arthritis
- Rheumatoid vasculitis (eg, skin ulcers, vasculitic neuropathy, and pericarditis)
- Osteoporosis
- Cushing syndrome from corticosteroids

Prognosis
- Excess mortality is largely due to cardiovascular disease

9. When to Refer and When to Admit

When to Refer
- Early referral to a rheumatologist is essential for appropriate diagnosis and the timely introduction of effective therapy

When to Admit
- At diagnosis sometimes to exclude other entities
- Superimposed septic arthritis
- Rheumatoid vasculitis
- Severe ocular inflammatory disease (eg, impending corneal melt)

SUGGESTED REFERENCES

Aletaha D et al. 2010 Rheumatoid arthritis classification criteria: an American College of Rheumatology/ European League Against Rheumatism collaborative initiative. *Arthritis Rheum.* 2010 Sep;62(9): 2569–2581. [PMID: 20872595]

Lee EB et al. ORAL Start Investigators. Tofacitinib versus methotrexate in rheumatoid arthritis. *N Engl J Med.* 2014 Jun 19;370(25):2377–2386. [PMID: 24941177]

O'Dell JR et al. CSP 551 RACAT Investigators. Therapies for active rheumatoid arthritis after methotrexate failure. *N Engl J Med.* 2013 Jul 25;369(4):307–318. [PMID: 23755969]

O'Dell JR et al. TEAR Trial Investigators. Validation of the methotrexate-first strategy in patients with early, poor-prognosis rheumatoid arthritis: results from a two-year randomized, double-blind trial. *Arthritis Rheum.* 2013 Aug;65(8):1985–1994. [PMID: 23686414]

Smolen JS et al. Adjustment of therapy in rheumatoid arthritis on the basis of achievement of stable low disease activity with adalimumab plus methotrexate or methotrexate alone: the randomized controlled OPTIMA trial. *Lancet.* 2014 Jan 25;383(9914):321–332. [PMID: 24168956]

Systemic Lupus Erythematosus

46

A 22-year-old African American woman reports intermittent joint pain in her right knee and the joints of the fingers of her right hand, especially the proximal interphalangeal joints, as well as a rash on her cheeks and nose that appears after sun exposure. On review of systems, she reports chest pain with deep breaths. On physical examination, she has painless oral ulcers on her palate, a pleural friction rub, and a facial rash sparing the nasolabial folds. The urine dipstick reveals 3+ protein, and laboratory testing reveals a white blood cell count of 3400/μL, a platelet count of 89,000/μL, positive rapid plasma reagin test, a positive antinuclear antibody (ANA) test with a titer of 1:320, and a positive anti-Smith (anti-Sm) antibody test.

LEARNING OBJECTIVES

► Learn the clinical manifestations and objective findings of systemic lupus erythematosus (SLE)

► Know the diagnostic criteria for SLE

► Understand the laboratory tests involved in the diagnosis of SLE

► Know the differential diagnosis of SLE

► Learn the treatment options for SLE

QUESTIONS

1. What are the salient features of this patient's problem?

2. How do you think through her problem?

3. What are the key features, including essentials of diagnosis, general considerations, and demographics, of SLE?

4. What are the symptoms and signs of SLE?

5. What is the differential diagnosis of SLE?

6. What are laboratory and procedural findings in SLE?

7. What are the treatments for SLE?

8. What are the outcomes, including complications and prognosis, of SLE?

9. When should patients with SLE be referred to a specialist and admitted to the hospital?

ANSWERS

1. Salient Features

Young African American woman; symmetric, intermittent arthritis involving the fingers and knee; malar rash that spares the nasolabial folds; photosensitivity; symptoms and signs of pleuritis (chest pain, friction rub); oral ulcers; renal involvement (proteinuria); leukopenia and thrombocytopenia; false-positive syphilis test; positive ANA with high titer; positive anti-Sm test

2. How to Think Through

Which populations are most affected by lupus? What is the typical timing and pattern of progression in lupus? What features of lupus are found on history? (Recall the common symptoms by building a mental image of the affected areas of the body—cognition, conjunctivitis/vision change, hair loss, sicca symptoms, oral ulcers, malar rash, photosensitivity, pleuritis, pericarditis, GI symptoms, joint pain, and Raynaud phenomenon.) How might you assess involvement of the kidneys? (Urinalysis, renal biopsy.) What are the important serologies for lupus? (ANA is 99% positive but is nonspecific; anti-Sm and anti-double-stranded DNA have low sensitivity but high specificity.) How is the complete blood count useful? Will complement levels be elevated or decreased?

What features of lupus and rheumatoid arthritis (RA) overlap? (Arthritis, pleural inflammation, and leukopenia.) How can you differentiate them? (The arthritis in RA more often affects the small joints of the hands and feet, is symmetrical, shows evidence of inflammation on examination (rubor [redness], dolor [pain], calor [warmth], tumor [swelling]), and shows erosions on radiographs.)

3. Key Features

Essentials of Diagnosis

- Multiple system involvement
- Occurs mainly in young women, more common in young and African American women
- Rash over areas exposed to sunlight
- Joint symptoms in 90% of patients
- Anemia, leukopenia, and thrombocytopenia
- ANA with high titer to double-stranded DNA

General Considerations

- SLE is an inflammatory autoimmune disorder that affects multiple organ systems
- The clinical course is marked by spontaneous remission and relapses
- Drug-induced lupus must be considered and is distinguished from SLE in four ways
  - The sex ratio is nearly equal
  - It typically presents with fever, arthralgia, myalgia, and serositis but not nephritis and central nervous system (CNS) features
  - Hypocomplementemia and antibodies to double-stranded DNA are absent
  - The clinical features and most laboratory abnormalities usually revert toward normal when the offending drug is withdrawn

Demographics

- Among patients affected by SLE, females greatly outnumber males: 85% are women
- SLE occurs in 1:1000 white women but in 1:250 black women

4. Symptoms and Signs

- Fever, anorexia, malaise, and weight loss
- **Skin** lesions
  - Occur in most patients at some time
  - The characteristic "butterfly" rash affects < 50%
  - Alopecia is common

- **Raynaud** phenomenon (20% of patients) often antedates other symptoms
- **Joint** symptoms, with or without active synovitis
  — Occur in > 90% and are often the earliest manifestation
  — The arthritis can lead to reversible swan neck deformities
- **Ocular**
  — Conjunctivitis
  — Photophobia
  — Blurring of vision
  — Transient or permanent monocular blindness
- **Pulmonary**
  — Pleurisy
  — Pleural effusion
  — Bronchopneumonia
  — Pneumonitis
  — Restrictive lung disease
- **Cardiac**
  — Pericarditis
  — Myocarditis
  — Arrhythmias
  — The typical verrucous endocarditis of Libman–Sacks is usually clinically silent but can produce acute or chronic valvular regurgitation—most commonly mitral regurgitation
- **Mesenteric vasculitis**
  — Occasionally occurs and may resemble polyarteritis nodosa, including the presence of aneurysms in medium-sized blood vessels
  — Abdominal pain (particularly postprandial), ileus, peritonitis, and perforation may result
- **Neurologic**
  — Psychosis
  — Cognitive impairment
  — Seizures
  — Peripheral and cranial neuropathies
  — Transverse myelitis
  — Strokes
  — Severe depression and psychosis may be exacerbated by the administration of large doses of corticosteroids
- **Glomerulonephritis (GN):** several forms may occur, including mesangial, focal and diffuse proliferative, and membranous

5. Differential Diagnosis

- Drug-induced lupus (Table 46-1) (especially procainamide, hydralazine, and isoniazid)
- Scleroderma
- RA
- Inflammatory myopathy, especially dermatomyositis
- Rosacea
- Vasculitis, eg, polyarteritis nodosa
- Endocarditis
- Lyme disease

6. Laboratory and Procedural Findings

Laboratory Tests
- Production of many different autoantibodies (Tables 46-2 and 46-3)
- ANA tests are sensitive for systemic lupus but are not specific—ie, they are positive in low titer in up to 20% of healthy adults and also in many patients with nonlupus conditions such as RA, autoimmune thyroid disease, scleroderma, and Sjögren syndrome

Table 46-1. Drugs associated with lupus erythematosus.

Definite Association	Minocycline
Chlorpromazine	Procainamide
Hydralazine	Quinidine
Isoniazid	
Methyldopa	
Possible Association	Nitrofurantoin
β-Blockers	Penicillamine
Captopril	Phenytoin
Carbamazepine	Propylthiouracil
Cimetidine	Sulfasalazine
Ethosuximide	Sulfonamides
Levodopa	Trimethadione
Lithium	
Methimazole	
Unlikely Association	Penicillin
Allopurinol	Reserpine
Chlorthalidone	Streptomycin
Gold salts	Tetracyclines
Griseofulvin	
Methysergide	
Oral contraceptives	

Modified and reproduced, with permission, from Hess EV et al. Drug-related lupus. *Bull Rheum Dis*. 1991;40(4):1–8.

- Antibodies to double-stranded DNA and to Sm are specific for SLE but not sensitive, since they are present in only 60% and 30% of patients, respectively
- Depressed serum complement—a finding suggestive of disease activity—often returns toward normal in remission
- Three types of antiphospholipid antibodies occur (Table 46-2)
  — The first causes the biologic false-positive tests for syphilis
  — The second is lupus anticoagulant, a risk factor for venous and arterial thrombosis and miscarriage
  — The third is anticardiolipin antibody

Table 46-2. Frequency (%) of laboratory abnormalities in systemic lupus erythematosus.

Anemia	60%
Leukopenia	45%
Thrombocytopenia	30%
Biologic false-positive tests for syphilis	25%
Antiphospholipid antibodies	
Lupus anticoagulant	7%
Anticardiolipin antibody	25%
Direct Coombs-positive	30%
Proteinuria	30%
Hematuria	30%
Hypocomplementemia	60%
ANA	95%–100%
Anti-native DNA	50%
Anti-Sm	20%

ANA, antinuclear antibody; anti-Sm, anti-Smith antibody.

Modified and reproduced, with permission, from Hochberg MC et al. Systemic lupus erythematosus: a review of clinicolaboratory features and immunologic matches in 150 patients with emphasis on demographic subsets. *Medicine (Baltimore)*. 1985;64(5):285–295.

Table 46-3. Criteria for the classification of SLE. (A patient is classified as having SLE if any ≥ 4 of 11 criteria are met.)

1. Malar rash
2. Discoid rash
3. Photosensitivity
4. Oral ulcers
5. Arthritis
6. Serositis
7. Kidney disease
   a. > 5 g/d proteinuria, or
   b. ≥ 3$^+$ dipstick proteinuria, or
   c. Cellular casts
8. Neurologic disease
   a. Seizures, or
   b. Psychosis (without other cause)
9. Hematologic disorders
   a. Hemolytic anemia, or
   b. Leukopenia (< 4000/μL), or
   c. Lymphopenia (< 1500/μL), or
   d. Thrombocytopenia (< 100 000/μL)
10. Immunologic abnormalities
   a. Positive LE cell preparation, or
   b. Antibody to native DNA, or
   c. Antibody to Sm, or
   d. False-positive serologic test for syphilis
11. Positive ANA

ANA, antinuclear antibody; SLE, systemic lupus erythematosus.

Modified and reproduced, with permission, from Tan EM et al. The 1982 revised criteria for the classification of systemic lupus erythematosus. *Arthritis Rheum.* 1982;25(11):1271–1277.

• Abnormality of urinary sediment is almost always found in association with renal lesions. Red blood cells, with or without casts, and mild proteinuria are frequent

Diagnostic Procedures
• The diagnosis of SLE can be made with reasonable probability if 4 of the 11 criteria set forth in Table 46-3 are met. These criteria should be viewed as rough guidelines that do not supplant clinical judgment in its diagnosis
• Renal biopsy is useful in deciding whether to treat with cyclophosphamide, and to rule out SLE-related end-stage renal disease that may no longer benefit from treatment

7. Treatments

Medications
• Skin lesions often respond to the local administration of corticosteroids
• Minor joint symptoms can usually be alleviated by rest and nonsteroidal anti-inflammatory drugs
• Antimalarials (hydroxychloroquine)
  — May be helpful in treating lupus rashes or joint symptoms
  — Appear to reduce the incidence of severe disease flares
  — Dose of hydroxychloroquine is 200 or 400 mg/d orally and should not exceed 6.5 mg/kg/d
  — Annual monitoring for retinal changes is recommended
• Corticosteroids are required for the control of certain serious complications, such as
  — Thrombotic thrombocytopenic purpura
  — Hemolytic anemia
  — Myocarditis
  — Pericarditis
  — GN
  — Alveolar hemorrhage
  — CNS involvement

- Immunosuppressive agents such as cyclophosphamide, chlorambucil, and azathioprine are used in cases resistant to corticosteroids
  — Cyclophosphamide improves renal survival
  — Overall patient survival, however, is no better than in the prednisone-treated group
- Systemic corticosteroids are not usually given for minor arthritis, skin rash, leukopenia, or the anemia associated with chronic disease
- Belimumab
  — Monoclonal antibody that inhibits the activity of a B-cell growth factor
  — For treatment of antibody-positive SLE patients with active disease who have not responded to standard therapies (eg, NSAIDs, antimalarials, or immunosuppressive therapies)
  — However, precise indications for its use have not been defined
  — Its efficacy in severe disease activity is unknown
  — Appears less effective in blacks

Therapeutic Procedures

- Avoid sun exposure and use sunscreen

8. Outcomes

Complications

- Thrombocytopenic purpura
- Hemolytic anemia
- Myocarditis
- Pericarditis
- GN
- Alveolar hemorrhage
- CNS involvement

Prognosis

- Ten-year survival rate exceeds 85%
- In most patients, the illness pursues a relapsing and remitting course
- In some patients, the disease pursues a virulent course, leading to serious impairment of vital structures such as lung, heart, brain, or kidneys, and even death
- Accelerated atherosclerosis attributed, in part, to corticosteroid use, has been responsible for a rise in late deaths due to myocardial infarction

9. When to Refer and When to Admit

When to Refer

- Most patients should be monitored in consultation with a rheumatologist
- Severity of organ involvement dictates referral to other subspecialties, such as a nephrologist and pulmonologist

When to Admit

- Rapidly progressive glomerulonephritis, pulmonary hemorrhage, transverse myelitis, and other severe organ-threatening manifestations of lupus usually require inpatient assessment and management
- Severe infections, particularly in the setting of immunosuppressant therapy, should prompt admission

SUGGESTED REFERENCES

Hahn BH. Belimumab for systemic lupus erythematosus. *N Engl J Med.* 2013 Apr 18;368(16):1528–1535 [PMID: 23594005]

Maneiro JR et al. Maintenance therapy of lupus nephritis with mycophenolate or azathioprine: systematic review and meta-analysis. *Rheumatology (Oxford).* 2014 May;53(5):834–838. [PMID: 24369416]

Murphy G et al. Systemic lupus erythematosus and other autoimmune rheumatic diseases: challenges to treatment. *Lancet.* 2013 Aug 31;382(9894):809–818. [PMID: 23972423]

Skaggs BJ et al. Accelerated atherosclerosis in patients with SLE—mechanisms and management. Nat Rev *Rheumatol.* 2012 Feb 14;8(4):214–223. [PMID: 22331061]

Tsokos GC. Systemic lupus erythematosus. *N Engl J Med.* 2011 Dec 1;365(22):2110–2121. [PMID: 22129255]

Walsh M et al. Mycophenolate mofetil or intravenous cyclophosphamide for lupus nephritis with poor kidney function: a subgroup analysis of the Aspreva Lupus Management Study. *Am J Kidney Dis.* 2013 May;61(5):710–715. [PMID: 23375819]

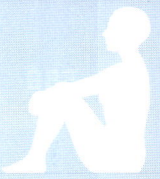

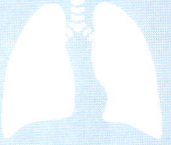

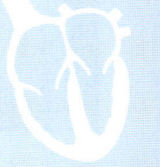

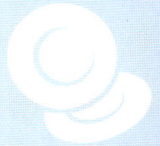

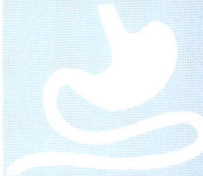

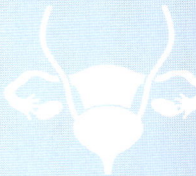

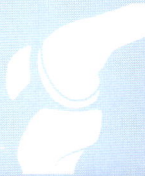

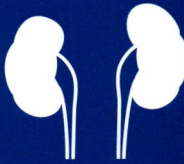

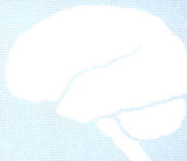

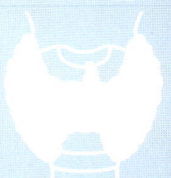

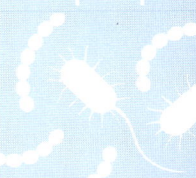

47

Glomerulonephritis

A 61-year-old woman presents to the emergency room with 3 days of shortness of breath and lower extremity swelling. Previously healthy, she had no history of heart disease. Two weeks ago, she had been treated in hospital for pneumonia and group A streptococcus bacteremia, from which she recovered. On physical examination now, her blood pressure is 170/100 mm Hg, she has crackles in both lower lung fields, a normal cardiac examination, and 2+ pitting edema in both lower extremities. Her urinalysis shows proteinuria and hematuria. Microscopic examination reveals many dysmorphic red blood cells with some red blood cell casts. An echocardiogram shows normal systolic function.

LEARNING OBJECTIVES

▶ Learn the clinical manifestations and objective findings of glomerulonephritis (GN)
▶ Understand the diseases that are associated with development of GN
▶ Know the different causes of GN and how they differ in presentation and diagnostic testing
▶ Learn the various treatments for GN, which depend on its cause

QUESTIONS

1. What are the salient features of this patient's problem?
2. How do you think through her problem?
3. What are the key features, including essentials of diagnosis and general considerations, of GN?
4. What are the symptoms and signs of GN?
5. What is the differential diagnosis of GN?
6. What are laboratory, imaging, and procedural findings in GN?
7. What are the treatments for GN?
8. What are the outcomes, including prognosis, follow-up and complications, of GN?
9. When should patients with GN be referred to a specialist or admitted to the hospital?

ANSWERS

1. Salient Features

Lower extremity edema and volume overload; hypertension; mild proteinuria, hematuria, and RBC casts; normal cardiac function; recent streptococcal infection suggesting possible postinfectious GN

2. How to Think Through

When a patient presents with new edema, it is important to consider causes other than heart failure. Fortunately, the clinician here obtained a urinalysis, which is an easy, affordable screening test for both hematuria and proteinuria. Given the abnormal result, microscopic evaluation of urine sediment, preferably by a nephrologist, should follow. What is the most serious cause of a case such as this? (Rapidly progressive glomerulonephritis [RPGN].) One cause of RPGN is poststreptococcal GN (suggested by this case). What laboratory studies help define the cause of RPGN? (Serum complement levels, antiglomerular basement membrane [anti-GBM] antibody, antinuclear antibody [ANA] titer, antineutrophil cytoplasmic antibodies [ANCA], cryoglobulins, hepatitis B virus surface antigen, hepatitis C virus [HCV] antibody.)

Complement levels help narrow the differential diagnosis of RPGN. Postinfectious GN, lupus nephritis, and cryoglobulinemia all consume complement by forming immune complexes. By contrast, normal complement levels are found in ANCA-associated ("pauci-immune"), anti-GBM (Goodpasture syndrome), and immunoglobulin A (IgA) nephropathy.

Renal biopsy is not always performed in patients with evidence of recent streptococcal infection. but can be helpful in poststreptococcal GN in demonstrating characteristic light microscopy, immunofluorescence, and electron microscopy findings. And, in this severe case, it could be considered if it would change treatment. Cases of RPGN can be treated with corticosteroids, other immunosuppressive medications, or, in the case of mixed cryoglobulinemia, plasmapheresis.

3. Key Features

Essentials of Diagnosis

- Acute kidney injury, dependent edema, and hypertension
- Hematuria, dysmorphic red cells, red cell casts, and mild proteinuria

General Considerations

- A relatively uncommon cause of acute kidney injury, ~5% of cases of hospitalized intrinsic renal failure
- Acute glomerulonephritis usually signifies an inflammatory process causing renal dysfunction over days to weeks that may or may not resolve
- Table 47-1 shows the classification, modes of presentations, associations, and serologic findings of glomerulonephritis
- See also Figure 47-1 for a display of the serologic findings of glomerulonephritis
- Inflammatory glomerular lesions include mesangioproliferative, focal and diffuse proliferative, and crescentic lesions
- Rapidly progressive acute glomerulonephritis can cause permanent damage to glomeruli if not identified and treated rapidly
- Postinfectious glomerulonephritis commonly appears after pharyngitis or impetigo with onset 1 to 3 weeks after infection (average 7–10 days)
  — Bacterial causes of postinfectious glomerulonephritis
    ⚬ Bacteremic states (especially with *Staphylococcus aureus)*
    ⚬ Bacterial pneumonias
    ⚬ Deep-seated abscesses

Table 47-1. Classification and findings in glomerulonephritis: Nephritic spectrum presentations.

	Typical Presentation	Association/Notes	Serology
Postinfectious glomerulonephritis	Children: abrupt onset of nephritic syndrome and acute kidney injury but can present anywhere in nephritic spectrum	Streptococci, other bacterial infections (eg, staphylococci, endocarditis, shunt infections)	Rising ASO titers, low complement levels
IgA nephropathy (Berger disease) and Henoch–Schönlein purpura, systemic IgA vasculitis	Classically: gross hematuria with upper respiratory tract infection; can present anywhere in nephritic spectrum; Henoch–Schönlein purpura with vasculitic rash and gastrointestinal hemorrhage	Abnormal IgA glycosylation in both primary (familial predisposition) and secondary disease (associated with cirrhosis, HIV, celiac disease) Henoch–Schönlein purpura in children after an inciting infection	No serologic tests helpful; complement levels are normal
Pauci-immune (granulomatosis with polyangiitis, Churg–Strauss, polyarteritis, idiopathic crescentic glomerulonephritis)	Classically as crescentic or RPGN, but can present anywhere in nephritic spectrum; may have respiratory tract/sinus symptoms in granulomatosis with polyangiitis	See Figure 47-1	ANCAs: MPO or PR3 titers high; complement levels normal
Antiglomerular basement membrane glomerulonephritis; Goodpasture syndrome	Classically as crescentic or RPGN, but can present anywhere in nephritic spectrum; with pulmonary hemorrhage in Goodpasture syndrome	May develop as a result of respiratory irritant exposure (chemicals or tobacco use)	Anti-GBM antibody titers high; complement levels normal
Cryoglobulin-associated glomerulonephritis	Often acute nephritic syndrome; often with systemic vasculitis including rash and arthritis	Most commonly associated with chronic hepatitis C; may occur with other chronic infections or some connective tissue diseases	Cryoglobulins positive; rheumatoid factor may be elevated; complement levels low
Idiopathic MPGN	Classically presents with acute nephritic syndrome, but can see nephrotic syndrome features in addition	Most patients are < 30 y old. Type I most common. Type II (dense deposit disease) associated with C3 nephritic factor	Low complement levels
Hepatitis C infection	Anywhere in nephritic spectrum	Can cause MPGN pattern of injury or cryoglobulinemic glomerulonephritis; membranous nephropathy pattern of injury uncommon	Low complement levels; positive hepatitis C serology; rheumatoid factor may be elevated
Systemic lupus erythematosus	Anywhere in nephritic spectrum, depending on pattern/severity of injury	Treatment depends on clinical course and International Society of Nephrology and Renal Pathology Society (ISN/RPS) classification on biopsy	High ANA and anti-double-stranded DNA titers; low complement levels

ANA, antinuclear antibody; ANCAs, antineutrophil cytoplasmic antibodies; ASO, antistreptolysin O; GBM, glomerular basement membrane; MPGN, membranoproliferative glomerulonephritis; MPO, myeloperoxidase; RPGN, rapidly progressive glomerulonephritis.

- ∘ Gram-negative infections
- ∘ Infective endocarditis
- ∘ Shunt infections
- — Viral, fungal, and parasitic causes of postinfectious glomerulonephritis
  - ∘ Hepatitis B or C
  - ∘ Human immunodeficiency virus (HIV)
  - ∘ Cytomegalovirus infection
  - ∘ Infectious mononucleosis
  - ∘ Coccidioidomycosis
  - ∘ Malaria
  - ∘ Mycobacteria
  - ∘ Syphilis
  - ∘ Toxoplasmosis
- Pauci-immune necrotizing glomerulonephritis is caused by granulomatosis with polyangiitis, microscopic polyangiitis, or Churg–Strauss syndrome
- Antineutrophil cytoplasmic antibody-associated glomerulonephritis can also present as a primary renal lesion without systemic involvement

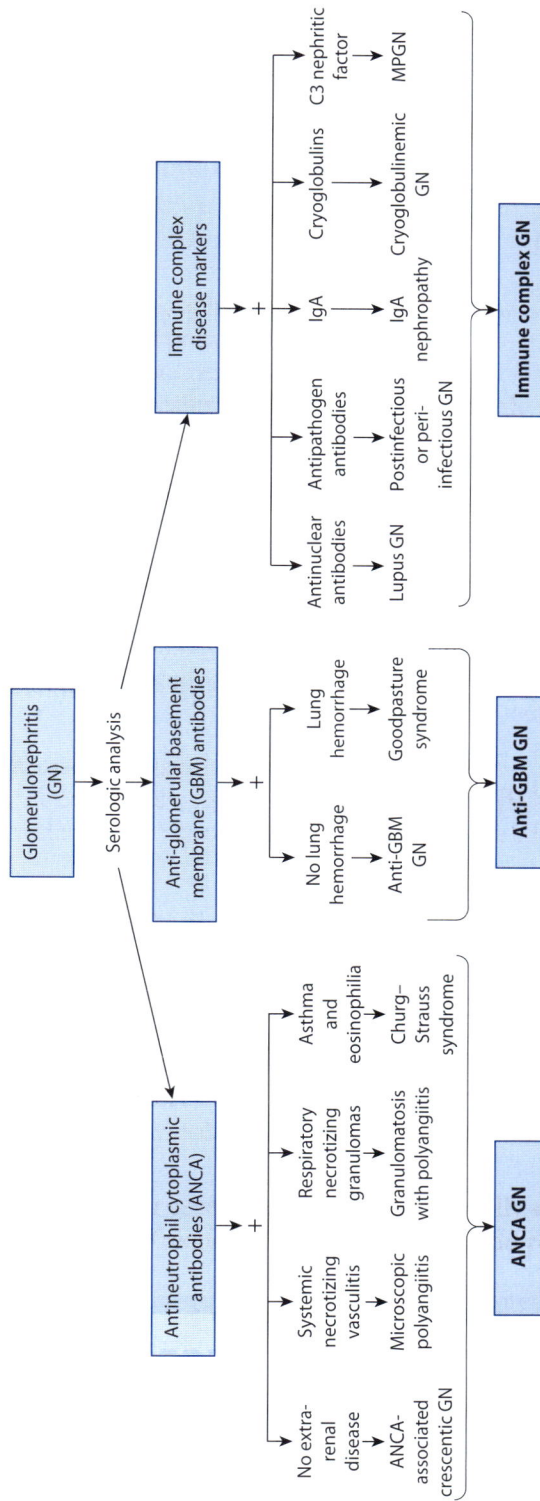

Figure 47-1. Serologic analysis of patients with glomerulonephritis. ANCA, antineutrophil cytoplasmic antibodies; GBM, glomerular basement membrane; MPGN, membranoproliferative glomerulonephritis. (Modified, with permission, from Greenberg A et al. Primer on Kidney Diseases. Academic Press; 1994; and Jennette JC, Falk RJ. Diagnosis and management of glomerulonephritis and vasculitis presenting as acute renal failure. *Med Clin North Am.* 1990;74(4):893–908. © Elsevier.).

- Membranoproliferative glomerulonephritis (MPGN) is an idiopathic renal disease that usually presents with nephritic features ranging from asymptomatic glomerular hematuria and proteinuria, to episodes of gross hematuria, to the acute nephritic syndrome
- MPGN patients are usually age < 30 years; MPGN may also present with the acute nephritic syndrome
- Essential (mixed) cryoglobulinemia is a disorder associated with cold-precipitable immunoglobulins (cryoglobulins); glomerular disease occurs from the precipitation of cryoglobulins in glomerular capillaries
  — Causes of cryoglobulinemia include hepatitis C infection (usual), hepatitis B or other occult viral, bacterial, fungal infections, and some connective tissue diseases

4. Symptoms and Signs

- Hypertension
- Edema, first in body parts with low tissue tension such as periorbital and scrotal regions
- Dark urine
- Hematuria
- Proteinuria
- Oliguria
- Cryoglobulinemia may have purpuric or necrotizing skin lesions, arthralgias, hepatosplenomegaly
- Pauci-immune cases may have fever, malaise, weight loss, hematuria, purpura, or mononeuritis multiplex
- In granulomatosis with polyangiitis (formerly Wegener granulomatosis), 90% have upper or lower respiratory tract lesions that bleed (presenting with hemoptysis)
- MPGN patients may have hypocomplementemia and, in about 50%, a recent history of upper respiratory tract infection

5. Differential Diagnosis

Causes of Glomerulonephritis

- IgA nephropathy (Berger disease)
- Peri-infectious or postinfectious GN
- Endocarditis
- Lupus nephritis
- Cryoglobulinemic GN (often associated with hepatitis C viral infection)
- MPGN
- Pauci-immune (ANCA-associated) GN
- Acute interstitial nephritis
- Acute tubular necrosis

6. Laboratory, Imaging, and Procedural Findings

Laboratory Tests

- Urinalysis
  — Dipstick: hematuria, moderate proteinuria (usually < 3 g/d)
  — Microscopic: abnormal urinary sediment with cellular elements such as RBCs, RBC casts, and white cells
- Obtain a 24-hour urine for protein excretion and creatinine clearance
- Serum creatinine can rise over days to months, depending on the rapidity of the underlying process
- BUN: creatinine ratio is not a reliable marker of renal function and is more reflective of the underlying volume status of the patient
- Urine creatinine clearance is an unreliable marker of glomerular filtration rate in cases of rapidly changing serum creatinine values

- Fractional excretion of sodium is usually low (< 1%), unless the renal tubulointerstitial space is affected and renal dysfunction is marked
- Serum complement levels (C3, C4, CH50), which are
  — Low in immune complex glomerulonephritis aside from IgA nephropathy
  — Normal in pauci-immune and antiglomerular basement membrane-related glomerulonephritis
- Other tests
  — Antistreptolysin O (ASO) titer, anti-GBM antibody level, ANA titer
  — Cryoglobulins
  — Hepatitis B surface antigen and HCV antibody
  — C3 nephritic factor
  — ANCA
- Postinfectious glomerulonephritis may have high ASO titer and low serum complement levels
- In pauci-immune disease, a cytoplasmic pattern of ANCA is specific for antiproteinase 3 antibodies, whereas a perinuclear pattern is specific for antimyeloperoxidase antibodies
- Most patients with granulomatosis with polyangiitis are C-ANCA positive; the remainder can have a P-ANCA pattern or rarely do not demonstrate ANCA serologically
- Microscopic angiitis has either a P-ANCA or C-ANCA pattern about 80% of the time
- In cryoglobulinemia, serum complement levels are low and rheumatoid factor often elevated
- There are 2 types of MPGN
  — In Type I, the classic complement pathway is activated, leading to low or normal serum C3 with low C4 levels
  — In Type II, the alternative complement pathway is activated and serum C3 level is low while C4 is normal; C3 nephritic factor, a circulating IgG antibody, is found in the serum

Imaging Studies
- Renal ultrasound

Diagnostic Procedures
- Renal biopsy: Type of glomerulonephritis can be categorized according to the light microscopy immunofluorescence pattern and electron microscopy appearance
- Postinfectious renal biopsy
  — Light microscopy shows diffuse proliferative glomerulonephritis
  — Immunofluorescence shows IgG and C3 in a granular pattern in the mesangium and along the capillary basement membrane
  — Electron microscopy shows large, dense subepithelial deposits or "humps"
- RPGN renal biopsy: necrotizing lesions and crescents
- MPGN renal biopsy
  — Type I
    ◦ Light microscopy shows glomerular basement membrane thickened by immune complex deposition, abnormal mesangial cell proliferation, and "splitting" or "tram-track" appearance to the capillary wall
    ◦ Electron microscopy shows subendothelial deposits
    ◦ Immunofluorescence shows IgG, IgM, and granular deposits of C3, C1q, and C4
  — Type II
    ◦ Light microscopy findings similar to type I
    ◦ However, electron microscopy shows ribbon-like deposit of homogeneous material replacing part of the glomerular basement membrane
    ◦ Pauci-immune GN renal biopsy: small vessels and glomeruli lack immune deposits on immunofluorescence

7. Treatments

Medications
- Specific therapy is aimed at the underlying cause
- Supportive measures include antihypertensive medications, salt restriction, diuretics, and antibiotics as indicated for infections
- Corticosteroids in high doses and cytotoxic agents such as cyclophosphamide may be required, depending on the nature and severity of disease

Therapeutic Procedures
- In pauci-immune disease, institute treatment early; prognosis depends mainly on extent of renal involvement before treatment is started
- Treatment of pauci-immune disease is high-dose corticosteroids (methylprednisolone, 1–2 g/d intravenously for 3 days, followed by prednisone, 1 mg/kg orally for 1 month, with a slow taper over the next 6 month) and cytotoxic agents (cyclophosphamide, 0.5–1.0 g/m² intravenously per month or 1.5–2 mg/kg orally for 3–6 months is followed by long-term azathioprine or mycophenolate mofetil)
  — Monitor ANCA levels to help determine efficacy of treatment
  — Patients receiving cyclophosphamide should receive prophylaxis for *Pneumocystis jiroveci,* such as double-strength trimethoprim-sulfamethoxazole orally 3 d/wk
- Treatment for MPGN is controversial, but there may be some role for corticosteroids, cyclophosphamide, cyclosporine, and mycophenolate mofetil
  — Children with nephrotic syndrome give prednisone 40 mg/m² every other day for a prolonged duration
  — Adults: less likely to respond
- Antiplatelet drugs are used in MPGN: aspirin, 500 to 975 mg/d orally, plus dipyridamole, 225 mg/d orally; efficacy of this regimen is not well proven
- Renal transplantation is an option in MPGN, but both types may recur thereafter in the transplanted kidney
- Plasma exchange has been used with mixed results to treat posttransplant recurrence of MPGN
- Cryoglobulinemia is treated by aggressive treatment of the underlying infection, including α-interferon for hepatitis C-related cryoglobulinemia in some patients, as well as pulse corticosteroids, plasma exchange, and cytotoxic agents
- Table 47-2 shows suitable actions for different stages of chronic kidney disease.

8. Outcomes

Prognosis
- In MPGN, in the past, 50% of patients progressed to end-stage renal disease in 10 years; fewer do so now with introduction of more aggressive therapy
  — Prognosis less favorable with type II disease, early renal insufficiency, hypertension, and persistent nephrotic syndrome

Follow-Up
- With nephrologist, as dictated by specific disease

Complications
- Chronic kidney disease

9. When to Refer and When to Admit

When to Refer
- Any evidence of possible glomerulonephritis

When to Admit
- Any acute or rapidly progressive symptoms (days to weeks) may be cause for admission depending on the disease

Table 47-2. Stages of chronic kidney disease: a clinical action plan.[a,b]

Stage[c]	Description	GFR (mL/min/1.73 m²)	Action
1	Kidney damage with normal or ↑↑ GFR	≥ 90	Diagnosis and treatment of underlying etiology if possible. Treatment of comorbid conditions. Estimate progression, work to slow progression. Cardiovascular disease risk reduction.
2	Kidney damage with mildly ↓ GFR	60–89	
3a	Mild-moderately ↓ GFR	45–59	As above, and evaluating and treating complications.
3b	Moderate-severely ↓ GFR	30–44	
4	Severely ↓ GFR	15–29	Preparation for ESRD
5	End-stage renal disease (ESRD)	< 15 (or dialysis)	Dialysis, transplant, or palliative care

[a]Based on National Kidney Foundation, KDOQI, and KDIGO Chronic Kidney Disease Guidelines.

[b]Chronic kidney disease is defined as either kidney damage or GFR < 60 mL/min/1.73 m² for ≥ 3 months. Kidney damage is defined as pathologic abnormalities or markers of damage, including abnormalities in blood or urine tests or imaging studies.

[c]At all stages, persistent albuminuria confers added risk for CKD progression and cardiovascular disease in the following gradations: < 30 mg/d = lowest added risk, 30–300 mg/d = mildly increased risk, > 300–1000 mg/d moderately increased risk, > 1000 mg/d = severely increased risk.

GFR, glomerular filtration rate.

Modified and reproduced from Kidney Disease: Improving Global Outcomes (KDIGO) CKD Work Group. KDIGO 2012 Clinical Practice Guideline for the Evaluation and Management of Chronic Kidney Disease. *Kidney Int.* 2013 Jan;3(1) (suppl):1–150.

SUGGESTED REFERENCES

Ad-hoc working group of ERBP; Fliser D et al. A European Renal Best Practice (ERBP) position statement on the Kidney Disease Improving Global Outcomes (KDIGO) clinical practice guidelines on acute kidney injury: part 1: definitions, conservative management and contrast-induced nephropathy. *Nephrol Dial Transplant.* 2012 Dec;27(12):4263–4272. [PMID: 23045432]

Hebert LA et al. Differential diagnosis of glomerular disease: a systematic and inclusive approach. *Am J Nephrol.* 2013;38(3):253–266. [PMID: 24052039]

Perazella MA. Diagnosing drug-induced AIN in the hospitalized patient: a challenge for the clinician. *Clin Nephrol.* 2014 Jun;81(6):381–388. [PMID: 24691017]

48

Hypokalemia

A 45-year-old woman presents to the emergency room after 5 days of nausea, vomiting, and diarrhea. She states she has only been able to drink water occasionally, and her vomiting and diarrhea have been profuse. On review of systems, she complains of fatigue and muscle cramps. Her past medical history includes hypertension, for which she takes hydrochlorothiazide (HCTZ). Physical examination reveals symmetric hyporeflexia of the extremities. An electrocardiogram (ECG) reveals broad and flattened T waves with a prominent U waves. Her serum K^+ is measured at 2.5 mEq/L.

LEARNING OBJECTIVES

▶ Learn the clinical manifestations and objective findings of hypokalemia
▶ Know the causes of hypokalemia and how to distinguish between them
▶ Understand the other electrolyte abnormalities that predispose to hypokalemia
▶ Learn the treatment options for mild and severe hypokalemia
▶ Know how to prevent hypokalemia in patients taking diuretic agents

QUESTIONS

1. What are the salient features of this patient's problem?
2. How do you think through her problem?
3. What are the key features, including essentials of diagnosis and general considerations, of hypokalemia?
4. What are the causes of hypokalemia?
5. What are the symptoms and signs of hypokalemia?
6. What are laboratory and procedural findings in hypokalemia?
7. What are the treatments for hypokalemia?
8. What are the outcomes, including follow-up, complications, and prognosis, of hypokalemia?
9. When should patients with hypokalemia be referred to a specialist or admitted to the hospital?

ANSWERS

1. Salient Features

Vomiting and diarrhea causing extrarenal potassium losses; fatigue and muscle cramps; thiazide diuretic use, causing kaliuresis; hyporeflexia on examination; ECG with flattened T waves and U waves; low serum potassium level

2. How to Think Through

The patient's symptom of fatigue can be attributed to her poor oral intake in the setting of acute illness. What factors in her history and physical examination prompt you to consider an electrolytes abnormality? (Protracted vomiting in combination with diarrhea, muscle cramps, and hyporeflexia.) Is the underlying cause of her hypokalemia intrarenal or extrarenal? (Both, but mainly extrarenal.) What diagnostic test can help differentiate between an intrarenal and extrarenal cause of the potassium loss? (Measurement of urine K^+ concentration and calculation of the transtubular potassium gradient [TTKG].) What role does the thiazide diuretic likely play here? (The gastrointestinal [GI]) losses are likely the primary cause of the potassium loss, with HCTZ limiting her ability to retain sufficient potassium to compensate. Given the combination of losses, measurement of urine K^+ and calculation of the TTKG are not necessary.) How should the patient be managed initially? (Oral repletion of potassium, reserving intravenous [IV] repletion [which can be dangerous] for the patient who does not tolerate oral potassium. Hydration intravenously or orally. Suspension of HCTZ until full recovery.) If her potassium level were to remain low after initial repletion, is there another electrolyte abnormality that should be explored? (Yes. Look for a low serum magnesium.)

3. Key Features

Essentials of Diagnosis
- Serum K^+ is < 3.5 mEq/L (< 3.5 mmol/L)
- Severe hypokalemia may induce dangerous arrhythmias and rhabdomyolysis
- TTKG can distinguish renal from nonrenal loss of potassium

General Considerations
- GI loss due to infectious diarrhea is most common cause
- Potassium shift into the cell is transiently stimulated by insulin and glucose and facilitated by β-adrenergic stimulation
- α-Adrenergic stimulation blocks potassium shift into the cell
- Aldosterone is an important regulator of body potassium, increasing potassium secretion in the distal renal tubule
- Magnesium is an important cofactor for potassium uptake and for maintenance of intracellular potassium levels
- Magnesium depletion should be suspected in persistent hypokalemia refractory to potassium repletion

4. Causes

- Potassium shift into cell
  - Insulin excess, eg, postprandial
  - Alkalosis
  - β-Adrenergic agonists
  - Trauma (via epinephrine release)
  - Hypokalemic periodic paralysis
  - Barium or cesium intoxication
- Renal potassium loss (urine $K^+ > 40$ mEq/L)
  - Increased aldosterone (mineralocorticoid) effects

- ○ Primary hyperaldosteronism
- ○ Secondary hyperaldosteronism (dehydration, heart failure)
- ○ Renovascular or malignant hypertension
- ○ Cushing syndrome
- ○ European licorice (inhibits cortisol)
- ○ Renin-producing tumor
- ○ Congenital abnormality of steroid metabolism (eg, adrenogenital syndrome, 17α-hydroxylase defect)
- — Increased flow of distal nephron
  - ○ Diuretics (furosemide, thiazides)
  - ○ Salt-losing nephropathy
- — Hypomagnesemia
  - ○ Diminished magnesium intake, eg, malabsorption, malnutrition
  - ○ Increased renal loss, eg, aminoglycoside, cetuximab, cisplatin, amphotericin B, pentamidine
- — Renal tubular acidosis (type I or II)
  - ○ Fanconi syndrome
  - ○ Interstitial nephritis
  - ○ Metabolic alkalosis (bicarbonaturia)
- — Genetic disorder of the nephron
  - ○ Bartter syndrome
  - ○ Liddle syndrome
- • Extrarenal potassium loss (urine K^+ < 20 mEq/L)
  - — Vomiting, diarrhea, and laxative abuse
  - — Villous adenoma, Zollinger–Ellison syndrome

5. Symptoms and Signs

- • Muscular weakness, fatigue, and muscle cramps are common in mild-to-moderate hypokalemia
- • Constipation or ileus may result from smooth muscle involvement
- • Flaccid paralysis, hyporeflexia, hypercapnia, tetany, and rhabdomyolysis may be seen in severe hypokalemia (serum K^+ < 2.5 mEq/L)
- • Hypertension may result from aldosterone or mineralocorticoid excess
- • Renal manifestations include nephrogenic diabetes insipidus and interstitial nephritis

6. Laboratory and Procedural Findings

Laboratory Tests

- • Serum K^+ < 3.5 mEq/L (< 3.5 mmol/L)
- • Urinary potassium concentration is low (< 20 mEq/L) as a result of extrarenal loss and inappropriately high (> 40 mEq/L) with renal loss
- • Calculating TTKG is a rapid method to evaluate net potassium secretion

$$- \text{TTKG} = \frac{\text{Urine } K^+/\text{Plasma } K^+}{\text{Urine osm}/\text{Plasma osm}}$$

- • Hypokalemia with a TTKG > 4 suggests renal potassium loss with increased distal K^+ secretion
  - — In such cases, plasma renin and aldosterone levels are helpful in differential diagnosis
  - — The presence of nonabsorbed anions, including bicarbonate, also increases the TTKG

Diagnostic Procedures

- • ECG can show
  - — Decreased amplitude and broadening of T waves
  - — Prominent U waves

— Premature ventricular contractions

— Depressed ST segments

7. Treatments

Medications

- Oral potassium is the safest way to treat mild-to-moderate deficiency
- Dietary potassium is almost entirely coupled to phosphate—rather than chloride—and does not correct potassium loss associated with chloride depletion, such as from diuretics or vomiting
- In the setting of abnormal kidney function and mild to moderate diuretic dosage
  — 20 mEq/d of oral potassium is generally sufficient to prevent hypokalemia
  — However, 40 to 100 mEq/d over a period of days to weeks is needed to treat hypokalemia and fully replete potassium stores
- Indications for IV potassium replacement
  — Severe, life-threatening hypokalemia
  — Inability to take oral supplementation
- For severe deficiency, potassium may be given through a peripheral IV line in a concentration that should not exceed 40 mEq/L at rates of up to 40 mEq/L/h
- Coexisting magnesium and potassium depletion can result in refractory hypokalemia despite potassium repletion if there is no magnesium repletion

8. Outcomes

Follow-Up

- Monitor ECG continuously when infusing IV potassium for severe hypokalemia
- Check serum potassium level every 3 to 6 hours

Complications

- Hypokalemia increases the likelihood of digitalis toxicity
- In patients with heart disease, hypokalemia induced by β_2-adrenergic agonists (eg, for asthma) and diuretics (eg, for hypertension) may impose a substantial risk

Prognosis

- Most hypokalemia will correct with replacement after 24 to 72 hours

9. When to Refer and When to Admit

When to Refer

- Patients with unexplained hypokalemia, refractory hyperkalemia, or clinical features suggesting alternative diagnoses (eg, aldosteronism or hypokalemic periodic paralysis) should be referred for endocrinology or nephrology consultation

When to Admit

- Patients with symptomatic or severe hypokalemia, especially with cardiac manifestations, require cardiac monitoring, frequent laboratory testing, and potassium supplementation

SUGGESTED REFERENCES

Asmar A et al. A physiologic-based approach to the treatment of a patient with hypokalemia. *Am J Kidney Dis*. 2012 Sep;60(3):492–497. [PMID: 22901631]

Marti G et al. Etiology and symptoms of severe hypokalemia in emergency department patients. *Eur J Emerg Med*. 2014 Feb;21(1):46–51. [PMID: 23839104]

Pepin J et al. Advances in diagnosis and management of hypokalemic and hyperkalemic emergencies. *Emerg Med Pract*. 2012 Feb;14(2):1–18. [PMID: 22413702]

Rastegar A. Attending rounds: patient with hypokalemia and metabolic acidosis. *Clin J Am Soc Nephrol*. 2011 Oct;6(10):2516–2521. [PMID: 21921151]

49

Hyponatremia

A 75-year-old man with terminal small cell carcinoma of the lung presents to the emergency department with altered mental status. The patient's wife, who cares for him at home, states that he is quite weak at baseline, requiring assistance with all activities of daily living. Over the last few days, he has become progressively more lethargic. She has been careful to adequately hydrate him, waking him every 2 hours to give him water to drink. His appetite has been poor, but he willingly ingests the water, consuming 2 to 3 quarts per day. He is taking morphine for pain and dyspnea. On examination, the patient is a cachectic man in mild respiratory distress. He is lethargic but arousable. He is oriented to person only. Vital signs reveal a temperature of 38°C, blood pressure of 110/60 mm Hg, heart rate of 88 bpm, respiratory rate of 18/min, and oxygen saturation of 96% on 3 L of oxygen. On head-neck examination, pupils are 3 mm and reactive, scleras are anicteric, and conjunctivas are pink. Mucous membranes are moist. Neck is supple. There are decreased breath sounds in the left lower posterior lung field and rales in the upper half. Cardiac examination shows a regular heartbeat without murmur, gallop, or rub. Abdomen is benign without masses. Extremities are without edema, cyanosis, or clubbing. Neurologic examination shows only bilateral positive Babinski reflexes and asterixis. Laboratory studies reveal a serum sodium of 118 mg/dL.

LEARNING OBJECTIVES

▶ Learn the clinical manifestations and objective findings of hyponatremia
▶ Understand the factors that predispose to hyponatremia
▶ Know the causes of hyponatremia
▶ Learn the treatments for hyponatremia
▶ Understand how to prevent complications from hyponatremia

QUESTIONS

1. What are the salient features of this patient's problem?
2. How do you think through his problem?

3. What are the key features, including essentials of diagnosis, general considerations, and demographics, of hyponatremia?

4. What are the symptoms and signs of hyponatremia?

5. What is the etiology of hyponatremia?

6. What are laboratory findings in hyponatremia?

7. What are the treatments for hyponatremia?

8. What are the outcomes, including follow-up, complication, and prognosis, of hyponatremia?

9. When should patients with hyponatremia be referred to a specialist or admitted to the hospital?

ANSWERS

1. Salient Features

Altered mental status; lethargy; increased free water intake; low serum sodium on laboratory results; a diagnosis (lung disease) associated with the syndrome of inappropriate antidiuretic hormone secretion (SIADH)

2. How to Think Through

In "true" hyponatremia (hypotonic hyponatremia), which hormone causes the problem? (ADH.) In normal physiology, how does the body regulate **osmolarity**? (By retaining water via ADH.) How does the body regulate intravascular **volume**? (By retaining sodium via the renin–angiotensin–aldosterone axis.) To assess hyponatremia, it is crucial to grasp that ADH can be a powerful regulator of volume as well. Why does ADH have the power to retain water to the degree that osmolarity falls? (Think of this ability as an "evolutionary emergency plan" to preserve intravascular volume in the setting of hypovolemia.) What laboratory characteristic is shared by all patients with true hyponatremia? (Urine osmolarity > serum osmolarity.) The task is to determine why the ADH is high.

How do we classically break down the differential diagnosis for true hyponatremia? (By volume status.) What are the indications of volume status mentioned in this case? (Blood pressure, heart rate, mucus membranes, and absence of edema.) What are the causes of euvolemic hyponatremia? (Water intoxication, SIADH.)

What disease states are associated with SIADH? Would you expect the patient's urine osmolarity to be greater or less than his serum osmolarity? (He is inappropriately concentrating his urine, so his urine will be greater than his serum osmolarity.) What is the appropriate treatment? (Free water restriction.) How quickly should his sodium level be corrected and what is the danger of too rapid correction?

3. Key Features

Essentials of Diagnosis
- Serum Na^+ < 135 mEq/L (< 135 mmol/L)
- Hyponatremia usually reflects excess water retention relative to sodium, rather than sodium deficiency
- Sodium concentration is not a measure of total body sodium
- Volume status and serum osmolality are essential to determine the cause
- Hypotonic fluids commonly cause hyponatremia in hospitalized patients

General Considerations
- Most cases reflect water imbalance and abnormal water handling, not sodium imbalance

Demographics
- Most common electrolyte abnormality observed in the general hospitalized population

4. Symptoms and Signs

- Mild hyponatremia (serum sodium 130–135 mEq/L) is usually asymptomatic
- As the serum sodium concentration drops, nausea and malaise progress to headache, lethargy, and disorientation
- The most serious symptoms of severe and rapidly developing hyponatremia are
  — Seizure
  — Coma
  — Permanent brain damage
  — Respiratory arrest
  — Brainstem herniation
  — Death

5. Etiology

- ADH plays a primary role in the pathophysiology of hyponatremia
- A diagnostic algorithm using serum osmolality and volume status separates the causes of hyponatremia into therapeutically useful categories (Figure 49-1)
- **Isotonic hyponatremia or pseudohyponatremia**
  — Severe hyperlipidemia or hyperproteinemia
  — Caused by lipids and proteins interfering with serum sodium measurement
  — Serum osmolality is isotonic because lipids and proteins do not affect osmolality measurement
  — Newer sodium assays using ion-specific electrodes do not produce pseudohyponatremia

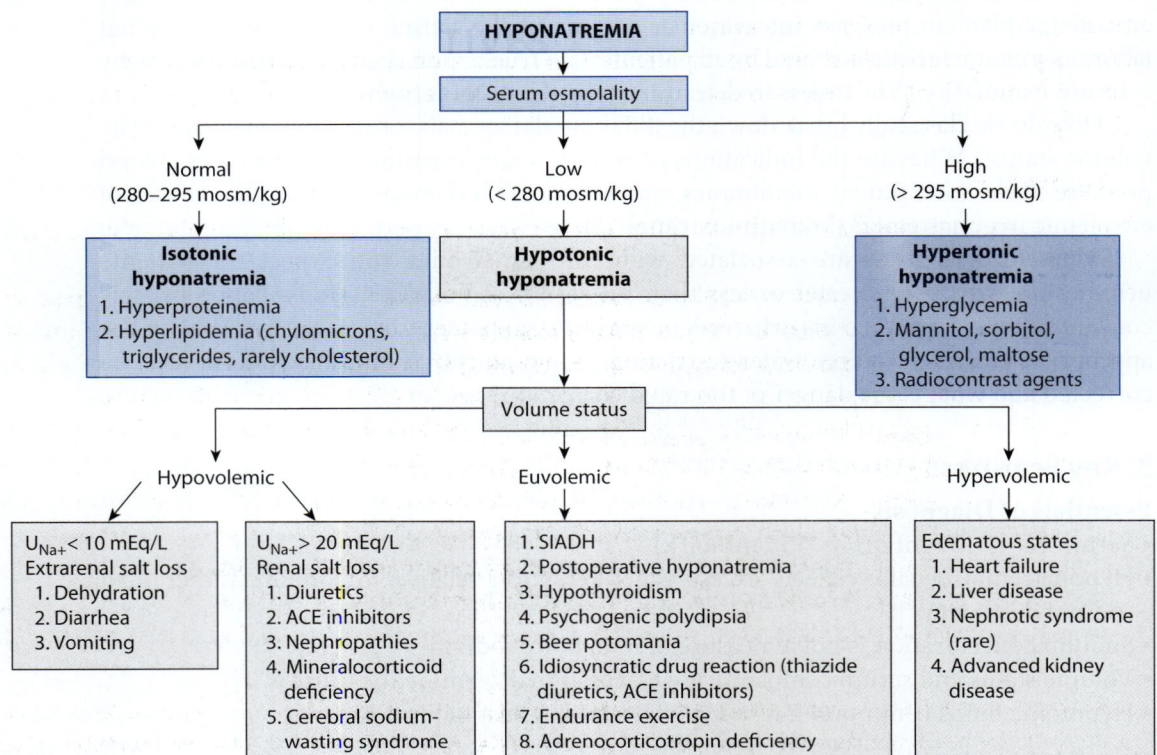

Figure 49-1. Evaluation of hyponatremia using serum osmolality and extracellular fluid volume status. ACE, angiotensin-converting enzyme; SIADH, syndrome of inappropriate antidiuretic hormone. (Adapted, with permission, from Narins RG et al. Diagnostic strategies in disorders of fluid, electrolyte and acid-base homeostasis. *Am J Med.* 1982;72(3):496–520.)

- **Hypotonic hyponatremia**
  — Hypovolemic
    ○ Occurs with renal or extrarenal volume loss and hypotonic fluid replacement
    ○ Total body sodium and total body water are decreased
    ○ Cerebral salt wasting in patients with intracranial disease; clinical features include refractory hypovolemia and hypotension
  — Euvolemic
    ○ SIADH (see Table 49-1)
    ○ Postoperative hyponatremia
    ○ Hypothyroidism
    ○ Adrenal insufficiency
    ○ Psychogenic polydipsia
    ○ Beer potomania
    ○ Idiosyncratic drug reaction (thiazides, angiotensin-converting enzyme inhibitors)
    ○ Endurance exercise
    ○ Reset osmostat
  — Hypervolemic (edematous states)
    ○ Heart failure
    ○ Cirrhosis
    ○ Nephrotic syndrome
    ○ Advanced kidney disease
- **Hypertonic hyponatremia**
  — Occurs in cases of hyperglycemia (eg, diabetic ketoacidosis and hyperosmolar hyperglycemic state) and with mannitol administration for increased intracranial pressure
  — Glucose and mannitol osmotically pull intracellular water into the extracellular space

6. Laboratory Findings

Laboratory Tests
- Serum Na^+ < 135 mEq/L (< 135 mmol/L)
- Obtain other serum electrolytes, serum creatinine, serum osmolality, and urine sodium
- Thyroid and adrenal function tests may occasionally be necessary to enable diagnosis of SIADH

7. Treatment

- There is no consensus about the optimal rate of sodium correction in symptomatic hyponatremic patients
- However, recent guidelines have introduced new recommendations
  — First, a relatively small increase of 4 to 6 mEq/L in the serum sodium may be all that is necessary to reverse the neurologic manifestations of symptomatic hyponatremia
  — Second, acute hyponatremia (eg, exercise-associated hyponatremia) with severe neurologic manifestations can be reversed rapidly with 100 mL of 3% hypertonic saline infused over 10 minutes (repeated twice as necessary)
  — Third, lower correction rates for chronic hyponatremia are recommended, as low as 4 to 8 mEq/L per 24 hours, in patients at high risk for demyelination
  — Fourth, chronic hyponatremic patients at high risk for demyelination who are corrected too rapidly are candidates for treatment with a combination of ddAVP and intravenous dextrose 5% to relower the serum sodium

Medications
- Regardless of volume status, restrict free water, and hypotonic fluid intake
- Free water intake from oral intake and intravenous (IV) fluids should generally be < 1 to 1.5 L/d
- For **hypovolemic** patients, adequate fluid resuscitation with isotonic fluids (either normal saline or lactated Ringer solution). For **cerebral salt wasting** patients, hypertonic saline or normal saline may prevent circulatory collapse; some may respond to fludrocortisone

Table 49-1. Causes of syndrome of inappropriate ADH secretion (SIADH).

Central Nervous System Disorders
Head trauma
Stroke
Subarachnoid hemorrhage
Hydrocephalus
Brain tumor
Encephalitis
Guillain–Barré syndrome
Meningitis
Acute psychosis
Acute intermittent porphyria
Pulmonary Lesions
Tuberculosis
Bacterial pneumonia
Aspergillosis
Bronchiectasis
Neoplasms
Positive pressure ventilation
Malignancies
Bronchogenic carcinoma
Pancreatic carcinoma
Prostatic carcinoma
Renal cell carcinoma
Adenocarcinoma of colon
Thymoma
Osteosarcoma
Malignant lymphoma
Leukemia
Drugs
Increased ADH production
Antidepressants: tricyclics, monoamine oxidase inhibitors, SSRIs
Antineoplastics: cyclophosphamide, vincristine
Carbamazepine
Methylenedioxymethamphetamine (MDMA; Ecstasy)
Clofibrate
Neuroleptics: thiothixene, thioridazine, fluphenazine, haloperidol, trifluoperazine
Potentiated ADH action
Carbamazepine
Chlorpropamide, tolbutamide
Cyclophosphamide
NSAIDs
Somatostatin and analogs
Amiodarone
Others
Postoperative
Pain
Stress
AIDS
Pregnancy (physiologic)
Hypokalemia

ADH, antidiuretic hormone; NSAIDs, nonsteroidal anti-inflammatory drugs; SSRIs, selective serotonin reuptake inhibitors.

- For **hypervolemic** patients, loop diuretics or dialysis, or both, may be required
- **Euvolemic** patients may respond to free water restriction alone
- **Demeclocycline** (300–600 mg twice daily orally)
  — Used for patients who cannot adequately restrict water intake or have an inadequate response to conservative measures
  — It inhibits the effect of ADH on the distal tubule

- **Vasopressin antagonists**
  — May revolutionize the treatment of euvolemic and hypervolemic hyponatremia, especially in persons with heart failure
  — V_2 receptors primarily mediate the diuretic effect of ADH
  — Tolvaptan
    ◦ Started at 15 mg orally daily
    ◦ Can be increased to 30 and 60 mg daily at 24-hour intervals if hyponatremia persists or if the increase in sodium concentration is < 5 mEq/L over the preceding 24 hours
  — Conivaptan
    ◦ Given as an intravenous loading dose of 20 mg delivered over 30 minutes, then as 20 mg continuously over 24 hours
    ◦ Subsequent infusions may be administered every 1 to 3 days at 20 to 40 mg/d by continuous infusion
  — The standard free water restriction for hyponatremic patients should be lifted for patients receiving vasopressin antagonists since the aquaresis can result in excessive sodium correction in a fluid-restricted patient
  — Frequent monitoring of the serum sodium is necessary

8. Outcomes

Follow-Up
- If symptomatic, measure serum Na+ about every 4 hours and observe the patient closely

Complication
- Iatrogenic cerebral osmotic demyelination
  — Most serious complication
  — Develops from overly rapid or inappropriate sodium correction
  — May occur outside the brainstem
  — May occur days after sodium correction or initial neurologic recovery from hyponatremia
  — Hypoxic episodes during hyponatremia may contribute to demyelination
  — Neurologic effects are generally catastrophic and irreversible

Prognosis
- Premenopausal women in whom hyponatremic encephalopathy develops are more likely than postmenopausal women to suffer permanent brain damage or die

9. When to Refer and When to Admit

When to Refer
- Nephrology or endocrinology consultation should be considered in severe, symptomatic, refractory, or complicated cases of hyponatremia
- Aggressive therapies with hypertonic saline, demeclocycline, vasopressin antagonists, or dialysis mandate specialist consultation
- Consultation may be necessary for patients with end-stage liver or heart disease

When to Admit
- Patients who are symptomatic or who require aggressive therapies for close monitoring and frequent laboratory testing

SUGGESTED REFERENCES

Lehrich RW et al. Role of vaptans in the management of hyponatremia. *Am J Kidney Dis.* 2013 Aug;62(2):364–376. [PMID: 23725974]

Leung AA et al. Preoperative hyponatremia and perioperative complications. *Arch Intern Med.* 2012 Oct 22;172(19):1474–1481. [PMID: 22965221]

Shchekochikhin D et al. Hyponatremia: an update on current pharmacotherapy. *Expert Opin Pharmacother.* 2013 Apr;14(6):747–755. [PMID: 23496346]

Spasovski G et al; Hyponatraemia Guideline Development Group. Clinical practice guideline on diagnosis and treatment of hyponatraemia. *Eur J Endocrinol.* 2014 Feb 25;170(3):G1–G47. Erratum in: *Eur J Endocrinol.* 2014 Jul;171(1):X1. [PMID: 24569125]

Verbalis JG et al. Diagnosis, evaluation, and treatment of hyponatremia: expert panel recommendations. *Am J Med.* 2013 Oct;126(10 suppl 1):S1–S42. [PMID: 24074529]

Acute Kidney Injury

A 36-year-old woman with diabetes mellitus sustained a fall onto her arm while at a construction site. She was brought to the emergency department where she received a computed tomography (CT) scan with contrast. She subsequently underwent pinning and reconstructive surgery of her arm, and received perioperative broad-spectrum antibiotics. Her blood pressure remained normal throughout her hospital course. On the second hospital day, there was a doubling of her serum creatinine, from 0.8 to 1.9 mg/dL. Her urine output dropped to 20 mL/h. Serum creatine kinase returned at 600 units/L (normal range 96–140 units/L).

LEARNING OBJECTIVES

▶ Learn the clinical manifestations, objective findings, and complications of acute kidney injury (AKI)

▶ Understand the definition of AKI and how to diagnose its cause

▶ Know the differential diagnosis of the causes of prerenal, intrinsic renal, and postrenal AKI

▶ Learn the treatment for AKI and the indications for dialysis

QUESTIONS

1. What are the salient features of this patient's problem?

2. How do you think through her problem?

3. What are the key features, including essentials of diagnosis and general considerations, of AKI?

4. What are the symptoms and signs of AKI?

5. What is the differential diagnosis of AKI?

6. What are laboratory, imaging, and procedural findings in AKI?

7. What are the treatments for AKI?

8. When should patients with AKI be referred to a specialist or admitted to the hospital?

ANSWERS

1. Salient Features

Increase in serum creatinine concentration; oliguria; traumatic injury and moderately elevated creatine kinase (CK); administration of iodinated contrast and antibiotics.

2. How to Think Through

Serum creatinine is an indirect measure of glomerular filtration rate (GFR). What are the limitations in the use of serum creatinine as a measure of GFR? (Serum creatinine accurately reflects GFR only when renal function is at a steady state.) What is the patient's true GFR if her creatinine rose from 0.8 to 1.9 mg/dL in 24 hours? (A 1-mg/dL rise per day indicates complete cessation of renal function—a GFR of 0.) Of the possible causes of AKI in this case, how would you rank the likely contributors? (Contrast nephropathy > rhabdomyolysis > acute tubular necrosis [ATN] due to antibiotics. Iodinated contrast can cause rapid onset of AKI, probably due to both ATN and vasoconstriction. Diabetes mellitus and underlying chronic kidney disease (CKD) increase the risk for contrast nephropathy. Rhabdomyolysis generally follows CK elevation into the several thousands, and is more often seen in acute stimulant abuse or with prolonged stasis, such as loss of consciousness due to excess alcoholism.) Could the antibiotics have caused ATN? (Possibly, but the onset is typically slower.) Could the antibiotics have caused acute interstitial nephritis (AIN)? (Again, the onset is too fast, and there was no evidence of fever, rash, or white blood cell casts.) What are the key elements of the workup for AKI? (Urinalysis with microscopic examination of the sediment for red cells, white blood cells, and casts. Urine protein, creatinine, and sodium. Renal ultrasonography.) What are the crucial aspects of management of AKI, regardless of etiology? (Daily weights, strict monitoring of electrolytes, volume status, intake and output. Adjustment of all medication dosing. Avoidance of nonsteroidal anti-inflammatory drugs [NSAIDs], angiotensin-converting enzyme inhibitors (ACEIs)/angiotensin II receptor blockers (ARBs), and diuretics. Low potassium diet.)

3. Key Features

Essentials of Diagnosis

- Defined as a rapid increase in serum creatinine
- Inability to maintain acid–base, fluid, and electrolyte balance and to excrete nitrogenous wastes
- Oliguria can be associated
- Symptoms and signs depend on cause

General Considerations

- 5% of hospital admissions and 30% of ICU admissions have AKI
- 25% of hospitalized patients develop AKI
- Serum creatinine concentration typically increases 1.0 to 1.5 mg/dL daily in the absence of functioning kidneys
- Three categories of AKI
  — Prerenal insults
  — Intrinsic renal disease
  — Postrenal causes

4. Symptoms and Signs

- Nausea, vomiting
- Malaise
- Hypertension
- Pericardial friction rub, effusions, and cardiac tamponade
- Arrhythmias

- Rales and volume overload
- Abdominal pain and ileus
- Bleeding secondary to platelet dysfunction
- Encephalopathy, altered sensorium, asterixis, and seizures
- Oliguria, defined as urinary output < 500 mL/d or < 20 mL/h

5. Differential Diagnosis

Prerenal Causes
- Dehydration
- Hemorrhage (eg, gastrointestinal bleeding)
- Heart failure
- Renal artery stenosis, including fibromuscular dysplasia
- NSAIDs, ACEIs, ARBs

Postrenal Causes
- Obstruction (eg, benign prostatic hyperplasia, bladder tumor)

Intrinsic Renal Disease
- ATN
  - Toxins
    - NSAIDs
    - Antibiotics
    - Contrast
    - Multiple myeloma
    - Rhabdomyolysis
    - Hemolysis
    - Chemotherapy
    - Hyperuricemia
    - Cyclosporine
  - Ischemia (eg, prolonged prerenal insults)
- Acute glomerulonephritis (AGN)
  - Immune complex
    - Immunoglobulin A nephropathy
    - Endocarditis
    - Systemic lupus erythematosus (SLE)
    - Cryoglobulinemia
    - Postinfectious
    - Membranoproliferative
  - Pauci-immune (ANCA$^+$)
    - Granulomatosis with polyangiitis (formerly Wegener granulomatosis)
    - Churg–Strauss syndrome
    - Microscopic polyarteritis
  - Antiglomerular basement membrane (anti-GBM)
    - Goodpasture disease
    - Anti-GBM glomerulonephritis
- Vascular
  - Malignant hypertension
  - Thrombotic thrombocytopenia purpura
  - Atheroembolism
- AIN
  - Drugs
    - β-Lactams
    - Sulfa
    - Diuretics

- NSAIDs
- Rifampin
- Phenytoin
- Allopurinol
— Infections
  - *Streptococcus*
  - Leptospirosis
  - Cytomegalovirus
  - Histoplasmosis
  - Rocky Mountain spotted fever
— Immune
  - SLE
  - Sjögren syndrome
  - Sarcoidosis
  - Cryoglobulinemia

6. Laboratory, Imaging, and Procedural Findings

Laboratory Tests
- Serum creatinine and BUN elevated
- BUN–creatinine ratio > 20:1 in prerenal and postrenal causes, and AGN; < 20:1 in ATN and AIN
- Hyperkalemia
- Anion gap metabolic acidosis
- Hyperphosphatemia
- Hypocalcemia
- Anemia
- Fractional excretion of sodium (FE_{Na}) can be useful in oliguric states
  — FE_{Na} = clearance of Na^+/GFR = clearance of Na^+/creatinine clearance
  — FE_{Na} = (urine Na^+/plasma Na^+)/(urine Cr/plasma Cr) × 100
- FE_{Na} low (< 1%) in prerenal insults; high (> 1%) in ATN; variable in postrenal causes, AIN, AGN

Imaging Studies
- Renal ultrasonography to exclude obstruction or other anatomic abnormalities; check renal size and echo texture
- CT or magnetic resonance imaging if retroperitoneal fibrosis from tumor or radiation is suspected

Diagnostic Procedures
- Electrocardiography: peaked T waves, PR prolongation, and QRS widening in hyperkalemia, long QT interval with hypocalcemia

7. Treatments

Therapeutic Procedures
- Prerenal insults
  — Treatment depends on cause
  — Maintain euvolemia
  — Monitor serum electrolytes
  — Avoid nephrotoxic drugs
- Postrenal causes: relief of obstruction if present
  — Place catheters or stents to treat obstruction
  — Catheterize the bladder if hydroureter and hydronephrosis are present with an enlarged bladder on ultrasonography

- Intrinsic renal disease: treatment depends on cause (see Acute Tubular Necrosis); hold offending agents
- Hemodialysis, peritoneal dialysis: indications include
  — Uremic symptoms such as pericarditis, encephalopathy, or coagulopathy
  — Fluid overload unresponsive to diuresis
  — Refractory hyperkalemia
  — Severe metabolic acidosis (pH < 7.20)
  — Neurologic symptoms such as seizures or neuropathy

8. When to Refer and When to Admit

When to Refer
- If a patient has signs of AKI that have not reversed over 1 to 2 weeks, but no signs of acute uremia, the patient can usually be referred to a nephrologist rather than admitted
- If a patient has signs of persistent urinary tract obstruction, the patient should be referred to a urologist

When to Admit
- The patient should be admitted if there is sudden loss of kidney function resulting in abnormalities that cannot be handled expeditiously in an outpatient setting (eg, hyperkalemia, volume overload, and uremia) or other requirements for acute dialysis

SUGGESTED REFERENCES

Kinsey GR et al. Pathogenesis of acute kidney injury: foundation for clinical practice. *Am J Kidney Dis.* 2011 Aug;58(2):291–301. [PMID: 21530035]

Okusa MD et al. Reading between the (guide)lines—the KDIGO practice guideline on acute kidney injury in the individual patient. *Kidney Int.* 2014 Jan;85(1):39–48. [PMID: 24067436]

Walther CP et al. Summary of clinical practice guidelines for acute kidney injury. *Hosp Pract (1995).* 2014 Feb;42(1):7–14. [PMID: 24566591]

51

Chronic Kidney Disease

A 58-year-old obese woman with hypertension, type 2 diabetes mellitus, and chronic kidney disease (CKD) is admitted to hospital after a right femoral neck fracture sustained in a fall. Recently, she has been complaining of fatigue and was started on epoetin alfa subcutaneous injections. Her other medications include an angiotensin-converting enzyme (ACE) inhibitor, a β-blocker, a diuretic, calcium supplementation, and insulin. On review of systems, she reports mild tingling in her lower extremities. On examination, her blood pressure is 148/60 mm Hg. She is oriented and able to answer questions appropriately. There is no evidence of jugular venous distention or pericardial friction rub. Her lungs are clear, and her right lower extremity is in Buck's traction in preparation for surgery. Asterixis is absent.

LEARNING OBJECTIVES

- ► Learn the clinical manifestations and objective findings of uremia and CKD
- ► Understand the epidemiology of CKD in the United States
- ► Know the primary and secondary causes of CKD
- ► Learn the pharmacologic and nonpharmacologic approaches to the treatment of CKD
- ► Know when to initiate dialysis in patients with CKD

QUESTIONS

1. What are the salient features of this patient's problem?
2. How do you think through her problem?
3. What are the key features, including essentials of diagnosis and general considerations, of CKD?
4. What are the symptoms and signs of CKD?
5. What is the differential diagnosis of CKD?
6. What are laboratory, imaging, and procedural findings in CKD?
7. What are the treatments for CKD?
8. What is the outcome, including the prognosis, of CKD?
9. When should patients with CKD be referred to a specialist or admitted to the hospital?

ANSWERS

1. Salient Features

Hypertension; diabetes mellitus; anemia, responsive to epoetin alfa injections; lower extremity tingling suggestive of neuropathy

2. How to Think Through

What are the likely contributors to this patient's CKD? (Hypertension, leading to glomerulosclerosis and/or to renal artery stenosis, along with diabetic nephropathy, both likely contribute. Obesity-related kidney disease presents a third, independent possibility.) What studies would be appropriate? (Urinalysis with microscopy, urine protein measurement, renal ultrasound.) How can urine protein be estimated? (The ratio of spot urine protein to urine creatinine approximates the number of grams of protein lost per day. A ratio > 3.5 indicates nephrotic range proteinuria, which would be unexpectedly high for the above causes.) Is a renal biopsy needed? (No. In the absence of unexpected findings on the above studies, or an unexpected course, the diagnosis of CKD is based upon epidemiological risk factors.) What treatments are known to slow the progression of CKD? (ACEI or angiotensin receptor blocker [ARB]; control of hypertension with a goal systolic blood pressure of ≤ 130 mm Hg; optimal control of diabetes.) What are the important aspects of management of this patient's CKD while she is in the hospital? (Adjustment of all medication dosing. Monitoring of electrolytes, weight, volume status, input and output. Avoidance of nonsteroidal anti-inflammatory drugs.)

3. Key Features

Essentials of Diagnosis
- Decline in the glomerular filtration rate (GFR) over months to years
- Persistent proteinuria or abnormal renal morphology may be present
- Symptoms and signs of uremia when nearing end-stage disease
- Hypertension in most cases
- Bilateral small or echogenic kidneys on ultrasonogram in advanced disease

General Considerations
- Progressive decline in renal function
- Rarely reversible
- Affects > 13 million Americans, most of whom are unaware
- Over 70% of cases of late-stage CKD (stage 5 CKD and end-stage renal disease [ESRD]) in the United States are due to diabetes mellitus or hypertension/vascular disease
- Glomerulonephritis, cystic diseases, chronic tubulointerstitial diseases, and other urologic diseases account for the remainder (Table 55-1)
- Genetic polymorphisms of the *APOL-1* gene have been shown to be associated with an increased risk of the development of CKD in African Americans

4. Symptoms and Signs

- Symptoms develop slowly with the progressive decline in GFR and are nonspecific
- Patient can be asymptomatic until kidney disease is far advanced (GFR < 5–10 mL/min/1.73 m^2)
- General symptoms of uremia (Table 51-2).
  - Hypertension is the most common sign
  - Fatigue, and weakness
  - Anorexia, nausea, vomiting, pruritus, and a metallic taste in the mouth are also common
  - Generalized pruritus without rash

Table 51-1. Major causes of chronic kidney disease.

Glomerular Diseases

Primary Glomerular Diseases
Focal and segmental glomerulosclerosis
Membranoproliferative glomerulonephritis
IgA nephropathy
Membranous nephropathy
Alport syndrome (hereditary nephritis)
Secondary Glomerular Diseases
Diabetic nephropathy
Amyloidosis
Postinfectious glomerulonephritis
HIV-associated nephropathy
Collagen-vascular diseases (eg, SLE)
HCV-associated membranoproliferative glomerulonephritis

Tubulointerstitial Nephritis

Drug hypersensitivity
Heavy metals
Analgesic nephropathy
Reflux/chronic pyelonephritis
Sickle-cell nephropathy
Idiopathic

Cystic Diseases

Polycystic kidney disease
Medullary cystic disease

Obstructive Nephropathies

Prostatic disease
Nephrolithiasis
Retroperitoneal fibrosis/tumor
Congenital

Vascular Diseases

Hypertensive nephrosclerosis
Renal artery stenosis

HCV, hepatitis C virus; SLE, systemic lupus erythematosus.

Table 51-2. Symptoms and signs of uremia.

Organ System	Symptoms	Signs
General	Fatigue, weakness	Sallow appearing, chronically ill
Skin	Pruritus, easy bruisability	Pallor, ecchymoses, excoriations, edema, xerosis
ENT	Metallic taste in mouth, epistaxis	Urinous breath
Eye		Pale conjunctiva
Pulmonary	Shortness of breath	Rales, pleural effusion
Cardiovascular	Dyspnea on exertion, retrosternal pain on inspiration (pericarditis)	Hypertension, cardiomegaly, friction rub
Gastrointestinal	Anorexia, nausea, vomiting, hiccups	
Genitourinary	Nocturia, erectile dysfunction	Isosthenuria
Neuromuscular	Restless legs, numbness and cramps in legs	
Neurologic	Generalized irritability and inability to concentrate, decreased libido	Stupor, asterixis, myoclonus, peripheral neuropathy

— Irritability, memory impairment, insomnia, subtle memory defects, restless legs, paresthesias, and twitching
— Pleuritic chest pain can occur with pericarditis (rare)
• Renal osteodystrophy (osteitis fibrosa cystica), osteomalacia, and adynamic bone disease

5. Differential Diagnosis

• Primary glomerular diseases (eg, focal and segmental glomerulosclerosis, IgA nephropathy) (Table 51-1)
• Secondary glomerular diseases (eg, diabetic nephropathy, amyloidosis, sickle cell nephropathy, HIV-associated nephropathy)
• Tubulointerstitial nephritis (eg, drug hypersensitivity, analgesic nephropathy, chronic pyelonephritis)
• Hereditary disease (eg, polycystic kidney disease, Alport syndrome, medullary cystic disease)
• Obstructive nephropathies (eg, prostatic disease, nephrolithiasis, congenital)
• Vascular diseases (eg, hypertensive nephrosclerosis, renal artery stenosis)

6. Laboratory, Imaging, and Procedural Findings

Laboratory Tests

• Abnormal GFR persisting for at least 3 months
• Plot of the inverse of serum creatinine ($1/S_{Cr}$) versus time if three or more prior measurements are available helps estimate time to ESRD
• Anemia
• Platelet dysfunction, bleeding time prolongation
• Metabolic acidosis
• Hyperphosphatemia, hypocalcemia
• Hyperkalemia
• Urinary sediment: broad waxy casts
• Proteinuria may be present

Imaging Studies

• Renal ultrasonogram for anatomic abnormalities, kidney size, and echogenicity

Diagnostic Procedures

• Possible renal biopsy if cause is unclear

7. Treatments

• Control of diabetes should be aggressive in early CKD; risk of hypoglycemia increases in advanced CKD, and glycemic targets may need to be relaxed to avoid this dangerous complication
• Blood pressure control is vital to slow progression of all forms of CKD; agents that block the renin–angiotensin–aldosterone system are particularly important in proteinuric disease
• Several small studies suggest a possible benefit of oral alkali therapy in slowing CKD progression when acidemia is present (see above)
• There is also theoretic value in lowering uric acid levels in those with concomitant hyperuricemia, but clinical data regarding benefit are still lacking
• Management of traditional cardiovascular risk factors should also be emphasized
• Management of acid–base disorders is important as chronic acidosis can result in muscle protein catabolism, and may accelerate progression of CKD

Medications

• Acute hyperkalemia: calcium chloride or gluconate intravenously, insulin administration with glucose intravenously, bicarbonate intravenously, and ion exchange resin (sodium polystyrene sulfonate) orally or per rectum, cardiac monitoring

- Chronic hyperkalemia: dietary potassium restriction, sodium polystyrene sulfonate, 15 to 30 g once daily orally in juice or sorbitol
- Acid–base disorders: sodium bicarbonate 20 to 30 mmol/d divided into two doses, titrated to maintain serum bicarbonate at > 21 mmol/L.
- Hypertension
  — Salt and water restriction, weight loss, and decreased salt diet (2–3 g/d)
  — Diuretics nearly always needed
  — Thiazides work in early CKD
  — However, loop diuretics are more effective in patients with GFR < 30 mL/min/1.73 m^2
  — In addition to diuretics, initial drug therapy should include ACE inhibitors or ARBs in patients with proteinuria
  — Second-line antihypertensive agents include calcium channel blockers and β-blockers
- Heart failure
  — Salt and water restriction, loop diuretics
  — ACE inhibitors can be used with close monitoring if serum creatinine > 3 mg/dL
- Anemia
  — Recombinant erythropoietin, 50 units/kg (3000–4000 units/dose) one or two times weekly intravenously or subcutaneously
  — Darbepoetin is started at 0.45 μg/kg and can be administered every 2 to 4 weeks intravenously or subcutaneously
  — Ferrous sulfate, 325 mg 1× to 3× daily if serum ferritin < 100 ng/mL or if iron saturation < 20% to 25%
- Coagulopathy
  — Dialysis
  — Desmopressin, 25 μg every 8 to 12 hours intravenously for two doses prior to surgery
  — Conjugated estrogens, 2.5 to 5 mg orally for 5 to 7 days, may have an effect for several weeks but is very seldom used
- Renal osteodystrophy, osteomalacia
  — Dietary phosphorus restriction
  — Oral phosphorus-binding agents such as calcium carbonate (650 mg/tablet) or calcium acetate (667 mg/capsule) block absorption of dietary phosphorus in the gut and are given thrice daily with meals. Phosphorus-binding agents that do not contain calcium are sevelamer (800–3200 mg) and lanthanum (500–1000 mg)
  — Newer iron-based, non-calcium-containing phosphorus binders for long-term use include ferric citrate and sucroferric oxyhydroxide
  — Vitamin D or vitamin D analogs (if iPTH > 2× to 3× normal), correction of serum phosphate and calcium toward normal values
  — Calcitriol 0.25 to 0.5 μg once daily or every other day

Nonpharmacologic Approach
Diet
- Benefits of protein restriction in slowing decline of GFR must be weighed against the risk of cachexia upon the initiation of dialysis
- Salt and water restriction
  — 2 g/d of sodium for nondialysis patient approaching ESRD
  — Daily fluid restriction to 2 L may be needed if volume overload is present
- Potassium restriction to < 50 to 60 mEq/d
- Phosphorus restriction to 800 to 1000 mg/d
- Magnesium-containing laxatives and antacids contraindicated

Therapeutic Procedures
- Kidney transplantation
  — Care for transplant recipients includes treatment of CV risk factors, bone health (maintenance of normal vitamin D, periodic bone densitometry, and treatment of residual

hyperparathyroidism), annual dermatologic screening for skin cancers, scrutiny of the medication list for adverse drug–drug interactions, and regular vaccinations.
- Indications for hemodialysis, peritoneal dialysis
  — Uremic symptoms (eg, pericarditis, encephalopathy, and coagulopathy)
  — Fluid overload unresponsive to diuresis
  — Refractory hyperkalemia
  — Severe metabolic acidosis (pH < 7.20)
  — Dialysis initiation should be considered when GFR is < 10 mL/min/1.73 m^2

8. Outcome

Prognosis

- Roughly 80% and 90% of patients with CKD die, primarily of CVD, before reaching the need for dialysis.
- Mortality is higher for patients receiving dialysis than for those receiving a kidney transplant versus healthy age-matched controls
- Patients undergoing dialysis have an average life expectancy of 3 to 5 years, but survival for as long as 25 years is seen depending on the disease entity
- Overall 5-year survival on dialysis is currently estimated at 40%, with survival rates dependent on the underlying disease
- Dialysis should be carefully weighed in patients with a short life expectancy and very elderly persons, with some studies showing a decrease in functional status in the first year of such treatment.
- Common causes of death
  — Cardiac disease (50%)
  — Infection
  — Cerebrovascular disease
  — Malignancy
- Other significant mortality predictors
  — Diabetes mellitus
  — Advanced age
  — Low serum albumin
  — Lower socioeconomic status
  — Inadequate dialysis

9. When to Refer and When to Admit

When to Refer

- A patient with stage 3 to 5 CKD should be referred to a nephrologist for management in conjunction with the primary care clinician
- A patient with other forms of CKD such as those with significant proteinuria (> 1 g/d) or polycystic kidney disease should be referred to a nephrologist at earlier stages

When to Admit

- Patients with decompensation of problems related to CKD, such as worsening of acid–base status, electrolyte abnormalities, volume status that cannot be appropriately treated in the outpatient setting
- Patient needs to start dialysis, and is not stable for outpatient initiation

SUGGESTED REFERENCES

Baldwin MD. The primary care physician/nephrologist partnership in treating chronic kidney disease. *Prim Care*. 2014 Dec;41(4):837–856. [PMID: 25439537]

Bhan I. Phosphate management in chronic kidney disease. *Curr Opin Nephrol Hypertens*. 2014 Mar;23(2): 174–179. [PMID: 24445424]

Casey JR et al. Patients' perspectives on hemodialysis vascular access: a systematic review of qualitative studies. *Am J Kidney Dis*. 2014 Dec;64(6):937–953. [PMID: 25115617]

Davies SJ. Peritoneal dialysis—current status and future challenges. *Nat Rev Nephrol*. 2013 Jul;9(7): 399–408. [PMID: 23689122]

Delanaye P et al. Outcome of the living kidney donor. *Nephrol Dial Transplant*. 2012 Jan;27(1):41–50. [PMID:22287701]

Dobre M et al. Current status of bicarbonate in CKD. *J Am Soc Nephrol*. 2015 Mar;26(3):515–523. [PMID: 25150154]

Gansevoort RT et al. Chronic kidney disease and cardiovascular risk: epidemiology, mechanisms, and prevention. *Lancet*. 2013 Jul 27;382(9889):339–352. [PMID: 23727170]

Himmelfarb J et al. Hemodialysis. *N Engl J Med*. 2010 Nov 4;363(19):1833–1845. [PMID: 21047227]

Jain N et al. Effects of dietary interventions on incidence and progression of CKD. *Nat Rev Nephrol*. 2014 Dec;10(12):712–724. [PMID: 25331786]

James PA et al. 2014 evidence-based guideline for the management of high blood pressure in adults: report from the panel members appointed to the Eighth Joint National Committee (JNC 8). *JAMA*. 2014 Feb 5;311(5):507–520. [PMID: 24352797]

Jha V et al. Chronic kidney disease: global dimension and perspectives. *Lancet*. 2013 Jul 20;382(9888): 260–272. [PMID: 23727169]

Ketteler M et al. Use of phosphate binders in chronic kidney disease. *Curr Opin Nephrol Hypertens*. 2013 Jul;22(4):413–420. [PMID: 23736841]

Knight J et al. Optimal targets for blood pressure control in chronic kidney disease: the debate continues. *Curr Opin Nephrol Hypertens*. 2014 Nov;23(6):541–546. [PMID: 25295958]

Komenda P et al. Estimated glomerular filtration rate and albuminuria: diagnosis, staging and prognosis. *Curr Opin Nephrol Hypertens*. 2014 May;23(3):251–257. [PMID: 24675138]

Kovesdy CP et al. Blood pressure and mortality in U.S. veterans with chronic kidney disease: a cohort study. *Ann Intern Med*. 2013 Aug 20;159(4):233–242. [PMID: 24026256]

Kumar S et al. Why do young people with chronic kidney disease die early? *World J Nephrol*. 2014 Nov 6;3(4):143–155. [PMID: 25374808]

McGill RL et al. Transplantation and the primary care physician. *Adv Chronic Kidney Dis*. 2011 Nov;18(6):433–438. [PMID: 22098662]

Palmer SC et al. Dietary and fluid restrictions in CKD: a thematic synthesis of patient views from qualitative studies. *Am J Kidney Dis*. 2015 Apr;65(4):559–573. [PMID: 25453993]

Palmer SC et al. Erythropoesis-stimulating agents for anaemia in adults with chronic kidney disease: a network meta-analysis. *Cochrane Database Syst Rev*. 2014 Dec 8;12:CD010590. [PMID: 25486075]

Palmer SC et al. HMG CoA reductase inhibitors (statins) for persons with chronic kidney disease not requiring dialysis. *Cochrane Database Syst Rev*. 2014 May 31;5:CD007784. [PMID: 24880031]

Parsa A et al. *APOL1* risk variants, race and progression of chronic kidney disease. *N Engl J Med*. 2013 Dec 5;369(23):2183–2196. [PMID: 24206458]

Qaseem A et al. Screening, monitoring, and treatment of stage 1 to 3 chronic kidney disease: a clinical practice guideline from the American College of Physicians. *Ann Intern Med*. 2013 Dec 17;159(12): 835–847. [PMID: 24145991]

Rivas Velasquez KM et al. Evaluation and management of the older patient with chronic kidney disease. *Prim Care*. 2014 Dec;41(4):857–874. [PMID: 25439538]

Segall L et al. Heart failure in patients with chronic kidney disease: a systematic integrative review. *Biomed Res Int*. 2014;2014:937398. [PMID: 24959595]

Sinnakirouchenan R et al. Role of sodium restriction and diuretic therapy for "resistant" hypertension in chronic kidney disease. *Semin Nephrol*. 2014;34(5):514–519. [PMID: 25416660]

Snyder S et al. Obesity-related kidney disease. *Prim Care*. 2014 Dec;41(4):875–893. [PMID: 25439539]

Sprangers B et al. Recurrence of glomerulonephritis after renal transplantation. *Transplant Rev (Orlando)*. 2013 Oct;27(4):126–134. [PMID: 23954034]

Stevens PE et al. Evaluation and management of chronic kidney disease: synopsis of the Kidney Disease: Improving Global Outcomes 2012 Clinical Practice Guideline. *Ann Intern Med*. 2013 Jun 4;158(11):825–830. [PMID: 23732715]

Streja E et al. Controversies in timing of dialysis initiation and the role of race and demographics. *Semin Dial*. 2013 Nov–Dec;26(6):658–666. [PMID: 24102770]

Thiruchelvam PT et al. Renal transplantation. *BMJ*. 2011 Nov 14;343:d7300. [PMID: 22084316]

Tong A. Thematic synthesis of qualitative studies on patient and caregiver perspectives on end-of-life care in CKD. *Am J Kidney Dis*. 2014 Jun;63(6):913–927. [PMID: 24411716]

Wu HM et al. Oral adsorbents for preventing or delaying progression of chronic kidney disease. *Cochrane Database Syst Rev*. 2014 Oct 15;10:CD007861. [PMID: 25317905]

Zuber K et al. Medication dosing in patients with chronic kidney disease. *JAAPA*. 2013 Oct;26(10): 19–25. [PMID: 24201917]

Kidney Stone Disease

52

A 48-year-old man presents to the emergency department with severe, colicky right flank pain. He denies dysuria or fever. He does report significant nausea without vomiting. He has never experienced anything like this before. On examination he is afebrile, his blood pressure is 160/80 mm Hg, and his pulse rate 110/min. He is writhing on the gurney, unable to find a comfortable position. His right flank is mildly tender to palpation, and abdominal examination is benign. Urinalysis is significant for 1+ blood, and microscopy reveals 10 to 20 red blood cells per high-power field. Nephrolithiasis is suspected, and the patient is intravenously hydrated and given pain medication with temporary relief.

LEARNING OBJECTIVES

▶ Learn the clinical manifestations and objective findings of kidney stone disease
▶ Understand the different types of urinary stones and the factors that predispose to them
▶ Learn how to diagnose the different types of hypercalciuria
▶ Know the differential diagnosis of kidney stone disease
▶ Learn the treatment for kidney stone disease depending on the type of stone
▶ Understand which patients require surgical intervention

QUESTIONS

1. What are the salient features of this patient's problem?
2. How do you think through his problem?
3. What are the key features, including essentials of diagnosis and general considerations, of kidney stone disease?
4. What are the symptoms and signs of kidney stone disease?
5. What is the differential diagnosis of kidney stone disease?
6. What are laboratory and imaging findings in kidney stone disease?
7. What are the treatments for kidney stone disease?
8. What is the outcome, including prevention, of kidney stone disease?
9. When should patients with kidney stone disease be referred to a specialist or admitted to the hospital?

ANSWERS

1. Salient Features

Severe flank pain; first episode in fourth decade of life; nausea and vomiting; writhing in discomfort; afebrile; flank tender to palpation; benign abdominal examination; hematuria

2. How to Think Through

The colicky pain with the hematuria suggests nephrolithiasis. The patient also has demographic risk factors. (Stones occur in men > women, ages 30–50.) What feature in this case makes nephrolithiasis more likely than an acute abdomen? (The patient is moving continually.) Why is he hypertensive and tachycardic? (Most likely due to pain.) What is the most common type of renal calculi? (Calcium oxalate.) While serum and urine studies can help ascertain the type of stone, as can radiographic lucency and appearance, analysis of a recovered stone is best. Which stones are radiolucent on plain abdominal film? (Uric acid stones.) What radiographic study is preferred? (Noncontrast helical computed tomography [CT].)

The largest stone that can pass spontaneously is 6 mm. Are there medications that can facilitate the passage of a stone? (α-Blockers and calcium channel blockers.) Pain control with nonsteroidal anti-inflammatory drugs and opioids is the other key component of treatment. What developments in this case would serve as indications for further intervention? (Failure to pass the stone; intractable pain and nausea; fever.) What are some of the interventions available? (Extracorporeal shock wave or percutaneous lithotripsy.) Treatment and dietary interventions vary based on the type of stone. What dietary modification should be recommended to prevent recurrence? (Low-salt diet; decreased animal protein intake; increased fluid intake.)

3. Key Features

Essentials of Diagnosis

- Severe flank pain
- Nausea and vomiting
- Identification on noncontrast helical CT scan or ultrasonography

General Considerations

- Affects 240,000 to 720,000 Americans per year
- Males > females (2.5:1)
- Initial presentation predominates between the third and fourth decades
- Incidence is greatest during hot summer months
- Contributing factors to urinary stone formation
  — Geographic factors
    ◦ High humidity
    ◦ Elevated temperatures
  — Genetic factors
    ◦ Cystinuria
    ◦ Distal renal tubular acidosis
  — Dietary and other factors
    ◦ High protein and high salt intake
    ◦ Persons in sedentary occupations have a higher incidence than manual laborers
- Increasing evidence is revealing that urinary stone disease may be a precursor to subsequent cardiovascular disease
- Five major types of urinary stones
  — Calcium oxalate
  — Calcium phosphate
  — Struvite (magnesium ammonium phosphate)

— Uric acid

— Cystine

• Most urinary stones contain calcium (85%) and are radiopaque; uric acid stones are radiolucent

• **Hypercalciuric calcium nephrolithiasis** (> 250 mg/24 h) can be caused by absorptive, resorptive, and renal disorders (Table 52-1)

   — **Absorptive hypercalciuria**
      › Secondary to increased absorption of calcium at the level of the small bowel, predominantly in the jejunum
      › Can be further subdivided into types I, II, and III
      › Type I: Independent of calcium intake. There is increased urinary calcium on a regular or even a calcium-restricted diet
      › Type II: Diet dependent
      › Type III: Secondary to a renal phosphate leak, which results in increased vitamin D synthesis and secondarily increased small bowel absorption of calcium

   — **Resorptive hypercalciuria**
      › Secondary to hyperparathyroidism
      › Hypercalcemia, hypophosphatemia, hypercalciuria, and an elevated serum parathyroid hormone level are found

   — **Renal hypercalciuria**
      › Occurs when the renal tubules are unable to efficiently reabsorb filtered calcium
      › Hypercalciuria and secondary hyperparathyroidism result

• **Hyperuricosuric calcium nephrolithiasis** is secondary to dietary excesses or uric acid metabolic defects

• **Hyperoxaluric calcium nephrolithiasis** is usually due to primary intestinal disorders, including chronic diarrhea, inflammatory bowel disease, or steatorrhea

• **Hypocitraturic calcium nephrolithiasis** is secondary to disorders associated with metabolic acidosis including chronic diarrhea, type I (distal) renal tubular acidosis, and long-term hydrochlorothiazide treatment

• **Uric acid calculi**: Contributing factors include
   — Low urinary pH
   — Myeloproliferative disorders
   — Malignancy with increased uric acid production
   — Abrupt and dramatic weight loss
   — Uricosuric medications

• **Struvite calculi** (magnesium–ammonium–phosphate, "staghorn" calculi)

Table 52-1. Diagnostic criteria of different types of hypercalciuria.

	Absorptive Type I	Absorptive Type II	Absorptive Type III	Resorptive	Renal
Serum					
Calcium	N	N	N	↑	N
Phosphorus	N	N	↓	↓	N
PTH	N	N	N	↑	↑
Vitamin D	N	N	↑	↑	↑
Urinary Calcium					
Fasting	N	N	↑	↑	↑
Restricted	↑	N	↑	↑	↑
After calcium load	↑	↑	↑	↑	↑

PTH, parathyroid hormone; ↑, elevated; ↓, low; N, normal.

— Occur with recurrent urinary tract infections with urease-producing organisms, including *Proteus*, *Pseudomonas*, *Providencia*, and, less commonly, *Klebsiella*, *Staphylococcus,* and *Mycoplasma spp.* (but not *Escherichia coli*)
— Urine pH ≥ 7.2
• **Cystine calculi**: Inherited disorder with recurrent stone disease

4. Symptoms and Signs

• Colicky pain in the flank, usually severe
• Nausea and vomiting
• Patients constantly moving—in sharp contrast to those with an acute abdomen
• Pain episodic and radiates anteriorly over the abdomen
• With stone in the ureter, pain may be referred into the ipsilateral groin
• With stone at the ureterovesical junction, marked urinary urgency and frequency; pain may radiate to the tip of the penis
• After the stone passes into the bladder, there typically is minimal pain with passage through the urethra
• Stone size does not correlate with severity of symptoms

5. Differential Diagnosis

• Cholecystitis
• Appendicitis
• Diverticulitis
• Epididymitis
• Pyelonephritis
• Prostatitis
• Pancreatitis
• Lower lobe pneumonia
• Abdominal aortic aneurysm
• Musculoskeletal pain

6. Laboratory and Imaging Findings

Laboratory Tests
• Urinalysis
— Microscopic or gross hematuria (~90%)
— Absence of microhematuria does not exclude urinary stones
• Urinary pH
— Persistent urinary pH < 5.5 is suggestive of uric acid or cystine stones
— Persistent urinary pH ≥ 7.2 is suggestive of a struvite infection stone
— Urinary pH between 5.5 and 6.8 typically indicates calcium-based stones
• Metabolic evaluation
— Stone analysis on recovered stones
— Patients with uncomplicated first-time stones: serum calcium, electrolytes, and uric acid
— For patients with recurrent stones or patients with a family history of stone disease
  ◦ Sodium intake and animal protein intake should be reduced
  ◦ Adequate fluid should be ingested
  ◦ After these changes have been made, obtain 24-hour urine collection for urinary volume, pH, calcium, uric acid, oxalate, phosphate, sodium, and citrate excretion
— Serum parathyroid hormone, calcium, uric acid, electrolytes (including bicarbonate), and creatinine and blood urea nitrogen should also be obtained

Imaging Studies
• Plain film of the abdomen (KUB, kidney–ureter–bladder) and renal ultrasonography will diagnose most stones
• Spiral CT is often first-line tool in evaluating flank pain

- All stones whether radiopaque or radiolucent on KUB are visible on noncontrast CT, except the rare calculi due to indinavir therapy

7. Treatments

Medications

- **Type I absorptive hypercalciuria**
  - Thiazide diuretics decrease renal calcium excretion (they may lose their hypocalciuric effect after 5 years of continued therapy)
  - Cellulose phosphate, 10 to 15 g in three divided doses given with meals to decrease bowel absorption of calcium
  - Follow-up metabolic surveillance every 6 to 8 months to exclude hypomagnesemia, secondary hyperoxaluria, and recurrent calculi
- **Type II absorptive hypercalciuria**
  - Decrease calcium intake by 50% (to approximately 400 mg once daily)
  - There is no specific medical therapy
- **Type III absorptive hypercalciuria**: orthophosphates (250 mg three times daily) to inhibit vitamin D synthesis
- **Renal hypercalciuria**: thiazides (effective long term)
- **Hyperuricosuric calcium nephrolithiasis**
  - Most cases (85%) can be treated with dietary purine restrictions
  - Those cases not reversed with dietary restriction, allopurinol, 300 mg once daily orally
- **Hyperoxaluric calcium nephrolithiasis**
  - Measures to curtail the diarrhea or steatorrhea
  - Oral calcium supplements with meals
- **Hypocitraturic calcium nephrolithiasis**
  - Potassium citrate, 60 mEq total daily intake, divided either into three times daily as tablets or twice daily as the crystal formulations dissolved in water (it is also available as a solution)
  - Alternatively, oral lemonade has been shown to increase urinary citrate by about 150 mg/24 h
- **Uric acid calculi**
  - Increasing the urinary pH > 6.2 increases uric acid solubility
  - Potassium citrate, 20 mEq (two 10-mEq waxed tablets) three or four times daily or 30 mEq of crystal formulations in water twice daily
  - Patients should monitor their urinary alkalinization with nitrazine pH paper with the goal urinary pH between > 6.2 and < 6.5
  - If hyperuricemia is present, allopurinol, 300 mg once daily orally
- **Struvite calculi**
  - After stone extraction, consider suppressive antibiotics
  - Acetohydroxamic acid, an effective urease inhibitor, is poorly tolerated
- **Cystine calculi**
  - Difficult to manage medically
  - Prevention by increased fluid intake, alkalinization of the urine above pH 7.0 (monitored with nitrazine pH paper), penicillamine, and tiopronin

Surgery

- **Resorptive hypercalciuria, primary hyperparathyroidism**: surgical resection of the parathyroid adenoma
- **Infection with ureteral obstruction**: a medical emergency requiring both antibiotics and prompt drainage by a ureteral catheter or a percutaneous nephrostomy tube
- **Ureteral stones**
  - Stones < 5 to 6 mm in diameter will usually pass spontaneously
  - Active medical expulsive therapy with appropriate pain medications is appropriate for first few weeks

— Medical expulsive therapy (eg, tamsulosin, 0.4 mg orally once daily, plus ibuprofen, 600 mg orally three times per day with a full stomach, with or without a short course of a low-dose oral corticosteroid, [such as prednisone 10 mg orally daily for 3–5 days) increases rate of spontaneous stone passage

— Therapeutic intervention required if spontaneous passage does not occur or if patient has intolerable pain or persistent nausea and vomiting

— Indications for earlier intervention include
   ◦ Severe pain unresponsive to medications
   ◦ Fever
   ◦ Persistent nausea and vomiting requiring intravenous hydration

— Distal ureteral stones: ureteroscopic stone extraction or in situ extracorporeal shock wave lithotripsy (SWL)

— Proximal and midureteral stones can be treated with SWL or ureteroscopic extraction, and a double-J ureteral stent to ensure adequate drainage

- **Renal calculi**
— Conservative observation for patients presenting without pain, urinary tract infections, or obstruction
— Intervention if calculi become symptomatic or grow in size
— For renal stones < 1.5 cm, treat by SWL
— For stones in the inferior calix or those > 3 cm, treat by percutaneous nephrolithotomy
— Perioperative antibiotics as indicated by preoperative urine cultures

Therapeutic Procedures
- Forced intravenous fluid diuresis is not productive and exacerbates pain

8. Outcome

Prevention
- Increased fluid intake to void 1.5 to 2.0 L/d to reduce stone recurrence
- Patients are encouraged to ingest fluids during meals, 2 hours after each meal, prior to going to sleep in the evening, and during the night
- Reduce sodium intake
- Reduce animal protein intake during individual meals

9. When to Refer and When to Admit

When to Refer
- Evidence of urinary obstruction
- Urinary stone with associated flank pain
- Anatomic abnormalities or solitary kidney
- Concomitant pyelonephritis or recurrent infection

When to Admit
- Intractable nausea/vomiting or pain
- Obstructing stone with signs of infection (eg, fever)

SUGGESTED REFERENCES
Gul Z et al. Medical and dietary therapy for kidney stone prevention. Korean *J Urol.* 2014 Dec;55(12):775–779. [PMID: 25512810]

Qaseem A et al. Dietary and pharmacologic management to prevent recurrent nephrolithiasis in adults: a clinical practice guideline from the American College of Physicians. *Ann Intern Med.* 2014 Nov 4;161(9):659–667. [PMID: 25364887]

Richman K et al. The growing prevalence of kidney stones and opportunities for prevention. *R I Med J.* 2014 Dec 2;97(12):31–34. [PMID: 25463625]

Tseng TY et al. Kidney stones. *Clin Evid (Online).* 2011 Nov 10;2011. [PMID: 22075544]

Metabolic Acidosis

53

A 43-year-old man with severe depression is brought into the emergency department after being found collapsed at home. His family states he had been recently despondent and they had not heard from him for 3 days. On physical examination, he is unresponsive and tachypneic with a respiratory rate of 41 breaths/min despite a normal lung examination. His chest radiograph is unremarkable. An arterial blood gas (ABG) shows a pH of 6.93, $Paco_2$ of 20 mm Hg, Pao_2 of 100 mm Hg, and a HCO_3^- of 4 mEq/L. Serum electrolyte tests show an anion gap of 35.

LEARNING OBJECTIVES

▶ Learn the clinical manifestations and objective findings of metabolic acidosis and how the clinical scenario helps elucidate the cause of the acidosis

▶ Understand the factors that predispose to metabolic acidosis

▶ Learn how to calculate the serum anion gap and how to differentiate anion gap metabolic acidosis from nonanion gap metabolic acidosis

▶ Learn how to calculate the urinary anion gap and thus to distinguish gastrointestinal (GI) from renal causes of metabolic acidosis

▶ Learn the treatment for metabolic acidosis depending upon its cause

QUESTIONS

1. What are the salient features of this patient's problem?

2. How do you think through his problem?

3. What are the key features, including essentials of diagnosis and general considerations, of metabolic acidosis?

4. What are the symptoms and signs of metabolic acidosis?

5. What is the differential diagnosis of metabolic acidosis?

6. What are laboratory findings in metabolic acidosis?

7. What are the treatments for metabolic acidosis?

8. What are the outcomes, including complications, prognosis, and prevention, of metabolic acidosis?

9. When should patients with metabolic acidosis be referred to a specialist or admitted to the hospital?

ANSWERS

1. Salient Features

Severe depression with risk for suicide attempt; tachypnea without evidence of lung disease; acidemia with decreased $Paco_2$ and increased anion gap

2. How to Think Through

The emergency department team has obtained the most crucial test for a nonresponsive, tachypneic patient: the ABG. ABG interpretation is complex, and the test is typically obtained during inherently stressful clinical circumstances, necessitating a systematic approach. Is the patient hypoxic? (No.) Is he acidemic or alkalemic? (Acidemic.) Is the primary cause metabolic or respiratory? (Metabolic. He is hyperventilating, effectively reducing the $Paco_2$ well below the normal value of 40 mm Hg.) Is there an anion gap? (Yes, the anion gap is 35.) The disorder can now be named: anion gap metabolic acidosis with compensatory respiratory alkalosis. What is the differential diagnosis of this disorder? (Diabetic or alcoholic ketoacidosis, uremia, lactic acidosis, ethylene glycol or methanol ingestion, salicylate or paraldehyde intoxication, isoniazid or iron overdose.)

The history of depression raises the concern for a suicide attempt by an ingestion. Which of the above should be prioritized and what should be the next diagnostic steps? (An osmol gap would support methanol or ethylene glycol ingestion. A serum salicylate level should also be checked.) What is the treatment for methanol or ethylene glycol ingestion? (Fomepizole, a competitive inhibitor of alcohol dehydrogenase; hemodialysis.)

When ingestion of any substance is suspected, coingestion should be considered (eg, a serum acetaminophen level should always be checked).

3. Key Features

Essentials of Diagnosis

- Metabolic acidosis can be classified as either an increased or normal or decreased anion gap
- Anion gap $= Na^+ - (HCO_3^- + Cl^-)$
- The hallmark of increased anion gap metabolic acidosis is that the low HCO_3^- is associated with normochloremia (normal serum Cl^-), so that the anion gap increases
- In contrast, in a normal (non-) anion gap metabolic acidosis, the low HCO_3^- is associated with hyperchloremia, so that the anion gap remains normal
- A decreased HCO_3^- is seen also in respiratory alkalosis, but the pH distinguishes between the two disorders

General Considerations

- Calculation of the anion gap is useful in determining the cause of the metabolic acidosis
- Normochloremic (increased anion gap) metabolic acidosis
  - Generally results from addition to the blood of organic acids such as lactate, acetoacetate, β-hydroxybutyrate, and exogenous toxins
  - Uremia produces an increased anion gap metabolic acidosis via unexcreted organic acids and anions

4. Symptoms and Signs

- Symptoms are mainly those of the underlying disorder
- Compensatory hyperventilation may be misinterpreted as a primary respiratory disorder
- When severe, Kussmaul respirations (deep, regular, and sighing respirations indicating intense stimulation of the respiratory center) occur

5. Differential Diagnosis

Etiology of Increased Anion Gap Metabolic Acidosis

- Lactic acidosis
  - Type A: cardiogenic, septic, or hemorrhagic shock; carbon monoxide or cyanide poisoning

— Type B: metabolic causes (eg, diabetes mellitus, ketoacidosis, liver disease, kidney disease, infection, leukemia, or lymphoma); toxins (eg, ethanol, methanol, salicylates, isoniazid, or metformin); nucleoside analog reverse transcriptase inhibitors
• Diabetic ketoacidosis
• Alcoholic ketoacidosis
  — Acid–base disorders in alcoholism are frequently mixed (10% have triple acid–base disorder)
  — Three types of metabolic acidoses: ketoacidosis, lactic acidosis, and hyperchloremic acidosis from bicarbonate loss in urine from ketonuria
  — Metabolic alkalosis from volume contraction and vomiting
  — Respiratory alkalosis from alcohol withdrawal, pain, sepsis, or liver disease
• Uremic acidosis (usually at glomerular filtration rate < 15–30 mL/min)
• Ethylene glycol toxicity
• Methanol toxicity
• Salicylate toxicity (mixed metabolic acidosis with respiratory alkalosis)

Etiology of Normal (Non-) Anion Gap Metabolic Acidosis
• Most common causes of nonanion gap acidosis
  — Gastrointestinal (GI) HCO_3^- loss
  — Defects in renal acidification (renal tubular acidoses)

Renal Tubular Acidosis (RTA)
• Hyperchloremic acidosis with a normal anion gap and normal or near normal glomerular filtration rate, in the absence of diarrhea
• Three major types of RTA can be differentiated by the clinical setting: urinary pH, urinary anion gap (see below), serum K^+ level
• **Type I (distal H^+ secretion defect)**
  — Due to selective deficiency in H^+ secretion in the distal nephron
  — Low serum K^+
  — Despite acidosis, urinary pH cannot be acidified (urine pH > 5.5)
  — Associated with autoimmune disease, hypercalcemia
• **Type II (proximal HCO_3^- reabsorption defect)**
  — Due to a selective defect in the proximal tubule's ability to adequately reabsorb filtered HCO_3^-
  — Low serum K^+
  — Urine pH < 5.5
  — Associated with multiple myeloma and nephrotoxic drugs
• **Type IV (hyporeninemic hypoaldosteronism)**
  — Only RTA characterized by hyperkalemic, hyperchloremic acidosis
  — Defect is aldosterone deficiency or antagonism, which impairs distal nephron Na^+ reabsorption and K^+ and H^+ excretion
  — Urine pH < 5.5
  — Renal salt wasting is frequently present
  — Most common in diabetic nephropathy, tubulointerstitial renal diseases, acquired immunodeficiency syndrome, and hypertensive nephrosclerosis

6. Laboratory Findings

Laboratory Tests
• See Tables 53-1 and 53-2
• Blood pH, serum HCO_3^-, and P_{CO_2} are decreased
• Anion gap is increased (normochloremic), normal or decreased (hyperchloremic)
• Hyperkalemia may be seen
• In lactic acidosis, lactate levels are at least 4 to 5 mEq/L but commonly 10 to 30 mEq/L
• The diagnosis of alcoholic ketoacidosis is supported by the absence of a diabetic history and no evidence of glucose intolerance after initial therapy

Table 53-1. Primary acid–base disorders and expected compensation.

Disorder	Primary Defect	Compensatory Response	Magnitude of Compensation
Respiratory acidosis			
Acute	$\uparrow P_{CO_2}$	$\uparrow HCO_3^-$	$\uparrow HCO_3^-$ 1 mEq/L per 10 mm Hg $\uparrow P_{CO_2}$
Chronic	$\uparrow P_{CO_2}$	$\uparrow HCO_3^-$	$\uparrow HCO_3^-$ 3.5 mEq/L per 10 mm Hg $\uparrow P_{CO_2}$
Respiratory alkalosis			
Acute	$\downarrow P_{CO_2}$	$\downarrow HCO_3^-$	$\downarrow HCO_3^-$ 2 mEq/L per 10 mm Hg $\downarrow P_{CO_2}$
Chronic	$\downarrow P_{CO_2}$	$\downarrow HCO_3^-$	$\downarrow HCO_3^-$ 5 mEq/L per 10 mm Hg $\downarrow P_{CO_2}$
Metabolic acidosis	$\downarrow HCO_3^-$	$\downarrow P_{CO_2}$	$\downarrow P_{CO_2}$ 1.3 mm Hg per 1 mEq/L $\downarrow HCO_3^-$
Metabolic alkalosis	$\uparrow HCO_3^-$	$\uparrow P_{CO_2}$	$\uparrow P_{CO_2}$ 0.7 mm Hg per 1 mEq/L $\uparrow HCO_3^-$

- Urinary anion gap from a random urine sample (urine $[Na^+ + K^+] - Cl^-$) reflects the ability of the kidney to excrete NH_4Cl as in the following equation:
  — $Na^+ + K^+ + NH_4^+ = Cl^- + 80$

  where 80 is the average value for the difference in the urinary anions and cations other than Na^+, K^+, NH_4^+, and Cl^-
- Urinary anion gap is equal to $80 - NH_4^+$; this gap aids in the distinction between GI and renal causes of hyperchloremic (normal or non-anion gap) acidosis
  — If the cause of the metabolic acidosis is GI
    ◦ HCO_3^- loss (diarrhea) is responsible
    ◦ Renal acidification ability remains normal
    ◦ NH_4Cl excretion increases in response to the acidosis
    ◦ Urinary anion gap is negative (eg, −30 mEq/L)
  — If the cause is distal RTA
    ◦ The kidney is unable to excrete H^+ and thus unable to increase NH_4Cl excretion
    ◦ Therefore, urinary anion gap is positive (eg, +25 mEq/L)
  — In type II (proximal) RTA
    ◦ The kidney has defective HCO_3^- reabsorption, leading to increased HCO_3^- excretion rather than decreased NH_4Cl excretion
    ◦ Thus, the urinary anion gap is often negative
- Urinary pH may not as readily differentiate between renal and GI etiologies

Table 53-2. Hyperchloremic, normal anion gap metabolic acidoses.

	Renal Defect	Serum [K⁺]	Distal H⁺ Secretion — Urinary NH₄⁺ Plus Minimal Urine pH	Titratable Acid	Urinary Anion Gap	Treatment
Gastrointestinal HCO_3^- loss	None	$\downarrow$	< 5.5	$\uparrow\uparrow$	Negative	Na^+, K^+, and HCO_3^- as required
Renal tubular acidosis						
I. Classic distal	Distal H^+ secretion	$\downarrow$	> 5.5	$\downarrow$	Positive	$NaHCO_3$ (1–3 mEq/kg/d)
II. Proximal secretion	Proximal H^+	$\downarrow$	< 5.5	Normal	Positive	$NaHCO_3$ or $KHCO_3$ (10–15 mEq/kg/d), thiazide
IV. Hyporeninemic hypoaldosteronism	Distal Na^+ reabsorption, K^+ secretion, and H^+ secretion	$\uparrow$	< 5.5	$\downarrow$	Positive	Fludrocortisone (0.1–0.5 mg/d), dietary K^+ restriction, furosemide (40–160 mg/d), $NaHCO_3$ (1–3 mEq/kg/d)

Modified and reproduced, with permission, from Cogan MG. *Fluid and Electrolytes: Physiology and Pathophysiology*. McGraw-Hill, 1991.

7. Treatments

Medications

- Supplemental HCO_3^- is indicated for treatment of hyperkalemia but is controversial for treatment of increased anion gap metabolic acidosis
- Administration of large amounts of HCO_3^- may have deleterious effects, including
  — Hypernatremia
  — Hyperosmolality
  — Volume overload
  — Worsening of intracellular acidosis
- In salicylate intoxication, alkali therapy must be started (unless blood pH is already alkalinized by respiratory alkalosis), because the increment in pH converts salicylate to more impermeable salicylic acid and thus prevents central nervous system damage
- The amount of HCO_3^- deficit can be calculated as follows
  — Amount of HCO_3^- deficit $= 0.5 \times$ body weight $\times (24 - HCO_3^-)$
  — Half of the calculated deficit should be administered within the first 3 to 4 hours to avoid overcorrection and volume overload
- In methanol intoxication, inhibition of alcohol dehydrogenase (the enzyme that metabolizes methanol to formaldehyde) by fomepizole is the standard of care; though ethanol is a competitive substrate for alcohol dehydrogenase and can also be administered
- Treatment of RTA is mainly achieved by administration of alkali (either as bicarbonate or citrate) to correct metabolic abnormalities and prevent nephrocalcinosis and chronic kidney disease
- Large amounts of alkali (10–15 mEq/kg/d) may be required to treat proximal RTA because most of the alkali is excreted into the urine, which exacerbates hypokalemia
- Thus, a mixture of sodium and potassium salts is preferred
- The addition of thiazides may reduce the amount of alkali required, but hypokalemia may develop
- Correction of type 1 distal RTA requires
  — Less alkali (1–3 mEq/kg/d) than proximal RTA
  — Potassium supplementation as necessary
- For the treatment of type IV RTA
  — Dietary potassium restriction may be needed and potassium-retaining drugs should be withdrawn
  — Fludrocortisone may be effective in cases with hypoaldosteronism, but should be used with care, preferably in combination with loop diuretics
  — In some cases, oral alkali supplementation (1–3 mEq/kg/d) may be required

Therapeutic Procedures

- Treatment is aimed at the underlying disorder, such as insulin and volume resuscitation to restore tissue perfusion
- Lactate will later be metabolized to produce HCO_3^- and increase pH

8. Outcomes

Complications

- In type IV RTA, the hyperkalemia can be exacerbated by drugs, including
  — Angiotensin-converting enzyme inhibitors
  — Aldosterone receptor blockers, such as spironolactone
  — Nonsteroidal anti-inflammatory drugs

Prognosis

- The mortality rate of lactic acidosis exceeds 50%

Prevention

- To prevent lactic acidosis, avoid metformin use if there is tissue hypoxia or acute kidney injury

- Acute kidney injury can occur rarely with the use of radiocontrast agents in patients receiving metformin therapy; metformin should be temporarily halted on the day of the test and for 2 days after injection of radiocontrast agents to avoid potential lactic acidosis if renal failure occurs

9. When to Refer and When to Admit

When to Refer

- Most clinicians will refer patients with renal tubular acidoses to a nephrologist for evaluation and possible alkali therapy

When to Admit

- Because of the high mortality rate, all patients with lactic acidosis should be admitted
- Other patients with significant metabolic acidosis are almost always admitted, particularly those resulting from diabetic ketoacidosis, alcoholic ketoacidosis, uremic acidosis, or ethylene glycol, methanol, or salicylate toxicity

SUGGESTED REFERENCES

Emmett M. Acetaminophen toxicity and 5-oxoproline (pyroglutamic acid): a tale of two cycles, one an ATP-depleting futile cycle and the other a useful cycle. *Clin J Am Soc Nephrol.* 2014 Jan;9(1):191–200. [PMID: 24235282]

Kraut JA et al. Differential diagnosis of nongap metabolic acidosis: value of a systematic approach. *Clin J Am Soc Nephrol.* 2012 Apr;7(4):671–679. [PMID: 22403272]

Kraut JA et al. The serum anion gap in the evaluation of acid-base disorders: what are its limitations and can its effectiveness be improved? *Clin J Am Soc Nephrol.* 2013 Nov;8(11):2018–2024. [PMID: 23833313]

Rice M et al. Approach to metabolic acidosis in the emergency department. *Emerg Med Clin North Am.* 2014 May;32(2):403–420. [PMID: 24766940]

Vichot AA et al. Use of anion gap in the evaluation of a patient with metabolic acidosis. *Am J Kidney Dis.* 2014 Oct;64(4):653–657. [PMID: 25132207]

Nephrotic Syndrome

54

A 40-year-old woman with Hodgkin lymphoma is admitted to the hospital because of anasarca. She has no known history of renal, liver, or cardiac disease. Her serum creatinine level is slightly elevated at 1.4 mg/dL. Serum albumin level is 2.8 g/dL. Liver test results are normal. Urinalysis demonstrates no red or white blood cell casts, but 4+ protein is noted and a 24-hour urine collection shows a protein excretion of 4 g/24 h. She is diagnosed with nephrotic syndrome, and renal biopsy suggests minimal change disease (MCD). Corticosteroids and diuretics are instituted, with gradual improvement of edema. Her hospital course is complicated by a deep venous thrombosis of the left calf and thigh that requires anticoagulation.

LEARNING OBJECTIVES

▶ Learn the clinical manifestations and objective findings of nephrotic syndrome
▶ Understand the most common lesions that cause nephrotic syndrome
▶ Know the differential diagnosis of nephrotic syndrome
▶ Learn the treatments for nephrotic syndrome and which patients need renal biopsy
▶ Know the complications associated with nephrotic syndrome

QUESTIONS

1. What are the salient features of this patient's problem?
2. How do you think through her problem?
3. What are the key features, including essentials of diagnosis and general considerations, of nephrotic syndrome?
4. What are the symptoms and signs of nephrotic syndrome?
5. What is the differential diagnosis of nephrotic syndrome?
6. What are laboratory and procedural findings in nephrotic syndrome?
7. What are the treatments for nephrotic syndrome?
8. What are the outcomes, including complications and prognosis, of nephrotic syndrome?
9. When should patients with nephrotic syndrome be referred to a specialist or admitted to the hospital?

ANSWERS

1. Salient Features

Anasarca; elevated serum creatinine; hypoalbuminemia; bland urine sediment; proteinuria > 3 g/d; renal biopsy showing MCD; resolution with corticosteroid therapy; associated thrombosis from hypercoagulability

2. How to Think Through

The urinalysis is an important tool for recognizing possible nephritic or nephrotic syndromes in a patient with new edema. What is the criterion for nephrotic range proteinuria? (> 3.5 g/d.) Along with proteinuria, what are the other components of nephrotic syndrome? (Hypoalbuminemia < 3.0 g/dL; anasarca, including periorbital edema, pulmonary edema, and pleural effusion; hyperlipidemia with fat bodies in the urine; thrombophilia.) Acute kidney injury (AKI) does not always accompany nephrotic syndrome and a normal serum creatinine should not halt investigation.

What are the four most common causes of nephrotic syndrome? (MCD; membranous nephropathy [MN]; focal glomerular glomerulosclerosis; membranoproliferative glomerulonephropathy [MPGN].) What common medications may precipitate nephrotic syndrome, mimic MCD, and increase the chance of AKI? (Nonsteroidal anti-inflammatory drugs.) Patients with nephrotic syndrome have impaired immune defenses, and a significant fraction have a thrombotic event. While the pathophysiology of these phenomena are not fully understood, urinary loss of proteins (immunoglobulin G, antithrombin [AT] and plasminogen likely plays a role in both.)

Was renal biopsy needed in this case? (Yes. Diabetic nephropathy is sometimes presumed in a diabetic patient. In this case, a firm diagnosis is needed to choose the correct treatment pathway.) With the biopsy result, how should she be managed? (Corticosteroid treatment leads to remission in the vast majority of cases of MCD, and it is tapered over several months. Also, treat with a diuretic, angiotensin-converting enzyme [ACE] inhibitor, warfarin, low-sodium diet.)

3. Key Features

Essentials of Diagnosis

- Bland urine sediment with few if any cells or casts
- Proteinuria > 3 g/d
- Serum albumin < 3 g/dL
- Edema
- Hyperlipidemia is typical
- Oval fat bodies in the urine

General Considerations

- One-third of patients will have a systemic disease such as diabetes mellitus (DM), amyloidosis, or systemic lupus erythematosus (SLE)
- Four most common lesions (Table 54-1)
  — MCD
  — MN
  — Focal glomerular glomerulosclerosis
  — MPGN

4. Symptoms and Signs

- Peripheral edema with serum albumin < 3 g/dL
- Edema is initially dependent, but may become generalized and include periorbital edema
- Dyspnea caused by pulmonary edema, pleural effusions, and diaphragmatic compromise with ascites

Table 54-1. Classification and findings in glomerulonephritis: Nephrotic spectrum presentations.

Disease	Typical Presentation	Association/Notes
Minimal change disease (nil disease; lipoid nephrosis) (MCD)	Child with sudden onset of full nephrotic syndrome	Children: associated with allergy or viral infection Adults: associated with Hodgkin disease, NSAIDs
Membranous nephropathy (MN)	Anywhere in nephrotic spectrum, but nephrotic syndrome not uncommon; particular predisposition to hypercoagulable state	Primary (idiopathic) MN may be associated with antibodies to PLA_2R Associated with non-Hodgkin lymphoma, carcinoma (gastrointestinal, renal, bronchogenic, thyroid), gold therapy, penicillamine, SLE, chronic hepatitis B or C infection
Focal and segmental glomerulosclerosis	Anywhere in nephrotic spectrum; children with congenital disease have nephrotic syndrome	Children: congenital disease with podocyte gene mutation, or in spectrum of disease with minimal change disease Adults: Associated with heroin abuse, HIV infection, reflux nephropathy, obesity, pamidronate, podocyte protein mutations
Membranoproliferative glomerulonephropathy (MPGN)	Can present with nephrotic syndrome, but usually with nephritic features as well (glomerular hematuria)	Most patients are < 30 years old Type I most common Type II (dense deposit disease) associated with C3 nephritic factor Low complement levels
Amyloidosis	Anywhere in nephrotic spectrum	AL: plasma cell dyscrasia with Ig light chain overproduction and deposition; check SPEP and UPEP AA: serum amyloid protein A overproduction and deposition in response to chronic inflammatory disease (rheumatoid arthritis, inflammatory bowel disease, chronic infection)
Diabetic nephropathy	High GFR (hyperfiltration)→microalbuminuria→frank proteinuria→decline in GFR	Diabetes diagnosis precedes nephropathy diagnosis by years
HIV-associated nephropathy	Heavy proteinuria, often nephrotic syndrome, progresses to ESRD relatively quickly	Usually seen in antiviral treatment-naïve patients (rare in HAART era), predilection for those of African descent (*APOL1* mutation)

ESRD, end-stage renal disease; GFR, glomerular filtration rate; HAART, highly active antiretroviral therapy; NSAIDs, nonsteroidal anti-inflammatory drugs; PLA_2R, phospholipase A2 receptor; SLE, systemic lupus erythematosus; SPEP/UPEP: serum and urine protein electrophoresis.

- Abdominal distention from ascites
- Increased susceptibility to infection because of urinary loss of immunoglobulins and complement
- Increased risk of venous thrombosis secondary to urinary loss of anticoagulant factors

Etiologies
- DM
- Lupus nephritis
- Amyloidosis
- HIV-associated nephropathy
- Multiple myeloma
- Idiopathic
  — MCD
  — MN
  — Focal segmental glomerulosclerosis
  — MPGN

5. Differential Diagnosis
- Heart failure
- Cirrhosis
- Venous insufficiency

- Protein-losing enteropathy
- Malnutrition
- Hypothyroidism

6. Laboratory and Procedural Findings

Laboratory Tests

- Serum creatinine may or may not be abnormal at time of presentation depending on severity and chronicity of disease
- Urinalysis: proteinuria; few cellular elements or casts
- Oval fat bodies appear as "grape clusters" under light microscopy and "Maltese crosses" under polarized light
- Serum albumin < 3 g/dL, serum total protein < 6 g/dL
- Urine spot protein-to-creatinine ratio gives an approximation of grams of protein excreted per day
- Elevated hemoglobin A_{1C} in diabetics
- Hyperlipidemia
- Elevated erythrocyte sedimentation rate
- Obtain serum complement levels, serum and urine protein electrophoresis, antinuclear antibodies, and serologic tests for hepatitis (as indicated)

Diagnostic Procedures

- Renal biopsy indicated in adults with new-onset idiopathic nephrotic syndrome if a primary renal disease is suspected that may require drug therapy
- If creatinine levels are high, damage may be irreversible, making kidney biopsy less useful
- In the setting of long-standing diabetes mellitus, renal biopsy is rarely performed unless there is reason to suspect a different etiology

7. Treatments

Medications

- Loop and thiazide diuretics in combination—often requiring large doses
- ACE inhibitors and angiotensin receptor blockers (ARBs) (except in the setting of AKI)
- Combination ACE inhibitor and ARB therapy is not supported by the evidence
- Antilipidemic agents; avoid combining gemfibrozil with statins since the combination increases risk for rhabdomyolysis, especially in patients with chronic kidney disease (CKD)
- Glucose and blood pressure control in diabetic nephropathy
- Corticosteroids, cytotoxic agents as indicated for primary renal lesion
- Patients with frequent relapses may require cyclophosphamide or rituximab
- Patients are hypercoagulable from urinary loss of AT, protein C, and protein S. Treat all patients with thrombosis with warfarin for at least 3 to 6 months; recurrent thrombosis requires lifelong anticoagulation

Therapeutic Procedures

- In those with subnephrotic proteinuria or mild nephrotic syndrome, dietary protein restriction may be helpful in slowing progression of renal disease
- In those with very heavy proteinuria (> 10 g/d), protein malnutrition may occur and daily protein intake should replace daily urinary protein losses
- Salt restriction helps edema

8. Outcomes

Complications

- Increased infections from immunoglobulin loss
- Thrombosis from associated hypercoagulability
- CKD

Prognosis

• Depends on underlying renal pathology

9. When to Refer and When to Admit

When to Refer

• Any patient noted to have nephrotic syndrome should be referred immediately to a nephrologist for aggressive volume and blood pressure management, assessment for renal biopsy, and treatment of the underlying disease. Proteinuria of > 1 g/d without the nephrotic syndrome also merits nephrology referral, though with less urgency.

When to Admit

• Patients with edema refractory to outpatient therapy or rapidly worsening kidney function that may require inpatient interventions should be admitted.

SUGGESTED REFERENCES

Barbano B. Thrombosis in nephrotic syndrome. *Semin Thromb Hemost.* 2013 Jul;39(5):469–476. [PMID: 23625754]

Cadnapaphornchai MA et al. The nephrotic syndrome: pathogenesis and treatment of edema formation and secondary complications. *Pediatr Nephrol.* 2014 Jul;29(7):1159–1167. [PMID: 23989393]

Gbadegesin RA et al. Genetic testing in nephrotic syndrome—challenges and opportunities. *Nat Rev Nephrol.* 2013 Mar;9(3):179–184. [PMID: 23321566]

Glassock RJ. Attending rounds: an older patient with nephrotic syndrome. *Clin J Am Soc Nephrol.* 2012 Apr;7(4):665–670. [PMID: 22403277]

Glassock RJ et al. Nephrotic syndrome redux. *Nephrol Dial Transplant.* 2015 Jan;30(1):12–17. [PMID: 24723546]

Sharma SG et al. The modern spectrum of renal biopsy findings in patients with diabetes. *Clin J Am Soc Nephrol.* 2013 Oct;8(10):1718–1724. [PMID: 23886566]

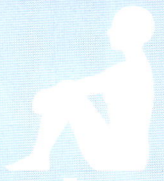
Skin Disorders

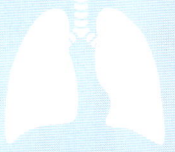
Pulmonary/Ear, Nose, & Throat Disorders

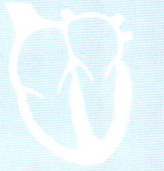
Heart/Hypertension/Lipid Disorders

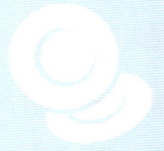
Hematologic Disorders

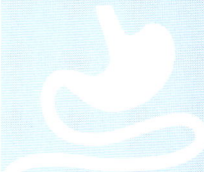
Gastrointestinal/Liver/Pancreas Disorders

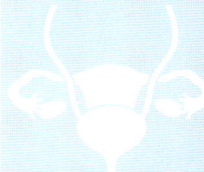
Gynecologic/Urologic Disorders

Musculoskeletal Disorders

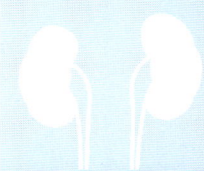
Kidney/Electrolyte Disorders

Nervous System/Psychiatric Disorders

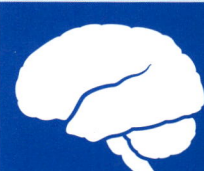

Endocrine/Metabolic Disorders

Infectious Disorders

55

Altered Mental Status

An 82-year-old woman with mild dementia is hospitalized in the intensive care unit (ICU) for urosepsis and treated with intravenous antibiotics. On hospital day 3, despite improvement of her sepsis, she becomes acutely confused. Her other medications include opioids for pain and diphenhydramine for insomnia. On physical examination, she is alert and can remember her name, but has poor attention and believes that she is in a grocery store and that the year is 1952. Her neurologic examination is otherwise normal. She appears agitated and has been aggressive with the nursing staff. On subsequent examination later in the day, her symptoms are significantly better.

LEARNING OBJECTIVES

▶ Learn the clinical manifestations and objective findings of altered mental status (AMS) and how to distinguish delirium, stupor, and coma

▶ Understand the factors that predispose to the development of delirium

▶ Know the differential diagnosis of AMS

▶ Learn the emergency treatment for acute AMS

▶ Know how to treat delirium due to alcohol withdrawal and other medical causes

▶ Understand how to prognosticate early in the course of coma

QUESTIONS

1. What are the salient features of this patient's problem?

2. How do you think through her problem?

3. What are the key features, including essentials of diagnosis and general considerations, of AMS?

4. What are the symptoms and signs of AMS?

5. What is the differential diagnosis of AMS?

6. What are laboratory, imaging, and procedural findings in AMS?

7. What are the treatments for AMS?

8. What is the outcome, including prognosis, of AMS?

9. When should patients with AMS be referred to a specialist or admitted to the hospital?

ANSWERS

1. Salient Features

Elderly woman with underlying dementia; ICU admission; confusion despite appropriate treatment of underlying disease; opioid and anticholinergic use; disoriented with poor attention; nonfocal neurologic examination; agitation; waxing and waning course

2. How to Think Through

AMS is common among patients, disarming for clinicians, and alarming to families. A patient in the emergency room with AMS requires a broad diagnostic approach. We have more information about this hospitalized patient. What is the term for her constellation of features? (Delirium.) What are the defining features of delirium? How is attention assessed? (Serial 7s or spelling WORLD backward.)

What are common risk factors that predispose patients to delirium? (Baseline cognitive impairment, older age, severe illness, pain, presence of a Foley catheter, use of restraints, and polypharmacy.) What are the three most common medicine classes that contribute to delirium in the elderly? (Benzodiazepines, opioids, and anticholinergics.)

How should this patient be managed? (Discontinue medications with central nervous system [CNS] activity where possible. Nonpharmacologic interventions are the mainstay: frequent reorientation of patient; family involvement; darkness and quiet at night, minimizing vital signs and other disruptions; manual tasks for distraction during daytime. Use of neuroleptic medications is controversial [due to increased mortality] and so is limited to patients with agitation that places them at risk of harm or that causes distress.)

3. Key Features

Essentials of Diagnosis
- AMS broadly refers to a change in level of consciousness, sensorium, memory, and/or attention and can include delirium or acute confusional state, psychosis, stupor, and coma
- Delirium is an acute, fluctuating disturbance of consciousness, associated with a change in cognition or development of perceptual disturbances, is typically precipitated by a systemic problem (eg, drugs, infection, hypoxemia, or metabolic derangement) in the setting of underlying risk factors (causes are listed in Table 55-1)
- Delirium is defined as (1) acute onset and fluctuating course and (2) inattention and either (3) disorganized thinking or (4) altered level of consciousness
- Stuporous patients respond only to repeated vigorous stimuli
- Comatose patients are unarousable and unresponsive

General Considerations
- Delirium can coexist with dementia and should be considered a syndrome of acute brain dysfunction analogous to acute kidney injury
- Delirium features can be quickly assessed using the 3D-CAM tool and the CAM-S tool is useful in assessing delirium severity
- Terminal delirium occurs commonly at the end of life
  — May be related to multiple medical causes, including organ failure
  — May be unrecognized
- Coma is a major complication of serious CNS disorders and can result from seizures, hypothermia, metabolic disturbances, or structural lesions causing bilateral cerebral hemispheric dysfunction or a disturbance of the brainstem reticular activating system
- A mass lesion involving one cerebral hemisphere may cause coma by compressing the brainstem
- Abrupt onset of coma suggests
  — Subarachnoid hemorrhage (SAH)
  — Brainstem stroke
  — Intracerebral hemorrhage (ICH)

Table 55-1. Etiology of delirium and other cognitive disorders.

Disorder	Possible Causes
Intoxication	Alcohol, sedatives, bromides, analgesics (eg, pentazocine), psychedelic drugs, stimulants, and household solvents
Drug withdrawal	Withdrawal from alcohol, sedative-hypnotics, corticosteroids
Long-term effects of alcohol	Wernicke–Korsakoff syndrome
Infections	Septicemia; meningitis and encephalitis due to bacterial, viral, fungal, parasitic, or tuberculous organisms or to central nervous system syphilis; acute and chronic infections due to the entire range of microbiologic pathogens
Endocrine disorders	Thyrotoxicosis, hypothyroidism, adrenocortical dysfunction (including Addison disease and Cushing syndrome), pheochromocytoma, insulinoma, hypoglycemia, hyperparathyroidism, hypoparathyroidism, panhypopituitarism, diabetic ketoacidosis
Respiratory disorders	Hypoxia, hypercapnia
Metabolic disturbances	Fluid and electrolyte disturbances (especially hyponatremia, hypomagnesemia, and hypercalcemia), acid–base disorders, hepatic disease (hepatic encephalopathy), kidney failure, porphyria
Nutritional deficiencies	Deficiency of vitamin B_1 (beriberi), vitamin B_{12} (pernicious anemia), folic acid, nicotinic acid (pellagra); protein–calorie malnutrition
Trauma	Subdural hematoma, subarachnoid hemorrhage, intracerebral bleeding, concussion syndrome
Cardiovascular disorders	Myocardial infarctions, cardiac arrhythmias, cerebrovascular spasms, hypertensive encephalopathy, hemorrhages, embolisms, and occlusions indirectly causing decreased cognitive function
Cancer and other neoplasms	Primary or metastatic lesions of the central nervous system, malignant hypercalcemia
Seizure disorders	Ictal, interictal, and postictal dysfunction
Collagen-vascular and immunologic disorders	Autoimmun disorders, including systemic lupus erythematosus, Sjögren syndrome, and AIDS
Degenerative neurologic diseases	Alzheimer disease, Pick disease, multiple sclerosis, parkinsonism, Huntington chorea, normal pressure hydrocephalus
Medications	Anticholinergic medications, antidepressants, H_2-blocking agents, digoxin, salicylates (long-term use), and a wide variety of other over-the-counter and prescribed medications

- A slower onset and progression of coma occur with other structural or mass lesions; a metabolic cause is likely with a preceding intoxicated state or agitated delirium

Demographics
- Alcohol or substance withdrawal is the most common cause of delirium in the general hospital

4. Symptoms and Signs

- Level of consciousness, attention, and cognition
  — Delirium onset is usually rapid, there is a marked deficit of memory and recall, and anxiety and irritability are common
  — The mental status in delirium fluctuates (impairment is usually least in the morning), with varying inability to concentrate, maintain attention, and sustain purposeful behavior
  — "Sundowning"—mild-to-moderate delirium at night
    ◦ More common in patients with preexisting dementia
    ◦ May be precipitated by hospitalization, drugs, and sensory deprivation
  — Amnesia is retrograde (impaired recall of past memories) and anterograde (inability to recall events after the onset of the delirium)
  — Orientation problems follow the inability to retain information
  — Perceptual disturbances (often visual hallucinations) and psychomotor restlessness with insomnia are common
  — Autonomic changes include tachycardia, dilated pupils, and sweating
  — Physical findings vary according to the cause

- Response to painful stimuli in patients with altered mental status
  - Purposive limb withdrawal from painful stimuli implies that sensory pathways from and motor pathways to the stimulated limb are functionally intact
  - Unilateral absence of responses to stimuli to both sides of the body implies
    - A corticospinal lesion
  - Bilateral absence of responses suggests brainstem involvement
    - Bilateral pyramidal tract lesions
    - Psychogenic unresponsiveness
  - Decorticate posturing occurs
    - With lesions of the internal capsule and rostral cerebral peduncle
    - With dysfunction or destruction of the midbrain and rostral pons
    - In the arms accompanied by flaccidity or slight flexor responses in the legs in patients with extensive brainstem damage extending down to the pons at the trigeminal level
- Pupillary response
  - Hypothalamic disease processes may lead to unilateral Horner syndrome
  - Bilateral diencephalic involvement or destructive pontine lesions leads to small but reactive pupils
  - Ipsilateral pupillary dilation with no response to light occurs with compression of the third cranial nerve, eg, with uncal herniation
  - Pupils are slightly smaller than normal but responsive to light in many metabolic encephalopathies
  - Pupils may be fixed and dilated following overdosage with atropine or scopolamine
  - Pupils may be pinpoint (but responsive) with opioids
  - Pupillary dilation for several hours after cardiopulmonary arrest implies a poor prognosis
- Eye movements
  - Conjugate deviation to the side suggests the presence of an ipsilateral hemispheric lesion or a contralateral pontine lesion
  - A mesencephalic lesion leads to downward conjugate deviation
  - Dysconjugate ocular deviation in coma implies a structural brainstem lesion (or preexisting strabismus)
- Oculomotor responses to passive head turning
  - In response to brisk rotation, flexion, and extension of the head, conscious patients with open eyes do not exhibit contraversive conjugate eye deviation (doll's head eye response) unless there is voluntary visual fixation or bilateral frontal pathology
  - With cortical depression in lightly comatose patients, a brisk doll's head eye response is seen
  - With brainstem lesions, this oculocephalic reflex becomes impaired or lost, depending on the lesion site
- Oculovestibular reflex
  - Tested by caloric stimulation using irrigation with ice water
  - In normal persons, jerk nystagmus is elicited for about 2 or 3 minutes, with the slow component toward the irrigated ear
  - In unconscious patients with an intact brainstem, the fast component of the nystagmus disappears, so that the eyes tonically deviate toward the irrigated side for 2 to 3 minutes before returning to their original position
  - With impairment of brainstem function, the response is perverted and disappears
  - In metabolic coma, oculocephalic and oculovestibular reflex responses are preserved, at least initially
- Respiratory patterns
  - Cheyne–Stokes respiration may occur with bihemispheric or diencephalic disease or in metabolic disorders
  - Hyperventilation occurs with lesions of the brainstem tegmentum
  - Apneustic breathing (prominent end-inspiratory pauses) suggests damage at the pontine level

— Atactic breathing (completely irregular pattern, with deep and shallow breaths occurring randomly): associated with lesions of the lower pons (pontine tegmentum) and medulla

5. Differential Diagnosis

- Drugs
  - Opioids
  - Alcohol
  - Sedatives
  - Antipsychotics
- Metabolic
  - Hypoxia
  - Hypoglycemia or hyperglycemia
  - Hypercalcemia
  - Hyponatremia or hypernatremia
  - Uremia
  - Hepatic encephalopathy
  - Hypothyroidism or hyperthyroidism
  - Vitamin B_{12} or thiamine deficiency
  - Carbon monoxide poisoning
  - Wilson disease
- Infectious
  - Meningitis
  - Encephalitis
  - Bacteremia
  - Urinary tract infections
  - Pneumonia
  - Neurosyphilis
- Environmental
  - Hypothermia
  - Heat stroke
- Psychiatric
  - Schizophrenia
  - Depression
  - ICU psychosis
- Neurovascular
  - Stroke
  - SAH
  - Hypertensive encephalopathy
  - CNS vasculitis
  - Thrombotic thrombocytopenic purpura
  - Disseminated intravascular coagulation
  - Hyperviscosity
- Other neurologic disorders
  - Space-occupying lesion, eg, brain tumor, subdural hematoma, hydrocephalus
  - Seizure
  - Brain death
  - Persistent vegetative state
  - Locked-in syndrome

6. Laboratory, Imaging, and Procedural Findings

Laboratory Tests

- Comprehensive physical examination including a search for neurologic abnormalities, infection, or hypoxia

- Routine laboratory tests may include
  — Serum electrolytes
  — Serum glucose
  — Serum creatinine and blood urea nitrogen
  — Liver tests
  — Thyroid function tests
  — Arterial blood gases
  — Complete blood count
  — Serum calcium, phosphorus, magnesium, vitamin B_{12}, folate
  — Blood cultures
  — Urinalysis
  — Cerebrospinal fluid analysis
- See Table 55-1

Imaging Studies
- Urgent noncontrast computed tomography (CT) scanning of the head to identify
  — ICH
  — Brain herniation
  — Structural (mass) lesion
- Electroencephalography (EEG) may be helpful for identifying seizures and generalized slowing of delirium and metabolic encephalopathy
- Magnetic resonance imaging can help identify abnormalities not seen on CT

Diagnostic Procedures
- The diagnostic workup of the comatose patient must proceed concomitantly with management
- Lumbar puncture (if CT scan reveals no structural lesion) to exclude SAH or meningitis

7. Treatments

Medications
- The aim of treatment is to identify and correct the underlying causal medical problem
- Discontinue nonessential drugs that may be contributing to the problem, such as
  — Analgesics
  — Corticosteroids
  — Cimetidine
  — Lidocaine
  — Anticholinergic drugs
  — CNS depressants
  — Mefloquine
- Two indications for medication in delirious states
  — Behavioral control (eg, pulling out lines)
  — Subjective distress (eg, pronounced fear due to hallucinations)
  — If these indications are present, antipsychotic agents (eg, haloperidol, 0.5–1 mg orally, or quetiapine, 25 mg orally, at bedtime or twice daily) are the medication of choice
  — Caution should be used with antipsychotic medications, including checking the QTc interval, eliminating other QTc prolonging medications, and correcting any electrolyte abnormalities.
- Benzodiazepines should be avoided except in the circumstance of alcohol or benzodiazepine withdrawal
- If there is a suggestion of alcohol or substance withdrawal, a benzodiazepine such as lorazepam (1–2 mg every hour) can be given
- If there is little likelihood of withdrawal syndrome, haloperidol may be used in doses of 1 to 10 mg every hour in delirium
- Once the underlying condition has been identified and treated, adjunctive medications can be tapered

- Dextrose 50% (25 g), naloxone (0.4–1.2 mg), and thiamine (100 mg) are given intravenously without delay in patients with stupor or coma

Therapeutic Procedures

- Treatment depends on underlying cause
- For delirium, a pleasant, comfortable, nonthreatening, and physically safe environment with adequate nursing or attendant services should be provided
- Emergency measures for unstable patients or those with coma and stupor
  - Supportive therapy for respiration or blood pressure is initiated as needed
  - In hypothermia, all vital signs may be absent; all such patients should be rewarmed before the prognosis is assessed
  - The patient is positioned on one side with the neck partly extended, dentures removed, and secretions cleared by suction
  - If necessary, the patency of the airway is maintained by an oropharyngeal airway
- Decompressive craniectomy may reduce otherwise refractory intracranial hypertension in some cases of traumatic brain injury, but it does not improve neurologic outcome
- Hypothermic therapy is controversial

8. Outcome

Prognosis

- The prognosis is good for recovery of mental functioning in delirium when the underlying condition is reversible
- In coma because of cerebral ischemia and hypoxia, the absence of pupillary light reflexes at the time of initial examination implies little chance of regaining independence
- By contrast, preserved pupillary light responses, the development of spontaneous eye movements (roving, conjugate, or better), and extensor, flexor, or withdrawal responses to pain at this early stage imply a relatively good prognosis

9. When to Refer and When to Admit

When to Refer

- All patients

When to Admit

- All patients with stupor or coma to an ICU

SUGGESTED REFERENCES

Barr J et al. American College of Critical Care Medicine. Clinical practice guidelines for the management of pain, agitation, and delirium in adult patients in the intensive care unit. *Crit Care Med.* 2013 Jan;41(1):263–306. [PMID: 23269131]

Carr DB et al. The older adult driver with cognitive impairment: "It's a very frustrating life". *JAMA.* 2010 April 28;303(16):1632–1641. [PMID: 20424254]

Gitlin LN et al. Nonpharmacologic management of behavioral symptoms in dementia. *JAMA.* 2012 Nov 21;308(19):2020–2029. [PMID: 23168825]

Lin JS et al. Screening for cognitive impairment in older adults: a systematic review for the U.S. Preventive Services Task Force. *Ann Intern Med.* 2013 Nov 5;159(9):601–612. [PMID: 24145578]

Nasreddine ZS et al. The Montreal Cognitive Assessment, MoCA: a brief screening tool for mild cognitive impairment. *J Am Geriatr Soc.* 2005 April;53(4):695–699. [PMID: 15817019]

Porsteinsson AP et al. Effect of citalopram on agitation in Alzheimer disease: the CitAD randomized clinical trial. *JAMA.* 2014 Feb 19;311(7):682–691. [PMID: 24549548]

Russ TC et al. Cholinesterase inhibitors for mild cognitive impairment. *Cochrane Database Syst Rev.* 2012 Sep 12;9:CD009132. [PMID: 22972133]

Torpy JM et al. JAMA patient page. Dementia. *JAMA.* 2009 Aug 12;302(6):704. [PMID: 19671914]

Widera E et al. Finances in the older patient with cognitive impairment: "He didn't want me to take over". *JAMA.* 2011 Feb 16;305(7):698–706. [PMID: 21325186]

Dementia

56

A 73-year-old man is brought in by his wife with concerns about his worsening memory. He is a retired engineer who has recently been getting lost in the neighborhood where he has lived for 30 years. He has been found wandering and has often been brought home by neighbors. When asked about this, he becomes upset and defensive and states that he was just trying to get some exercise. He has also had trouble dressing himself and balancing his checkbook. A physical examination is unremarkable, except that he scores 18 points out of 30 on the Mini-Mental State Examination, a test of cognitive function. A metabolic workup is normal. A computed tomography (CT) scan of the head shows generalized brain atrophy, though perhaps only what would be expected for his age. He is diagnosed with dementia, likely from Alzheimer disease (AD).

LEARNING OBJECTIVES

- ▶ Learn the clinical manifestations and objective findings of dementia
- ▶ Know the different types of dementia and how to distinguish them
- ▶ Understand how to screen for dementia and how to confirm the diagnosis
- ▶ Know the differential diagnosis of dementia
- ▶ Learn the medical treatment for dementia and strategies for caregivers

QUESTIONS

1. What are the salient features of this patient's problem?

2. How do you think through his problem?

3. What are the key features, including essentials of diagnosis, general considerations, and demographics, of dementia?

4. What are the symptoms and signs of dementia?

5. What is the differential diagnosis of dementia?

6. What are laboratory, imaging, and procedural findings in dementia?

7. What are the treatments for dementia?

8. What are the outcomes, including follow-up, complications, and prognosis, of dementia?

9. When should patients with dementia be referred to a specialist or admitted to the hospital?

ANSWERS

1. Salient Features

Age > 65 years; worsening memory; wandering; loss of abilities in activities of daily living; abnormal objective cognitive function testing; normal metabolic workup; brain atrophy on imaging studies without focal lesion

2. How to Think Through

Impaired cognitive function and personality change are often seen in both inpatient and outpatient settings. Before a diagnosis of dementia can be made, there are important causes to exclude, such as delirium. What are the distinguishing features of delirium versus dementia? (Delirium is acute in onset, waxing and waning, with inattention, and either an altered level of consciousness or disorganized thinking. Dementia is marked by progressive decline in short-term memory and at least one other cognitive domain.) What are other mimics of dementia? (Medication toxicities, depression and psychotic disorders, thyroid disease, vitamin B_{12} deficiency, HIV, syphilis, malignancy.) What are the major causes of dementia and their defining characteristics? (See below.)

Once a diagnosis of AD is made, how should the patient be treated? (The effectiveness of cholinesterase inhibitors is modest at best. Close attention to the patient's level of function and safety become paramount, with activities of daily living [ADL] and instrumental activities of daily living [I-ADL] assistance, and emphasis on structure and routine.) The use of antipsychotic medications to control difficult behavioral symptoms is controversial. What are two key toxicities of these medicines in patients with dementia? (Arrhythmia due to prolonged QT interval and stroke.) Complications such as anorexia, dysphagia, and aspiration are associated with end-stage dementia, and hospice care is often appropriate at this stage.

3. Key Features

Essentials of Diagnosis
- Progressive decline of intellectual function
- Loss of short-term memory and at least one other cognitive deficit
- Deficit severe enough to cause impairment of function
- No delirium (absence of waxing and waning in level of consciousness) and no psychiatric disease

General Considerations
- Defined as a progressive, acquired impairment in multiple cognitive domains, at least one of which is memory
- The deficits must represent a decline in function significant enough to interfere with work or social life
- "Mild cognitive impairment" describes a decline that has not resulted in a change in the level of function
- Dementia frequently coexists with depression and delirium
- Patients have little cognitive reserve and can have acute cognitive or functional decline with a new medical illness

Demographics
- Prevalence of AD in the United States doubles every 5 years in the older population, reaching 30% to 50% at age 85
- Women suffer disproportionately, as patients (even after age adjustment) and as caregivers
- AD accounts for two-thirds of cases of dementia in the United States, with vascular dementia (either alone or combined with AD) accounting for much of the rest
- Risk factors
  — Older age
  — Family history

— Lower educational level
— Female sex

4. Symptoms and Signs

• Memory impairment with at least one or more of the following
  — Aphasia (typically, word finding difficulty)
  — Apraxia (inability to perform previously learned tasks)
  — Agnosia (inability to recognize objects)
  — Impaired executive function (poor abstraction, mental flexibility, planning, and judgment)
• AD
  — Typical earliest deficits are in memory and visuospatial abilities
  — Social graces may be retained despite advanced cognitive decline
  — Personality changes and behavioral difficulties (wandering, inappropriate sexual behavior, aggression) may develop as the disease progresses
  — Hallucinations, delusions, and symptoms of depression often occur as dementia worsens
  — End-stage disease characterized by
    ◦ Near-mutism
    ◦ Inability to sit up
    ◦ Inability to hold up the head
    ◦ Inability to track objects with the eyes
    ◦ Difficulty with eating and swallowing
    ◦ Weight loss
    ◦ Bowel or bladder incontinence
    ◦ Recurrent respiratory or urinary infections
• "Subcortical" dementias
  — Psychomotor slowing
  — Reduced attention
  — Early loss of executive function
  — Personality changes
• Lewy body dementia
  — May be confused with delirium, as fluctuating cognitive impairment is frequently observed
  — Rigidity and bradykinesia are primarily noted; tremor is rare
  — Hallucinations—classically visual and bizarre—may occur
• Frontotemporal dementias
  — Personality change (euphoria, disinhibition, and apathy) and compulsive behaviors (often peculiar eating habits or hyperorality)
  — In contrast to AD, visuospatial function is relatively preserved
• Dementia with motor findings, such as extrapyramidal features or ataxia, may represent a less-common disorder (eg, progressive supranuclear palsy, corticobasal ganglionic degeneration, olivopontocerebellar atrophy)

5. Differential Diagnosis

• Depression (so-called pseudodementia)
• Mild cognitive impairment
• Delirium
• Medication side effects
• Neurodegenerative disease
• Infection or inflammatory disease
• Neoplasm or a paraneoplastic condition
• Endocrine or metabolic disease
• Normal pressure hydrocephalus

- For rapidly progressive dementia, also consider
  — Prion disease
  — Infections
  — Toxins
  — Neoplasms
- Autoimmune and inflammatory diseases, including corticosteroid-responsive (Hashimoto) encephalopathy and antibody-mediated paraneoplastic syndromes
- See Table 56-1

6. Laboratory, Imaging, and Procedural Findings

Laboratory Tests
- Recommended tests include
  — Complete blood count
  — Serum thyroid-stimulating hormone
  — Serum vitamin B_{12} level
  — Serum electrolytes

Table 56-1. Common causes of age-related dementia.

Disorder	Pathology	Clinical Features
Alzheimer disease	Plaques containing β-amyloid peptide, and neurofibrillary tangles containing tau protein, occur throughout the neocortex	• Most common age-related neurodegenerative disease; incidence doubles every 5 years after age 60 • Short-term memory impairment is early and prominent in most cases • Variable deficits of executive function, visuospatial function, and language
Vascular dementia	Multifocal ischemic change	• Stepwise or progressive accumulation of cognitive deficits in association with repeated strokes • Symptoms depend on localization of strokes
Dementia with Lewy bodies	Histologically indistinguishable from Parkinson disease: α-synuclein-containing Lewy bodies occur in the brainstem, midbrain, olfactory bulb, and neocortex. Alzheimer pathology may coexist.	• Cognitive dysfunction, with prominent visuospatial and executive deficits • Psychiatric disturbance, with anxiety, visual hallucinations, and fluctuating delirium • Parkinsonian motor deficits with or after other features • Cholinesterase inhibitors lessen delirium; poor tolerance of many psychoactive medications, including neuroleptics and dopaminergics
Frontotemporal dementia (FTD)	Neuropathology is variable and defined by the protein found in intraneuronal aggregates. Tau protein, TAR DNA-binding protein 43 (TDP-43), or fused-in-sarcoma (FUS) protein account for most cases.	• Peak incidence in the sixth decade; approximately equal to Alzheimer disease as a cause of dementia in patients under 60 years old. • Familial cases result from mutations in genes for tau, progranulin, or others Behavioral variant FTD • Deficits in empathy, social comportment, insight, abstract thought, and executive function • Behavior is disinhibited, impulsive, and ritualistic, with prominent apathy and increased interest in sex or sweet/fatty foods • Relative preservation of memory • Focal right frontal atrophy • Association with amyotrophic lateral sclerosis Semantic variant primary progressive aphasia • Deficits in word-finding, single word comprehension, object and category knowledge, and face recognition • Behaviors may be rigid, ritualistic, or similar to behavioral variant FTD • Focal, asymmetric temporal pole atrophy Nonfluent/agrammatic variant primary progressive aphasia • Speech is effortful with dysarthria, phonemic errors, sound distortions, and poor grammar • Focal extrapyramidal signs and apraxia of the right arm and leg are common • On a diagnostic and pathological continuum with corticobasal degeneration • Focal left frontal atrophy

— Serum creatinine

— Serum glucose

— Serum calcium

— Serum total cholesterol, HDL cholesterol, LDL cholesterol, triglycerides

— Serum tests for HIV antibody, syphilis (eg, fluorescent treponemal antibody [FTA] test), liver tests,

— Lyme serology, paraneoplastic autoimmune antibodies, ceruloplasmin, urine heavy metal screen, CSF protein and cultures, and ApoE genotyping may be informative but not considered routine

Imaging Studies

• Magnetic resonance imaging is beneficial for

— Younger patients

— Persons who have, acute or subacute onset or focal neurologic signs, seizures, or gait abnormalities

• Noncontrast CT is sufficient in older patients with more classic picture of AD

• Positron-emission tomography (PET)

— Labeled with fluorodeoxyglucose (FDG)

› May identify particular brain structures that are hypometabolic and thus likely to harbor pathology

› May be useful in discriminating between Alzheimer disease and frontotemporal dementia

— Labeled with ligand for β-amyloid

› Is highly sensitive to amyloid pathology

› May help provide positive evidence for Alzheimer disease in a patient with cognitive decline

› However, after age 60 or 70, amyloid plaques can accumulate in the absence of cognitive impairment; thus, the specificity of a positive amyloid scan diminishes with age

— Labeling with ligands for tau, a pathogenic protein in Alzheimer disease, progressive supranuclear palsy, and some forms of frontotemporal dementia, has entered clinical trials and may help refine premortem diagnostic accuracy

Diagnostic Procedures

• Evaluate for deficits related to cardiovascular accidents, parkinsonism, or peripheral neuropathy

• The "mini-cog"—a combination of the "clock draw" test (in which the patient is asked to sketch a clock face, with all the numerals placed properly, the two clock hands positioned at a specified time) and the "three-item recall" at 1 minute—is a fairly quick and good screen; an abnormally drawn clock markedly increases the probability of dementia

• When patients fail either of these screening tests, further testing with the Montreal Cognitive Assessment (MoCA) questionnaire, neurocognitive testing, or other instruments (eg, the Folstein Mini-Mental State Examination questionnaire) is warranted

• Examine for comorbid conditions that may aggravate the disability

7. Treatments

Medications

• Acetylcholinesterase inhibitors (eg, donepezil, galantamine, rivastigmine, memantine) are first-line therapy for Alzheimer disease and dementia with Lewy bodies

— Modest improvements in cognitive function in mild to moderate dementia

— May be modestly beneficial in improving neuropsychiatric symptoms

— Do not appear to prevent progression of disability or institutionalization

— Starting dosages

› Donepezil, 5 mg orally daily (maximum 10 mg daily)

› Galantamine, 4 mg orally twice daily (maximum 12 mg twice daily); a once-daily extended-release formulation is also available

○ Rivastigmine, 1.5 mg orally twice daily (maximum 6 mg twice daily) or 4.6, 9.5, or 13.3 mg/24 hours transdermally daily
○ Memantine, 5 mg orally daily (maximum 10 mg twice daily)
— Increase doses gradually as tolerated
— Side effects include nausea, diarrhea, anorexia, weight loss, and syncope
• Choose other medications based on symptoms—depression, anxiety, psychosis
• "Typical" antipsychotic agents (eg, haloperidol)
— May modestly reduce aggression, but not agitation
— Significant adverse effects including risk of sudden death
• "Atypical" antipsychotic agents (eg, risperidone, olanzapine, quetiapine, aripiprazole, clozapine, ziprasidone)
— Better tolerated than older agents
— However, should be avoided in patients with vascular risk factors due to an increased risk of weight gain, stroke, and sudden death
— Associated with hyperglycemia in diabetic patients
— Considerably more expensive than haloperidol
• In several short-term trials and one long-term trial, both typical and atypical antipsychotics increased mortality compared with placebo when used to treat elderly demented patients with behavioral disturbances
• Food and Drug Administration has issued black box warning about the risk of QTc prolongation and torsades de pointes on electrocardiogram, and thus the potential for sudden death, with both haloperidol and atypical antipsychotic agents in treatment of depression-related psychosis
• Starting and target neuroleptic dosages are low (eg, haloperidol 0.5–2.0 mg; risperidone 0.25–2 mg)
• Selective serotonin reuptake inhibitors
— Generally safe and well-tolerated in elderly, cognitively impaired patients
— May be efficacious for the treatment of depression, anxiety, or agitation
— Citalopram has been shown in a randomized placebo-controlled trial to improve symptoms of agitation; doses greater than 40 mg daily carry a risk of dysrhythmia from QT interval prolongation; the maximum recommended dose is 20 mg daily in patients > 60 years,
— Paroxetine should be avoided because it has anticholinergic effects
— Bupropion or venlafaxine may also be tried
• Insomnia is common
— Trazodone (25–50 mg orally at bedtime as needed) can be safe and effective
— Avoid over-the-counter antihistamine hypnotics, along with benzodiazepines, because of their tendency to worsen cognition and precipitate delirium

Therapeutic Procedures
• Provide structure and routine
• Discontinue all nonessential drugs and correct, if possible, any sensory (visual, hearing) deficits
• Exclude unrecognized delirium, pain, urinary obstruction, or fecal impaction
• Caregivers should speak simply to the patient, break down activities into simple component tasks, and use a "distract, not confront" approach

8. Outcomes

Follow-Up
• Federal regulations require drug reduction efforts at least every 6 months if antipsychotic agents are used in a nursing home patient
• Drivers with dementia are at an increased risk for motor vehicle accidents; however, many patients continue to drive safely well beyond the time of diagnosis

— There is no clear-cut evidence to suggest a single best approach to determining a patient's risk

— There is no accepted "gold standard" test of incapability

— Therefore, clinicians must consider several factors when forming a recommendation about whether a patient should continue driving

• Often early in the course of dementia, patients start having difficulty managing their financial affairs

— Clinicians should have some proficiency to address financial concerns

— No gold standard test is available to identify when a patient with dementia no longer has financial capacity

— However, the clinician should be on the lookout for signs that a patient is either at risk for or actually experiencing financial incapacity

— Clinicians should be able to educate about the need for advance financial planning and to recommend that patients complete a durable power of attorney for finance matters when the capacity to do so still exists

Complications

• Clinicians should be alert for signs of elder abuse when working with stressed caregivers

Prognosis

• Rapidly progressive dementia (eg, Jakob–Creutzfeldt disease) is defined as obvious decline over a few weeks to a few months

• Life expectancy with AD is typically 3 to 15 years

• Other neurodegenerative dementias, such as Lewy body dementia, show more rapid decline

• Hospice care is often appropriate for patients with end-stage dementia

9. When to Refer and When to Admit

When to Refer

• Referral for neurocognitive and psychological testing may be helpful to distinguish dementia from depression, to diagnose dementia in persons of poor education or very high premorbid intellect, and to aid diagnosis when cognitive impairment is mild

When to Admit

• Dementia complicates other medical problems, and the threshold for admission should be lower

• Dementia alone is not an indication for admission, but admission is sometimes necessary when a superimposed delirium poses safety risks at home

SUGGESTED REFERENCES

Donaghy PC et al. The clinical characteristics of dementia with Lewy bodies and a consideration of prodromal diagnosis. *Alzheimers Res Ther*. 2014 Jul 21;6(4):46. [PMID: 25484925]

Galasko D. The diagnostic evaluation of a patient with dementia. *Continuum* (Minneap Minn). 2013 Apr;19(2):397–410. [PMID: 23558485]

Paterson RW et al. Diagnosis and treatment of rapidly progressive dementias. *Neurol Clin Pract*. 2012 Sep;2(3):187–200. [PMID: 23634367]

Pressman PS et al. Diagnosis and management of behavioral variant frontotemporal dementia. *Biol Psychiatry*. 2014 Apr 1;75(7):574–581. [PMID: 24315411]

Reitz C et al. Alzheimer disease: epidemiology, diagnostic criteria, risk factors and biomarkers. *Biochem Pharmacol*. 2014 Apr 15;88(4):640–651. [PMID: 24398425]

Schwarz S et al. Pharmacological treatment of dementia. *Curr Opin Psychiatry*. 2012 Nov;25(6): 542–550. [PMID: 22992546]

57

Depression

A 57-year-old woman presents to her primary care clinician complaining of insomnia for 4 months. She reports that she can often fall asleep, but awakens very early in the morning and cannot get back to sleep. She also has a lack of interest in things that she previously enjoyed, frequent feelings of guilt and hopelessness, decreased energy, and occasional thoughts of "ending it all." Her symptoms are making it hard for her to perform well at her place of employment. She denies any drug use or alcoholism. A physical examination, including thyroid examination, is normal. Laboratory tests including a thyroid-stimulating hormone (TSH) are normal.

LEARNING OBJECTIVES

▶ Learn the clinical manifestations and objective findings of depression
▶ Understand the different ways that depression can present
▶ Know the differential diagnosis of depression, including related diseases
▶ Learn the treatments for depression, and options after initial treatment failure
▶ Know how to prevent suicide in patients with depression

QUESTIONS

1. What are the salient features of this patient's problem?

2. How do you think through her problem?

3. What are the key features, including essentials of diagnosis, general considerations, and demographics, of depression?

4. What are the symptoms and signs of depression?

5. What is the differential diagnosis of depression?

6. What are laboratory findings in depression?

7. What are the treatments for depression?

8. What are the outcomes, including follow-up, complications, prevention, and prognosis, of depression?

9. When should patients with depression be referred to a specialist or admitted to the hospital?

ANSWERS

1. Salient Features

Sleep disturbance with early awakening; anhedonia; decreased energy; guilt and hopelessness; suicidal ideation; symptoms causing functional disturbance; normal examination and laboratory results; not due to a substance use disorder

2. How to Think Through

The prevalence of depression is high; unaddressed depression is a significant cause of morbidity and impediment to successful management of other chronic diseases. This patient's initial complaint is sleep disturbance, which is common. What are her other symptoms and signs of depression? (Loss of interest, dysphoria, decreased energy, suicidal ideation.) When considering depression, what are the other crucial psychiatric diagnoses to consider? (Bipolar disorder, adjustment disorder, dysthymia, seasonal affective disorder [SAD], and substance abuse/dependence.) What medical disorder most commonly causes symptoms that mimic depression? (Hypothyroidism.) What are the treatment options? (Psychotherapy and pharmacotherapy are equivalent in efficacy; combination of the two is superior to either alone.) What are the classes of pharmacotherapy? (Selective serotonin reuptake inhibitors [SSRIs], serotonin–norepinephrine reuptake inhibitors (SNRIs), tricyclics, and monoamine oxidase inhibitors [MAOIs].) What is most serious potential adverse effect of these medications? (Serotonin syndrome may occur when SSRIs, SNRIs or atypical antidepressants are taken in conjunction with MAOIs or selegiline or with other serotonergic agents.) What are the common side effects of SSRIs? (Headache, nausea, tinnitus, insomnia, nervousness, and sexual dysfunction.) While monitoring treatment, one must screen for suicidal ideation.

3. Key Features

Essentials of Diagnosis

- In most depressions
  - Mood varies from mild sadness to intense guilt, worthlessness, and hopelessness
  - Difficulty in thinking and concentration, with rumination and indecision
  - Loss of interest, with diminished involvement in activities
  - Somatic complaints
  - Disrupted, reduced, or excessive sleep
  - Loss of energy, appetite, and sex drive
  - Anxiety
- In some severe depressions
  - Psychomotor disturbance: retardation or agitation
  - Delusions of a somatic or persecutory nature
  - Withdrawal from activities
  - Suicidal ideation

General Considerations

- Sadness and grief are normal responses to loss; depression is not
- Unlike grief, depression is marked by a disturbance of self-esteem, with a sense of guilt and worthlessness
- Dysthymia is a chronic depressive disturbance with symptoms generally milder than in a major depressive episode

Demographics

- Up to 30% of primary care patients have depressive symptoms
- Under recognized among the elderly: major depressive disorder occurs in up to 5% of community-dwelling older adults, while clinically significant depressive symptoms are present in up to 16% of older adults.

4. Symptoms and Signs

- Anhedonia
- Withdrawal from activities
- Feelings of guilt
- Poor concentration and cognitive dysfunction
- Anxiety
- Chronic fatigue and somatic complaints
- Diurnal variation with improvement as the day progresses
- Vegetative signs
  — Insomnia
  — Anorexia
  — Constipation
- Occasionally, severe agitation and psychotic ideation
- Atypical features
  — Hypersomnia
  — Overeating
  — Lethargy
  — Mood reactivity

5. Differential Diagnosis

- Bipolar disorder or cyclothymia
- Adjustment disorder with depressed mood
- Dysthymia
- Premenstrual dysphoric disorder
- Major depression with postpartum onset: usually 2 weeks to 6 months postpartum
- Seasonal affective disorder
- Carbohydrate craving
  — Lethargy
  — Hyperphagia
  — Hypersomnia

6. Laboratory Findings

Laboratory Tests

- Tests to be completed to exclude medical causes of depression include
  — Complete blood cell count
  — Serum TSH
  — Red blood cell folate
  — Toxicology screen (when indicated)

7. Treatments

Medications

- See Table 57-1 and Figure 57-1
- SSRIs, SNRIs, and atypical antidepressants
  — Generally lack anticholinergic or cardiovascular side effects
  — Most are activating and should be given in the morning
  — Some patients may experience sedation with paroxetine, fluvoxamine, and mirtazapine
  — Clinical response varies from 2 to 6 weeks
  — Common side effects are headache, nausea, tinnitus, insomnia, nervousness
  — Sexual dysfunction is very common and may respond to sildenafil or related agents
  — "Serotonin syndrome" may occur when taken in conjunction with MAOIs or selegiline
  — With the exception of paroxetine, SSRIs should be tapered over weeks to months to avoid a withdrawal syndrome

Table 57-1. Commonly used antidepressants.

Drug	Usual Daily Dose (mg)	Daily Maximum Dose (mg)	Sedative Effects[a]	Anticholinergic Effects[a]
SSRIs				
Citalopram (Celexa)	20	40	< 1	1
Escitalopram (Lexapro)	10	20	< 1	1
Fluoxetine (Prozac, Sarafem)	5–40	80	< 1	< 1
Fluvoxamine (Luvox)	100–300	300	1	< 1
Nefazodone (Serzone)	300–600	600	2	< 1
Paroxetine (Paxil)	20–30	50	1	1
Sertraline (Zoloft)	50–150	200	< 1	< 1
Vilazodone (Viibryd)	40	40	< 1	< 1
SNRIs				
Desvenlafaxine (Pristiq)	50	100	1	< 1
Duloxetine (Cymbalta)	40	60	2	3
Levomilnacipran (Fetzima)	40	120	1	1
Milnacipran (Savella)	100	200	1	1
Venlafaxine XR (Effexor)	150–225	225	1	< 1
Tricyclic and clinically similar compounds				
Amitriptyline (Elavil)	150–250	300	4	4
Amoxapine (Asendin)	150–200	400	2	2
Clomipramine (Anafranil)	100	250	3	3
Desipramine (Norpramin)	100–250	300	1	1
Doxepin (Sinequan)	150–200	300	4	3
Imipramine (Tofranil)	150–200	300	3	3
Maprotiline (Ludiomil)	100–200	300	4	2
Nortriptyline (Aventyl, Pamelor)	100–150	150	2	2
Protriptyline (Vivactil)	15–40	60	1	3
Trimipramine (Surmontil)	75–200	200	4	4
Monoamine oxidase inhibitors				
Phenelzine (Nardil)	45–60	90	…	…
Selegiline transdermal (Emsam)	6 (skin patch)	12	…	…
Tranylcypromine (Parnate)	20–30	50	…	…
Other compounds				
Bupropion SR (Wellbutrin SR)	300	400[c]	< 1	< 1
Bupropion XL (Wellbutrin XL)	300[d]	450[d]	< 1	< 1
Mirtazapine (Remeron)	15–45	45	4	2
Trazodone (Desyrel)	100–300	400	4	< 1
Vortioxetine (Brintellix)	10	20	<1	< 1

SSRIs, serotonin selective reuptake inhibitors.

[a]1, weak effect; 4, strong effect.

[b]Average wholesale price (AWP, for AB-rated generic when available) for quantity listed. Source: *Red Book Online, 2014, Truven Health Analytics, Inc.*, Inc. AWP may not accurately represent the actual pharmacy cost because wide contractual variations exist among institutions.

[c]200 mg twice daily.

[d]Wellbutrin XL is a once-daily form of bupropion. Bupropion is still available as immediate release, and, if used, no single dose should exceed 150 mg.

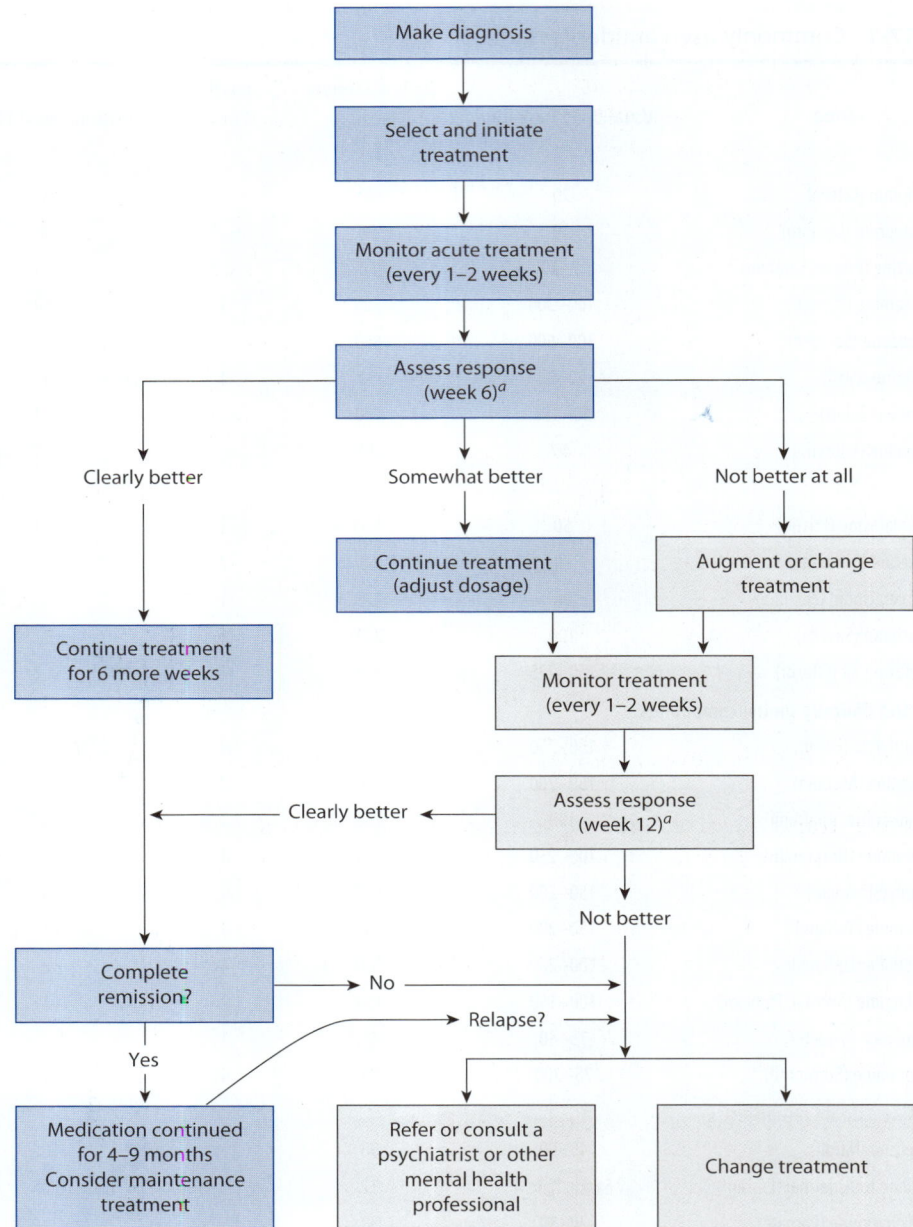

ªTimes of assessment (weeks 6 and 12) rest on very modest data. It may be necessary to revise the treatment plan earlier for patients not responding at all.

FIGURE 57-1. Overview of treatment for depression. (Reproduced from Agency for Health Care Policy and Research. Depression in Primary Care. Vol. 2: Treatment of Major Depression. United States Department of Health and Human Services, 1993.)

— SNRIs block reuptake of norepinephrine in addition to serotonin and include duloxetine, venlafaxine, and desvenlafaxine
— Atypical antidepressants include bupropion and mirtazapine
— Fluoxetine, fluvoxamine, sertraline, and venlafaxine appear to be safe in pregnancy; paroxetine carries a black box warning for possible teratogenicity
— Their use should be weighed against the risks of an untreated depression in the mother
• Tricyclic antidepressants
— Mainstay of treatment before SSRIs
— Start at low dose and increase by 25 mg weekly to avoid sedation and anticholinergic side effects
— Overdose can be serious

- MAOIs
  - Commonly cause orthostatic hypotension and sympathomimetic effects
  - Third-line agents due to dietary restrictions and drug–drug interactions
  - However, with the availability of selegiline, which is a skin patch, dietary restrictions are not necessary in the lowest dosage strength (6 mg/24 h)
- Potential for withdrawal syndromes requires gradual tapering
- Drug selection should be influenced by any history of prior responses
- If response is inadequate, can either switch to a second agent or augment the first agent with lithium (600–900 mg/d orally), buspirone (30–60 mg/d orally), or liothyronine (25–50 µg/d orally), according to the STAR*D study, or a second-generation antipsychotic such as aripiprazole (5–15 mg/d) or olanzapine (5–15 mg/d).
- Stimulants such as dextroamphetamine (5–30 mg/d) or methylphenidate (10–45 mg/d) can be used for short-term treatment of medically ill and geriatric patients or in refractory cases
- Ketamine infusion
  - Leads to rapid improvement in depressive symptoms
  - However, effects of a single treatment are short lived

Therapeutic Procedures

- Electroconvulsive therapy is the most effective (70%–85%) treatment for severe depression
  - Indications are contraindications to medications or depression refractory to medications
  - Most common side effects are headache and memory disturbances, which are usually short lived
- Vagus nerve stimulation is approved for treatment of extremely refractory depression, though there is limited clinical experience
- Repetitive transcranial magnetic stimulation is approved by the Food and Drug Administration for individuals who have failed one trial of an antidepressant and is being evaluated for wider application
- Deep brain stimulation (DBS) continues to be explored for the treatment of refractory depression but controlled studies have not shown success to date.
- Psychological
  - Medication and psychotherapy together are more effective than either modality alone
  - Psychotherapy is seldom possible in the acute phase of severe depression
- Social
  - In depressions involving alcoholism, early involvement in recovery programs is important to future success
  - Family, employers, and friends can help mobilize a recently depressed patient

8. Outcomes

Follow-Up

- Medication trials should be monitored every 1 to 2 weeks until 6 weeks, when the effectiveness of the medication can be assessed
- If successful, medications should be continued for 6 to 12 months before tapering is considered
- Medications should be continued indefinitely in patients with their first episode before age 20, >2 episodes after age 40, or a single episode after age 50
- Tapering of medications should occur gradually over several months

Complications

- A lifetime risk of 10% to 15% of suicide among patients with depression
- Four major groups who attempt suicide
  - Those who are overwhelmed by problems in living
  - Those who are clearly attempting to control others
  - Those with severe depressions
  - Those with psychotic illness

Prevention

- Patients at risk for suicide should receive medications in small amounts
- Guns and drugs should be removed from the patient's house
- High-risk patients should be asked not to drive

Prognosis

- Patients frequently respond well to a full trial of drug treatment

9. When to Refer and When to Admit

When to Refer

- When depression is refractory to antidepressant therapy
- When depression is moderate to severe
- When suicidality or significant loss of function is present
- With active psychosis or history of mania

When to Admit

- Patients at risk for suicide
- Complex treatment modalities are required

SUGGESTED REFERENCES

Ansari A et al. The psychopharmacology algorithm project at the Harvard South Shore Program: an update on bipolar depression. *Harv Rev Psychiatry*. 2010;18(1):36–55. [PMID: 20047460]

Banerjee S et al. Sertraline or mirtazapine for depression in dementia (HTA-SADD): a randomised, multicentre, double-blind, placebo-controlled trial. *Lancet*. 2011 Jul 30;378(9789):403–411. [PMID: 21764118]

Battes LC et al. Beta blocker therapy is associated with reduced depressive symptoms 12 months post percutaneous coronary intervention. *J Affect Disord*. 2012 Feb;136(3):751–757. [PMID: 22032873]

Chad L et al. Update on antidepressant use during breastfeeding. *Can Fam Physician*. 2013 Jun;59(6):633–634. [PMID: 23766044]

Connolly KR et al. Emerging drugs for major depressive disorder. *Expert Opin Emerg Drugs*. 2012 Mar;17(1):105–126. [PMID: 22339643]

George MS et al. The expanding evidence base for rTMS treatment of depression. *Curr Opin Psychiatry*. 2013 Jan;26(1):13–18. [PMID: 23154644]

Gibbons RD et al. Suicidal thoughts and behavior with antidepressant treatment: reanalysis of the randomized placebo-controlled studies of fluoxetine and venlafaxine. *Arch Gen Psychiatry*. 2012 Jun;69(6):580–587. [PMID: 22309973]

Grady MM et al. Novel agents in development for the treatment of depression. *CNS Spectr*. 2013 Dec;18(suppl 1):37–40. [PMID: 24252548]

Kok RM et al. Continuing treatment of depression in the elderly: a systematic review and meta-analysis of double-blinded randomized controlled trials with antidepressants. *Am J Geriatr Psychiatry*. 2011 March;19(3):249–255. [PMID: 21425505]

Kéri S et al. Blood biomarkers of depression track clinical changes during cognitive-behavioral therapy. *J Affect Disord*. 2014 Aug;164:118–122. [PMID: 24856564]

Mojtabai R. Diagnosing depression in older adults in primary care. *N Engl J Med*. 2014 Mar 27;370(13):1180–1182. [PMID: 24670164]

Phillips ML et al. Bipolar disorder diagnosis: challenges and future directions. *Lancet*. 2013 May 11;381(9878):1663–1671. [PMID: 23663952]

Prina AM et al. Association between depression and hospital outcomes among older men. *CMAJ*. 2013 Feb 5;185(2):117–123. [PMID: 23228999]

Stewart DE. Clinical practice. Depression during pregnancy. *N Engl J Med*. 2011 Oct 27;365(17):1605–1611. [PMID: 22029982]

Taylor WD. Clinical practice. Depression in the elderly. *N Engl J Med*. 2014 Sep 25;371(13):1228–1236. [PMID: 25251617]

Epilepsy

58

A middle-aged man is transported to the emergency department unconscious and accompanied by a nurse from the medical floor. The nurse states that the patient was in line in front of her in the hospital cafeteria when he suddenly fell to the floor. He then had a "generalized tonic–clonic seizure." She called for assistance and accompanied him to the emergency department. No other historical information is available. On physical examination, the patient is confused and unresponsive to commands. He is breathing adequately and has oxygen in place via nasal prongs. His vital signs are as follows: temperature, 38°C; blood pressure, 170/90 mm Hg; heart rate, 105 bpm; respiratory rate, 18/min. Oxygen saturation is 99% on 2 L of oxygen. Neurologic examination is notable for reactive pupils of 3 mm, intact gag reflex, decreased movement of the left side of the body, and positive Babinski signs bilaterally. Examination is otherwise unremarkable.

LEARNING OBJECTIVES

▶ Learn the clinical manifestations and objective findings of epilepsy
▶ Understand how to identify the underlying and potentially reversible causes of seizures and epilepsy
▶ Know the differential diagnosis of epilepsy
▶ Learn how to select a medication for the treatment of epilepsy
▶ Know the public health and safety implications for physicians in the treatment of epilepsy

QUESTIONS

1. What are the salient features of this patient's problem?
2. How do you think through his problem?
3. What are the key features, including essentials of diagnosis, general considerations, and demographics, of epilepsy?
4. What are the symptoms and signs of epilepsy?
5. What is the differential diagnosis of epilepsy?
6. What are laboratory, imaging, and procedural findings in epilepsy?
7. What are the treatments for epilepsy?
8. What are the outcomes, including follow-up, complications, and prognosis, of epilepsy?
9. When should patients with epilepsy be referred to a specialist or admitted to the hospital?

ANSWERS

1. Salient Features

Witnessed seizure activity; postictal confusion; immediately after the seizure, neurologic examination abnormalities; otherwise unremarkable examination

2. How to Think Through

Can a syncopal event include myoclonic seizure-like movements? (Yes. Syncope—lack of sufficient blood flow to the brain, which is a definition that distinctly does not include seizure—can be associated with myoclonic jerks.) What features help identify this event as a seizure? (Postictal confusion and drowsiness, transient abnormal neurologic examination consistent with Todd paralysis. Tongue biting and incontinence are also commonly seen with seizure and not with syncope.) Knowing nothing about this patient's history, what are the primary causes of seizure to consider? (Hypoglycemia, hyponatremia, alcohol or benzodiazepine withdrawal, medication or illicit sympathomimetic toxicity [eg, cocaine], mass effect from tumor, trauma, stroke, and central nervous system [CNS] infection.) How should he be managed upon arrival in the emergency department? (First, review the ABCs. Establish intravenous access. Empiric thiamine and glucose are often administered. A complete blood count [CBC] and serum electrolytes, glucose, and calcium should be sent. Pending the history and clinical course, CNS imaging should be considered.)

What defines epilepsy? (Recurrent seizures.) What features constitute a tonic–clonic seizure? Can a patient have a bilateral tonic–clonic seizure and remain conscious? (No. Both hemispheres are involved.) How are seizures classified? (See Table 58-1.) What are common anticonvulsants? (See Table 58-2.)

Table 58-1. Seizure classification.

Seizure Type	Key Features	Other Associated Features
Focal seizures	Involvement of only a restricted part of brain; may evolve to a bilateral, convulsive seizure	
Without impairment of consciousness		Observable focal motor or autonomic symptoms, or subjective sensory or psychic symptoms may occur
With impairment of consciousness		Above symptoms may precede, accompany, or follow the period of altered responsiveness
Generalized seizures	Diffuse involvement of brain at onset	
Absence (petit mal)	Consciousness impaired briefly; patient often unaware of attacks	May have clonic, tonic, or atonic (ie, loss of postural tone) components; autonomic components (eg, enuresis); or accompanying automatisms Almost always begin in childhood and frequently cease by age 20
Atypical absences	May be more gradual in onset and termination than typical absence	More marked changes in tone may occur
Myoclonic	Single or multiple myoclonic jerks	
Tonic–clonic (grand mal)	Tonic phase: Sudden loss of consciousness, with rigidity and arrest of respiration, lasting < 1 min Clonic phase: Jerking occurs, usually for < 2–3 min Flaccid coma: Variable duration	May be accompanied by tongue biting, incontinence, or aspiration; commonly followed by postictal confusion variable in duration
Status epilepticus	Repeated seizures without recovery between them; a fixed and enduring epileptic condition lasting ≥ 30 min	

Table 58-2. Drug treatment for seizures in adults.

Drug	Usual Adult Daily Oral Dose	Minimum No. of Daily Doses	Time to Steady State Drug Levels	Optimal Drug Level	Selected Side Effects and Idiosyncratic Reactions
Generalized or Focal Seizures					
Phenytoin	200–400 mg	1	5–10 d	10–20 µg/mL	Nystagmus, ataxia, dysarthria, sedation, confusion, gingival hyperplasia, hirsutism, megaloblastic anemia, blood dyscrasias, skin rashes, fever, systemic lupus erythematosus, lymphadenopathy, peripheral neuropathy, dyskinesias
Carbamazepine extended-release (ER) formulation	400–1600 mg ER	2	3–4 d	4–8 µg/mL	Nystagmus, dysarthria, diplopia, ataxia, drowsiness, nausea, blood dyscrasias, hepatotoxicity, hyponatremia. May exacerbate myoclonic seizures
Valproic acid	1500–2000 mg	2–3	2–4 d	50–100 µg/mL	Nausea, vomiting, diarrhea, drowsiness, alopecia, weight gain, hepatotoxicity, thrombocytopenia, tremor, pancreatitis
Phenobarbital	100–200 mg	1	14–21 d	10–40 µg/mL	Drowsiness, nystagmus, ataxia, skin rashes, learning difficulties, hyperactivity
Primidone	750–1500 mg	3	4–7 d	5–15 µg/mL	Sedation, nystagmus, ataxia, vertigo, nausea, skin rashes, megaloblastic anemia, irritability
Lamotrigine[a,b,e]	100–500 mg	2	4–5 d	?	Sedation, skin rash, visual disturbances, dyspepsia, ataxia
Topiramate[a–d]	200–400 mg	2	4 d	?	Somnolence, nausea, dyspepsia, irritability, dizziness, ataxia, nystagmus, diplopia, glaucoma, renal calculi, weight loss, hypohidrosis, hyperthermia
Oxcarbazepine[a,c]	900–1800 mg	2	2–3 d	?	As for carbamazepine
Levetiracetam[a,b]	1000–3000 mg	2	2 d	?	Somnolence, ataxia, headache, behavioral changes
Zonisamide[a]	200–600 mg	1	14 d	?	Somnolence, ataxia, anorexia, nausea, vomiting, rash, confusion, renal calculi. Do not use in patients with sulfonamide allergy
Tiagabine[a]	32–56 mg	2	2 d	?	Somnolence, anxiety, dizziness, poor concentration, tremor, diarrhea
Pregabalin[a]	150–300 mg	2	2–4 d	?	Somnolence, dizziness, poor concentration, weight gain, thrombocytopenia, skin rashes, anaphylactoid reactions
Gabapentin[a]	900–3600 mg	3	1 d	?	Sedation, fatigue, ataxia, nystagmus, weight loss
Felbamate[a,c,f]	1200–3600 mg	3	4–5 d	?	Anorexia, nausea, vomiting, headache, insomnia, weight loss, dizziness, hepatotoxicity, aplastic anemia
Lacosamide[a]	100–400 mg	2	3 d	?	Vertigo, diplopia, nausea, headache, fatigue, ataxia, tremor, anaphylactoid reactions, PR interval prolongation on electrocardiogram (ECG), cardiac dysrhythmia, suicidality
Ezogabine[a]	300–1200 mg	3	2–3 d	?	Dizziness, somnolence, confusion, vertigo, nausea, ataxia, psychiatric disturbances
Absence Seizures					
Ethosuximide	100–1500 mg	2	5–10 d	40–100 µg/mL	Nausea, vomiting, anorexia, headache, lethargy, unsteadiness, blood dyscrasias, systemic lupus erythematosus, urticaria, pruritus
Valproic acid	1500–2000 mg	3	2–4 d	50–100 µg/mL	See above
Clonazepam	0.04–0.2 mg/kg	2	?	20–80 ng/mL	Drowsiness, ataxia, irritability, behavioral changes, exacerbation of tonic–clonic seizures
Myoclonic Seizures					
Valproic acid	1500–2000 mg	3	2–4 d	50–100 µg/mL	See above
Clonazepam	0.04–0.2 mg/kg	2	?	20–80 ng/mL	See above

[a]Approved as adjunctive therapy for focal-onset seizures.

[b]Approved as adjunctive therapy for primary generalized tonic–clonic seizures.

[c]Approved as initial monotherapy for focal-onset seizures.

[d]Approved as initial monotherapy for primary generalized tonic–clonic seizures.

[e]Approved as monotherapy (after conversion from another drug) in focal-onset seizures.

[f]Not to be used as a first-line drug; when used, blood counts should be performed regularly (every 2–4 weeks). Should be used only in selected patients because of risk of aplastic anemia and hepatic failure. It is advisable to obtain written informed consent before use.

3. Key Features

Essentials of Diagnosis

- Recurrent seizures
- Epilepsy should not be diagnosed on the basis of a solitary seizure
- Characteristic electroencephalographic (EEG) changes may occur
- Postictal confusion or focal neurologic deficits may follow and last hours

General Considerations

- The most likely cause relates to the age of onset
- Genetic epilepsy onset ranges from the neonatal period to adolescence or even later in life
- Metabolic disorders may cause seizures
- Trauma is an important cause of seizures
  — Seizures in the first week after head injury do not imply that they will persist
  — Prophylactic anticonvulsant drugs have not been proven to reduce the incidence of posttraumatic epilepsy
- Tumors and other space-occupying lesions result in seizures that are often focal, and most likely with frontal, parietal, or temporal lesions
- Vascular disease is the leading cause in patients aged ≥ 60
- Alzheimer disease (AD) and other neurodegenerative disorders can cause seizures in later life
- CNS infections (meningitis, encephalitis, or brain abscess) must be considered in all age groups as potentially reversible causes of seizures
- Causes of secondary seizures
  — CNS vasculitis, eg, systemic lupus erythematosus
  — Metabolic disorders, including withdrawal from alcohol or other CNS depressant drugs, hypoglycemia, hyperglycemia, uremia, and hyponatremia
  — Trauma
  — CNS infection
  — Neurodegenerative disease, eg, AD
  — Febrile seizures in children younger than 5 years

Demographics

- Epilepsy affects approximately 0.5% of the US population

4. Symptoms and Signs

- Nonspecific prodrome in some (headache, mood alterations, lethargy, myoclonic jerking)
- Aura may precede a generalized seizure by a few seconds or minutes and is itself a part of the attack, arising locally from a restricted region of the brain
- The type of aura depends on the cerebral site of origin of the seizure, eg, gustatory or olfactory hallucinations or visual hallucinations with temporal or occipital lesions, respectively
- In most patients, seizures occur unpredictably
- Fever, sleep loss, alcohol, stress, or flashing lights may precipitate seizures
- Clinical examination may be normal interictally unless there is a structural cause for the seizures
- Immediately postictally, there may be a focal deficit (Todd paresis) or bilateral positive Babinski signs (extensor plantar responses)
- Focal signs postictally suggest focal CNS abnormality
- Seizures may be classified as shown in Table 58-1

5. Differential Diagnosis

- Syncope
- Cardiac arrhythmia

- Stroke or transient ischemic attack
- Pseudoseizure
- Panic attack
- Migraine
- Narcolepsy

6. Laboratory Tests, Imaging, and Procedural Findings

Laboratory Tests

- Hematologic and biochemical screening tests
  — CBC
  — Serum glucose
  — Serum electrolytes
  — Serum creatinine
  — Serum calcium, magnesium
  — Liver biochemical tests
- Lumbar puncture may be necessary (consider computed tomography [CT] first)
  — When any sign of infection is present
  — To evaluate new-onset seizures

Imaging Studies

- MRI on all patients with new-onset seizure disorders has been common but may be unnecessary
- MRI is indicated in all patients with
  — Focal neurologic symptoms or signs
  — Focal seizures, or electroencephalographic findings of a focal disturbance
  — New onset of seizures after the age of 20 years because of the possibility of an underlying neoplasm
- CT may be used when MRI is contraindicated (eg, in a patient with a metallic implant); however, it is generally less sensitive than MRI

Diagnostic Procedures

- History is key, including eyewitness accounts
- EEG
  — May support clinical diagnosis of epilepsy (paroxysmal spikes or sharp waves)
  — May guide prognosis
  — May help classify the seizure disorder
  — Important in evaluating candidates for surgical treatment
- Repeated Holter monitoring may be necessary to establish the diagnosis of cardiac arrhythmia

7. Treatments

Medications

- Anticonvulsant drug treatment is generally not required for
  — A single seizure unless further attacks occur or investigations reveal some underlying untreatable pathology
  — Alcohol withdrawal seizures, which are self-limited
- Patients with alcohol withdrawal seizures should be observed in hospital for at least 24 hours
- Anticonvulsant drug dose is gradually increased until seizures are controlled or side effects occur
- If seizures continue despite treatment at the maximal tolerated dose, a second drug is added and the first drug is then gradually withdrawn
- In most patients, control can be achieved with a single anticonvulsant drug
- Discontinue the anticonvulsant only when the patient is seizure-free for at least 2 years

- Dose reduction should be gradual over a period of weeks or months
  — If seizures recur, treatment is reinstituted with same drugs used previously
- A seizure recurrence after the medication is discontinued is more likely if
  — The patient did not respond to therapy initially
  — Focal or multiple types of seizures
  — EEG abnormalities persist
- Consider the teratogenic potential when initiating any anticonvulsant
- See Table 58-2 for a summary of drug treatments for seizures by type

Surgery
- Surgical resection is most efficacious when there is a single well-defined seizure focus, particularly in the temporal lobe
- Bilateral deep brain stimulation of the anterior thalamus for medically refractory focal-onset seizures may be of benefit, and there is an evolving role for electrical stimulation of other cortical and subcortical targets.

Therapeutic Procedures
- Advise patients to avoid situations that may be dangerous or life-threatening if they have a seizure
- State laws may require clinicians to report to the public health department or department of motor vehicles any patients with seizures or other episodic lapses of consciousness

8. Outcomes

Follow-Up
- Dosing should not be based simply on serum levels because some patients require levels that exceed the therapeutic range ("toxic levels") but tolerate these without ill effect
- In general, the dose of an antiepileptic agent is increased depending on clinical response, not serum drug level
- The trough drug level is then measured to provide a reference point for the maximum tolerated dose
- Measure serum drug levels when another drug is added to the therapeutic regimen and to assess compliance in poorly controlled patients
- Certain antiepileptic drugs may be teratogenic; epileptic women of childbearing potential require special care

Complications
- Status epilepticus
- Residual encephalopathy after prolonged seizures or poor control of seizures

Prognosis
- The risk of seizure recurrence in different series varies between about 30% and 70%
- Among well-chosen patients who undergo surgical resection, up to 70% remain seizure-free after extended follow-up

9. When to Refer and When to Admit

When to Refer
- Behavioral episodes are of uncertain nature
- Seizures are difficult to control or have focal features
- There are accompanying neurologic signs
- There is a progressive neurologic disorder
- Status epilepticus is suspected

When to Admit
- If status epilepticus
- If psychogenic nonepileptic seizures are suspected
- If surgery is contemplated

SUGGESTED REFERENCES

Angus-Leppan H. First seizures in adults. *BMJ*. 2014 Apr 15;348:g2470. [PMID: 24736280]

Berg AT et al. Revised terminology and concepts for organization of seizures and epilepsies: report of the ILAE Commission on Classification and Terminology, 2005–2009. *Epilepsia*. 2010 Apr;51(4): 676–685. [PMID: 20196795]

Englot DJ et al. Rates and predictors of long-term seizure freedom after frontal lobe epilepsy surgery: a systematic review and meta-analysis. *J Neurosurg*. 2012 May;116(5):1042–1048. [PMID: 22304450]

Fisher RS et al. Electrical brain stimulation for epilepsy. *Nat Rev Neurol*. 2014 May;10(5):261–270. [PMID: 24709892]

Glauser T et al. Updated ILAE evidence review of antiepileptic drug efficacy and effectiveness as initial monotherapy for epileptic seizures and syndromes. *Epilepsia*. 2013 Mar;54(3):551–563. [PMID: 23350722]

Moshé SL et al. Epilepsy: new advances. *Lancet*. 2015 Mar 7;385(9971):884-898. [PMID: 25260236]

Nowell M et al. Advances in epilepsy surgery. *J Neurol Neurosurg Psychiatry*. 2014 Nov;85(11): 1273–1279. [PMID: 24719180]

Prasad M et al. Anticonvulsant therapy for status epilepticus. *Cochrane Database Syst Rev*. 2014 Sep 10;9:CD003723. [PMID: 25207925]

59

Bacterial Meningitis

A 19-year-old freshman living in a college dormitory presents to the emergency room with 1 day of fever and headache. On presentation, she complains of anorexia, lethargy, nausea, and vomiting, as well as muscle aches and neck stiffness. On physical examination, her temperature is 39.1°C, and heart rate 124/min. She appears toxic. Her neck is stiff and there are small, purple, and nonblanching petechiae on both of her legs. She is slightly confused about the day's events. Lumbar puncture (LP) is performed and the opening pressure is elevated. Cerebrospinal fluid (CSF) examination shows elevated protein, pleocytosis, low glucose, and intracellular gram-negative diplococci (GNDC) on Gram-stained smear.

LEARNING OBJECTIVES

► Learn the clinical manifestations and objective findings of bacterial meningitis, and the differences between the two most common causes of the disease in adults, pneumococcal and meningococcal meningitis

► Understand the factors that predispose to meningitis

► Know the differential diagnosis of meningitis

► Learn about empiric antibiotic treatment for meningitis, depending on demographic factors, and how to narrow therapy after culture results return

► Understand how to interpret results of CSF analysis

QUESTIONS

1. What are the salient features of this patient's problem?

2. How do you think through her problem?

3. What are the key features, including essentials of diagnosis, general considerations, and demographics of meningitis?

4. What are the symptoms and signs of meningitis?

5. What is the differential diagnosis of meningitis?

6. What are laboratory, imaging, and procedural findings in meningitis?

7. What are the treatments for meningitis?

8. What are the outcomes, including follow-up, complications, prevention, and prognosis of meningitis?

9. When should patients with meningitis be referred to a specialist or admitted to the hospital?

ANSWERS

1. Salient Features

Young adult living in a crowded situation; headache, confusion, muscle aches; meningismus; fever and tachycardia; toxic appearance; petechial rash; CSF with elevated opening pressure, pleocytosis, elevated protein, low glucose, and intracellular organisms consistent with meningococcus on smear

2. How to Think Through

Fever, headache, nausea, and myalgias are a common constellation of nonspecific symptoms, usually caused by viral infection such as influenza. The challenge is to identify those few patients with a serious infection, such as bacterial endocarditis or meningitis. Clinicians should always query patients with acute headache about neck stiffness or pain, and about photophobia. On physical examination, the commonly cited Kernig and Brudzinski signs are not sensitive tests, and their absence does not rule out meningitis. The jolt test, in which headache worsens with rapid horizontal rotation, may be more sensitive. This patient's heart rate is commensurate with fever, but could also indicate the onset of shock, and her blood pressure should be carefully monitored. Her petechial rash is the crucial physical finding. Where should the examiner search for petechiae? (The entire skin and mucosa of the soft palate should be examined.)

While there is a broad differential diagnosis for a petechial rash, meningococcal meningitis is an emergency, and this finding should spur rapid additional evaluation and treatment. She should be placed on isolation precautions. What complications could occur? (Shock, disseminated intravascular coagulation [DIC], altered mental status, seizures, coma, and death.) How should she be managed? (Rapid initiation of antibiotics. Corticosteroids improve outcomes in pneumococcal meningitis, and when adrenal infarction complicates meningococcal meningitis with meningococcemia (so-called Waterhouse Friderichsen syndrome). Fluid resuscitation is vital.

3. Key Features

Essentials of Diagnosis
- Fever, headache, vomiting, confusion, delirium, convulsions
- Petechial rash of skin and mucous membranes
- Neck and back stiffness (meningismus)
- Purulent spinal fluid with bacteria on Gram stain—eg, gram-negative intracellular and extracellular diplococci (*Neisseria meningitidis*) or gram-positive diplococci (*Streptococcus pneumoniae*) or gram-positive rod (*Listeria monocytogenes*)
- Culture of CSF, blood, or aspirates of petechial lesions confirms the diagnosis

General Considerations
- Bacterial meningitis is a central nervous system infection that is a medical emergency
- Immediate diagnostic steps must be instituted to establish the specific cause
- *S pneumoniae* (pneumococcus) is the most common cause of meningitis in adults and the second most common cause of meningitis in children over the age of 6 years
- *N meningitidis* (meningococcus) of groups A, B, C, Y, W-135, and others is transmitted by droplets and may take the form of meningococcemia (a fulminant form of septicemia) without meningitis, meningococcemia with meningitis, or predominantly meningitis
- Chronic recurrent meningococcemia with fever, rash, and arthritis can occur, particularly in those with terminal complement deficiencies

Demographics
- College freshmen—particularly those living in dormitories—and men who have sex with men have been shown to have an increased risk of invasive meningococcal disease

- Until 2000, *S pneumoniae* infections caused 100,000 to 135,000 hospitalizations for pneumonia, 6 million cases of otitis media, and 60,000 cases of invasive disease, including 3300 cases of meningitis; disease figures are now changing due to introduction of the conjugate vaccine

4. Symptoms and Signs

- High fever, chills, and headache; back, abdominal, and extremity pains; and nausea and vomiting are typical
- In severe cases, rapidly developing confusion, delirium, seizures, and coma occur
- Nuchal and back rigidity are typical
- A petechial rash, often first appearing in the lower extremities and at pressure points, is found in meningococcemia
- Petechiae may vary from pinhead sized to large ecchymoses or even areas of skin gangrene that may later slough if the patient survives
- Compared with meningitis caused by the meningococcus, pneumococcal meningitis
  — Lacks a rash
  — Has focal neurologic deficits, cranial nerve palsies, and obtundation as more prominent features
  — May present simultaneously with pneumococcal pneumonia (and sometimes endocarditis, the so-called "Osler triad")

5. Differential Diagnosis

- Meningitis due to other bacteria, eg, *L monocytogenes*, or to viruses, eg, echovirus causing an "aseptic" meningitis
- Subarachnoid hemorrhage
- Encephalitis
- Petechial rash due to
  — Gonococcemia
  — Infective endocarditis
  — Thrombotic thrombocytopenic purpura
  — Rocky Mountain spotted fever
  — Viral exanthem
  — Rickettsial or echovirus infection
  — Other bacterial infections (eg, staphylococcal infections, scarlet fever)
- "Neighborhood reaction" causing abnormal CSF, such as
  — Brain abscess
  — Epidural abscess
  — Vertebral osteomyelitis
  — Mastoiditis
  — Sinusitis
  — Brain tumor
- Dural sinus thrombosis
- Noninfectious meningeal irritation
  — Carcinomatous or lymphomatous meningitis
  — Sarcoidosis
  — Systemic lupus erythematosus
  — Drugs (eg, nonsteroidal anti-inflammatory drugs, trimethoprim–sulfamethoxazole)

6. Laboratory, Imaging, and Procedural Findings

Laboratory Tests

- The organism is usually found by smear or culture of the CSF, oropharynx, blood, or aspirated petechiae
- Prothrombin time and partial thromboplastin time are prolonged, fibrin dimers are elevated, serum fibrinogen level is low, and platelet count is depressed if disseminated DIC is present

Table 59-1. Typical cerebrospinal fluid findings in meningitis and entities in its differential diagnosis.

Diagnosis	Cells/µL	Glucose (mg/dL)	Protein (mg/dL)	Opening Pressure
Normal	0–5 lymphocytes	45–85[a]	15–45	70–180 mm H$_2$0
Purulent meningitis (bacterial)[b], community-acquired	200–20,000 polymorphonuclear neutrophils	Low (< 45)	High (> 50)	Markedly elevated
Granulomatous meningitis (mycobacterial, fungal)[c]	100–1000, mostly lymphocytes[c]	Low (< 45)	High (> 50)	Moderately elevated
Spirochetal meningitis	100–1000, mostly lymphocytes[c]	Normal	Moderately high (> 50)	Normal to slightly elevated
Aseptic meningitis, viral or meningoencephalitis[d]	25–2000, mostly lymphocytes[c]	Normal or low	High (> 50)	Slightly elevated
"Neighborhood reaction"[e]	Variably increased	Normal	Normal or high	Variable

[a]Cerebrospinal fluid glucose must be considered in relation to blood glucose level. Normally, cerebrospinal fluid glucose is 20–30 mg/dL lower than blood glucose, or 50% to 70% of the normal value of blood glucose.

[b]Organisms in smear or culture of cerebrospinal fluid; counterimmunoelectrophoresis or latex agglutination may be diagnostic.

[c]Polymorphonuclear neutrophils may predominate early.

[d]Viral isolation from cerebrospinal fluid early; antibody titer rise in paired specimens of serum; polymerase chain reaction for herpesvirus.

[e]May occur in mastoiditis, brain abscess, epidural abscess, sinusitis, septic thrombus, brain tumor. Cerebrospinal fluid culture results usually negative.

- CSF (see Table 59-1 for interpretation)
  — Elevated opening pressure
  — Elevated white blood cell count (typically > 1000/µL), with a predominance of polymorphonuclear leukocytes
  — Glucose concentration is < 40 mg/dL, or < 50% of the simultaneous serum concentration
  — Protein usually exceeds 150 mg/dL
  — Gram stain shows gram-positive cocci in up to 80% to 90% of cases of pneumococcal meningitis or GNDC in meningococcal meningitis
  — The absence of organisms in a Gram-stained smear does not rule out the diagnosis
- In untreated cases, blood or CSF cultures are almost always positive
- Bacteremia is common
- Antigen detection tests for pneumococcus may occasionally be helpful in establishing the diagnosis in the patient who has been partially treated and in whom cultures and stains are negative

Imaging Studies
- If there are any neurologic defects or signs of elevated intracranial pressure (ICP), magnetic resonance imaging (MRI) or computed tomography (CT) imaging should be done to exclude a mass lesion before LP to prevent herniation (*although after blood cultures are obtained, antibiotic administration should not be delayed to obtain imaging studies*)

Diagnostic Procedures
- LP and CSF examination are essential to the diagnosis

7. Treatments
Medications
- Table 59-2 summarizes initial empiric antibiotics to be administered in cases of suspected or confirmed bacterial meningitis for the common causative organisms by patient age
- Table 59-3 provides examples of initial empiric antibiotics to be administered to acutely ill, hospitalized adults with various types of suspected meningitis

Table 59-2. Initial antimicrobial therapy for purulent meningitis of unknown cause.

Population	Common Microorganisms	Standard Therapy
18–50 y	*Streptococcus pneumoniae, Neisseria meningitidis*	Vancomycin[a] **plus** cefotaxime or ceftriaxone[b]
Over 50 y	*S pneumoniae, N meningitidis, Listeria monocytogenes,* gram-negative bacilli	Vancomycin[a] **plus** ampicillin,[c] **plus** cefotaxime or ceftriaxone[b]
Impaired cellular immunity	*L monocytogenes,* gram-negative bacilli, *S pneumoniae*	Vancomycin[a] **plus** ampicillin[c] **plus** cefepime[d]
Postsurgical or posttraumatic	*Staphylococcus aureus, S pneumoniae,* gram-negative bacilli	Vancomycin[a] **plus** cefepime[d]

[a]The dose of vancomycin is 15 mg/kg/dose intravenously every 6 h.

[b]The usual dose of cefotaxime is 2 g intravenously every 6 h and that of ceftriaxone is 2 g intravenously every 12 h. If the organism is sensitive to penicillin, 3 to 4 million units intravenously every 4 h is given.

[c]The dose of ampicillin is usually 2 g intravenously every 4 h.

[d]Cefepime is given in a dose of 2 to 3 g intravenously every 8 h.

- *Intravenous antimicrobial therapy should be started immediately after blood cultures are obtained in all acutely ill patients* and before proceeding with imaging studies, if these are indicated
- If LP must be delayed (eg, while awaiting results of an imaging study to exclude a mass lesion), ceftriaxone, 4 g intravenously, should be given after blood cultures (positive in 50% of cases) have been obtained
- If Gram-positive diplococci are present on the Gram stain, then vancomycin, 30 mg/kg/d intravenously in two divided doses, should be administered in addition to ceftriaxone until the isolate is confirmed not to be penicillin-resistant
- In those patients age > 50 or age < 2 years, empiric treatment for *L monocytogenes* should be added with ampicillin 2 g intravenously every 4 hours
- Once susceptibility to penicillin has been confirmed, penicillin, 24 million units daily intravenously in six divided doses, or ceftriaxone, 4 g/d as a single dose or as two divided doses, is recommended
- Chloramphenicol, 1 g every 6 hours, is an alternative in the severely penicillin- or cephalosporin-allergic patient
- The best therapy for penicillin-resistant strains depends upon susceptibility testing
  — If the minimum inhibitory concentration (MIC) of ceftriaxone or cefotaxime is ≤ 0.5 μg/mL, single-drug therapy with either of these cephalosporins is likely to be effective
  — When the MIC is ≥ 1 μg/mL, treatment with a combination of ceftriaxone, 2 g every 12 hours, plus vancomycin, 30 mg/kg/d in two divided doses, is recommended

Table 59-3. Examples of initial antimicrobial therapy for acutely ill, hospitalized adults with meningitis pending identification of causative organism.

Suspected Clinical Diagnosis	Likely Etiologic Diagnosis	Drugs of Choice
Meningitis, bacterial, community-acquired	Pneumococcus,[a] meningococcus	Cefotaxime,[b] 2–3 g intravenously every 6 h; **or** ceftriaxone, 2 g intravenously every 12 h plus vancomycin, 15 mg/kg intravenously every 8 h
Meningitis, bacterial, age > 50, community acquired	Pneumococcus, meningococcus, *Listeria monocytogenes,*[c] gram-negative bacilli	Ampicillin, 2 g intravenously every 4 h, plus cefotaxime, 2–3 g intravenously every 6 h; or ceftriaxone, 2 g intravenously every 12 h plus vancomycin, 15 mg/kg intravenously every 8 h
Meningitis, postoperative (or posttraumatic)	*S aureus,* gram-negative bacilli (pneumococcus, in posttraumatic)	Vancomycin, 15 mg/kg intravenously every 8 h, plus cefepime, 3 g intravenously every 8 h

[a]Some strains may be resistant to penicillin.

[b]Most studies on meningitis have been with cefotaxime or ceftriaxone.

[c]TMP-SMZ can be used to treat *Listeria monocytogenes* in patients allergic to penicillin in a dosage of 15–20 mg/kg/d of TMP in three or four divided doses.

- Duration of therapy is 10 to 14 days in documented cases of bacterial meningitis
  — Give dexamethasone (0.6 mg/kg/d divided into four divided doses, or 10 mg) intravenously immediately prior to or concomitantly with the first dose of appropriate antibiotic and every 6 hours thereafter for a total of 4 days if pneumococcal meningitis is suspected (eg, if gram-positive diplococci are seen on CSF gram stain); similarly, treat *immediately* with hydrocortisone 100 to 300 mg intravenously, then 50 mg intravenously every 6 hours, if adrenal infarction is suspected in meningococcal meningitis with meningococcemia (eg, gram-negative diplococci are seen on CSF gram stain; petechiae; shock).

Therapeutic Procedures
- LP
  — Should be performed in all patients with suspected meningitis
  — Obtain MRI or CT imaging to exclude a mass lesion before LP to prevent herniation if papilledema, other evidence of increased ICP, or focal neurologic deficits are present

8. Outcomes

Follow-Up
- If a patient with a penicillin-resistant organism has not responded to a third-generation cephalosporin, repeat LP is indicated to assess the bacteriologic response

Complications
- Obtundation or deterioration in mental status may result from cerebral edema and increased ICP
- With meningococcal meningitis
  — DIC
  — Ischemic necrosis of digits, distal extremities
- With pneumococcal meningitis
  — Hearing loss
  — Residual neurologic deficit

Prevention
- For meningococcal meningitis, effective polysaccharide vaccines for meningococcus groups A, C, Y, and W-135 are available (see *Current Medical Diagnosis and Treatment 2016,* Table 30-7)
- The Advisory Committee on Immunization Practices recommends immunization with a dose of MCV4 for preadolescents ages 11–12 with a booster at age 16
- For ease of program implementation, persons aged 21 years or younger should have documentation of receipt of a dose of MCV4 not more than 5 years before enrollment in college
- If the primary dose was administered before the 16th birthday, a booster dose should be administered before enrollment
- Vaccine is also recommend as a two-dose primary series administered 2 months apart for
  — Persons aged 2 through 54 years with persistent complement deficiency
  — Persons with functional or anatomic asplenia
  — Adolescents with HIV infection
- All other persons at increased risk for meningococcal disease (eg, military recruits, microbiologists, or travelers to an epidemic or highly endemic country) should receive a single dose
- Outbreaks in closed populations are best controlled by eliminating nasopharyngeal carriage of meningococci
  — Rifampin is the drug of choice, in a dosage of 600 mg twice daily orally for 2 days
  — Ciprofloxacin, 500 mg orally once or ceftriaxone, 250 mg intramuscularly once is also effective in adults
- For prevention of pneumococcal meningitis, pneumococcal vaccine is recommended (see *Current Medical Diagnosis and Treatment 2016,* Table 30-7)

- In particular, pneumococcal vaccine is recommended for patients with
  — Asplenia
  — Sickle cell disease
  — Chronic illnesses (eg, cardiopulmonary disease, alcoholism, cirrhosis, chronic kidney disease, nephrotic syndrome, CSF leaks)
  — Asthma
  — Immunocompromise (eg, patients with Hodgkin disease, lymphoma, chronic lymphocytic leukemia, multiple myeloma, congenital immunodeficiency, asymptomatic or symptomatic HIV infection, organ or bone marrow transplant recipients)
  — Patients who receive immunosuppressive therapy or smoke cigarettes, and all Alaskan Natives should also receive the vaccine
  — Because of the apparent increased risk of developing pneumococcal meningitis following cochlear implants, patients receiving these implants should be vaccinated

Prognosis
- Mortality is < 5% with early therapy of patients with meningitis
- Meningococcemia is associated with a 20% mortality
- Patients presenting with depressed levels of consciousness have a worse outcome
- Dexamethasone administered with antibiotic to adults with pneumococcal meningitis has been associated with a 60% reduction in mortality and a 50% reduction in unfavorable outcome

9. When to Refer and When to Admit

When to Refer
- All patients with suspected bacterial meningitis

When to Admit
- All patients in whom bacterial meningitis is suspected should be admitted for empiric therapy and observation

SUGGESTED REFERENCES

Campsall PA et al. Severe meningococcal infection: a review of epidemiology, diagnosis, and management. *Crit Care Clin*. 2013 Jul;29(3):393–409. [PMID: 23830646]

Cohn AC et al. Centers for Disease Control and Prevention (CDC). Prevention and control of meningococcal disease: recommendations of the Advisory Committee on Immunization Practices (ACIP). *MMWR Recomm Rep*. 2013 Mar 22;62(RR-2):1–28. [PMID: 23515099]

Erdem H et al. Mortality indicators in pneumococcal meningitis: therapeutic implications. *Int J Infect Dis*. 2014 Feb;19:13–19. [PMID: 24211227]

Mandal S et al. Prolonged university outbreak of meningococcal disease associated with a serogroup B strain rarely seen in the United States. *Clin Infect Dis*. 2013 Aug;57(3):344–348. [PMID: 23595832]

McIntyre PB et al. Effect of vaccines on bacterial meningitis worldwide. *Lancet*. 2012 Nov 10;380(9854):1703–1711. [PMID: 23141619]

Simon MS et al. Invasive meningococcal disease in men who have sex with men. *Ann Intern Med*. 2013 Aug 20;159(4):300–301. [PMID: 23778867]

van de Beek D et al. Advances in treatment of bacterial meningitis. *Lancet*. 2012 Nov 10;380(9854):1693–1702. [PMID: 23141618]

Zheteyeva Y et al. Safety of meningococcal polysaccharide-protein conjugate vaccine in pregnancy: a review of the Vaccine Adverse Event Reporting System. *Am J Obstet Gynecol*. 2013 Jun;208(6):478.e1–e6. [PMID: 23453881]

Myasthenia Gravis

60

A 35-year-old woman presents to the clinic with a chief complaint of double vision. She reports intermittent and progressively worsening double vision for approximately 2 months, rarely at first but now everyday. She works as a computer programmer, and the double vision increases the longer she stares at the computer screen. In addition, she has noted a drooping of her eyelids, which seems to worsen with prolonged computer work. Both symptoms subside with rest. She is generally fatigued but has noted no other weakness or neurologic symptoms. Her medical history is unremarkable. Physical examination is notable only for the cranial nerve examination, which shows impaired lateral movement of the right eye and bilateral ptosis, both of which worsen with repetitive eye movements. Motor, sensory, and reflex examinations are otherwise unremarkable.

LEARNING OBJECTIVES

▶ Learn the clinical manifestations and objective findings of myasthenia gravis (MG), including which muscle groups are most likely to be affected

▶ Understand the factors that predispose to developing MG, and diseases associated with it

▶ Know the differential diagnosis of MG

▶ Understand the ability of laboratory and muscle testing to diagnose MG

▶ Learn the treatments for MG including which patients should be referred for thymectomy

QUESTIONS

1. What are the salient features of this patient's problem?

2. How do you think through her problem?

3. What are the key features, including essentials of diagnosis, general considerations, and demographics, of MG?

4. What are the symptoms and signs of MG?

5. What is the differential diagnosis of MG?

6. What are laboratory, imaging, and procedural findings in MG?

7. What are the treatments for MG?

8. What are the outcomes, including complications and prognosis, of MG?

9. When should patients with MG be referred to a specialist or admitted to the hospital?

ANSWERS

1. Salient Features

Young woman with double vision (diplopia) and drooping of the eyelids (ptosis); intermittent, but progressive symptoms; fatigable voluntary muscle weakness and improvement with rest; bilateral ptosis on examination, which worsens with repetitive eye movements

2. How to Think Through

Diplopia should always be carefully evaluated. While it has many possible etiologies, what serious causes should be considered on initial evaluation? (Intracranial structural lesion or bleeding, temporal arteritis, thyroid ophthalmopathy, botulism, and others.) What is the pattern of symptoms seen in MG? (Daily fatigability, fluctuation of severity over weeks.) In addition to young adult women, what other demographic group is most often diagnosed with MG? (Older adult men.) What other comorbid and familial diseases occur with MG, which might strengthen a suspicion of it? (Autoimmune diseases such as rheumatoid arthritis [RA], systemic lupus erythematosus [SLE], Hashimoto thyroiditis, and Graves disease.) What muscle groups should be examined? (Ocular, bulbar [dysphagia, dysarthria], respiratory, and limb muscles.) Does MG affect the pupils? (No. This can help distinguish MG from botulism and third cranial nerve compression.) Can MG affect the sensory system? (No.) What causes muscle weakness in MG? (Autoantibodies to acetylcholine receptors [AChR] or to muscle-specific receptor tyrosine kinase [MuSK].) How can we confirm the diagnosis? (AChR antibody testing; electrophysiologic testing including repetitive nerve stimulation and electromyography [EMG].)

It is important to consider diseases of the thymus gland when MG is diagnosed. Thymic hyperplasia is present in 85% of patients with MG, and thymoma, in 15%. Resection of a thymoma can improve symptoms, even in the absence of radiologically identifiable thymoma. What is the pharmacologic mainstay of treatment? (Anticholinesterase [AChEI] drugs.)

3. Key Features

Essentials of Diagnosis

- Fluctuating weakness of voluntary muscles, producing symptoms such as
  — Diplopia
  — Ptosis
  — Difficulty in swallowing
- Activity increases weakness of affected muscles
- Short-acting AChEIs transiently improve the weakness

General Considerations

- MG occurs at all ages, but is most common in young women with HLA-DR3 and in older men, sometimes in association with thymoma MG is also associated with
  — Thyrotoxicosis
  — RA
  — SLE
- Onset is usually insidious, but the disorder is sometimes unmasked by a coincidental infection
- Exacerbations may occur before the menstrual period and during or shortly after pregnancy
- Symptoms are due to blockage of neuromuscular transmission caused by autoantibodies binding to AChR
- The external ocular muscles and certain other cranial muscles, including the masticatory, facial, and pharyngeal muscles, are especially likely to be affected
- The respiratory and limb muscles may also be involved

Demographics
- Most common in young women with HLA-DR3
- If thymoma is associated, older men are more commonly affected

4. Symptoms and Signs
- Initial symptoms
  - Ptosis
  - Diplopia
  - Difficulty in chewing or swallowing
  - Respiratory difficulties
  - Limb weakness
  - Some combination of these problems
- Weakness
  - May remain localized to a few muscle groups, especially the extraocular muscles
  - May become generalized
- Symptoms often fluctuate in intensity during the day
- This diurnal variation is superimposed on a tendency to longer-term spontaneous relapses and remissions that may last for weeks
- Clinical examination confirms the weakness and fatigability of affected muscles
- Extraocular palsies and ptosis, often asymmetric, are common
- Pupillary responses are normal
- The bulbar and limb muscles are often weak, but the pattern of involvement is variable
- Sustained activity of affected muscles increases the weakness, which improves after a brief rest
- Sensation is normal
- Usually no reflex changes

5. Differential Diagnosis
- Lambert–Eaton myasthenic syndrome (usually paraneoplastic)
- Botulism
- Aminoglycoside-induced neuromuscular weakness

6. Laboratory, Imaging, and Procedural Findings

Laboratory Tests
- Elevated level of serum AChR antibodies
  - Test has a sensitivity of 80% to 90%
- Certain patients have an elevated level of serum antibodies to MuSK
  - These patients are more likely to have facial, respiratory, and proximal muscle weakness than those with antibodies to AChR

Imaging Studies
- Computed tomography of the chest with and without contrast
  - Should be obtained to demonstrate a coexisting thymoma
  - However, normal studies do not exclude this possibility

Diagnostic Procedures
- Electrophysiology
  - Demonstration of a decrementing muscle response to repetitive 2- or 3-Hz stimulation of motor nerves indicates a disturbance of neuromuscular transmission
  - Such an abnormality may even be detected in clinically strong muscles with certain provocative procedures
- Needle EMG
  - Shows a marked variation in configuration and size of individual motor unit potentials in affected muscles
  - Single-fiber EMG reveals an increased jitter, or variability, in the time interval between two muscle fiber action potentials from the same motor unit

7. Treatments

Medications

- Drugs, such as aminoglycosides, that may exacerbate MG should be avoided
- AChEI drugs provide symptomatic benefit without influencing the course of the disease
- Neostigmine, pyridostigmine, or both can be used
  — Dose is determined on an individual basis
  — Usual dose of neostigmine, 7.5 to 30 mg four times daily orally (average, 15 mg)
  — Usual dose of pyridostigmine, 30 to 180 mg four times daily orally (average, 60 mg)
  — Overmedication may temporarily increase weakness
- Corticosteroids
  — Indicated if there has been a poor response to AChEI drugs and the patient has had thymectomy
  — Start while the patient is in the hospital, since weakness may initially be aggravated
  — Dose is determined on an individual basis
  — An initial high daily dose (eg, prednisone, 60–100 mg orally) can gradually be tapered to a relatively low maintenance level as improvement occurs; total withdrawal is, however, difficult
- Azathioprine
  — May also be effective
  — Usual dose, 2 to 3 mg/kg/d orally after a lower initial dose
- Mycophenolate mofetil or cyclosporine is typically reserved for more refractory cases or as a strategy to reduce the corticosteroid dose
- Plasmapheresis or intravenous immunoglobulin therapy
  — May be helpful in patients with major disability
  — May also be useful for managing acute crisis and for stabilizing patients before thymectomy
  — Have similar efficacy

Surgery

- Thymectomy
  — Usually leads to symptomatic benefit or remission
  — Should be considered in all patients younger than age 60, unless weakness is restricted to the extraocular muscles
- If the disease is of recent onset and only slowly progressive, operation is sometimes delayed for a year or so, in the hope that spontaneous remission will occur

8. Outcomes

Complications

- Aspiration pneumonia
- Life-threatening exacerbations of myasthenia (so-called myasthenic crisis) may lead to respiratory muscle weakness requiring immediate admission to the intensive care unit

Prognosis

- The disorder follows a slowly progressive course and may have a fatal outcome owing to respiratory complications such as aspiration pneumonia

9. When to Refer and When to Admit

When to Refer

- Refer all patients with a new diagnosis of MG to a neurologist

When to Admit

- Patients with acute exacerbation or respiratory muscle involvement
- Patients requiring plasmapheresis
- Patients who are starting corticosteroid therapy
- For thymectomy

SUGGESTED REFERENCES

Diaz A et al. Is thymectomy in non-thymomatous myasthenia gravis of any benefit? *Interact Cardiovasc Thorac Surg.* 2014 Mar;18(3):381–389. [PMID: 24351507]

Sieb JP. Myasthenia gravis: an update for the clinician. *Clin Exp Immunol.* 2014 Mar;175(3):408–418. [PMID: 24117026]

61

Parkinson Disease

A 63-year-old man comes to the clinic with a several month history of difficulty with his gait and coordination. He finds walking difficult and has almost fallen on a number of occasions, especially when trying to change directions. He has also found that using his hands is difficult, and other people have noticed that his hands shake. Physical examination is notable for a resting tremor in the hands that disappears with intentional movement. He has a shuffling gait with difficulty turning. There is "cogwheeling" rigidity in his arms, a jerky sensation with passive flexion and extension of the arms.

LEARNING OBJECTIVES

▶ Learn the clinical manifestations and objective findings of Parkinson disease (PD), including the primary attributes of parkinsonian tremor and gait

▶ Understand the secondary causes of PD

▶ Know the differential diagnosis for PD

▶ Learn the medication classes, combination therapies, and surgical options used in the treatment for PD

▶ Know what the complications of treatment for PD are, and how to manage them

QUESTIONS

1. What are the salient features of this patient's problem?

2. How do you think through his problem?

3. What are the key features, including essentials of diagnosis, general considerations, and demographics, of PD?

4. What are the symptoms and signs of PD?

5. What is the differential diagnosis of PD?

6. What are procedural findings in PD?

7. What are the treatments for PD?

8. What is the outcome, including complications, of PD?

9. When should patients with PD be referred to a specialist or admitted to the hospital?

ANSWERS

1. Salient Features

Gait disturbance; difficulty in changing directions; resting tremor without intention tremor; shuffling gait; cogwheeling rigidity of the limbs on physical examination

2. How to Think Through

This patient has several characteristic physical findings of parkinsonism. What other findings are commonly seen in PD and should be explored here? (Name as many as possible, then see Symptoms and Signs.) Before concluding that this patient has idiopathic PD, what other processes should be considered? (Extrapyramidal side effects of neuroleptic medications; multisystem atrophy, characterized in part by dysautonomia; normal pressure hydrocephalus [NPH], characterized by difficulty initiating gait and incontinence; progressive supranuclear palsy [PSP].) What neurodegenerative process is associated with PD? (Dementia with Lewy bodies, characterized by paranoia, visual hallucinations, waxing and waning mental status, sometimes resembling delirium.)

Once a diagnosis of idiopathic PD is made, how should the patient be treated? What are the pharmacologic classes employed? (Anticholinergics, amantadine, carbidopa/levodopa, and other dopaminergic agonists, see Treatment.) Why might we delay treatment with levodopa and use other agents initially? (While levodopa is the most effective treatment for PD, it can cause both dyskinesias as well as response fluctuations—the "on–off" phenomenon—in which bradykinesia alternates unpredictably with dyskinesias.) What nonpharmacologic interventions are available? (Deep brain stimulation. Additionally, all patients should have physical therapy, home safety evaluation, and mobility aids as needed.)

3. Key Features

Essentials of Diagnosis

- Motor disturbances including tremor, rigidity, bradykinesia, and progressive postural instability
- Depression and anxiety are common, as are anosmia, constipation, and sleep disturbances
- Cognitive impairment is sometimes prominent

General Considerations

- Risk factors
  — Age
  — Family history
  — Male sex
  — Ongoing herbicide/pesticide exposure
  — Significant prior head trauma
- Dopamine depletion due to degeneration of the dopaminergic nigrostriatal system leads to an imbalance of dopamine and acetylcholine
- Exposure to toxins and certain medications can lead to parkinsonism
  — Manganese dust
  — Carbon disulfide
  — Severe carbon monoxide poisoning
  — 1-Methyl-4-phenyl-1,2,5,6-tetrahydropyridine (a recreational drug)
  — Neuroleptic drugs
  — Reserpine
  — Metoclopramide
- Postencephalitic parkinsonism is becoming increasingly rare
- Only rarely is hemiparkinsonism the presenting feature of a space-occupying lesion

Demographics

- Common disorder that occurs in all ethnic groups, with an approximately equal sex distribution
- The most common variety, idiopathic PD, begins most often in people between ages 45 and 65 years
- May rarely occur on a familial basis

4. Symptoms and Signs

- Cardinal features
  — Tremor
  — Rigidity
  — Bradykinesia
  — Postural instability
- Tremor
  — Four to six cycles per second
  — Most conspicuous at rest
  — Enhanced by stress
  — Often less severe during voluntary activity
  — Commonly confined to one limb or to one side for months or years before becoming more generalized
  — May be present about mouth and lips
  — May be absent in some patients
- Rigidity causes the flexed posture
- Bradykinesia is the most disabling symptom, ie, a slowness of voluntary movement and a reduction in automatic movements such as swinging of the arms while walking
- Immobility of the facial muscles with
  — Widened palpebral fissures
  — Infrequent blinking
  — Fixity of facial expression
  — Seborrhea of face and scalp
- Mild blepharoclonus
- Repetitive tapping (about twice per second) over the bridge of the nose producing a sustained blink response (Myerson sign)
- Other findings
  — Saliva drooling from the mouth
  — Soft and poorly modulated voice
  — Variable rest tremor and rigidity in some or all of the limbs
  — Slowness of voluntary movements
  — Impairment of fine or rapidly alternating movements
  — Micrographia
- No muscle weakness and no alteration in the tendon reflexes or plantar responses
- Difficulty rising from a sitting position and beginning to walk
- Gait
  — Small shuffling steps and a loss of the normal automatic arm swing
  — Unsteadiness on turning, difficulty in stopping, and a tendency to fall
- Decline in intellectual function
- Depression and anxiety
- Anosmia
- Constipation
- Sleep disturbances

5. Differential Diagnosis

- Essential tremor
- Depression

- Wilson disease
- Huntington disease
- NPH
- Multisystem atrophy (previously called Shy–Drager syndrome)
- PSP
- Corticobasal ganglionic degeneration
- Jakob–Creutzfeldt disease
- Other causes of parkinsonism, eg, drugs
  — Antipsychotic agents
  — Reserpine
  — Metoclopramide

6. Procedural Findings

Diagnostic Procedures
- Primarily a clinical diagnosis

7. Treatments

Medications
- Amantadine (100 mg twice daily orally)
  — May improve all of the clinical features of parkinsonism
  — Ameliorates dyskinesias resulting from prolonged levodopa therapy
- Sinemet
  — A combination of carbidopa and levodopa in a fixed ratio (1:10 or 1:4)
  — Start with small dose, eg, 1 tablet of Sinemet 25/100 (containing 25 mg of carbidopa and 100 mg of levodopa) three times daily orally, and gradually increase depending on the response
- Sinemet carbidopa–levodopa (CR)
  — A controlled-release formulation (containing 25 or 50 mg of carbidopa and 100 or 200 mg of levodopa)
  — Sometimes helpful in reducing fluctuations in clinical response and in reducing the frequency with which medication must be taken
- Stalevo is a commercial preparation of levodopa combined with both carbidopa and entacapone
  — Stalevo 50 (12.5 mg of carbidopa, 50 mg of levodopa, and 200 mg of entacapone)
  — Stalevo 100 (25 mg of carbidopa, 100 mg of levodopa, and 200 mg of entacapone)
  — Stalevo 150 (37.5 mg of carbidopa, 150 mg of levodopa, and 200 mg of entacapone)
- Pramipexole and Ropinirole
  — Newer dopamine agonists that is not an ergot derivative
  — Effective in both early and advanced stages of Parkinson disease
  — Often started either before the introduction of levodopa or with a low dose of Sinemet when dopaminergic therapy is first introduced
  — Pramipexole dosing:
    › Start with 0.125 mg, doubled after 1 week, and again after another week
    › Daily dose is then increased by 0.75 mg at weekly intervals depending on response and tolerance
    › Most patients require between 0.5 and 1.5 mg three times daily orally
  — Ropinirole dosing:
    › Start with 0.25 mg three times daily orally
    › Total daily dose is increased at weekly intervals by 0.75 mg until the fourth week and increased by 1.5 mg thereafter
    › Most patients require between 2 and 8 mg three times daily orally
- Rotigotine is a dopamine agonist absorbed transdermally from a skin patch; it is started at 2 mg once daily and increasing weekly by 2 mg daily until achieving an optimal response, up to a maximum of 8 mg daily

- Rasagiline and selegiline
  - Selective monoamine oxidase B inhibitors
  - Rasagiline (1 mg/d orally taken in morning) may slow progression of disease
  - Selegiline (5 mg orally with breakfast and lunch) is sometimes used instead as adjunctive treatment; improves fluctuations or declining response to levodopa
  - Although it is sometimes advised that tyramine-rich foods be avoided when either of these agents is taken because of the theoretical possibility of a hypertensive ("cheese") effect, there is no clinical evidence to support the need for such dietary precautions when they are taken at the recommended dosage
- Entacapone and tolcapone, two catecholamine-O-methyltransferase inhibitors, may be used as an adjunct to Sinemet when there are response fluctuations or inadequate responses
  - Entacapone is given as 200 mg orally with each dose of Sinemet
  - Entacapone is generally preferred over tolcapone
  - Tolcapone is given in a dosage of 100 or 200 mg three times daily orally
  - Tolcapone should be avoided in patients with preexisting liver disease because of rare cases of fulminant hepatic failure following its use
  - With either preparation, the dose of Sinemet taken concurrently may have to be reduced by up to one-third to avoid side effects
- Anticholinergics (see Table 61-1) are more helpful for tremor and rigidity than bradykinesia
  - Start with a small dose
  - Common side effects include dryness of the mouth, nausea, constipation, palpitations, cardiac arrhythmias, urinary retention, confusion, agitation, restlessness, drowsiness, mydriasis, increased intraocular pressure, and defective accommodation
  - Contraindicated in patients with prostatic hypertrophy, narrow-angle glaucoma, or obstructive intestinal disease
  - Often tolerated poorly by the elderly
  - Should be avoided when cognitive impairment or a predisposition to delirium exists
- Confusion and psychotic symptoms often respond to atypical antipsychotic agents
  - Olanzapine
  - Quetiapine
  - Risperidone
  - Clozapine
- Clozapine may rarely cause marrow suppression, and weekly blood cell counts are therefore necessary
  - Starting dose, 6.25 mg at bedtime orally
  - Dose is increased to 25 to 100 mg/d as needed
  - In low doses, clozapine may also improve iatrogenic dyskinesias
- Bromocriptine is not widely used in the United States because of side effects
- Pergolide has been withdrawn from the US market after two studies showed that serious cardiac valvular abnormalities developed in some patients taking the drug

Table 61-1. Some anticholinergic antiparkinsonian drugs.

Drug	Usual Daily Dose
Benztropine mesylate (Cogentin)	1–6 mg
Biperiden (Akineton)	2–12 mg
Orphenadrine (Disipal, Norflex)	150–400 mg
Procyclidine (Kemadrin)	7.5–30 mg
Trihexyphenidyl (Artane)	6–20 mg

Modified, with permission, from Aminoff MJ. Pharmacologic management of parkinsonism and other movement disorders. In: Katzung BG, ed. *Basic & Clinical Pharmacology*. 11th ed. New York: McGraw-Hill; 2009.

Surgery

- High-frequency bilateral stimulation of the subthalamic nuclei or globus pallidus internus may benefit all of the major features of the disease, and it has a lower morbidity than lesion surgery

Therapeutic Procedures

- Drug therapy may not be required early
- Physical and speech therapy and simple aids to daily living may help
  — Rails or banisters placed strategically about the home
  — Special table cutlery with large handles
  — Nonslip rubber table mats
  — Devices to amplify the voice
- Gene therapy
  — Injections of adeno-associated viruses encoding various human genes have been made into the subthalamic nucleus or putamen in various Phase I and Phase II trials of gene therapy
  — Results have been disappointing except that transfer of the gene for glutamic acid decarboxylase into the subthalamic nucleus seems to improve motor function
  — Trials are continuing but the procedure appears to be safe

8. Outcome

Complications

- Levodopa-induced dyskinesias may take any form
  — Chorea
  — Athetosis
  — Dystonia
  — Tremor
  — Tics
  — Myoclonus
- Later complications of the drug include response fluctuations (the "on–off phenomenon")
  — Abrupt but transient fluctuations in the severity of parkinsonism occur unpredictably but frequently during the day
  — The "off" period of marked bradykinesia has been shown to relate in some instances to falling plasma levels of levodopa
  — During the "on" phase, dyskinesias are often conspicuous but mobility is increased
  — Because of this complication, levodopa therapy should be postponed and dopamine agonists used instead, except in the elderly

9. When to Refer and When to Admit

When to Refer

- Refer all patients with PD to a neurologist

When to Admit

- Admit all patients requiring neurosurgical treatment

SUGGESTED REFERENCES

Athauda D et al. The ongoing pursuit of neuroprotective therapies in Parkinson disease. *Nat Rev Neurol*. 2015 Jan;11(1):25–40. [PMID: 25447485]

Connolly BS et al. Pharmacological treatment of Parkinson disease: a review. *JAMA*. 2014 Apr 23–30;311(16):1670–1683. [PMID: 24756517]

Kalia SK et al. Deep brain stimulation for Parkinson's disease and other movement disorders. *Curr Opin Neurol*. 2013 Aug;26(4):374–3480. [PMID: 23817213]

LeWitt PA et al. AAV2-GAD gene therapy for advanced Parkinson's disease: a double-blind, sham-surgery controlled, randomised trial. *Lancet Neurol*. 2011 Apr;10(4):309–319. [PMID: 21419704]

Williams DR et al. Parkinsonian syndromes. *Continuum (Minneap Minn)*. 2013 Oct;19(5):1189–1212. [PMID: 24092286]

62 Stroke

An 82-year-old woman with atrial fibrillation came to the emergency room after the acute onset of difficulty in moving her right arm and leg 1 hour before presentation. Her past medical history includes a transient ischemic attack (TIA), hypertension, and diabetes mellitus. She had been taking warfarin, but discontinued it 3 months prior after a mechanical fall, and now takes no medications. On physical examination, she has weakness in, and sensory neglect of, her right upper and lower extremities. Her neurologic examination further reveals a global aphasia with deficits in comprehension and object naming. Complete blood count including platelets and coagulation panels are normal. A noncontrast computed tomography (CT) of the brain shows no intracranial bleeding. Intravenous (IV) recombinant tissue plasminogen activator is administered.

LEARNING OBJECTIVES

▶ Learn the clinical manifestations and objective findings of ischemic, lacunar, and hemorrhagic stroke syndromes
▶ Understand the factors that predispose to stroke and how to prevent them
▶ Know the differential diagnosis of stroke
▶ Learn the treatment for ischemic and hemorrhagic stroke
▶ Know the indications and contraindications for tissue-type plasminogen activator use in ischemic stroke

QUESTIONS

1. What are the salient features of this patient's problem?
2. How do you think through her problem?
3. What are the key features, including essentials of diagnosis, general considerations, and demographics of stroke?
4. What are the symptoms and signs of stroke?
5. What is the differential diagnosis of stroke?
6. What are laboratory, imaging, and procedural findings in stroke?
7. What are the treatments for stroke?

8. What are the outcomes, including follow-up, prognosis and prevention, of stroke?

9. When should patients with stroke be referred to a specialist or admitted to the hospital?

ANSWERS

1. Salient Features

Elderly patient; acute onset aphasia, right-sided hemiplegia, and neglect; presentation within 4.5 hours of onset of symptoms; risk factors of atrial fibrillation, hypertension, diabetes mellitus, and previous TIA; not on anticoagulant medication; no intracranial bleeding

2. How to Think Through

Stroke is a leading cause of death in the Western world and is a major cause of morbidity. What are the likely causes of this patient's stroke? (Atrial fibrillation leading to cardioembolic stroke; hypertension and diabetes mellitus leading to carotid atherosclerosis or intracranial small vessel disease and thrombotic stroke.) What is her CHADS2 score? (This decision aid is used to assess risk of embolic stroke in patients with atrial fibrillation. She receives 1 point each for hypertension, age > 75 years, and diabetes, plus 2 points for prior TIA, for a total of 5 points. This confers a 6.9% risk of stroke per year, without anticoagulation.) Based on her examination, what vascular territory is involved? (Left middle cerebral artery.) How can the examiner differentiate aphasia from dysarthria? (Repetition of simple words is intact in most cases of aphasia, and demonstrates intelligible speech production.)

What factors must be assessed prior to thrombolysis? (*Absence* of: hemorrhage on non-contrast CT scan; stroke or head trauma in prior 3 months; recent major surgery or major bleeding; duration of symptoms > 4.5 hours; blood pressure > 185/110; international normalized ratio [INR] > 1.7; platelets < 100, 000/μL.) If the patient is in atrial fibrillation the day following the stroke, should cardioversion be considered to reduce risk of a second stroke? (No! Cardioversion in a patient with atrial fibrillation and recent stroke elderly, cerebral amyloid angiopathy who is not on anticoagulation can precipitate an embolic stroke.)

3. Key Features

Essentials of Diagnosis

- **Ischemic stroke** is a thrombotic or embolic occlusion of a major vessel leading to cerebral infarction
- **Intracerebral hemorrhage** is usually caused by hypertension and occurs suddenly, often during activity
- With both of these types of stroke, the resulting deficit depends on the particular vessel involved and the extent of any collateral circulation
- **Lacunar strokes** are small lesions (usually < 5 mm in diameter) that occur in the distribution of short penetrating arteries in the basal ganglia, pons, cerebellum, internal capsule, thalamus, or deep cerebral white matter (less common)
- Risk factors for lacunar strokes include poorly controlled hypertension and diabetes mellitus

General Considerations

- Strokes are traditionally subdivided into infarcts (thrombotic or embolic) and hemorrhages, but clinical distinction may not be possible
- A previous stroke is a risk factor for a subsequent stroke

Demographics

- Stroke is the third leading cause of death in the United States, despite a general decline in its incidence in the last 30 years

4. Symptoms and Signs

- Table 62-1 displays features of the major stroke subtypes
- Onset is usually abrupt

Table 62-1. Features of the major stroke subtypes.

Stroke Type and Subtype	Clinical Features	Diagnosis	Treatment
Ischemic Stroke			
Lacunar infarct	Small (< 5 mm) lesions in the basal ganglia, pons, cerebellum, or internal capsule; less often in deep cerebral white matter; prognosis generally good; clinical features depend on location, but may worsen over first 24–36 h	MRI with diffusion-weighted sequences usually defines the area of infarction; CT is insensitive acutely but can be used to exclude hemorrhage	Aspirin; long-term management is to control risk factors (hypertension and diabetes mellitus)
Carotid circulation obstruction	See text—signs vary depending on occluded vessel	Noncontrast CT to exclude hemorrhage but findings may be normal during first 6–24 hr of an ischemic stroke; diffusion-weighted MRI is gold standard for identifying acute stroke; electrocardiography, echocardiography, blood glucose, complete blood count, and tests for hypercoagulable states, hyperlipidemia are indicated; Holter monitoring in selected instances; carotid duplex ultrasound, CTA, MRA, or conventional angiography in selected cases	Select patients for intravenous thrombolytics or intraarterial mechanical thrombolysis; aspirin is first-line therapy; anticoagulation with heparin for cardioembolic strokes when no contraindications exist
Vertebrobasilar occlusion	See text—signs vary based on location of occluded vessel	As for carotid circulation obstruction	As for carotid circulation obstruction
Hemorrhagic Stroke			
Spontaneous intracerebral hemorrhage	Commonly associated with hypertension; also with bleeding disorders, amyloid angiopathy Hypertensive hemorrhage is located commonly in the basal ganglia and less commonly in the pons, thalamus, cerebellum, or cerebral white matter	Noncontrast CT is superior to MRI for detecting bleeds of < 48-h duration; laboratory tests to identify bleeding disorder: angiography may be indicated to exclude aneurysm or AVM. Do not perform lumbar puncture	Most managed supportively, but cerebellar bleeds or hematomas with gross mass effect may require urgent surgical evacuation
Subarachnoid hemorrhage	Present with sudden onset of worst headache of life, may lead rapidly to loss of consciousness; signs of meningeal irritation often present; etiology usually aneurysm or AVM, but 20% have no source identified	CT to confirm diagnosis, but may be normal in rare instances; if CT negative and suspicion high, perform lumbar puncture to look for red blood cells or xanthochromia; angiography to determine source of bleed in candidates for treatment	See sections on AVM and aneurysm
Intracranial aneurysm	Most located in the anterior circle of Willis and are typically asymptomatic until subarachnoid bleed occurs; 20% rebleed in first 2 wk	CT indicates subarachnoid hemorrhage, and angiography then demonstrates aneurysms; angiography may not reveal aneurysm if vasospasm present	Prevent further bleeding by clipping aneurysm or coil embolization; nimodipine helps prevent vasospasm; reverse vasospasm by intravenous fluids and induced hypertension after aneurysm has been obliterated, if no other aneurysms are present; angioplasty may also reverse symptomatic vasospasm
AVMs	Focal deficit from hematoma or AVM itself	CT reveals bleed, and may reveal the AVM; may be seen by MRI. Angiography demonstrates feeding vessels and vascular anatomy	Surgery indicated if AVM has bled or to prevent further progression of neurologic deficit; other modalities to treat nonoperable AVMs are available at specialized centers

AVMs, arteriovenous malformations; CTA, computed tomography angiography; MRA, magnetic resonance angiography.

- Examine the heart for murmur or arrhythmia and the carotid and subclavian arteries for bruits
- In hemiplegia of pontine origin, the eyes often deviate toward the paralyzed side
- In a hemispheric lesion, the eyes commonly deviate away from the hemiplegic side
- Symptoms and signs depend on structures involved

Thrombotic or Embolic Occlusion (Ischemic Stroke)

Carotid Circulation

- Ophthalmic artery occlusion
  - Symptomless in most
  - May produce transient monocular blindness (amaurosis fugax)
- Anterior cerebral artery occlusion distal to junction with anterior communicating artery
  - Weakness and cortical sensory loss in the contralateral leg and sometimes mild proximal arm weakness
  - May see contralateral grasp reflex, paratonic rigidity, and abulia (lack of initiative) or frank confusion
  - Urinary incontinence is not uncommon
  - Bilateral infarction is likely to cause marked behavioral changes and memory disturbances
  - Unilateral occlusion proximal to the junction with the anterior communicating artery is generally well tolerated because of the collateral supply from the other side
- Middle cerebral artery occlusion
  - Contralateral hemiplegia, hemisensory loss, and homonymous hemianopia (ie, bilaterally symmetric loss of vision in half of the visual fields), with the eyes deviated to the side of the lesion
  - If the dominant hemisphere is involved, global aphasia is present
  - May be impossible to distinguish from occlusion of the internal carotid artery
  - May see considerable swelling of the hemisphere, leading to drowsiness, stupor, and coma
- Occlusion of the anterior branch of the middle cerebral artery
  - Expressive dysphasia
  - Contralateral paralysis and loss of sensations in the arm, the face, and, to a lesser extent, the leg
- Occlusion of the posterior branch of the middle cerebral artery
  - Receptive (Wernicke) aphasia
  - Homonymous visual field defect

Vertebrobasilar Circulation

- Posterior cerebral artery occlusion may lead to
  - Thalamic syndrome of sensory loss
  - Ipsilateral facial, ninth and tenth cranial nerve lesions
  - Limb ataxia and numbness
  - Horner syndrome, combined with contralateral sensory loss of the limb
- Occlusion of both vertebral arteries or the basilar artery
  - Coma with pinpoint pupils
  - Flaccid quadriplegia
  - Sensory loss
  - Variable cranial nerve abnormalities
- Partial basilar artery occlusion
  - Diplopia
  - Visual loss
  - Vertigo
  - Dysarthria
  - Ataxia
  - Weakness or sensory disturbances in some or all of the limbs
  - Discrete cranial nerve palsies
- Occlusion of any major cerebellar artery
  - Vertigo
  - Nausea
  - Vomiting

— Nystagmus
— Ipsilateral limb ataxia
— Contralateral spinothalamic sensory loss in the limbs
— Massive cerebellar infarction may lead to coma, tonsillar herniation, and death

Hemorrhage (Hemorrhagic Stroke)

Hypertensive Intracerebral Hemorrhage

• Spontaneous, nontraumatic intracerebral hemorrhage in patients with no angiographic evidence of an associated vascular anomaly (eg, aneurysm or angioma) is usually due to hypertension
• Likely pathologic basis is microaneurysms that develop on perforating vessels 100 to 300 μm in diameter in hypertensive patients
• Occurs most frequently in the basal ganglia and less commonly in the pons, thalamus, cerebellum, and cerebral white matter
• Extension into the ventricular system or subarachnoid space may cause signs of meningeal irritation
• In the elderly, cerebral amyloid angiopathy is an important and frequent cause of hemorrhage
  — It is usually lobar in distribution and sometimes recurrent
  — It is associated with a better prognosis than hypertensive hemorrhage

Other Causes of Intracranial Hemorrhage

• May occur with
  — Hematologic and bleeding disorders (eg, leukemia, thrombocytopenia, hemophilia, or disseminated intravascular coagulation)
  — Anticoagulant therapy
  — Liver disease
  — High alcohol intake
  — Primary or secondary brain tumors
• There is also an association with advancing age, and male sex
• Bleeding from an intracranial aneurysm or arteriovenous malformation is primarily into the subarachnoid space, but it may also be partly intraparenchymal
• In some cases, no specific cause for cerebral hemorrhage can be identified

Hemorrhage into the Cerebral Hemisphere

• Consciousness is initially lost or impaired in about 50% of patients
• Vomiting is frequent at the onset, and headache is sometimes present
• Focal symptoms and signs follow, depending on the site of the bleed
• With hypertensive hemorrhage, there is generally a rapidly evolving neurologic deficit with hemiplegia or hemiparesis
• A hemisensory disturbance occurs with more deeply placed lesions
• With lesions of the putamen, loss of conjugate lateral gaze may be present
• With thalamic hemorrhage, there may be a loss of upward gaze, downward or skew deviation of the eyes, lateral gaze palsies, and pupillary inequalities

Cerebellar Hemorrhage

• Sudden onset of nausea and vomiting, dysequilibrium, headache, and loss of consciousness that may be fatal within 48 hours
• Less commonly, the onset is gradual and episodic or slowly progressive, suggesting an expanding cerebellar lesion
• Onset and course can be intermediate
  — Lateral conjugate gaze palsies to the side of the lesion
  — Small reactive pupils
  — Contralateral hemiplegia; peripheral facial weakness
  — Ataxia of gait, limbs, or trunk
  — Periodic respiration
  — Some combination of these findings

Lacunar Strokes

- There are several clinical syndromes
  - Contralateral pure motor or pure sensory deficit
  - Ipsilateral ataxia with crural paresis
  - Dysarthria with clumsiness of the hand
- Deficits may progress over 24 to 36 hours before stabilizing

5. Differential Diagnosis

- Hypoglycemia
- TIA
- Focal seizure (Todd paralysis)
- Migraine
- Peripheral causes of vertigo (Ménière disease)
- Ischemic stroke
- Subarachnoid hemorrhage
- Subdural or epidural hemorrhage

6. Laboratory, Imaging, and Procedural Findings

Laboratory Tests

- Complete blood cell count, erythrocyte sedimentation rate, blood glucose, and serologic tests for syphilis
- Screening for hypercoagulable disorders is indicated if suspected clinically (eg, in a young patient without apparent risk factors for stroke)
  - Antiphospholipid antibodies (lupus anticoagulants and anticardiolipin antibodies)
  - Activated protein C resistance/Factor V Leiden mutation
  - Serum protein C, protein S, or antithrombin deficiency
  - Hyperprothrombinemia (prothrombin gene G20210A mutation)
  - Serum homocysteine level
- Serum total cholesterol, HDL cholesterol, LDL cholesterol, triglycerides: elevated serum cholesterol and other lipids may indicate an increased risk of thrombotic stroke
- A predisposing cause of hemorrhage may be revealed by
  - Complete blood cell count
  - Platelet count
  - Bleeding time
  - Prothrombin and partial thromboplastin times
  - Liver and kidney function tests
- ECG or continuous cardiac monitoring for at least 24 hours to help exclude a cardiac arrhythmia or recent myocardial infarction that might be a source of embolization
- Blood cultures if endocarditis is suspected
- Echocardiography (bubble contrast study) if heart disease is a concern
- Cerebrospinal fluid examination
  - Not always necessary but may be helpful if cerebral vasculitis or another inflammatory or infectious cause of stroke is suspected
  - Should be delayed until after CT or magnetic resonance imaging (MRI) to exclude any risk of herniation due to mass lesion or mass effect
  - Contraindicated in large hemorrhage because it may cause herniation

Imaging Studies (Table 62-1)

- CT scan of the head (noncontrast)
  - Should be performed immediately in all acute strokes, before the administration of aspirin or other antithrombotic agents, to exclude cerebral hemorrhage
  - Relatively insensitive to acute ischemic stroke
  - Important in hemorrhage for confirming and determining the size and site of the

— hematoma
— Sometimes show lacunar infarcts as small, punched-out, hypodense areas, but in other patients no abnormality is seen
  ◦ In some instances, patients with a clinical syndrome suggestive of lacunar infarction are found to have a severe hemispheric infarct on CT scanning
- Subsequent MRI with perfusion-weighted sequences should be performed
  — To define the distribution and extent of infarction and to outline any additional areas at risk
  — To exclude tumor, posterior fossa lesions, or other differential considerations
  — CT is superior to MRI for detecting intracranial hemorrhage of < 48 hours' duration
- Imaging of the cervical vasculature (carotid duplex ultrasonography, magnetic resonance or CT angiography, or conventional catheter angiography) is indicated as part of the workup to identify the source of the stroke, and may guide further intervention in hemorrhage if it reveals an aneurysm or arteriovenous malformation

Diagnostic Procedures
- Telemetry and Holter monitoring if paroxysmal cardiac arrhythmia is suspected and echocardiography (bubble contrast study) if valvular heart disease or patent foramen ovale is suspected as a cause of embolic stroke

7. Treatments

Medications
- Indications for antiplatelet therapy with aspirin, 325 mg orally daily, beginning immediately is indicated in patients not eligible for thrombolytic therapy and without CT evidence of intracranial hemorrhage
- For ischemic stroke, anticoagulant therapy
  — Should be started without delay in the setting of atrial fibrillation or other source of cardioembolism if CT scan shows no evidence of hemorrhage and the cerebrospinal fluid is clear
  — Treatment is with warfarin (target INR 2.0–3.0) or new (novel) oral anticoagulants (rivaroxaban, apixaban, and dabigatran); bridging with heparin is not necessary, but some advocate treatment with aspirin until the INR becomes therapeutic
  — Aspirin should not continue after achieving therapeutic anticoagulation, because of an increased risk of hemorrhage.
- For ischemic stroke, IV thrombolytic therapy with recombinant tissue plasminogen activator (rtPA)
  — 0.9 mg/kg to a maximum of 90 mg, with 10% given as a bolus over 1 minute and the remainder over 1 hour
  — Effective in reducing the neurologic deficit in selected patients who have no CT evidence of intracranial hemorrhage when given as soon as possible, but not > 4.5 hours after the onset of symptoms
- Contraindications to thrombolytic therapy
  — Recent hemorrhage (eg, CNS, GI tract, or elsewhere)
  — Increased risk of hemorrhage (eg, treatment with anticoagulants), arterial puncture at a noncompressible site
  — Systolic blood pressure (BP) above 185 mm Hg or diastolic pressure above 110 mm Hg

Surgery
- In cerebellar hemorrhage, prompt surgical evacuation of the hematoma is appropriate
- Decompression is helpful when a superficial hematoma in cerebral white matter is causing mass effect and herniation
- Ventricular drainage may be required in patients with intraventricular hemorrhage and acute hydrocephalus

Therapeutic Procedures

- Early management consists of general supportive measures
- Elevated intracranial pressure is managed by head elevation and osmotic agents such as mannitol
- Alternative therapies include
  - Endovascular intra-arterial rtPA administration
  - Mechanical removal of an embolus or clot from an occluded cerebral artery
  - Decompressive hemicraniectomy
- In patients with elevated systemic BP
  - Avoid antihypertensive therapy during acute phase (ie, within 2 weeks), since there is loss of cerebral autoregulation
  - If systolic BP exceeds 220 mm Hg, it can be lowered to 170 to 200 mm Hg using intravenous labetalol or nicardipine with continuous monitoring
  - After 2 weeks, systolic BP can be reduced further to < 140/90 mm Hg
- Physical therapy with early mobilization and active rehabilitation are important
- Occupational therapy may improve morale and motor skills
- Speech therapy may be beneficial in patients with expressive dysphasia or dysarthria
- In hemorrhage, the treatment of underlying structural lesions or bleeding disorders depends on their nature
- Hemostatic therapy with recombinant activated factor VII has not improved survival or functional outcome in hemorrhage
- There is no specific treatment for cerebral amyloid angiopathy
- Control hypertension or diabetes mellitus and avoid tobacco use

8. Outcomes

Follow-Up

- Early mobilization and active rehabilitation
- Leg brace, toe spring, frame, or cane, as needed

Prognosis

- The prognosis for survival after cerebral infarction is better than after cerebral (or subarachnoid) hemorrhage
- Loss of consciousness after a cerebral infarct implies a poorer prognosis than otherwise
- The extent of the infarct governs the potential for rehabilitation
- Lacunar strokes generally have a good prognosis, with partial or complete resolution often occurring over 4 to 6 weeks
- Surgery for cerebellar hemorrhage may lead to complete resolution of the clinical deficit
- Untreated cerebellar hemorrhage can spontaneously deteriorate from brainstem herniation with a fatal outcome
- Follow-up imaging during the hospitalization may reveal hematoma expansion, a predictor of poor outcome

Prevention

- Patients who have had an ischemic cerebral infarct are at risk for further strokes and for myocardial infarcts
- Statin therapy to lower serum lipid levels may reduce this risk of ischemic stroke
- Antiplatelet therapy with aspirin (325 mg once daily orally) in ischemic stroke
  - Reduces the recurrence rate by 30% among patients who have no cardiac cause for the stroke and who are not candidates for carotid endarterectomy
  - Nevertheless, the cumulative risk of recurrence of noncardioembolic stroke is still 3% to 7% annually
- A 2-year comparison did not show benefit of warfarin (INRs in range 1.4–2.8) over aspirin (325 mg once daily orally) for ischemic stroke

• Higher doses of warfarin should be avoided because they lead to an increased incidence of major bleeding

9. When to Refer and When to Admit

When to Refer
• All patients

When to Admit
• All patients with new stroke, immediately (within 4.5 hours of symptom onset if IV thrombolytic therapy with rtPA is under consideration)

SUGGESTED REFERENCES

Biffi A et al. Statin treatment and functional outcome after ischemic stroke: case-control and meta-analysis. *Stroke*. 2011 May;42(5):1314–1319. [PMID: 21415396]

Grise EM et al. Blood pressure control for acute ischemic and hemorrhagic stroke. *Curr Opin Crit Care*. 2012 Apr;18(2):132–138. [PMID: 22322257]

Hofmeijer J et al. HAMLET investigators. Surgical decompression for space-occupying cerebral infarction (the Hemicraniectomy After Middle Cerebral Artery infarction with Life-threatening Edema Trial [HAMLET]): a multicentre, open, randomised trial. *Lancet Neurol*. 2009 Apr;8(4):326–333. [PMID: 19269254]

Jauch EC et al. Guidelines for the early management of patients with acute ischemic stroke: a guideline for healthcare professionals from the American Heart Association/American Stroke Association. *Stroke*. 2013 Mar;44(3):870–947. [PMID: 23370205]

Jin J. JAMA patient page. Warning signs of a stroke. *JAMA*. 2014 Apr 23–30;311(16):1704. [PMID: 24756530]

Lansberg MG et al. Efficacy and safety of tissue plasminogen activator 3 to 4.5 hours after acute ischemic stroke: a meta-analysis. *Stroke*. 2009 Jul;40(7):2438–2441. [PMID: 19478213]

Mackey J. Evaluation and management of stroke in young adults. *Continuum (Minneap Minn)*. 2014 Apr;20(2):352–369. [PMID: 24699486]

Micheli S et al. Lacunar versus non-lacunar syndromes. *Front Neurol Neurosci*. 2012;30:94–98. [PMID: 22377873]

Silver B et al. Stroke: diagnosis and management of acute ischemic stroke. *FP Essent*. 2014 May;420: 16–22. [PMID: 24818555]

Smoking Cessation

63

A 33-year-old man visits his primary care clinician for advice about how to quit cigarette smoking. The patient started smoking a half pack per day at age 16, but gradually increased over the next 6 years to 1 pack daily. He had one previous quit attempt at age 30 when he first got married, but he resumed smoking within several days. He has never used nicotine replacement or other medical therapies to help quit. Currently, he smokes within ½ hour of awakening and when forced to go without cigarettes for more than a few hours (eg, on coast-to-coast airplane flights) he begins to crave them, with restlessness and irritability. He says that smoking relaxes him and he likes to smoke when he drinks coffee or alcohol and after meals. Over the past year, he has had several respiratory infections, with prolonged cough. He and his wife have recently had their first child, and his wife and their pediatrician have asked him to avoid smoking around the infant inside the home or car, and to try to quit for good.

LEARNING OBJECTIVES

▶ Learn the clinical manifestations and objective findings of nicotine withdrawal

▶ Understand the health hazards associated with cigarette smoking

▶ Learn the pharmacologic and nonpharmacologic treatments for smoking cessation

▶ Know how to properly counsel and encourage patients to stop smoking

QUESTIONS

1. What are the salient features of this patient's problem?

2. How do you think through his problem?

3. What are the key features, including essentials of diagnosis and general considerations, of smoking cessation?

4. What are the symptoms and signs of smoking cessation?

5. What is the differential diagnosis of smoking cessation?

6. What are procedural findings in smoking cessation?

7. What are the treatments for smoking cessation?

8. What are the outcomes, including follow-up, prevention, complications, and prognosis, of smoking cessation?

9. When should patients with smoking cessation be referred to a specialist?

ANSWERS

1. Salient Features

At least 15-pack-year smoking history; previous quit attempt; has never used adjuvant therapies; addiction and withdrawal symptoms; relaxation function of cigarettes may require alternative relaxation strategy; adverse effects of smoking that have happened to the patient can be used as motivators

2. How to Think Through

Tobacco cessation is the most important of all modifiable disease risk factors. While the approach must be a tailored to each patient, smoking should be addressed by the clinician at every opportunity. The Transtheoretical Stages of Change model provides a means of establishing a patient's position on the continuum of readiness to quit smoking. If this patient reports he is "ready to quit," the clinician can facilitate development of a cessation plan. What are the elements of an effective, multidimensional plan? (A quit date is jointly chosen so that preparation can begin. Risks and benefits of pharmacologic aids, including nicotine replacement, bupropion and varenicline, must be discussed. Potential support from family, peers, groups, telephone quit lines, and behavioral medicine specialists are to be explored. Activities associated with smoking are best avoided, and identification of replacement rituals is crucial.)

At the other end of the spectrum, other patients with nicotine dependence are "precontemplators," with limited interest in quitting. A cessation plan is not appropriate in such individuals. What is an appropriate strategy in such cases? (Motivational interviewing, see Tables 63-1 and 63-2.) The birth of this patient's first child and his respiratory symptoms are ideal anchors for such a discussion.

3. Key Features

Essentials of Diagnosis

- Inquire about
- Tobacco use, dependence, previous quit attempts and withdrawal symptoms
- Willingness to quit
- History of use of nicotine replacement and other medications

General Considerations

- Most important cause of preventable morbidity and mortality; responsible for one in four deaths in the United States
- 6.3 million premature deaths worldwide attributed to smoking in 2010 alone
- Leading causes of death: cardiovascular disease (including acute myocardial infarction and stroke), chronic obstructive pulmonary disease, and lung cancer
- Also increases risk of cancers of head and neck, esophagus, colon, prostate, pancreas, kidney, bladder, breast, and cervix; leukemia; peptic ulcers; fractures of the hip, wrist, and vertebrae; cataracts and age-related macular degeneration; invasive pneumococcal disease; and Alzheimer disease
- Smokers die 5 to 8 years earlier than never smokers
- Nicotine is highly addictive
- Environmental exposure to tobacco (eg, second-hand smoke exposure of nonsmokers) is being increasingly recognized to have similar adverse effects on the cardiovascular and pulmonary systems, as well as increasing risk of cervical and perhaps breast cancers,
- Smoking cessation reduces the risks of death and disease and increases life expectancy, even when patients quit smoking late in life

- Tobacco use is undertreated; 70% of smokers see a physician each year and only 20% receive advice or assistance about quitting
- Almost 40% of smokers attempt to quit each year, but only 4% are successful; patients whose clinicians advise them to quit are 1.6 times more likely to attempt quitting

4. Symptoms and Signs

- Nicotine withdrawal
  - Intense cravings for nicotine
  - Anxiety, frustration, and irritability
  - Fatigue or insomnia
  - Depression
  - Increased caloric intake and weight gain
  - Difficulty concentrating
  - Headache
  - Nausea

5. Differential Diagnosis

- Depression
- Anxiety disorder
- Other psychiatric illness
- Other or coexisting substance abuse disorder

6. Procedural Findings

Diagnostic Procedures

- Clinician's assessment of willingness to quit and "stage of change" is important
  - Five stages of change have been postulated
    - **Precontemplation** is when smokers no intention to change smoking behavior in the foreseeable future
    - **Contemplation** is the stage when smokers are aware smoking is a problem and are seriously thinking about quitting but have not yet made a commitment to take action
    - **Preparation** is the stage when smokers are intending to take action to quit in the next month and have unsuccessfully tried to quit in the past year
    - **Action** is the stage when smokers modify their behavior, experiences, or environment in order to overcome their smoking problem
    - **Maintenance** is the stage when those who have successfully quit work to prevent **relapse**
- Have a system to identify which patients are smokers so that they can be targeted for intervention

7. Treatments

Medications

- Several effective interventions are available to promote smoking cessation, including counseling, pharmacotherapy, and combinations of the two
- All patients trying to quit who do not have contraindications should be offered pharmacotherapy
- Nicotine replacement with patch, gum, lozenges (over the counter), and nasal spray or inhalers (prescription) is effective
- Bupropion sustained-release 150 to 300 mg/d orally boosts dopamine and norepinephrine levels and is an effective agent for cessation; a seizure disorder is a contraindication
- Varenicline, a nicotinic acetylcholine-receptor agonist, has been shown to improve cessation rates; dose is 0.5 mg/d orally for 3 days, then 0.5 mg orally twice daily for 4 days, then 1 mg orally twice daily for 11 weeks. Neuropsychiatric symptoms, including increased thoughts of suicidality, have led to a Black Box warning; its use requires careful monitoring

Table 63-1. Actions and strategies for the primary care clinician to help patients quit smoking.

Action	Strategies for Implementation
Step 1. Ask—Systematically Identify All Tobacco Users at Every Visit	
Implement an officewide system that ensures that for *every* patient at *every* clinic visit, tobacco-use status is queried and documented*a*	Expand the vital signs to include tobacco use Data should be collected by the health care team The action should be implemented using preprinted progress note paper that includes the expanded vital signs, a vital signs stamp or, for computerized records, an item assessing tobacco-use status Alternatives to the vital signs stamp are to place tobacco-use status stickers on all patients' charts or to indicate smoking status using computerized reminder systems
Step 2. Advise—Strongly Urge All Smokers to Quit	
In a *clear, strong,* and *personalized* manner, urge every smoker to quit	Advice should be **Clear:** "I think it is important for you to quit smoking now, and I will help you. Cutting down while you are ill is not enough" **Strong:** "As your clinician, I need you to know that quitting smoking is the most important thing you can do to protect your current and future health" **Personalized:** Tie smoking to current health or illness and/or the social and economic costs of tobacco use, motivational level/readiness to quit, and the impact of smoking on children and others in the household Encourage clinic staff to reinforce the cessation message and support the patient's quit attempt
Step 3. Attempt—Identify Smokers Willing to Make a Quit Attempt	
Ask every smoker if he or she is willing to make a quit attempt at this time	If the patient is willing to make a quit attempt at this time, provide assistance (see **Step 3**) If the patient prefers a more intensive treatment or the clinician believes more intensive treatment is appropriate, refer the patient to interventions administered by a smoking cessation specialist and follow up with him or her regarding quitting (see **Step 5**) If the patient clearly states he or she is not willing to make a quit attempt at this time, provide a motivational intervention
Step 4. Assist—Aid the Patient in Quitting	
A. Help the patient with a quit plan	**Set a quit date** Ideally, the quit date should be within 2 wk, taking patient preference into account **Help the patient prepare for quitting** The patient must: **Inform** family, friends, and coworkers of quitting and request understanding and support **Prepare the environment** by removing cigarettes from it. Prior to quitting, the patient should avoid smoking in places where he or she spends a lot of time (eg, home, car) **Review** previous quit attempts: What helped? What led to relapse? **Anticipate** challenges to the planned quit attempt, particularly during the critical first few weeks
B. Encourage nicotine replacement therapy except in special circumstances	Encourage the use of the nicotine patch or nicotine gum therapy for smoking cessation
C. Give key advice on successful quitting	**Abstinence:** Total abstinence is essential. Not even a single puff after the quit date **Alcohol:** Drinking alcohol is highly associated with relapse. Those who stop smoking should review their alcoholism and consider limiting or abstaining from alcohol during the quit process **Other smokers in the household:** The presence of other smokers in the household, particularly a spouse, is associated with lower success rates. Patients should consider quitting with their significant others and/or developing specific plans to maintain abstinence in a household where others still smoke
D. Provide supplementary materials	**Source:** Federal agencies, including the National Cancer Institute and the Agency for Health Care Policy and Research; nonprofit agencies (American Cancer Society, American Lung Association, American Heart Association); or local or state health departments **Selection concerns:** The material must be culturally, racially, educationally, and age appropriate for the patient **Location:** Readily available in every clinic office
Step 5. Arrange—Schedule Follow-Up Contact	
Schedule follow-up contact, either in person or via telephone*a*	**Timing:** Follow-up contact should occur soon after the quit date, preferably during the first week. A second follow-up contact is recommended within the first month. Schedule further follow-up contacts as indicated **Actions during follow-up:** Congratulate success. If smoking occurred, review the circumstances and elicit recommitment to total abstinence. Remind the patient that a lapse can be used as a learning experience and is not a sign of failure. Identify the problems already encountered and anticipate challenges in the immediate future. Assess nicotine replacement therapy use and problems. Consider referral to a more intense or specialized program

*a*Repeated assessment is not necessary in the case of adult who has never smoked or not smoked for many years and for whom the information is clearly documented in the medical record.

Adapted, with permission, from: The Agency for Health Care Policy and Research. Smoking Cessation Clinical Practice Guideline. *JAMA.* 1996;275(16):1270–1280. Copyright © 1996 American Medical Association. All rights reserved.

Therapeutic Procedures
- Table 63-1 summarizes ways in which physicians can help their patients quit smoking
- Table 63-2 summarizes common elements of supportive smoking treatments
- Advice to quit and pharmacotherapy should be tailored to patient's stage of readiness to change

Table 63-2. Common elements of supportive smoking treatments.

Component	Examples
Encouragement of the patient in the quit attempt	Note that effective cessation treatments are now available Note that half the people who have *ever* smoked have now quit Communicate belief in the patient's ability to quit
Communication of caring and concern	Ask how the patient feels about quitting Directly express concern and a willingness to help Be open to the patient's expression of fears of quitting, difficulties experienced, and ambivalent feelings
Encouragement of the patient to talk about the quitting process	Ask about • Reasons that the patient wants to quit • Difficulties encountered while quitting • Success the patient has achieved • Concerns or worries about quitting
Provision of basic information about smoking and successful quitting	Inform the patient about • The nature and time course of withdrawal • The addictive nature of smoking The fact that any smoking (even a single puff) increases the likelihood of full relapse

Adapted, with permission, from The Agency for Health Care Policy and Research. Smoking Cessation Clinical Practice Guideline. *JAMA.* 1996;275(16):1270–1280. Copyright © 1996 American Medical Association. All rights reserved.

- An intercurrent illness such as acute bronchitis or acute myocardial infarction may motivate even the most addicted smoker to quit
- Do not show disapproval of patients who have failed cessation or are not ready to attempt quitting
- Individualized or group counseling is cost-effective
- Cessation counseling by telephone ("quitlines") or text messaging are also effective
- Recommending that any smoking take place out of doors to limit the effects of passive smoke on housemates and coworkers can lead to smoking reduction and cessation
- e-cigarettes have become popular; some serve as a nicotine-delivery device, others deliver water vapor. Their efficacy in smoking cessation is disputed, and some users may find them addictive

8. Outcomes

Follow-Up
- Scheduling follow-up with patients attempting to quit is important for their successful cessation

Prevention
- Public policies, including higher cigarette taxes and more restrictive public smoking laws, have also been shown to encourage cessation, as have financial incentives directed to patients.

Complications
- Weight gain occurs in most (80%) of patients who quit smoking; 10% to 15% of those patients have major weight gain over 13 kg
- Planning for the possibility of weight gain, and means of mitigating it, may help with maintenance of cessation

Prognosis
- Rules against smoking in the home, older age, and higher education are factors associated with successful cessation

9. When to Refer

- All patients who would like help with smoking cessation should be referred to a quit line for support

SUGGESTED REFERENCES

Cahill K et al. Pharmacological interventions for smoking cessation: an overview and network meta-analysis. *Cochrane Database Syst Rev.* 2013 May 31;5:CD009329. [PMID: 23728690]

Carson KV et al. Training health professionals in smoking cessation. *Cochrane Database Syst Rev.* 2012 May 16;5:CD000214. [PMID: 22592671]

Free C et al. Smoking cessation support delivered via mobile phone text messaging (txt2stop): a single-blind, randomised trial. *Lancet.* 2011 Jul 2;378(9785):49–55. [PMID: 21722952]

Holford TR et al. Tobacco control and the reduction in smoking-related premature deaths in the United States, 1964–2012. *JAMA.* 2014 Jan 8;311(2):164–171. [PMID: 24399555]

Jamal A et al. Current cigarette smoking among adults—United States, 2005–2013. *MMWR Morb Mortal Wkly Rep.* 2014 Nov 28;63(47):1108–1112. [PMID: 25426653]

Lim SS et al. A comparative risk assessment of burden of disease and injury attributable to 67 risk factors and risk factor clusters in 21 regions, 1990–2010: a systematic analysis for the Global Burden of Disease Study 2010. *Lancet.* 2012 Dec 15;380(9859):2224–2260. [PMID: 23245609]

Lindson-Hawley N et al. Reduction versus abrupt cessation in smokers who want to quit. *Cochrane Database Syst Rev.* 2012 Nov 14;11:CD008033. [PMID: 23152252]

National Center for Chronic Disease Prevention and Health Promotion (US) Office on Smoking and Health. The Health Consequences of Smoking—50 Years of Progress: A Report of the Surgeon General. Atlanta (GA): Centers for Disease Control and Prevention (US); 2014. [PMID: 24455788]

Oza S et al. How many deaths are attributable to smoking in the United States? Comparison of methods for estimating smoking-attributable mortality when smoking prevalence changes. *Prev Med.* 2011 Jun;52(6):428–433. [PMID: 21530575]

Pierce JP et al. What public health strategies are needed to reduce smoking initiation? *Tob Control.* 2012 Mar;21(2): 258–264. [PMID: 22345263]

Rigotti NA et al. Interventions for smoking cessation in hospitalised patients. *Cochrane Database Syst Rev.* 2012 May 16;5:CD001837. [PMID: 22592676]

Rigotti NA et al. Sustained care intervention and postdischarge smoking cessation among hospitalized adults: a randomized clinical trial. *JAMA.* 2014 Aug 20;312(7):719–728. [PMID: 25138333]

Stead LF et al. Combined pharmacotherapy and behavioural interventions for smoking cessation. *Cochrane Database Syst Rev.* 2012 Oct 17;10:CD008286. [PMID: 23076944]

Sugerman DT. JAMA patient page. e-Cigarettes. *JAMA.* 2014 Jan 8;311(2):212. [PMID: 24399571]

Tahiri M et al. Alternative smoking cessation aids: a meta-analysis of randomized controlled trials. *Am J Med.* 2012 Jun;125(6):576–584. [PMID: 22502956]

Whittaker R et al. Mobile phone-based interventions for smoking cessation. *Cochrane Database Syst Rev.* 2012 Nov 14;11:CD006611. [PMID: 23152238]

Substance Abuse

64

A 32-year-old unemployed man presents to the emergency department with right lower quadrant abdominal pain of 17 hours duration. He has a fever of 38.9°C, rebound tenderness over MacBurney's point, and white blood cell of 18, 900/μL (with 13, 500 leukocytes/μL). He denies cigarette or substance use, but says he drinks alcohol "socially" ("a glass or two of wine with dinner"). He undergoes emergency appendectomy. On postoperative day 2, he becomes anxious, restless, and diaphoretic, with tachycardia (heart rate 125 beat/min) and hypertension (blood pressure 164/95 mm Hg), and he begins to pick at his intravenous line. When he becomes tremulous and begins to hallucinate about "bugs," his girlfriend admits that, since losing his job 1 and 1/2 years ago, he has been depressed and drinking "almost continuously," up to 3 or 4 bottles of wine daily. Over the next 72 hours, he develops mental confusion, sensory hyperacuity, and both hypokalemia and hypomagnesemia.

LEARNING OBJECTIVES

▶ Learn the clinical manifestations and objective findings of acute intoxication and withdrawal from substances of abuse

▶ Understand how to effectively screen for substance abuse disorders

▶ Know the differential diagnosis of substance abuse and the common comorbid conditions

▶ Learn the treatments for substance abuse in the acute intoxication, withdrawal, and maintenance phases of addiction

QUESTIONS

1. What are the salient features of this patient's problem?

2. How do you think through his problem?

3. What are the key features, including essentials of diagnosis and general considerations, of such substance abuse?

4. What are the symptoms and signs of substance abuse?

5. What is the differential diagnosis of substance abuse?

6. What are laboratory, imaging, and procedural findings in substance abuse?

7. What are the treatments for substance abuse?

8. What is the outcome, including complications, of substance abuse?

9. When should patients with substance abuse be referred to a specialist or admitted to the hospital?

ANSWERS

1. Salient Features

Difficult social situation (unemployment); heavy alcoholism with abstinence for 48 to 72 hours; tremulousness; visual hallucinations; vital sign abnormalities; diaphoresis; anxiety; confusion; hypokalemia and hypomagnesemia.

2. How to Think Through

Tachycardia and confusion in this postoperative patient requires a broad approach—infection, pain, pulmonary embolism, medication side effect, and delirium should all be considered. Substance use disorders are stratified as "at risk," "substance abuse," and "substance dependence." The symptoms and signs of withdrawal in this case are consistent with a diagnosis of alcohol dependence. The interval since the patient's last alcohol intake should be ascertained if possible, so that complications of its withdrawal can be anticipated.

What are the risks of untreated alcohol withdrawal? (Hallucinations [12–48 hours since last intake]; seizures [12–48 hours]; tremor, autonomic instability, delirium tremens [DTs] [48–96 hours]; other: falls, danger to staff, need for restraints and, in rare cases, mortality. Delirium tremens is characterized by a clouded sensorium, which this patient manifests; it is distinguished from alcoholic hallucinations by time of onset and signs of autonomic instability.) How should he be managed? (Benzodiazepine [BZD] administration is the mainstay for treatment of hallucinations and autonomic signs; thiamine; hydration; and management of electrolyte abnormalities.) When dysautonomia is controlled by BZDs, but hallucinations and agitation are not, haloperidol is often used. Oversedation is a major management challenge since BZDs accumulate, and it can require endotracheal intubation to avoid aspiration.

3. Key Features

Essentials of Diagnosis

- Psychological dependence: craving and behavior involved in procurement of the drug
- Physiologic dependence: withdrawal symptoms on discontinuance of the drug
- Tolerance: the need to increase the dose to obtained the desired effects
- Addiction: impairment in social and occupational functioning
- Associated illnesses such as alcoholic liver disease, cerebellar degeneration

General Considerations

- Alcohol and opioids are the most commonly abused substances
- Together, these are major public health problems
- In the United States, 51% of adults are current regular drinkers (at least 12 drinks in the past year)
- Maximum recommended alcohol consumption for adult women is ≤ 3 drinks per day (and 7 total per week), and for adult men is ≤ 4 drinks per day (and 14 total per week)
- The spectrum of alcohol misuse includes
  — Risky drinking, alcohol consumption above the recommended daily, weekly, or per occasion amounts
  — Harmful use, a pattern causing damage to health
  — Alcohol abuse, a pattern leading to clinically significant impairment or distress
  — Alcohol dependence, which includes three or more of the following: tolerance, withdrawal, increased consumption, desire to cut down use, giving up social activities, increased time using alcohol or recovering from use, continued use despite known adverse effects.

- Alcohol dependence and illegal drug abuse often coexist with other substance abuse disorders and psychiatric disorders
- Underdiagnosis and undertreatment of substance abuse are substantial, both because of patient denial and clinician lack of detection of clues
- At-risk drinking is repetitive use of alcohol, often to alleviate emotional problems; alcohol addiction is characterized by recurrent use despite difficulties in social, occupational, or legal arenas
- Clinician identification of abuse improves chances of recovery but only a quarter of alcohol-dependent patients have ever been treated
- Lifetime prevalence of illegal drug use is approximately 8% and is generally greater among men, young and unmarried individuals, Native Americans, and those of lower socioeconomic status
- The lifetime treatment rate for drug abuse is low (8%). Recognition of drug abuse presents special problems and requires that the clinician actively consider the diagnosis

4. Symptoms and Signs

- Acute alcohol intoxication: drowsiness, psychomotor dysfunction, disinhibition, dysarthria, ataxia, nystagmus; severe overdosage leads to respiratory depression, stupor, coma
- Acute alcohol withdrawal (within 12–48 hours of last drink): anxiety, decreased cognition, tremulousness, vital sign abnormalities, hallucinations, seizures
- DTs (usually 24–72 hours after last drink, but may occur up to 7–10 days later): mental confusion, tremor, sensory hyperacuity, visual hallucinations, diaphoresis, dehydration, seizures, cardiovascular abnormalities
- Alcoholic stigma: alcoholic odor on breath, tremor, peripherally neuropathy
- Stigmata of cirrhosis: eg, spider angiomas, ascites, palmar erythema, gynecomastia, caput medusa
- Opioid intoxication: euphoria, drowsiness, nausea, meiosis
- Opioid overdosage: respiratory depression, peripheral vasodilatation, pinpoint pupils, pulmonary edema, coma, and death
- Opioid withdrawal (in increasing severity): craving and anxiety; yawning, lacrimation, rhinorrhea, perspiration; mydriasis, piloerection, anorexia, tremors, hot and cold flashes, aching; fever, vital sign abnormalities; nausea, vomiting, diarrhea, weight loss

5. Differential Diagnosis

- Coexisting diseases with alcoholism
  — Anxiety disorders
  — Depression or bipolar disorder
  — Posttraumatic stress disorder
  — Personality disorders
- Alcohol withdrawal differential diagnosis
  — Paranoid schizophrenia
  — Hypoglycemia
  — Delirium or chronic brain disorder, eg, dementia
  — Acute intoxication with another substance, eg, an amphetamine
- Coexisting diseases with illicit drug use
  — Personality disorders
  — Anxiety disorders
  — Posttraumatic stress disorder
  — Other illicit substance use disorders
- Associations of use of anabolic-androgenic steroids
  — Use of other illicit drugs, alcohol, and cigarettes
  — Violence and criminal behavior.

6. Laboratory or Procedural Findings

Laboratory Tests

- Ethanol can produce an osmol gap
- Alcoholic patients may have elevated serum liver tests, uric acid, and triglycerides; decreased serum potassium, magnesium, and albumin; and coagulopathy
- Urinalysis with toxicology screening can be valuable, though watersoluble drugs such as alcohol, stimulants, and opioids are quickly eliminated
- Hair follicle testing can determine drug use over longer periods of time

Diagnostic Procedures

- The USPSTF recommends screening adults aged 18 years and older for alcohol misuse with brief behavioral counseling for those with a positive screening test
- Evidence-based screening questionnaires such as the AUDIT (Alcohol Use Disorder Identification Test) can identify those patients with alcohol abuse disorders
- The AUDIT questionnaire is a cost-effective and efficient diagnostic tool for routine screening of alcohol use disorders in primary care settings. The questionnaire (Table 64-1)

Table 64-1. Screening for alcohol abuse using the Alcohol Use Disorder Identification Text (AUDIT).[a]

(Scores for response categories are given in parentheses. Scores range from 0 to 40, with a cutoff score of ≥ 5 indicating hazardous drinking, harmful drinking, or alcohol dependence.)

1. How often do you have a drink containing alcohol?

(0) Never	(1) Monthly or less	(2) Two to four times a month	(3) Two or three times a week	(4) Four or more times a week

2. How many drinks containing alcohol do you have on a typical day when you are drinking?

(0) 1 or 2	(1) 3 or 4	(2) 5 or 6	(3) 7 to 9	(4) 10 or more

3. How often do you have six or more drinks on one occasion?

(0) Never	(1) Less than monthly	(2) Monthly	(3) Weekly	(4) Daily or almost daily

4. How often during the past year have you found that you were not able to stop drinking once you had started?

(0) Never	(1) Less than monthly	(2) Monthly	(3) Weekly	(4) Daily or almost daily

5. How often during the past year have you failed to do what was normally expected of you because of drinking?

(0) Never	(1) Less than monthly	(2) Monthly	(3) Weekly	(4) Daily or almost daily

6. How often during the past year have you needed a first drink in the morning to get yourself going after a heavy drinking session?

(0) Never	(1) Less than monthly	(2) Monthly	(3) Weekly	(4) Daily or almost daily

7. How often during the past year have you had a feeling of guilt or remorse after drinking?

(0) Never	(1) Less than monthly	(2) Monthly	(3) Weekly	(4) Daily or almost daily

8. How often during the past year have you been unable to remember what happened the night before because you had been drinking?

(0) Never	(1) Less than monthly	(2) Monthly	(3) Weekly	(4) Daily or almost daily

9. Have you or has someone else been injured as a result of your drinking?

(0) No	(2) Yes, but not in the past year	(4) Yes, during the past year

10. Has a relative or friend or a doctor or other health worker been concerned about your drinking or suggested you cut down?

(0) No	(2) Yes, but not in the past year	(4) Yes, during the past year

[a]Adapted, with permission, from BMJ Publishing Group Ltd. and Piccinelli M et al. Efficacy of the alcohol use disorders identification test as a screening tool for hazardous alcohol intake and related disorders in primary care: a validity study. *BMJ*. 1997 Feb 8;314 (7078):420–424.

consists of questions on the quantity and frequency of alcohol consumption, on alcohol dependence symptoms, and on alcohol-related problems

- May also use one-item screening: "How many times in the past year have you had X or more drinks in a day?" (X is 5 for men and 4 for women, and a response of > 1 is considered positive)

7. Treatments

Medications

- In acute alcohol detoxification, long-acting BZDs such as diazepam, lorazepam, or chlordiazepoxide are preferred and can be given on a a fixed schedule or through "front-loading" or "symptom-triggered" regimens
- Adjuvant sympatholytic medications can be used to treat hyperadrenergic symptoms that persist despite adequate sedation
- Alcohol dependence can be treated with
  — Disulfiram, an aversive agent that causes severe side effects in patients that consume alcohol; difficulty with compliance makes effective treatment difficult
  — Naltrexone reduces cravings, can lower the risk of treatment withdrawal in alcohol-dependent patients, and decreases alcoholism relapse; a long-acting intramuscular formulation of naltrexone is well-tolerated and reduces drinking significantly among treatment-seeking alcoholics
  — Acamprosate has not been shown to be effective
  — Topiramate is not Food and Drug Administration-approved for alcohol dependence, but may be more effective even than naltrexone in decreasing alcohol intake and cravings
- Multivitamins, thiamine, and vitamin B_{12} should be supplemented
- Methadone therapy for opioid dependence given orally at a dosage of 40 to 120 mg daily reduces relapses
- Buprenorphine, a partial opiate agonist, can ameliorate the symptoms and signs of withdrawal from opioids with a lower risk of overdose than methadone and may assist in enabling patients in coming off methadone maintenance
- Naloxone intravenously can quickly reverse the effects of opioid overdosage, but has a short duration of action and may require observation and readministration

Therapeutic Procedures

- Use of screening procedures such as the AUDIT questionnaire or single-question screening test employed along with brief intervention methods can produce a 10 to 30% reduction in long-term alcohol use and alcohol-related problems
- Brief advice and counseling without regular follow-up and reinforcement cannot sustain significant long-term reductions in unhealthy drinking behaviors
- Table 64-2 outlines basic steps clinicians can use in counseling their alcoholic patients

Table 64-2. Basic counseling steps for patients who abuse alcohol.

Establish a therapeutic relationship
Make the medical office or clinic off-limits for substance abuse
Present information about negative health consequences
Emphasize personal responsibility and self-efficacy
Convey a clear message and set goals
Involve family and other supports
Establish a working relationship with community treatment resources
Provide follow-up

Reproduced from the United States Department of Health & Human Services, U.S. Public Health Service. Office of Disease Prevention and Health Promotion. Clinician's Handbook of Preventive Services: Put Prevention Into Practice. U.S. Government Printing Office, 1994.

- Cognitive behavior therapy, contingency management, couples and family therapy and other behavioral treatments are effective interventions for drug addiction

8. Outcome

Complications

- Significant social and legal impairments
- Chronic alcoholic brain syndromes such as Wernicke–Korsakoff syndrome or general organic brain injury
- Alcoholic hallucinosis
- Peripheral neuropathy
- Cirrhosis, esophageal varices, and hepatic failure
- Fetal alcohol syndrome

9. When to Refer and When to Admit

When to Refer

- Patients who wish treatment should be referred to community resources for substance abuse treatment

When to Admit

- Some patients who wish treatment benefit from inpatient substance abuse rehabilitation
- Patients with severe alcohol withdrawal symptoms should be admitted
- Patients with opioid overdose often require admission for monitoring

SUGGESTED REFERENCES

Flórez G et al. Topiramate for the treatment of alcohol dependence: comparison with naltrexone. *Eur Addict Res*. 2011;17(1):29–36. [PMID: 20975274]

Garcia AM. State laws regulating prescribing of controlled substances: balancing the public health problems of chronic pain and prescription painkiller abuse and overdose. *J Law Med Ethics*. 2013 Mar;41(Suppl 1):42–45. [PMID: 23590739]

Kahan M et al. Buprenorphine: new treatment of opioid addiction in primary care. *Can Fam Physician*. 2011 Mar;57(3):281–289. [PMID: 21402963]

Manubay JM et al. Prescription drug abuse: epidemiology, regulatory issues, chronic pain management with narcotic analgesics. *Prim Care*. 2011 Mar;38(1):71–90. [PMID: 21356422]

Moyer VA; Preventive Services Task Force. Screening and behavioral counseling interventions in primary care to reduce alcohol misuse: U.S. Preventive Services Task Force recommendation statement. *Ann Intern Med*. 2013 Aug 6;159(3):210–218. [PMID: 23698791]

National Institute on Drug Abuse. DrugFacts: Prescription and over-the-counter medications—Revised November 2014. http://www.drugabuse.gov/publications/drugfacts/prescription-over-counter-medications

Schiller JS et al. Summary health statistics for U.S. adults: National Health Interview Survey, 2010, Table 27. *Vital Health Stat 10*. 2012 Jan;(252):94–96. [PMID: 22834228]

Smith PC et al. Primary care validation of a single-question alcohol screening test. *J Gen Intern Med*. 2009 July;24(7):783–788. [PMID: 19247718]

Soyka M et al. Emerging drugs to treat alcoholism. *Expert Opin Emerg Drugs*. 2010 Dec;15(4):695–711. [PMID: 20560783]

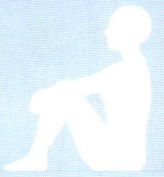

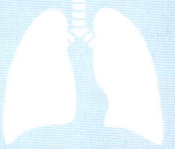

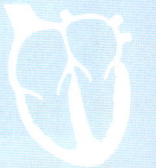

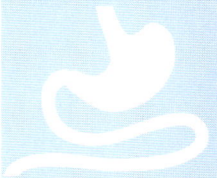

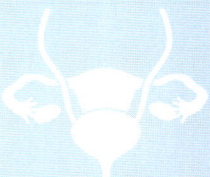

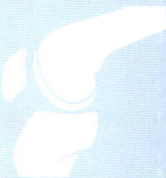

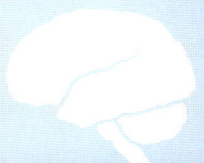

Endocrine/Metabolic Disorders

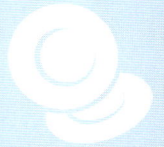

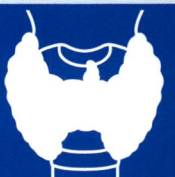

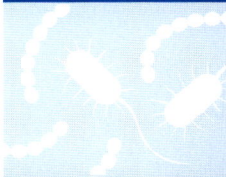

65 Adrenocortical Insufficiency

A 28-year-old man presents to the emergency room with headache, stiff neck, and fever. He is admitted to the intensive care unit after a lumbar puncture and is diagnosed with meningococcal meningitis. On hospital day 3, despite antibiotic treatment, he continues to be hypotensive and in shock, and complains of new abdominal pain when he is awake. On physical examination, he has multiple areas of purpura on his skin. Serum testing reveals hyponatremia, hyperkalemia, and hypoglycemia.

LEARNING OBJECTIVES

▶ Learn the clinical manifestations and objective findings of chronic and acute adrenocortical insufficiency

▶ Understand the factors and illnesses that predispose to adrenocortical insufficiency

▶ Know the differential diagnosis of adrenocortical insufficiency

▶ Learn the treatments for chronic and acute adrenocortical insufficiency and how they differ

▶ Understand the follow-up and testing required after an episode of acute adrenocortical insufficiency

▶ Know how to alter treatment in patients with chronic adrenocortical insufficiency who become acutely ill

QUESTIONS

1. What are the salient features of this patient's problem?

2. How do you think through his problem?

3. What are the key features, including essentials of diagnosis and general considerations, of adrenocortical insufficiency?

4. What are the symptoms and signs of adrenocortical insufficiency?

5. What is the differential diagnosis of adrenocortical insufficiency?

6. What are laboratory, and imaging findings in adrenocortical insufficiency?

7. What are the treatments for adrenocortical insufficiency?

8. What is the outcome, including follow-up, complications, and prognosis, of adrenocortical insufficiency?

9. When should patients with adrenocortical insufficiency be referred to a specialist or admitted to the hospital?

ANSWERS

1. Salient Features

Meningococcal meningitis with purpura; hypotension and shock; abdominal pain; hyponatremia, hyperkalemia, hypoglycemia

2. How to Think Through

This case shows the importance of keeping the full differential diagnosis in mind when treating a patient in shock. This patient has a known infection, but what other causes of hypotension, beyond septic shock, could be at play? (Cardiogenic shock, anaphylactic shock, neurogenic shock, and adrenal insufficiency.) How should adrenal function be evaluated? (AM plasma cortisol level < 3 mg/dL is diagnostic of adrenal insufficiency. Cosyntropin stimulation test indicates primary adrenal insufficiency if the rise in cortisol is < 20 µg/dL 30 to 60 minutes after administration of cosyntropin. Test is less reliable in the setting of acute illness and thus empiric treatment is often warranted.)

If adrenal insufficiency is suspected, what are possible causes? (Previously undetected primary adrenal insufficiency [Addison disease]; indolent adrenal infection such as tuberculosis; secondary [pituitary level] or tertiary [hypothalamic] lesions are possible, but rare. The most likely diagnoses here are a history of chronic glucocorticoid use [none evident] and bilateral hemorrhagic adrenal infarction.) What is the eponym for adrenal infarction in the setting of meningococcemia? (Waterhouse–Friderichsen syndrome.)

How do hyponatremia and hyperkalemia help localize the problem? (Only primary adrenal disease will impact production of aldosterone.) Is imaging indicated? (Yes. Computed tomography [CT] scan of the abdomen may show adrenal hemorrhage.) How should he be treated? (As soon as a plasma cortisol level is drawn, intravenous [IV] hydrocortisone for hypocortisolism and D50W for hypoglycemia should be started empirically.)

3. Key Features

Essentials of Diagnosis

- Weakness, fatigue, anorexia, weight loss; nausea and vomiting, diarrhea, abdominal pain, muscle and joint pains; amenorrhea
- Sparse axillary hair; increased skin pigmentation, especially of creases, pressure areas, and nipples
- Hypotension, dehydration, small heart
- Serum sodium may be low; potassium, calcium, and urea nitrogen may be elevated
- Neutropenia, mild anemia, eosinophilia, and relative lymphocytosis may be present
- Cosyntropin (ACTH 1–24) administration is unable to stimulate an increase in serum cortisol to > 20 µg/dL
- Plasma adrenocorticotropic hormone (ACTH) level elevated

General Considerations

- Adrenocortical insufficiency can be **chronic** or **acute**

Chronic Adrenocortical Insufficiency

- Addison disease refers to primary chronic adrenocortical insufficiency caused by dysfunction or absence of the adrenal cortices; it is distinct from secondary chronic adrenocortical insufficiency caused by deficient secretion of ACTH
- The prevalence of chronic adrenocortical insufficiency is about 140 per million, with an annual incidence of about 4 per million in the United States
- Characterized by chronic deficiency of cortisol, with consequent elevation of serum ACTH and α-melanocyte stimulating hormone (α-MSH), causing skin pigmentation that can be subtle or strikingly dark
- Causes of chronic adrenocortical insufficiency
  — Autoimmune adrenal destruction of adrenal glands is most common cause in the United States

— May be associated with
  ○ Autoimmune thyroid disease
  ○ Hypoparathyroidism
  ○ Type 1 diabetes mellitus
  ○ Vitiligo
  ○ Alopecia areata
  ○ Celiac disease (gluten enteropathy)
  ○ Primary ovarian failure
  ○ Testicular failure
  ○ Pernicious anemia
— Combination of Addison disease and hypothyroidism is Schmidt syndrome
— May occur in polyglandular autoimmunity (PGA-1 and PGA-2)
— Infection
  ○ Tuberculosis in areas of high prevalence; now rare in the United States
  ○ Coccidioidomycosis and histoplasmosis are rare but should be considered in immunosuppressed patients; cytomegalovirus can be a cause in HIV infection
— Bilateral adrenal hemorrhage may occur spontaneously, or with
  ○ Sepsis
  ○ Heparin-associated thrombocytopenia or anticoagulation
  ○ Antiphospholipid antibody syndrome
  ○ Surgery (postoperatively) or trauma
• Rare causes of chronic adrenocortical insufficiency
— Lymphoma
— Metastatic carcinoma
— Syphilitic gummas
— Scleroderma
— Amyloid disease
— Hemochromatosis
• Congenital causes of chronic adrenocortical insufficiency
— Familial glucocorticoid deficiency
— Allgrove syndrome (associated with achalasia, alacrima, and neurologic disease)
— X-linked adrenal leukodystrophy
— Congenital adrenal hypoplasia or hyperplasia

Acute Adrenocortical Insufficiency

• *Acute adrenocortical insufficiency is an emergency* caused by insufficient cortisol
• Causes of acute adrenocortical insufficiency
— May occur in patients treated for chronic adrenal insufficiency or as its presenting manifestation
— More common in primary adrenal insufficiency (adrenal gland disorder; Addison disease) than secondary adrenocortical hypofunction (pituitary gland disorder)
— Stress, eg, trauma, surgery, infection, hyperthyroidism, or prolonged fasting, in patient with latent or treated adrenal insufficiency
— Withdrawal of adrenocortical hormone replacement in patient with chronic adrenal insufficiency or temporary insufficiency related to withdrawal of exogenous corticosteroids
— Bilateral adrenalectomy or removal of a functioning adrenal tumor that had suppressed the other adrenal
— Injury to both adrenals by trauma, hemorrhage, anticoagulant therapy, thrombosis, infection, or, rarely, metastatic carcinoma
— Pituitary necrosis, or when thyroid hormone replacement is given to a patient with adrenal insufficiency
— Following etomidate, which is used intravenously for rapid anesthesia induction or intubation

— Meningococcemia may cause adrenal insufficiency secondary to adrenal infarction (Waterhouse–Friderichsen syndrome)

4. Symptoms and Signs

Chronic Adrenal Insufficiency

- Symptom onset is usually gradual and the diagnosis is often delayed since many early symptoms are nonspecific
- Muscle weakness and fatigue
- Fever
- Anorexia, nausea and vomiting, weight loss
- Anxiety, mental irritability, and emotional changes
- Patients usually have significant pain
  - Arthralgias
  - Myalgias
  - Chest pain
  - Abdominal pain
  - Back pain
  - Leg pain
  - Headache
- Skin
  - Diffuse tanning over nonexposed and exposed skin or multiple freckles
  - Hyperpigmentation, especially knuckles, elbows, knees, posterior neck, palmar creases, nail beds, pressure areas, and new scars
  - Vitiligo (10%)
- Hypoglycemia, when present, may worsen weakness and mental functioning, rarely leading to coma
- In diabetics, increased insulin sensitivity and hypoglycemic reactions
- Other autoimmune disease manifestations
- Hypotension and orthostasis is typical
  - Ninety percent have systolic blood pressure (SBP) < 110 mm Hg
  - SBP > 130 mm Hg is rare
- Small heart
- Scant axillary and pubic hair (especially in women, if hypogonadism also present)
- Neuropsychiatric symptoms, sometimes without adrenal insufficiency, in adult-onset adrenoleukodystrophy

Acute Adrenal Insufficiency

- Headache, lassitude, nausea and vomiting, abdominal pain, and diarrhea
- Confusion or coma
- Fever, as high as 40.6°C or more
- Dehydration, hypotension, and shock
- Recurrent hypoglycemia and reduced insulin requirements in patients with preexisting type 1 diabetes mellitus
- Meningococcemia is associated with purpura and adrenal insufficiency secondary to adrenal infarction (Waterhouse–Friderichsen syndrome)

5. Differential Diagnosis

- Other cause of hypotension or shock
  - Medications
  - Sepsis
  - Cardiogenic
  - Hypovolemic
  - Anaphylaxis

- Hyperkalemia due to other cause
  — Chronic kidney disease
    ◦ Gastrointestinal bleeding
  — Rhabdomyolysis
  — Hyperkalemic paralysis
  — Angiotensin-converting enzyme inhibitors and angiotensin receptor blockers
  — Spironolactone
- Hyponatremia due to other cause
  — Hypothyroidism
  — Diuretic use
  — Heart failure
  — Cirrhosis
  — Vomiting
  — Diarrhea
  — Severe illness
  — Major surgery
- Abdominal pain due to other cause
- Hyperpigmentation due to other cause, eg, hemochromatosis
- Isolated hypoaldosteronism
- Occult cancer
- Low serum cortisol-binding globulin in critical illness, causing low total serum cortisol; serum-free cortisol levels normal
- Secondary adrenal insufficiency (hypopituitarism)

6. Laboratory and Imaging Findings

Laboratory Tests

- Moderate neutropenia, lymphocytosis, and total eosinophil count > 300/μL
- Hyponatremia (90%), hyperkalemia (65%). (Patients with diarrhea may not be hyperkalemic)
- Fasting blood glucose may be low
- Hypercalcemia may be present
- Blood, sputum, or urine culture may be positive if bacterial infection is precipitating acute cause
- Plasma cortisol level < 3 mg/dL (< 83 nmol/L) at 8 AM is diagnostic, especially if accompanied by simultaneous elevated ACTH (usually > 200 pg/mL [> 44 pmol/L])
- Cosyntropin stimulation test
  — Synthetic ACTH 1 to 24 (cosyntropin), 0.25 mg, given intramuscularly
  — Serum cortisol obtained 45 minutes later
  — Normally, cortisol rises to ≥ 20 μg/dL
  — For patients taking corticosteroids, hydrocortisone must not be given for at least 8 hours before the test
  — Other corticosteroids (such as dexamethasone) do not interfere with specific assays for cortisol
- Plasma ACTH markedly elevated (generally > 200 pg/mL) if patient has primary adrenal disease
- Serum dehydroepiandrosterone (DHEA) > 1000 ng/mL excludes the diagnosis
- Antiadrenal antibodies detected in 50% of autoimmune Addison disease
- Antithyroid antibodies (45%) and other autoantibodies may be present in chronic disease
- Presence of serum antibodies to 21-hydroxylase help secure the diagnosis of autoimmune adrenocortical insufficiency
- Plasma very-long-chain fatty acid levels to screen for adrenoleukodystrophy in young men with idiopathic Addison disease
- Elevated levels of 17-OH progesterone diagnostic of salt-wasting congenital adrenal hyperplasia due to 21-hydroxylase deficiency

- Elevated plasma renin activity indicates
  — Depleted intravascular volume
  — The need for higher doses of fludrocortisone replacement
- Plasma epinephrine levels low
- Serum transferrin saturation elevated in cases of hemochromatosis (rare)

Imaging Studies

- Chest radiograph for tuberculosis, fungal infection, or cancer
- Abdominal CT shows small noncalcified adrenals in autoimmune Addison disease
  — Adrenals enlarged in about 85% of cases of metastatic or granulomatous disease
  — Calcification noted in cases of tuberculosis (~50%), hemorrhage, fungal infection, pheochromocytoma, and melanoma

7. Treatments

Medications

Chronic Adrenal Insufficiency

- Corticosteroid and mineralocorticoid replacement required in most cases; hydrocortisone alone may be adequate in mild cases
- Hydrocortisone
  — Drug of choice
  — Usually 15 to 30 mg orally in two divided doses: two-thirds in morning and one-third in late night or early evening
- Plenadren is a once-daily dual-release preparation of hydrocortisone (usual dose range is 20 to 30 mg); not available in the United States
- Prednisone 2 to 4 mg orally every morning and 1 to 2 mg orally every night or evening is an alternative
- Dose adjusted according to clinical response; proper dose usually results in normal white blood cell differential
- Corticosteroid dose raised in case of infection, trauma, surgery, diagnostic procedures, or other stress
  — Maximum hydrocortisone dose for severe stress is 50 mg every 6 hours intravenously or intramuscularly
  — Lower doses, oral or parenteral, for lesser stress
  — Dose tapered to normal as stress subsides
- Fludrocortisone, 0.05 to 0.3 mg once daily orally or once every other day, required by many patients
  — Dosage *increased* for
    ◦ Postural hypotension
    ◦ Hyponatremia
    ◦ Hyperkalemia
    ◦ Fatigue
    ◦ Elevated plasma renin activity
  — Dosage *decreased* for
    ◦ Edema
    ◦ Hypokalemia
    ◦ Hypertension
  — In some women with adrenal insufficiency, DHEA, 50 mg orally every morning, improves sense of well-being, an increase in muscle mass, and a reversal in bone loss at the femoral neck

Acute Adrenal Insufficiency

- If acute adrenocortical insufficiency is suspected
  — Draw blood sample for electrolytes, cortisol, and ACTH determinations
  — Without waiting for results, treat *immediately* with hydrocortisone 100 to 300 mg intravenously and saline

— Then, continue hydrocortisone 50 mg every 6 hours intravenously for first day, every 8 hours the second day, and taper as clinically appropriate

— Infections should be treated immediately and vigorously; broad-spectrum antibiotics given empirically while waiting for initial culture results

- D50W to treat hypoglycemia with careful monitoring of serum electrolytes, blood urea nitrogen, and creatinine
- When patient is able to take oral medication
  — Give hydrocortisone, 10 to 20 mg every 6 hours orally, and taper to maintenance levels
  — Most require hydrocortisone twice daily: 10 to 20 mg every morning, 5 to 10 mg every night
- Mineralocorticoid therapy
  — Not needed when large amounts of hydrocortisone are being given
  — However, as the dose is reduced, may need to add fludrocortisone, 0.05 to 0.2 mg once daily orally
  — Some patients never require fludrocortisone or become edematous at doses > 0.05 mg once or twice weekly

Therapeutic Procedures
- In acute adrenocortical insufficiency, once the crisis is over, must assess degree of permanent adrenal insufficiency and establish cause if possible

8. Outcomes

Follow-Up
- Follow clinically and adjust corticosteroid and (if required) mineralocorticoid doses
- Fatigue in treated patients may indicate
  — Suboptimal dosing of medication
  — Electrolyte imbalance
  — Concurrent problems, such as hypothyroidism or diabetes mellitus
- Corticosteroid dose must be increased in case of physiologic stress (see above)
- In acute disease, repeat cosyntropin stimulation test to document resolution and rule out chronic disease

Complications
- Complications of underlying disease (eg, tuberculosis) are more likely
- Adrenal crisis may be precipitated by intercurrent infections
- Associated autoimmune diseases are common (see above)
- Fatigue often persists despite treatment
- Excessive corticosteroid replacement can cause Cushing syndrome
- Acute adrenocortical insufficiency can cause shock and death if untreated

Prognosis
- Most patients able to live fully active lives
- Life expectancy is normal if adrenal insufficiency is diagnosed and treated with appropriate doses of corticosteroids and (if required) mineralocorticoids
- However, associated conditions can pose additional health risks, eg, patients with adrenal tuberculosis may have serious systemic infection
- Corticosteroid and mineralocorticoid replacement must not be stopped
- Patients should wear medical alert bracelet or medal reading "Adrenal insufficiency—takes hydrocortisone"
- Higher doses of corticosteroids must be administered to patients with infection, trauma, or surgery to prevent adrenal crisis
- Acute adrenocortical insufficiency frequently unrecognized and untreated since manifestations mimic more common conditions
- Lack of treatment for acute adrenocortical insufficiency leads to shock that is unresponsive to volume replacement and vasopressors, resulting in death

9. When to Refer and When to Admit

When to Refer

• If abnormal cosyntropin stimulation test to establish degree of permanent adrenal insufficiency and to establish its cause if possible

When to Admit

• Patients presenting with shock suspected to be deriving from acute adrenal crisis
• Patients presenting with an acute abdomen to exclude acute adrenal insufficiency as its cause
• Patients threatened by acute adrenal crisis (eg, those with severe bacterial infections) requiring immediate IV hydrocortisone administration

SUGGESTED REFERENCES

Charmandari E et al. Adrenal insufficiency. *Lancet*. 2014 Jun 21;383(9935):2152–2167. [PMID: 24503135]

Finkielstain GP et al. Clinical characteristics of a cohort of 244 patients with congenital adrenal hyperplasia. *J Clin Endocrinol Metab*. 2012 Dec;97(12):4429–4438. [PMID: 22990093]

Husebye ES et al. Consensus statement on the diagnosis, treatment and follow-up of patients with primary adrenal insufficiency. *J Intern Med*. 2014 Feb;275(2):104–115. [PMID: 24330030]

Nilsson AG et al. Prospective evaluation of long-term safety of dual-release hydrocortisone replacement administered once daily in patients with adrenal insufficiency. *Eur J Endocrinol*. 2014 Sep;171(3):369–377. [PMID: 24944332]

Quinkler M et al. What is the best long-term management strategy for patients with primary adrenal insufficiency? *Clin Endocrinol (Oxf)*. 2012 Jan;76(1):21–25. [PMID: 21585418]

Tiemensma J et al. Psychological morbidity and impaired quality of life in patients with stable treatment for primary adrenal insufficiency: cross-sectional study and review of the literature. *Eur J Endocrinol*. 2014 Aug;171(2):171–182. [PMID: 24801589]

Yong SL et al. Supplemental perioperative steroids for surgical patients with adrenal insufficiency. *Cochrane Database Syst Rev*. 2012 Dec 12;12:CD005367. [PMID: 23235622]

Yuen KC et al. Adrenal insufficiency in pregnancy: challenging issues in diagnosis and management. *Endocrine*. 2013 Oct;44(2):283–292. [PMID: 23377701]

66 Cushing Syndrome

A 35-year-old woman has hypertension of recent onset. Review of systems reveals several months of weight gain and menstrual irregularity. On examination she is obese, with a plethoric appearance. The blood pressure is 165/98 mm Hg. There are prominent purplish striae over the abdomen and multiple bruises over both lower legs. The patient's clinician entertains a diagnosis of hypercortisolism (Cushing syndrome).

LEARNING OBJECTIVES

▶ Learn the clinical manifestations and objective findings of Cushing syndrome
▶ Understand the causes of Cushing syndrome and their epidemiology
▶ Know the differential diagnosis of Cushing syndrome
▶ Understand the diagnostic options for Cushing syndrome and how to interpret the test results
▶ Learn the medical and surgical treatments for Cushing syndrome based on the cause

QUESTIONS

1. What are the salient features of this patient's problem?

2. How do you think through her problem?

3. What are the key features, including essentials of diagnosis, general considerations, and demographics, of Cushing syndrome?

4. What are the symptoms and signs of Cushing syndrome?

5. What is the differential diagnosis of Cushing syndrome?

6. What are laboratory, imaging, and procedural findings in Cushing syndrome?

7. What are the treatments for Cushing syndrome?

8. What are the outcomes, including complications and prognosis, of Cushing syndrome?

9. When should patients with Cushing syndrome be referred to a specialist or admitted to the hospital?

ANSWERS

1. Salient Features

Hypertension; weight gain; and menstrual irregularity (indicating pituitary dysfunction); purple striae on the abdomen

2. How to Think Through

Is a complete workup for secondary causes of hypertension appropriate in every new hypertension diagnosis? (No; 30% of US adults have hypertension, and most have idiopathic "essential hypertension." Also, tests such as endocrine assays have imperfect sensitivity and specificity. Look for symptoms and signs of secondary causes, and then direct diagnostic workup accordingly. Evaluate fully all cases of early onset and refractory hypertension.) In this case, evidence gathered by history and physical examination points to a possible secondary cause. In addition to her cushingoid appearance, weight gain, irregular menses, striae, and bruising, what other manifestations of cortisol excess should be sought in this patient? (Proximal muscle weakness, mood lability, elevated fasting glucose.) How do we establish that she has elevated cortisol levels or Cushing syndrome? (24-hour urine-free cortisol. Low-dose dexamethasone suppression test.) What test establishes the categories of possible causes of Cushing syndrome? (Plasma adrenocorticotropic hormone [ACTH] level. ACTH levels are abnormally high in *ACTH-dependent* processes such as hypothalamic cortisol releasing hormone [CRH] hypersecretion, ACTH-producing pituitary adenoma, and ectopic ACTH-producing tumor. Plasma ACTH levels are low in *ACTH-independent* processes such as adrenal adenoma or exogenous corticosteroid use.) Which of these two types of processes is the cause of Cushing disease? (Cushing *disease* is most often an ACTH-producing pituitary adenoma.)

3. Key Features

Essentials of Diagnosis

- Central obesity, muscle wasting, thin skin, psychological changes, hirsutism, purple striae
- Osteoporosis, hypertension, poor wound healing
- Hyperglycemia, leukocytosis, lymphocytopenia, hypokalemia, glycosuria
- Elevated serum cortisol and urinary-free cortisol. Lack of normal suppression by dexamethasone

General Considerations

- Cushing syndrome refers to manifestations of excessive corticosteroids
  — Commonly due to supraphysiologic doses of corticosteroid drugs
  — ~40% of cases are due to Cushing "disease," ACTH hypersecretion by a pituitary adenoma, which is usually small and benign
  — ~10% due to nonpituitary neoplasms (eg, small-cell lung carcinoma) that produce excessive ectopic ACTH
  — ~15% due to ACTH from a source that cannot be initially located
  — ~30% due to excessive autonomous secretion of cortisol by the adrenals independent of ACTH (serum ACTH usually low). Usually due to unilateral adrenal tumor of three types
    ◦ Benign adrenal adenomas are generally small tumors that produce mostly cortisol
    ◦ Adrenocortical carcinomas usually large and can produce excessive androgens as well as cortisol
    ◦ ACTH-independent macronodular adrenal hyperplasia can also produce hypercortisolism
  — May result from excessive ingestion of gamma-hydroxybutyric acid (GHB); resolves when drug is stopped
- Impaired glucose tolerance results from insulin resistance

Demographics

- Spontaneous Cushing syndrome is rare: 2.6 new cases yearly per million population
- ACTH-secreting pituitary adenoma (Cushing "disease") > 3 times more common in women than men

4. Symptoms and Signs

- Central obesity with plethoric "moon face," "buffalo hump," supraclavicular fat pads, protuberant abdomen, and thin extremities

- Muscle atrophy causes weakness, with difficulty standing up from a seated position or climbing stairs
- Oligomenorrhea or amenorrhea (or erectile dysfunction in males)
- Backache, headache
- Hypertension
- Osteoporosis or avascular bone necrosis
- Skin
  — Acne
  — Superficial skin infections
  — Purple striae (especially around the thighs, breasts, and abdomen)
  — Easy bruising, impaired wound healing
- Thirst and polyuria (with or without glycosuria); renal calculi
- Glaucoma
- Mental symptoms range from diminished concentration to increased mood lability to psychosis
- Increased susceptibility to opportunistic (unusual bacterial or fungal) infections
- Hirsutism and virilization may occur with adrenal carcinomas

5. Differential Diagnosis

- Chronic alcoholism (alcoholic pseudo-Cushing syndrome)
- Diabetes mellitus
- Depression (may have hypercortisolism)
- Osteoporosis due to other cause
- Obesity due to other cause
- Primary hyperaldosteronism
- Anorexia nervosa (high urine-free cortisol)
- Striae distensae ("stress marks") seen in adolescence and in pregnancy
- Lipodystrophy from antiretroviral agents
- Adrenal incidentalomas

6. Laboratory, Imaging, and Procedural Findings

Laboratory Tests

- Hyperglycemia
- Leukocytosis; relative granulocytosis and lymphopenia
- Hypokalemia (not hypernatremia), particularly with ectopic ACTH secretion
- Biochemical evaluation for Cushing syndrome can be difficult as test results are often misleading or conflicting
- Easiest screening test involves dexamethasone suppression test
  — 1 mg is given orally at 11 PM and serum is collected for cortisol determination at about 8 AM the next morning
  — Cortisol level < 5 µg/dL (< 135 nmol/L, fluorometric assay) or < 1.8 µg/dL (< 49 nmol/L), high-performance liquid chromatography [HPLC] assay) excludes Cushing syndrome with some certainty
- Midnight serum cortisol level > 7.5 µg/dL is indicative of Cushing syndrome; the patient should take nothing by mouth for 3 hours and have an intravenous line established in advance for a blood draw
- Late-night salivary cortisol assays are useful due to the inconvenience of obtaining a midnight blood specimen and a relatively high sensitivity and specificity for Cushing syndrome, but false-positive and false-negative tests occur
  ◦ Late-night salivary cortisol levels that are consistently > 250 ng/dL (7.0 nmol/L) are considered very abnormal

- If hypercortisolism is not excluded, measure 24-hour urine for free cortisol and creatinine
  — High 24-hour urine-free cortisol (or free cortisol to creatinine ratio of > 95 µg cortisol/g creatinine) helps confirm hypercortisolism
  — Misleadingly high urine-free cortisol occurs with high fluid intake
- If hypercortisolism is confirmed
  — Plasma ACTH below ~20 pg/mL indicates probable adrenal tumor
  — High or normal ACTH indicates pituitary or ectopic tumors
  — Blood for ACTH assay must be collected in a plastic tube, placed on ice, and processed quickly to avoid falsely low results

Imaging Studies
- Pituitary magnetic resonance imaging (MRI) shows an adenoma in ~50% of cases of ACTH-dependent Cushing syndrome
- Computed tomography (CT) scanning
  — Of chest and abdomen can help locate source of ectopic ACTH in lungs (carcinoid or small-cell carcinomas), thymus, pancreas, or adrenals
  — Of adrenals can localize adrenal tumor in most cases of non-ACTH-dependent Cushing syndrome
  — However, CT fails to detect the source of ACTH in about 40% of patients with ectopic ACTH secretion
- ^{111}In-octreotide scanning is also useful in detecting occult tumors, but [18]FDG-PET scanning is not usually helpful
- Some ectopic ACTH-secreting tumors elude discovery, necessitating bilateral adrenalectomy

Diagnostic Procedures
- If pituitary MRI is normal or shows incidental irregularity, selective inferior petrosal venous sampling for ACTH is performed (with corticotropin-releasing hormone stimulation) where available to confirm pituitary ACTH source, distinguishing it from an occult nonpituitary tumor secreting ACTH
- In patients with ACTH-dependent Cushing syndrome
  — Chest masses may be the source of ACTH
  — However, opportunistic infections are common
  — Therefore, it is prudent to biopsy a chest mass to confirm the pathologic diagnosis prior to resection

7. Treatments

Medications
- Cabergoline, 0.5 to 3.5 mg orally twice weekly
  — Alternative for patients who do not have a remission (or who have a recurrence) after selective transsphenoidal resection of pituitary adenoma
  — Successful in 40% of patients in one small study
- Pasireotide, 600 to 900 µg subcutaneously twice daily
  — Potential treatment for refractory Cushing disease
  — Normalizes the urine free cortisol in at least 17% of patients with Cushing disease
- Ketoconazole
  ◦ Inhibits adrenal steroidogenesis when given in doses of about 200 mg orally every 6 hours
  ◦ However, it is marginally effective and can cause liver toxicity
- Mifepristone
  ◦ Given orally in doses of 300 to 1200 mg/d
  ◦ Antagonizes glucocorticoid receptors and can be used in patients with endogenous Cushing syndrome and diabetes mellitus or glucose intolerance
  ◦ Side effects are frequent and include nausea, headache, fatigue, hypokalemia, and adrenal insufficiency; most importantly, it is an abortifacient

- Hydrocortisone replacement required temporarily after resection of pituitary adenoma or adrenal adenoma (see above)
- Mitotane for adrenal carcinoma
  — Initial dosage: 0.5 g twice daily with meals and increasing to 1 g twice daily within 2 weeks
  — Doses are adjusted every 2 to 3 weeks ideally to reach serum levels of 14 to 20 μg/mL
  — However, only about half the patients can tolerate mitotane levels > 14 μg/mL
  — Side effects include central nervous system depression, lethargy, hypogonadism, hyper-cholesterolemia, hypocalcemia, hepatotoxicity, leukopenia, hypertension, nausea, rash, thyroid-stimulating hormone suppression with hypothyroidism, and primary adrenal insufficiency
  — Accelerates the metabolism of sunitinib, cortisol, calcium channel blockers, benzodiazepines, some statins, some opioids, and some macrolide antibiotics
- Replacement hydrocortisone (15 mg in morning and 10 mg in afternoon) or prednisone should be started when mitotane doses reach 2 g daily
- A combination of mitotane (3–5 g/24 h), ketoconazole (0.4–1/2 g/24 h), and metyrapone (3–4.5 g/24 h) often suppress hypercortisolism
- Octreotide LAR, 20–40 mg injected intramuscularly every 28 days, suppresses ACTH secretion in about one-third of such cases
- Bisphosphonates may be used to treat osteoporosis (see Osteoporosis)

Surgery

- Selective transsphenoidal resection of a pituitary adenoma indicated in Cushing disease, after which remainder of pituitary usually returns to normal function
  — However, corticotrophs require 6 to 36 months to recover normal function
  — Thus, hydrocortisone replacement is required temporarily
  — Remission rates range from 65% to 90%
- Bilateral laparoscopic adrenalectomy if no remission (or recurrence) after pituitary surgery
- Laparoscopic resection for benign adrenal adenomas
  ○ May be done if they are < 6 cm in diameter
  ○ Because contralateral adrenal is suppressed, postoperative hydrocortisone replacement is required until recovery
- Surgical resection of ectopic ACTH-secreting tumors

Therapeutic Procedures

- Stereotactic pituitary radiosurgery (gamma knife) is an option for patients with ACTH-secreting pituitary tumors that persist or recur after pituitary surgery
  — Normalizes urine free cortisol in two-thirds of patients within 12 months
  — Can also be used to treat Nelson syndrome, the progressive enlargement of ACTH-secreting pituitary tumors following bilateral adrenalectomy
- Radiation therapy is an option for patients with ACTH-secreting pituitary tumors that persist or recur after pituitary surgery
- Conventional radiation therapy cures 23%

8. Outcomes

Complications

- Complications of hypertension or diabetes mellitus
- Increased susceptibility to infections
- Nephrolithiasis
- Depression, dementia, psychosis
- Following bilateral adrenalectomy for Cushing disease, progressive enlargement of pituitary adenoma may cause local effects (eg, visual field impairment) and hyperpigmentation (Nelson syndrome)
- "Cortisol withdrawal syndrome," even when given replacement corticosteroids for adrenal insufficiency; manifestations include
  — Hypotension
  — Nausea

— Fatigue
— Arthralgias
— Myalgias
— Pruritus
— Flaking skin

• Patients with Cushing syndrome of any cause face a high complication rate after treatment and all patients require intensive clinical care and close follow-up

Prognosis

• Although manifestations regress with time, patients often have residual mild cognitive impairment, muscle weakness, osteoporosis, and sequelae from vertebral fractures
• Younger patients have a better chance for recovery and children with short stature may have catch-up growth following cure
• Continued impaired quality of life is more common in women than in men
• Patients with failed pituitary surgery may require pituitary radiation therapy, which has its own morbidity
• Patients with Cushing syndrome due to benign adrenal adenoma have
  — Five-year survival rate of 95%
  — Ten-year survival rate of 90% following successful adrenalectomy
• Patients with Cushing disease from pituitary adenoma have similar survival if pituitary surgery is successful
• Transsphenoidal surgery fails in ~10% to 20%
• Despite complete remission after transsphenoidal surgery, ~15% to 20% recur over 10 years
• Laparoscopic bilateral adrenalectomy
  — May be required
  — Recurrence of hypercortisolism may occur as a result of growth of adrenal remnant stimulated by high ACTH levels
• Prognosis with ectopic ACTH-producing tumors depends on aggressiveness and stage of tumor
• Patients with ACTH of unknown source have
  — Five-year survival rate of 65%
  — Ten-year survival rate of 55%
• Five-year survival rates in patients with adrenocortical carcinoma
  ○ Stage 1: 81%
  ○ Stage 2: 61%
  ○ Stage 3: 50%
  ○ Stage 4: 13%

9. When to Refer and When to Admit

When to Refer

• If abnormal dexamethasone suppression test

When to Admit

• For transsphenoidal hypophysectomy, adrenalectomy, resection of ectopic ACTH-secreting tumor

SUGGESTED REFERENCES

Arnaldi G et al. Advances in the epidemiology, pathogenesis, and management of Cushing's syndrome complications. *J Endocrinol Invest*. 2012 Apr;35(4):434–448. [PMID: 22652826]
Bertagna X et al. Approach to the Cushing's disease patient with persistent/recurrent hypercortisolism after pituitary surgery. *J Clin Endocrinol Metab*. 2013 Apr;98(4):1307–1318. [PMID: 23564942]

Elias PC et al. Late-night salivary cortisol has a better performance than urinary free cortisol in the diagnosis of Cushing's syndrome. *J Clin Endocrinol Metab*. 2014 Jun;99(6):2045–2051. [PMID: 24628557]

Fassnacht M et al. Update in adrenocortical carcinoma. *J Clin Endocrinol Metab*. 2013 Dec;98(12): 4551–4564. [PMID: 24081734]

Graversen D et al. Mortality in Cushing's syndrome: a systematic review and meta-analysis. *Eur J Intern Med*. 2012 Apr;23(3):278–282. [PMID: 22385888]

Juszczak A et al. The therapy of Cushing's disease in adults and children: an update. *Horm Metab Res*. 2013 Feb;45(2):109–117. [PMID: 23225246]

Lambert JK et al. Predictors of mortality and long-term outcomes in treated Cushing's disease: a study of 346 patients. *J Clin Endocrinol Metab*. 2013 Mar;98(3):1022–1030. [PMID: 23393167]

Oßwald A et al. Favorable long-term outcomes of bilateral adrenalectomy in Cushing's disease. *Eur J Endocrinol*. 2014 Aug;171(2):209–215. [PMID: 24975318]

Ragnarsson O et al. Cushing's syndrome: a structured short- and long-term management plan for patients in remission. *Eur J Endocrinol*. 2013 Oct 4;169(5):R139–R152. [PMID: 23985132]

Ritzel K et al. Clinical review: outcome of bilateral adrenalectomy in Cushing's syndrome: a systematic review. *J Clin Endocrinol Metab*. 2013 Oct;98(10):3939–3948. [PMID: 23956347]

Starkman MN. Neuropsychiatric findings in Cushing syndrome and exogenous glucocorticoid administration. *Endocrinol Metab Clin North Am*. 2013 Sep;42(3):477–488. [PMID: 24011881]

Tritos NA et al. Update on radiation therapy in patients with Cushing's disease. *Pituitary*. 2015 Apr;18(2):263–268. [PMID: 25359445]

Valassi E et al. Clinical consequences of Cushing's syndrome. *Pituitary*. 2012 Sep;15(3):319–329. [PMID: 22527617]

Type 1 Diabetes Mellitus

67

A 22-year-old woman with a history of poorly controlled type 1 diabetes mellitus presents to the emergency room with abdominal pain, nausea, and vomiting. She has been feeling ill with a cough, sore throat, and decreased appetite, and so she has skipped several doses of insulin. On physical examination, she is tachypneic and her abdomen is diffusely tender to palpation without rebound or guarding. Serum testing reveals a glucose level of 512 mg/dL and an anion gap of 23, and her arterial pH is 7.12. Her urine dipstick is positive for ketones as well as glucose. A serum β-hydroxybutyric acid level is elevated.

LEARNING OBJECTIVES

▶ Learn the diagnostic criteria for type 1 diabetes mellitus

▶ Understand the genetic and demographic factors that predispose to type 1 diabetes mellitus

▶ Know the differential diagnosis of type 1 diabetes mellitus

▶ Learn the treatments, including the different preparations of insulin, for type 1 diabetes mellitus

QUESTIONS

1. What are the salient features of this patient's problem?

2. How do you think through her problem?

3. What are the key features, including essentials of diagnosis, general considerations, and demographics, of type 1 diabetes mellitus?

4. What are the symptoms and signs of type 1 diabetes mellitus?

5. What is the differential diagnosis of type 1 diabetes mellitus?

6. What are laboratory findings in type 1 diabetes mellitus?

7. What are the treatments for type 1 diabetes mellitus?

8. What are the outcomes, including follow-up, complications, prognosis, and prevention, of type 1 diabetes mellitus?

9. When should patients with type 1 diabetes mellitus be referred to a specialist or admitted to the hospital?

ANSWERS

1. Salient Features

Young age; abdominal pain, nausea, vomiting; recent illness and insulin nonadherence; anion-gap metabolic acidosis with resulting tachypnea; elevated serum glucose; urine and serum ketosis

2. How to Think Through

What clinical evidence helps distinguish between type 1 and type 2 diabetes at the time of initial diagnosis of this young woman? (Weight loss rather than obesity; absence of acanthosis nigricans, dyslipidemia, hypertension, or polycystic ovaries. Onset of type 1 is typically in early childhood or early puberty. Autoantibody tests—see below.) With what symptoms did she most likely present at the time of diagnosis? (Polyuria, polydipsia, lethargy, and weight loss.) This patient now presents with the defining features of diabetic ketoacidosis (DKA). In DKA, it is crucial to identify the precipitating factor. What likely precipitated DKA in this case? (Cough and pharyngitis suggest she has an infection, along with nonadherence to insulin.) Is any additional testing warranted to establish the precipitating factor? (Chest X-ray, if history or examination suggests pneumonia, urinalysis, and in older patients, consider an electrocardiogram.) DKA is best managed using a protocol. What are the key clinical and laboratory factors to monitor? (Volume status, serum glucose, bicarbonate, anion gap, potassium, and corrected sodium.) How much volume repletion is typically needed in DKA? (4–6 L.)

3. Key Features

Essentials of Diagnosis

- Polyuria, polydipsia, and weight loss associated with random plasma glucose $\geq$ 200 mg/dL (11.1 mmol/L)
- Plasma glucose $\geq$ 126 mg/dL (7.0 mmol/L) after an overnight fast, documented on more than one occasion
- Ketonemia, ketonuria, or both

General Considerations

- Caused by pancreatic islet β-cell destruction
- Destruction is autoimmune in > 95% of cases (type 1a) and idiopathic in the remainder (type 1b)
- About 95% of type 1 patients possess either HLA-DR3 or HLA-DR4 compared with 45% to 50% of white controls. HLA-DQB1*0302 is an even more specific marker for susceptibility
- Most patients have circulating antibodies to islet cells (ICA), glutamic acid decarboxylase (GAD65), insulin (IAA), and tyrosine phosphatase IA2 (ICA-512) and zinc transporter 8 at diagnosis
- The rate of pancreatic β-cell destruction ranges from rapid to slow
- Prone to ketoacidosis
- Plasma glucagon is elevated
- C peptide levels do not reliably distinguish between type 1 and type 2 diabetes mellitus

Demographics

- Occurs at any age but most commonly arises in children and young adults with a peak incidence before school age and again at around puberty
- Incidence
  — Highest in Scandinavia: in Finland, yearly incidence in children 14 years old or younger is 40 per 100,000
  — Lowest incidence is < 1 per 100,000 per year in China and parts of South America
  — In the United States, average is 16 per 100,000
  — Incidences are higher in states densely populated with persons of Scandinavian descent such as Minnesota
  — The global incidence is increasing, with an annual increase of ~3%

- An estimated 25.8 million Americans have diabetes mellitus, of whom ~1 million have type 1 diabetes

4. Symptoms and Signs
- Increased thirst (polydipsia)
- Increased urination (polyuria)
- Increased appetite (polyphagia) with weight loss
- Ketoacidosis
- Paresthesias
- Recurrent blurred vision
- Vulvovaginitis or pruritus
- Nocturnal enuresis
- Postural hypotension from lowered plasma volume

5. Differential Diagnosis
- Type 2 diabetes mellitus
- Hyperglycemia resulting from other causes
  — Medications (high-dose corticosteroids, pentamidine)
  — Other endocrine conditions (Cushing syndrome, glucagonoma, acromegaly, pheochromocytoma)
- Metabolic acidosis of other causes (alcoholic ketoacidosis)
- Nondiabetic glycosuria (renal glycosuria)

6. Laboratory Findings
Laboratory Tests
- Fasting plasma glucose > 126 mg/dL (7 mmol/L) or > 200 mg/dL (11.1 mmol/L) 2 hours after glucose load (Table 67-1)
- Hemoglobin A1c (HbA1c) of at least 6.5%
- Urine glucose (Clinistix, Diastix)
- Urine or blood ketones (Acetest, Ketostix) or both
- Hemoglobin A_{1c} reflects glycemic control over preceding 8 to 12 weeks
- Serum fructosamine
  — Reflects glycemic control over preceding 2 weeks
  — Helpful in presence of abnormal hemoglobins or in ascertaining glycemic control at time of conception among diabetic women
- Lipoprotein abnormalities; unlike in type 2 diabetes, moderately deficient control of hyperglycemia in type 1 diabetes is associated with only slight elevation of low-density lipoprotein (LDL) cholesterol and serum triglycerides and minimal change in high-density lipoprotein cholesterol
- Plasma glucagon is elevated
- C peptide levels do not reliably distinguish between type 1 and type 2 diabetes mellitus

Table 67-1. Criteria for the diagnosis of diabetes.

	Normal Glucose Tolerance	Impaired Glucose Tolerance	Diabetes Mellitus[b]
Fasting plasma glucose mg/dL (mmol/L)	< 100 (5.6)	100–125 (5.6–6.9)	≥ 126 (7.0)
2 h after glucose load mg/dL (mmol/L)	< 140 (7.8)	≥ 140–199 (7.8–11.0)	≥ 200 (11.1)
HbA$_{1c}$ (%)	< 5.7	5.7–6.4	≥ 6.5

[a]Give 75 g of glucose dissolved in 300 mL of water after an overnight fast in persons who have been receiving at least 150 to 200 g of carbohydrate daily for 3 days before the test.

[b]A fasting plasma glucose ≥ 126 mg/dL (7.0 mmol/L) or HbA$_{1c}$ of ≥ 6.5% is diagnostic of diabetes if confirmed by repeat testing.

Table 67-2. Summary of bioavailability characteristics of the insulins.

Insulin Preparations	Onset of Action	Peak Action	Effective Duration
Insulins lispro, aspart, glulisine	5–15 min	1–1.5 h	3–4 h
Human regular	30–60 min	2 h	6–8 h
Human NPH	2–4 h	6–7 h	10–20 h
Insulin glargine	1.5 h	Flat	~24 h
Insulin detemir	1 h	Flat	17 h
Technosphere inhaled insulin	5–15 minutes	1 hour	3 h

NPH, neutral protamine Hagedorn.

7. Treatments

Medications
- See Tables 67-2, 67-3, and 67-4
- Regular insulin (a U500 concentration is available for use in patients who are very resistant)
- Rapidly acting insulin analogs: insulin lispro, insulin aspart, insulin glulisine
- Intermediate-acting insulin purified: neutral protamine Hagedorn (NPH)
- Premixed insulins
  — 70% NPH/30% regular (70/30 insulin)
  — 50% NPH/50% regular (50/50 insulin)
  — 70% neutral protamine lispro (NPL)/25% insulin lispro (Humalog Mix 75/25)
  — 50% NPL/50% insulin lispro (Humalog Mix 50/50)
  — 70% insulin aspart protamine/30% insulin aspart (Novolog Mix 70/30)
- Long-acting insulins purified: insulin glargine, insulin detemir
- Pramlintide (islet amyloid polypeptide analog)
- Inhaled Insulin
  — Dry-powder formulation of recombinant human regular insulin, delivered by inhalation (technosphere insulin, Afrezza) is approved for use in adults with diabetes
  — Rapidly absorbed with maximum effect at 1 hour, declining to baseline by about 3 hours
  — Combined with basal insulin was as effective in glucose lowering as rapid acting insulin analogs combined with basal insulin

Table 67-3. Insulin preparations available in the United States.[a]

Rapidly acting human insulin analogs
Insulin lispro (Humalog, Lilly)
Insulin aspart (Novolog, Novo Nordisk)
Insulin glulisine (Apidra, Sanofi Aventis)
Short-acting regular insulin
Regular insulin (Lilly, Novo Nordisk)
Technosphere inhaled regular insulin (Afrezza)
Intermediate-acting insulins
NPH insulin (Lilly, Novo Nordisk)
Premixed insulins
70% NPH/30% regular (70/30 insulin—Lilly, Novo Nordisk)
70% NPL/25% insulin lispro (Humalog Mix 75/25—Lilly)
50% NPL/50% insulin lispro (Humalog Mix 50/50—Lilly)
70% insulin aspart protamine/30% insulin aspart (Novolog Mix 70/30—Novo Nordisk)
Long-acting human insulin analogs
Insulin glargine (Lantus, Sanofi Aventis)
Insulin detemir (Levemir, Novo Nordisk)

NPH, neutral protamine Hagedorn; NPL, neutral protamine lispro.

[a]All insulins available in the United States are recombinant human or human insulin analog origin. All the above insulins are dispensed at U100 concentration. There is an additional U500 preparation of regular insulin.

Table 67-4. Examples of intensive insulin regimens using rapidly acting insulin analogs (insulin lispro, aspart, or glulisine) and insulin detemir, or insulin glargine in a 70-kg man with type 1 diabetes.[a,b,c]

	Pre-Breakfast	Pre-Lunch	Pre-Dinner	At Bedtime
Rapidly acting insulin analog	5 units	4 units	6 units	
Insulin detemir	6–7 units			8–9 units
OR				
Rapidly acting insulin analog	5 units	4 units	6 units	—
Insulin glargine		—		15–16 units

[a]Assumes that patient is consuming approximately 75 g carbohydrate at breakfast, 60 g at lunch, and 90 g at dinner.

[b]The dose of rapidly acting insulin can be raised by 1 or 2 units if extra carbohydrate (15–30 g) is ingested or if premeal blood glucose is > 170 mg/dL (9.4 mmol/L).

[c]Insulin glargine or insulin detemir must be given as a separate injection.

— Formulated as a single use cartridge delivering 4 or 8 units immediately before the meal
— The most common adverse reaction was cough affecting 27 % of subjects
— A small decrease in pulmonary function (forced expiratory volume in 1 second [FEV1]) was persistent at 2 years; spirometry recommended prior to initiation; contraindicated in smokers and patients with chronic lung disease

Surgery
• Infuse intraoperatively and in immediate postoperative period: D5 0.9% saline with 20 mEq KCl intravenously at 100 to 200 mL/h. Infuse regular human insulin (25 units/250 mL 0.9% saline) into intravenous tubing at 1 to 3 units/h
• Monitor blood glucose hourly and adjust infusion for target glucose levels 100 to 180 mg/dL
• Patients receiving simultaneous pancreas and kidney transplants have 83% chance of pancreatic graft survival at 1 year and 69% at 5 years
• Solitary pancreas transplant only for recurrent life-threatening metabolic instability
• Islet cell transplantation
  — Insulin independence for more than 5 years has been demonstrated in patients who got anti-CD3 antibody or anti-thymocyte globulin induction immunosuppression and calcineurin inhibitors, mTor inhibitors, and mycophenolate mofetil as maintenance immunosuppression
  — Long-term immunosuppression is necessary to prevent allograft rejection and to suppress the autoimmune process that led to the disease initially
  — One major limitation is the need for more than one islet infusion to achieve insulin independence

Therapeutic Procedures
• Eucaloric healthy diet. Limit cholesterol to 300 mg once daily and protein to 10% of total calories
• Treat microalbuminuria with angiotensin-converting enzyme inhibitor (ACEI) to retard diabetic nephropathy
• Treat hypertension and hyperlipidemia (reduce LDL to < 100 mg/dL)
• Attempts have been made to prolong the partial clinical remission ("honeymoon") using such drugs as cyclosporine, azathioprine, prednisone, and antithymocyte globulin

8. Outcomes
Follow-Up
• Patients who received intensive insulin (multiple-injection or pump) therapy to obtain a mean HbA_{1c} of 7.2% (normal: < 6%), experienced a 60% reduction in risk of diabetic retinopathy, nephropathy, and neuropathy, compared with patients who received conventional therapy

Complications

- DKA
- Hypoglycemia and altered awareness of hypoglycemia
- Diabetic retinopathy, cataracts
- Nephropathy
- Neuropathy
- Diabetic atherothrombosis (heart disease, peripheral vascular disease)
- Lipodystrophy at injection sites
- Diabetic cheiroarthropathy
- Adhesive capsulitis
- Carpal tunnel syndrome
- Dupuytren contractures

Prognosis

- The Diabetes Control and Complications Trial (DCCT) showed that the poor prognosis for 40% of patients with type 1 diabetes is markedly improved by optimal care
- Patients can have a full life
- Tight control (mean HbA_{1c} 7.2%, normal: < 6%) in the DCCT was associated with a threefold greater risk of serious hypoglycemia as well as greater weight gain. However, no deaths occurred because of hypoglycemia, and no evidence of posthypoglycemic cognitive damage was detected
- Subsequent end-stage kidney disease predicted by microalbuminuria > 30 μg/mg creatinine; risk decreased by treatment with ACEI

Prevention

- Acetylsalicylic acid (aspirin) 81 to 325 mg (enteric-coated) orally daily to reduce risk of diabetic atherothrombosis without increasing risk of gastrointestinal hemorrhage
- Instruction in personal hygiene, in particular, care of feet, skin, and teeth
- Yearly diabetic eye examination
- Patient self-management training
- Self-monitoring of blood glucose
- Exercise

9. When to Refer and When to Admit

When to Refer

- Team educational approach is critical. Enlist nutritionist
- Poorly controlled diabetes

When to Admit

- Altered mental status
- DKA
- Marked volume disorders
- Marked electrolyte disorders
- Unstable comorbid conditions

SUGGESTED REFERENCES

American Association of Diabetes Educators. https://www.diabeteseducator.org/

American Diabetes Association. http://www.diabetes.org/

American Diabetes Association. Standards of medical care in diabetes—2015. *Diabetes Care*. 2015 Jan;38(suppl):S8–S16. [PMID: 25537706]

American Dietetic Association. http://www.eatright.org

Atkinson MA et al. Type 1 diabetes. *Lancet*. 2014 Jan 4;383(9911):69–82. [PMID: 23890997]

Blumer I et al. Diabetes and pregnancy: an endocrine society clinical practice guideline. *J Clin Endocrinol Metab*. 2013 Nov;98(11):4227–4249. [PMID: 24194617]

Chin JA et al. Diabetes mellitus and peripheral vascular disease: diagnosis and management. *Clin Podiatr Med Surg*. 2014 Jan;31(1):11–26. [PMID: 24296015]

Cryer PE. Mechanisms of hypoglycemia-associated autonomic failure in diabetes. *N Engl J Med*. 2013 Jul 25;369(4):362–372. [PMID: 23883381]

Diabetes Prevention Trial—Type 1 Diabetes Study Group. Effects of insulin in relatives of patients with type 1 diabetes mellitus. *N Engl J Med*. 2002 May 30;346(22):1685–1691. [PMID: 12037147]

Haidar A et al. Comparison of dual-hormone artificial pancreas, single-hormone artificial pancreas, and conventional insulin pump therapy for glycaemic control in patients with type 1 diabetes: an open-label randomised controlled crossover trial. *Lancet Diabetes Endocrinol*. 2015 Jan;3(1):17–26. [PMID: 25434967]

Juvenile Diabetes Foundation. http://jdrf.org/

Kansagara D et al. Intensive insulin therapy in hospitalized patients: a systematic review. *Ann Intern Med*. 2011 Feb 15;154(4):268–282. [PMID: 21320942]

Nyenwe EA et al. Evidence-based management of hyperglycemic emergencies in diabetes mellitus. *Diabetes Res Clin Pract*. 2011 Dec;94(3):340–351. [PMID: 21978840]

Savage MW et al. Joint British Diabetes Societies guideline for the management of diabetic ketoacidosis. *Diabet Med*. 2011 May;28(5):508–15. [PMID: 21255074]

Singleton JR et al. The diabetic neuropathies: practical and rational therapy. *Semin Neurol*. 2012 Jul;32(3):196–203. [PMID: 23117944]

Stitt AW et al. Advances in our understanding of diabetic retinopathy. *Clin Sci (Lond)*. 2013 Mar 13;125(1):1–17. [PMID: 23485060]

Switzer SM et al. Intensive insulin therapy in patients with type 1 diabetes mellitus. *Endocrinol Metab Clin North Am*. 2012 Mar;41(1):89–104. [PMID: 22575408]

The Diabetes Control and Complications Trial Research Group. The effect of intensive treatment of diabetes on the development and progression of long-term complications in insulin-dependent diabetes mellitus. *N Engl J Med*. 1993 Sep 30;329(14):977–986. [PMID: 8366922]

Tooley JE et al. New and future immunomodulatory therapy in type 1 diabetes. *Trends Mol Med*. 2012 Mar;18(3):173–81. [PMID: 22342807]

Tuomi T et al. The many faces of diabetes: a disease with increasing heterogeneity. *Lancet*. 2014 Mar 22;383(9922):1084–1094. [PMID: 24315621]

Waanders F et al. Current concepts in the management of diabetic nephropathy. *Neth J Med*. 2013 Nov;71(9):448–458. [PMID: 24218418]

68

Type 2 Diabetes Mellitus

A 53-year-old man presents to his primary care clinician for a routine checkup. He complains of increased thirst and frequent urination for the past few months. On physical examination, he is an obese man and his blood pressure is 152/87 mm Hg. His urinalysis is positive for glucose. A random finger-stick blood glucose reading in the office is 352 mg/dL. Serum hemoglobin A$_{1c}$ level is 10.2%.

LEARNING OBJECTIVES

▶ Learn the clinical manifestations and objective findings of type 2 diabetes mellitus and how to screen for the disease

▶ Understand the factors that predispose to type 2 diabetes mellitus

▶ Know the differential diagnosis of type 2 diabetes mellitus

▶ Learn the medical treatments for type 2 diabetes mellitus and which patients require insulin therapy

QUESTIONS

1. What are the salient features of this patient's problem?

2. How do you think through his problem?

3. What are the key features, including essentials of diagnosis, general considerations, and demographics, of type 2 diabetes mellitus?

4. What are the symptoms and signs of type 2 diabetes mellitus?

5. What is the differential diagnosis of type 2 diabetes mellitus?

6. What are laboratory findings in type 2 diabetes mellitus?

7. What are the treatments for type 2 diabetes mellitus?

8. What are the outcomes, including follow-up, complications, prognosis, and prevention, of type 2 diabetes mellitus?

9. When should patients with type 2 diabetes mellitus be referred to a specialist or admitted to the hospital?

ANSWERS

1. Salient Features

Middle aged; obese, polyuria, and polydipsia; associated hypertension; glycosuria; random blood sugar > 200 mg/dL with symptoms; hemoglobin A$_{1c}$ level > 6.5%

2. How to Think Through

Factors that increase the risk to develop type 2 diabetes include obesity, as in this case. What other risk factors should be considered? (Family history, ethnicity; physical activity; fat distribution; smoking; and others—even sleep duration.)

Besides polyuria and polydipsia, what other symptoms are often present when diabetes is first recognized? (Fatigue, weight loss, candidal vaginitis, blurred vision, peripheral neuropathy.) Do blurred vision and peripheral neuropathy necessarily indicate prolonged undetected diabetes? (Blurred vision may be caused by acute hyperglycemia, rather than long-standing diabetic retinopathy, but neuropathy implies long-term hyperglycemia.) Glucosuria occurs above what serum glucose concentration? (Approximately 300 mg/dL.)

How should this patient be evaluated? (Full physical examination including ophthalmologic, neurologic, and foot examinations, complete blood count, serum electrolytes, creatinine, lipid panel, urine microalbumin test, and baseline electrocardiography.) What are the four treatment priorities to reduce his risk of macrovascular and microvascular complications? (Weight loss, blood pressure control, glucose control, and statin therapy aiming for a low-density lipoprotein [LDL] cholesterol of at least < 100 mg/dL, ideally < 70 mg/dL.) How should he be treated today? (Given the degree of glucose elevation, electrolytes and renal function should be assessed. Begin metformin, intensive lifestyle modification and patient education, and home glucose monitoring for additional data. Arrange close follow-up—a second agent will very likely be needed. An antihypertensive should be initiated if hypertension is confirmed at the next visit and statin therapy should follow.)

3. Key Features

Essentials of Diagnosis

- Typically > 40 years of age
- Obesity
- Polyuria and polydipsia
- Candidal vaginitis sometimes an initial manifestation
- Often few or no symptoms
- After an overnight fast, plasma glucose ≥ 126 mg/dL (7 mmol/L) more than once
- After 75 g oral glucose, diagnostic values are ≥ 200 mg/dL (11.1 mmol/L) 2 hours after the oral glucose
- Hemoglobin A_{1c} (HbA_{1c}) ≥ 6.5%
- Often associated with hypertension, dyslipidemia, and atherosclerosis

General Considerations

- Circulating endogenous insulin is sufficient to prevent ketoacidosis but inadequate to prevent hyperglycemia from tissue insensitivity
- Strong genetic influences
- High prevalence of obesity in type 2 diabetes mellitus
  — 30% in Chinese and Japanese
  — 60% to 70% in North Americans, Europeans, and Africans
  — Nearly 100% in Pima Indians and Pacific Islanders from Nauru or Samoa
- Abdominal fat, with an abnormally high waist–hip ratio, is generally associated with obesity in type 2 diabetes. This visceral obesity correlates with insulin resistance, whereas subcutaneous fat seems to have less of an association

Demographics

- ~22 million Americans have type 2 diabetes
- Traditionally occurred in middle-aged adults but now more frequently encountered in children and adolescents
- No gender predominance

4. Symptoms and Signs

- Polyuria
- Increased thirst (polydipsia)
- Weakness or fatigue
- Recurrent blurred vision
- Vulvovaginitis or anogenital pruritus or balanoposthitis
- Peripheral neuropathy
- Obesity
- Often asymptomatic

5. Differential Diagnosis

Hyperglycemia

- Endocrinopathies
  — Type 1 diabetes mellitus
  — Cushing syndrome
  — Acromegaly
  — Pheochromocytoma
  — Glucagonoma
  — Somatostatinoma
- Drugs
  — High-dose corticosteroids
  — Thiazides
  — Phenytoin
  — Niacin
  — Oral contraceptives
  — Pentamidine
- Pancreatic insufficiency
  — Subtotal pancreatectomy
  — Chronic pancreatitis
  — Hemochromatosis ("bronze diabetes")
  — Hemosiderosis
- Other
  — Gestational diabetes
  — Cirrhosis
  — Schmidt syndrome (polyglandular failure: Addison disease, autoimmune thyroiditis, diabetes)

Polyuria

- Diabetes insipidus
- Hypercalcemia
- Psychogenic polydipsia

Nondiabetic glycosuria (benign)

- Genetic
- Fanconi syndrome
- Chronic kidney disease
- Pregnancy

6. Laboratory Findings

Laboratory Tests

- Fasting plasma glucose $\geq$ 126 mg/dL (7 mmol/L) or $\geq$ 200 mg/dL (11.1 mmol/L) 2 hours after glucose load (Table 68-1)
- Urine glucose (Clinistix, Diastix)
- Urine ketones (sometimes without serum ketones) (Acetest, Ketostix)

Table 68-1. Criteria for the diagnosis of diabetes mellitus.

	Normal Glucose Tolerance	Impaired Glucose Tolerance	Diabetes Mellitus[b]
Fasting plasma glucose mg/dL (mmol/L)	< 100 (5.6)	100–125 (5.6-6.9)	≥ 126 (7.0)
2 hr after glucose load mg/dL[a] (mmol/L)	< 140 (7.8)	≥ 140–199 (7.8-11.0)	≥ 200 (11.1)
HbA$_{1c}$ (%)	< 5.7	5.7–6.4	≥ 6.5

[a]Give 75 g of glucose dissolved in 300 mL of water after an overnight fast in persons who have been receiving at least 150–200 g of carbohydrate daily for 3 days before the test.

[b]A fasting plasma glucose ≥ 126 mg/dL (7.0 mmol) or HbA$_{1c}$ of ≥ 6.5% is diagnostic of diabetes if confirmed by repeat testing.

- HbA$_{1c}$ > 6.5% reflects glycemic control over preceding 8 to 12 weeks
- Serum fructosamine > 270 μmol/L
  — Reflects glycemic control over preceding 2 weeks
  — Helpful in the presence of abnormal hemoglobins and in ascertaining glycemic control at time of conception among diabetic women
- Lipoprotein abnormalities in obese persons with type 2 diabetes include
  — High serum triglyceride (300–400 mg/dL)
  — Low high-density lipoprotein (HDL) cholesterol (< 30 mg/dL)
  — A qualitative change in LDL particles
- These abnormalities differ from type 1 diabetes, which is associated with only slight elevation of LDL cholesterol and serum triglycerides and minimal change in HDL cholesterol

7. Treatments

Medications
- Tables 68-2, 68-3, and 68-4
- Drugs that stimulate insulin secretion
  — Sulfonylureas (acetohexamide, chlorpropamide, gliclazide, glipizide, glyburide, tolazamide, tolbutamide)
  — Meglitinide analogs (meglitinide, repaglinide)
  — D-phenylalanine derivative (nateglinide)
- Drugs that primarily lower glucose levels by their actions on the liver, muscle, and adipose tissue
  — Biguanide (metformin)
  — Thiazolidinediones (pioglitazone, rosiglitazone)
- Drugs that principally affect glucose absorption: α-glucosidase inhibitors (acarbose, miglitol, voglibose)
- Drugs that mimic incretin
  — Oral glucose provokes a threefold higher insulin response than an equivalent dose of glucose given IV due to the release of gut hormones that amplify the insulin release (glucagon-like peptide 1 [GLP-1] and glucose-dependent insulinotropic polypeptide [GIP1]
  — This "incretin effect" is reduced in patients with type 2 diabetes
- Current GLP-1 receptor agonists:
  — **Exenatide:** fixed-dose pens (5 or 10 μg) injected 60 minutes before breakfast and dinner; not for patients with a GFR <30 mL/min; in patients already taking metformin, sulfonylurea, or both, lowered the HbA$_{1c}$ value by 0.4% to 0.6% over a 30-week trial; patients also experienced weight loss of 3 to 6 pounds; a once-weekly, long-acting formulation lowered the HbA$_{1c}$ level a little more than the twice daily dose
  — **Liraglutide** is a once-daily injection; trials lasting 26 and 52 weeks, adding liraglutide to the therapeutic regimen (metformin, sulfonylurea, thiazolidinedione) lowered the HbA1c by 0.6% to 1.5% with weight loss of 1 to 6 pounds

Table 68–2. Drugs for treatment of type 2 diabetes mellitus.

Drug	Tablet Size	Daily Dose	Duration of Action
Sulfonylureas			
Acetohexamide (Dymelor)	250 and 500 mg	0.25–1.5 g as single dose or in two divided doses	8–24 h
Chlorpropamide (Diabinese)	100 and 250 mg	0.1–0.5 g as single dose	24–72 h
Gliclazide (not available in United States)	80 mg	40–80 mg as single dose; 160–320 mg as divided dose	12 h
Glimepiride (Amaryl)	1, 2, and 4 mg	1–4 mg once a day is usual dose; 8 mg once a day is maximal dose	Up to 24 h
Glipizide			
(Glucotrol)	5 and 10 mg	2.5–40 mg as a single dose or in two divided doses 30 minutes before meals	6–12 h
(Glucotrol XL)	2.5, 5, and 10 mg	2.5–10 mg once a day is usual dose; 20 mg once a day is maximal dose	Up to 24 h
Glyburide			
(Dia Beta, Micronase)	1.25, 2.5, and 5 mg	1.25–20 mg as single dose or in two divided doses	Up to 24 h
(Glynase)	1.5, 3, and 6 mg	1.5–12 mg as single dose or in two divided doses	Up to 24 h
Tolazamide (Tolinase)	100, 250, and 500 mg	0.1–1 g as single dose or in two divided doses	Up to 24 h
Tolbutamide (Orinase)	250 and 500 mg	0.5–2 g in two or three divided doses	6–12 h
Meglitinide analogs			
Mitiglinide (available in Japan)	5 and 10 mg	5 or 10 mg three times a day before meals	2 h
Repaglinide (Prandin)	0.5, 1, and 2 mg	0.5 to 4 mg three times a day before meals	3 h
d-Phenylalanine derivative			
Nateglinide (Starlix)	60 and 120 mg	60 or 120 mg three times a day before meals	1.5 h
Biguanides			
Metformin (Glucophage)	500, 850, and 1000 mg	1–2.5 g; 1 tablet with meals two or three times daily	7–12 h
Extended-release metformin (Glucophage XR)	500 and 750 mg	500–2000 mg once a day	Up to 24 h
Thiazolidinediones			
Pioglitazone (Actos)	15, 30, and 45 mg	15–45 mg daily	Up to 24 h
Rosiglitazone (Avandia)	2, 4, and 8 mg	4–8 mg daily (can be divided)	Up to 24 h
Alfa-glucosidase inhibitors			
Acarbose (Precose)	50 and 100 mg	25–100 mg three times a day just before meals	4 h
Miglitol (Glyset)	25, 50, and 100 mg	25–100 mg three times a day just before meals	4 h
Voglibose (not available in United States)	0.2 and 0.3 mg	0.2–0.3 mg three times a day just before meals	4 h
GLP-1 receptor agonists			
Exenatide (Byetta)	1.2 and 2.4 mL prefilled pens containing 5 μg and 10 μg (subcutaneous injection)	5 μg subcutaneously twice a day within 1 hour of breakfast and dinner. Increase to 10 μg subcutaneously twice a day after about a month. Do not use if calculated creatinine clearance is < 30 mL/min.	6 h
Exenatide, long-acting release (Byetta LAR, Bydureon)	2 mg (powder)	Suspend in provided diluent and inject subcutaneously	1 wk
Liraglutide (Victoza)	Prefilled, multidose pen that delivers doses of 0.6, 1.2, or 1.8 mg	0.6 mg subcutaneously once a day (starting dose). Increase to 1.2 mg after a wk if no adverse reactions. Dose can be further increased to 1.8 mg, if necessary.	24 h
Albiglutide (Tanzeum)	30, 50 mg single dose pen (powder)	Mix with diluent and inject subcutaneously. 30 mg is usual dose. Dose can be increased to 50 mg if necessary	1 wk
Dulaglutide (Trulicity)	0.75, 1.5 mg single dose pen or prefilled syringe	0.75 mg subcutaneously. Dose can be increased to 1.5 mg if necessary	1 wk
DPP-4 inhibitors			
Alogliptin (Nesina)	6.25, 12.5, and 25 mg	25 mg once daily; dose is 12.5 mg daily if calculated creatinine clearance is 30–59 mL/min and 6.25 mg daily if clearance < 30 mL/min.	24 h
Saxagliptin (Onglyza)	2.5 and 5 mg	2.5 or 5 mg once daily. Use 2.5 mg dose if calculated creatinine clearance is ≤ 50 mL/min or if also taking drugs that are strong CYP3A4/5 inhibitors such as ketoconazole.	24 h

(continued)

Table 68–2. Drugs for treatment of type 2 diabetes mellitus. (continued)

Drug	Tablet Size	Daily Dose	Duration of Action
Sitagliptin (Januvia)	25, 50, and 100 mg	100 mg once daily is usual dose; dose is 50 mg once daily if calculated creatinine clearance is 30–50 mL/min and 25 mg once daily if clearance is < 30 mL/min.	24 h
Vildagliptin (Galvus) (not available in United States)	50 mg	50 mg once or twice daily. Contraindicated in patients with calculated creatinine clearance ≤ 60 mL/min or AST/ALT three times upper limit of normal	24 h
Linagliptin (Tradjenta)	5 mg	5 mg daily	24 h
SGLT2 inhibitors			
Canagliflozin (Invokana)	100 and 300 mg	100 mg daily is usual dose. Do not use if eGFR < 45 mL/min/1.72 m². 300 mg dose can be used if normal eGFR, resulting in lowering the HbA_{1c} an additional ~ 0.1–0.25%	24 h
Dapagliflozin (Farxiga)	5 and 10 mg	10 mg daily. Use 5 mg dose in hepatic failure	24 h
Empagliflozin (Jardiance)	10 and 25 mg	10 mg daily. 25 mg dose can be used if necessary	24 h
Others			
Bromocriptine (Cycloset)	0.8 mg	0.8 mg daily. Increase wkly by 1 tablet until maximal tolerated dose of 1.6–4.8 mg daily	24 h
Colesevelam (Welchol)	625 mg	3 tablets twice a day	24 h
Pramlintide (Symlin)	5 mL vial containing 0.6 mg/mL; also available as prefilled pens. Symlin pen 60 or Symlin pen 120 (subcutaneous injection)	For insulin-treated type 2 patients, start at 60 µg dose three times a day (10 units on U100 insulin syringe). Increase to 120 µg three times a day (20 units on U100 insulin syringe) if no nausea for 3–7 d. Give immediately before meal.	2 h
		For type 1 patients, start at 15 µg three times a day (2.5 units on U100 insulin syringe) and increase by increments of 15 µg to a maximum of 60 µg three times a day, as tolerated.	
		To avoid hypoglycemia, lower insulin dose by 50% on initiation of therapy.	

AST/ALT, aspartate aminotransferase/alanine aminotransferase; eGFR, estimated glomerular filtration rate.

— **Albiglutide** is a weekly subcutaneous injection; monotherapy and combination therapy lowers HbA1c by about 0.8% with less weight loss than with exenatide and liraglutide.
— **Dulaglutide** is a weekly subcutaneous injection; monotherapy and combination therapy lowered HbA1c by about 0.7 to 1.6% and weight loss ranged from 2 to 7 pounds.
— The most frequent adverse reactions of the GLP1 receptor agonists are nausea (11%–40%), vomiting (4%–13%), and diarrhea (9%–17%); albiglutide has the lowest rates of these reactions; all are associated with increased risk of pancreatitis; approximately 1.4 to 2.2 cases of pancreatitis per 1000 patient years versus 0.6 to 0.9 in controls
— Inhibition of the enzyme DPP-4, which degrades endogenous GLP-1 and GIP, is another means of harnessing the incretin effect

Table 68-3. Summary of bioavailability characteristics of the insulins.

Insulin Preparations	Onset of Action	Peak Action	Effective Duration
Insulins lispro, aspart, glulisine	5–15 min	1–1.5 h	3–4 h
Human regular	30–60 min	2 h	6–8 h
Human NPH	2–4 h	6–7 h	10–20 h
Insulin glargine	1.5 h	Flat	~24 h
Insulin detemir	1 h	Flat	17 h
Technosphere inhaled insulin	5–15 min	1 h	3 h

NPH, neutral protamine Hagedorn.

Table 68-4. Insulin preparations available in the United States.[a]

Rapidly acting human insulin analogs
Insulin lispro (Humalog, Lilly)
Insulin aspart (Novolog, Novo Nordisk)
Insulin glulisine (Apidra, Sanofi Aventis)
Short-acting regular insulin
Regular insulin (Lilly, Novo Nordisk)
Technosphere inhaled regular insulin (Afrezza)
Intermediate-acting insulins
NPH insulin (Lilly, Novo Nordisk)
Premixed insulins
70% NPH/30% regular (70/30 insulin—Lilly, Novo Nordisk)
70% NPL/25% insulin lispro (Humalog Mix 75/25—Lilly)
50% NPL/50% insulin lispro (Humalog Mix 50/50—Lilly)
70% insulin aspart protamine/30% insulin aspart (Novolog Mix 70/30—Novo Nordisk)
Long-acting human insulin analogs
Insulin glargine (Lantus, Sanofi Aventis)
Insulin detemir (Levemir, Novo Nordisk)

NPH, neutral protamine Hagedorn; NPL, neutral protamine lispro.

[a]All insulins available in the United States are recombinant human or human insulin analog origin. All the above insulins are dispensed at U100 concentration. There is an additional U500 preparation of regular insulin.

- Current DPP-4 inhibitors:
  — **Sitagliptin**, 100 mg orally once a day (reduced for lower GFR) improved HbA_{1c} from 0.5% to 1.4%. when used alone or in combination with metformin and pioglitazone; dose reduction needed in patients with reduced GFR; the main adverse effect appears to be a predisposition to nasopharyngitis or upper respiratory tract infection; reports of rare, serious allergic reactions
  — **Saxagliptin**, 2.5 mg or 5 mg orally once a day; lowered HbA_{1c} by about 0.6% when added to metformin or glyburide or thiazolidine in 24-week clinical trials; does not cause weight gain or loss; the main adverse reactions were upper respiratory tract infection, headache, and urinary tract infection.
  — **Linagliptin**, 5 mg orally daily, lowers HbA_{1c} by about 0.4% to 0.6% when added to metformin, sulfonylurea, or pioglitazone; adverse reactions include nasopharyngitis and hypersensitivity reactions (urticaria, angioedema, localized skin exfoliation, bronchial hyperreactivity)
  — **Vildagliptin**, 50 mg once or twice daily, lowers HbA_{1c} by 0.5% to 1% when added to the therapeutic regimen of patients with type 2 diabetes; adverse reactions include upper respiratory tract infections, dizziness, and headache; rare cases of hepatic dysfunction; liver function testing recommended quarterly during the first year
- SGLT2 inhibitors are oral agents that reduce the reabsorption of glucose in the proximal tubule, leading to glucosuria
- Dapagliflozin
  — Usual dose is 10 mg daily but 5 mg daily is the recommended initial dose in hepatic failure
  — Reduces HbA_{1c} levels by 0.5% to 0.8% when used alone or in combination with other oral agents or insulin
  — Results in modest weight loss of about 2 to 4 kg
  — Its efficacy is reduced in kidney failure
  — Main side effects are increased incidence of genital infections and urinary tract infections
  — Patients taking dapagliflozin had higher rates of breast cancer (9 cases vs none in comparator arms) and bladder cancer (10 cases vs 1 in placebo arm)
- Canagliflozin
  — Reduces the threshold for glycosuria from a plasma glucose threshold of ~180 mg/dL to 70–90 mg/dL

— Reduces HbA$_{1c}$ by 0.6% to 1% when used alone or in combination with other oral agents or insulin
— Results in modest weight loss of 2 to 5 kg
— Usual dose is 100 mg/d but up to 300 mg/d can be used in patients with normal kidney function
— Contraindicated in patients with estimated GFR < 45 mL/min/1.73 m^2
— Modest increase in upper limb fractures observed with canagliflozin therapy (it remains unclear if this is due to an effect on bone strength or related to falls due to glucosuria-induced reduction of intravascular volume and hypotension)

• Empagliflozin
— The usual dosage is 10 mg daily but a higher dose of 25 mg daily can be used.
— Reduces HbA$_{1c}$ levels by 0.5% to 0.7% when used alone or in combination with other oral agents or insulin
— Results in modest weight loss of about 2 to 3 kg
— Main side effects are increased incidence of genital infections and urinary tract infections

• Others: bromocriptine, colesevelam, pramlintide (islet amyloid polypeptide analog)
• Insulin: indicated for persons with type 2 diabetes with insulinopenia and hyperglycemia unresponsive to diet and oral hypoglycemic agents
• Preprandial rapid-acting insulin plus basal insulin replacement with an intermediate- or long-acting insulin used to attain acceptable control of blood glucose (Table 68-3)
• Inhaled Insulin
— Dry-powder formulation of recombinant human regular insulin, delivered by inhalation (technosphere insulin, Afrezza) is approved for use in adults with diabetes
— Rapidly absorbed with maximum effect at 1 hour, declining to baseline by about 3 hours
— Combined with basal insulin was as effective in glucose lowering as rapid acting insulin analogs combined with basal insulin
— Formulated as a single use cartridge delivering 4 or 8 units immediately before the meal
— The most common adverse reaction was cough affecting 27 % of subjects
— A small decrease in pulmonary function (forced expiratory volume in 1 second [FEV1]) was persistent at 2 years; spirometry recommended prior to initiation; contraindicated in smokers and patients with chronic lung disease

• Combination oral agents: several drug combinations of thiazolidinediones with metformin or sulfonylureas; sulfonylureas with metformin are available but these limit optimal dose adjustment of individual drugs
• See Figure 68-1

Nonpharmacologic Approach

Diet
• Limitations
— Cholesterol to 300 mg daily
— Protein intake to 10% of total calories

Surgery
• See Table 68-5
• Many patients with type 2 diabetes who are taking insulin do well perioperatively without insulin for a few hours
• Ideally, patients with diabetes should undergo surgery early in the morning

8. Outcomes

Follow-Up
• Self-monitoring
• HbA$_{1c}$ quarterly
• Screen for microalbuminuria annually
• Serum lipids

Weight loss + exercise + metformin

If HbA_{1c} target not reached
after ~ 3 months

Metforrmin + another agent

If HbA_{1c} target not reached
after ~ 3 months

Metformin + two other agents

If HbA_{1c} target not reached
after ~ 3 months

Metformin + more complex insulin
regimen ± other noninsulin agent

Seven main classes of agents
- Metformin
- Sulfonylureas (includes nateglinide, repaglinide)
- Pioglitazone
- GLP-1 receptor agonists
- DPP-4 inhibitors
- SGLT2 inhibitors
- Insulins

**Factors in Therapeutic Decision
(single agent or combination)**

Efficacy
- DPP-4 inhibitors are of moderate efficacy
- All other agents are of high efficacy

Hypoglycemic risk
- Sulfonylureas and insulins have increased
  risk of hypoglycemia

Effect on weight
- Metformin and DPP-4 inhibitors are weight neutral
- GLP-1 receptor agonists and SGLT2 inhibitors
  promote weight loss
- Sulfonylureas, insulins, and pioglitazone are
  associated with weight gain

Major side effects
- Metformin can cause lactic acidosis
- Pioglitazone is associated with fluid retention,
  fracture risk, and possibly bladder cancer
- GLP-1 receptor agonists are associated with
  nausea and vomiting and pancreatitis
- DPP-4 inhibitors may be associated with
  pancreatitis risk
- SGLT2 inhibitors can cause urinary tract infections;
  genital mycotic infections; dehydration; cannot
  use in renal impairment

Cost
- All agents except metformin and
  sulfonylureas are expensive
- Insulins are expensive if the additional cost
  of monitoring is taken into consideration

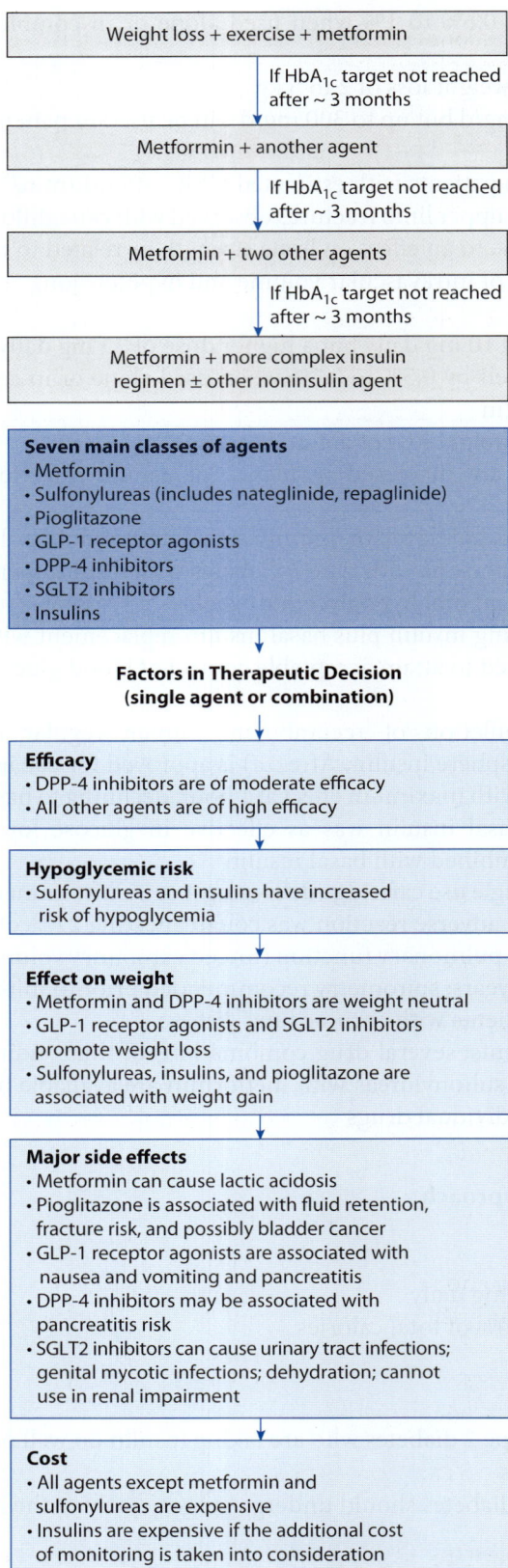

FIGURE 68-1. Algorithm for the treatment of type 2 diabetes based on the 2012 and 2015 recommendations of the consensus panel of the American Diabetes Association/European Association for the Study of Diabetes.

Table 68-5. Recommendations for management of insulin-treated diabetes during surgery.

Type of Diabetes	Minor Surgical Procedures (< 2 h; Eating Afterward)	Major Surgical Procedures (> 2 h; Invasion of Body Cavity; Not Eating Immediately After Recovery)
Type 2: Patients taking basal bolus insulin regimen; twice daily premixed insulin	No insulin on the day of operation. Start 5% dextrose infusion; monitor fingerstick blood glucose and give subcutaneous short-acting insulin every 4 or 6 h	Same regimen as minor procedure. If control is not satisfactory, then intravenous insulin infusion
Type 1: Patients taking basal bolus insulin regimen or using insulin pump	Patients using pump should discontinue the pump the evening before procedure and be given 24 h basal insulin. On day of procedure, start 5% dextrose; monitor blood glucose and give subcutaneous short-acting insulin every 4 or 6 h	Initiate insulin infusion on morning of procedure and transition back to usual regimen when eating

- Feet examination annually
- Diabetic eye examination annually
- Treatment goals
  — Self-monitored blood glucose, 80 to 120 mg/dL before meals; 100 to 140 mg/dL at bedtime; < 180 mg/dL 1.5 to 2.0 hours postprandially
  — $HbA_{1c} < 7.0\%$

Complications
- Hypoglycemia
- Ocular (diabetic cataracts and retinopathy)
- Diabetic nephropathy (microalbuminuria, progressive diabetic nephropathy)
- Gangrene of the feet
- Diabetic neuropathy
  — Peripheral neuropathy
  — Distal symmetric polyneuropathy
  — Isolated peripheral neuropathy
  — Painful diabetic neuropathy
  — Autonomic neuropathy
- Skin and mucous membranes
  — Pyogenic infections
  — Acanthosis nigricans
  — Eruptive xanthomas from hypertriglyceridemia associated with poor glucose control
  — Necrobiosis lipoidica diabeticorum
  — Shin spots
  — Intertriginous candida
  — Vulvovaginitis
- Bone and joint complications
  — Diabetic cheiroarthropathy, adhesive capsulitis, carpal tunnel syndrome, and dupuytren contractures
  — Nonvertebral fractures
  — Diffuse idiopathic skeletal hyperostosis
  — Hyperuricemia
  — Bursitis, particularly of shoulders and hips

Prognosis
- Antihypertensive control to a mean of 144/82 mm Hg had beneficial effects on all microvascular and all diabetes-related end points in the United Kingdom Prospective Diabetes Study

Prevention
- Goal of therapy is to prevent acute illness and reduce risk of long-term complications
- Lifestyle modifications can prevent or slow the development of diabetes

- Daily vigorous exercise prevents accumulation of visceral fat, which can prevent the development of diabetes
- Screen with fasting glucose at 3-year intervals beginning at age 45; screen earlier and more frequently if risk factors present

9. When to Refer and When to Admit

When to Refer

- Team-oriented educational approach, including a nutritionist, is critical
- Poorly controlled diabetes
- Patients should be referred to an ophthalmologist or optometrist for a dilated eye examination
- Patients with peripheral neuropathy or structural foot problems should be referred to a podiatrist
- Referrals to other specialists may be required for management of chronic complications of diabetes

When to Admit

- Altered mental status
- Diabetic ketoacidosis
- Marked volume disorders
- Marked electrolyte disorders
- Unstable comorbid conditions

SUGGESTED REFERENCES

ACCORD Study Group; Gerstein HC et al. Effects of intensive glucose lowering in type 2 diabetes. *N Engl J Med*. 2008 Jun 12;358(24):2545–2559. [PMID: 18539917]

ADVANCE Collaborative Group; Patel A et al. Intensive blood glucose control and vascular outcomes in patients with type 2 diabetes. *N Engl J Med*. 2008 Jun 12;358(24):2560–2572. [PMID: 18539916]

American Association of Diabetes Educators. https://www.diabeteseducator.org/

American Diabetes Association. http://www.diabetes.org

American Diabetes Association. Standards of medical care in diabetes—2015. *Diabetes Care*. 2015 Jan;38(suppl):S8–S16. [PMID: 25537706]

American Dietetic Association. http://www.eatright.org

Bennett WL et al. Comparative effectiveness and safety of medications for type 2 diabetes: an update including new drugs and 2-drug combinations. *Ann Intern Med*. 2011 May 3;154(9):602–613. Erratum in: *Ann Intern Med*. 2011 Jul 5;155(1):67–68. [PMID: 21403054]

Blumer I et al. Diabetes and pregnancy: an endocrine society clinical practice guideline. *J Clin Endocrinol Metab*. 2013 Nov;98(11):4227–4249. [PMID: 24194617]

Chin JA et al. Diabetes mellitus and peripheral vascular disease: diagnosis and management. *Clin Podiatr Med Surg*. 2014 Jan;31(1):11–26. [PMID: 24296015]

Cryer PE. Mechanisms of hypoglycemia-associated autonomic failure in diabetes. *N Engl J Med*. 2013 Jul 25;369(4):362–372. [PMID: 23883381]

Duckworth W et al; VADT Investigators. Glucose control and vascular complications in veterans with type 2 diabetes. *N Engl J Med*. 2009 Jan 8;360(2):129–139. [PMID: 19092145]

Gaede P et al. Effect of a multifactorial intervention on mortality in type 2 diabetes. *N Engl J Med*. 2008 Feb 7;358(6):580–591. [PMID: 18256393]

Holman RR et al. 10-year follow-up of intensive glucose control in type 2 diabetes. *N Engl J Med*. 2008 Oct 9;359(15):1577–1589. [PMID: 18784090]

Inzucchi SE et al. Management of hyperglycemia in type 2 diabetes, 2015: a patient-centered approach: update to a position statement of the American Diabetes Association and the European Association for the Study of Diabetes. *Diabetes Care*. 2015 Jan;38(1):140–149. [PMID: 25538310]

Juvenile Diabetes Foundation. http://jdrf.org/

Kansagara D et al. Intensive insulin therapy in hospitalized patients: a systematic review. *Ann Intern Med*. 2011 Feb 15;154(4):268–282. [PMID: 21320942]

Nyenwe EA et al. Evidence-based management of hyperglycemic emergencies in diabetes mellitus. *Diabetes Res Clin Pract*. 2011 Dec;94(3):340–351. [PMID: 21978840]

Savage MW et al. Joint British Diabetes Societies guideline for the management of diabetic ketoacidosis. *Diabet Med*. 2011 May;28(5):508–515. [PMID: 21255074]

Singleton JR et al. The diabetic neuropathies: practical and rational therapy. *Semin Neurol.* 2012 Jul;32(3):196–203. [PMID: 23117944]

Stitt AW et al. Advances in our understanding of diabetic retinopathy. *Clin Sci (Lond).* 2013 Mar 13;125(1):1–17. [PMID: 23485060]

The Diabetes Control and Complications Trial Research Group. The effect of intensive treatment of diabetes on the development and progression of long-term complications in insulin-dependent diabetes mellitus. *N Engl J Med.* 1993 Sep 30;329(14):977–986. [PMID: 8366922]

Turnbull FM et al. Intensive glucose control and macrovascular outcomes in type 2 diabetes. *Diabetologia.* 2009 Nov;52(11):2288–2298. [PMID: 19655124]

UK Prospective Diabetes Study (UKPDS) Group. Intensive blood-glucose control with sulphonylureas or insulin compared with conventional treatment and risk of complications in patients with type 2 diabetes (UKPDS 33). *Lancet.* 1998 Sep 12;352(9131):837–853. [PMID: 9742976]

UK Prospective Diabetes Study (UKPDS) Group. Tight blood pressure control and risk of macrovascular and microvascular complications in type 2 diabetes: UKPDS 38. *BMJ.* 1998 Sep 12;317(7160):703–713. [PMID: 9732337]

Waanders F et al. Current concepts in the management of diabetic nephropathy. *Neth J Med.* 2013 Nov;71(9):448–458. [PMID: 24218418]

69

Hyperaldosteronism (Aldosteronism)

A 42-year-old man presents for evaluation of newly diagnosed hypertension. He is currently taking no medications and offers no complaints. A careful review of systems reveals symptoms of fatigue, loss of stamina, and frequent urination, particularly at night. Physical examination is normal except for a blood pressure of 168/100 mm Hg. Serum electrolytes are: sodium, 152 mEq/L; potassium, 3.2 mEq/L; bicarbonate, 32 mEq/L; chloride, 112 mEq/L.

LEARNING OBJECTIVES

- ► Learn the clinical manifestations and objective findings of hyperaldosteronism that differentiate it from essential hypertension
- ► Understand which patients need screening for hyperaldosteronism
- ► Know the differential diagnosis of hyperaldosteronism
- ► Understand how to perform testing for hyperaldosteronism and interpret the plasma aldosterone:renin ratio
- ► Learn the treatments for hyperaldosteronism and their side effects

QUESTIONS

1. What are the salient features of this patient's problem?

2. How do you think through his problem?

3. What are the key features, including essentials of diagnosis, general considerations, and demographics, of hyperaldosteronism?

4. What are the symptoms and signs of hyperaldosteronism?

5. What is the differential diagnosis of hyperaldosteronism?

6. What are laboratory, imaging, and procedural findings in hyperaldosteronism?

7. What are the treatments for hyperaldosteronism?

8. What are the outcomes, including complications and prognosis, of hyperaldosteronism?

ANSWERS

1. Salient Features

Hypertension, including diastolic blood pressure elevation; fatigue; polyuria; hypernatremia; hypokalemia; elevated serum bicarbonate

2. How to Think Through

A complete diagnostic workup for secondary causes of hypertension is not necessary for every new diagnosis of high blood pressure, nor would it be feasible, given the prevalence of hypertension in the population. At the same time, secondary causes of hypertension, such as hyperaldosteronism, are under-recognized. What major factors should trigger a workup for secondary hypertension? (Onset at age < 50 years; symptoms suggestive of pheochromocytoma including headache, sweating, palpitations; hypertension refractory to three medications, one of which is a diuretic; physical examination findings such as abdominal bruit or cushingoid appearance.) This patient's age, his systolic blood pressure of > 160 mm Hg, and his diastolic pressure of 100 mm Hg are indications for investigation.

Serum sodium and potassium levels were appropriately checked and suggest a hyperactive renin–angiotensin–aldosterone axis. How can the problem be localized? (By obtaining an aldosterone:plasma renin activity ratio. If an elevated ratio is found, the next step is to document increased aldosterone secretion with a 24-hour urine aldosterone collection.)

Are his fatigue, poor stamina, and nocturia potentially attributable to this problem? (Yes, these may be due to the associated hypokalemia.) What are the two most likely causes of hyperaldosteronism? (Bilateral adrenal hyperplasia and unilateral adrenal adenoma [Conn syndrome].) How should he be treated? (An aldosterone blocking agent such as spironolactone or eplerenone. Laparoscopic adrenalectomy for adrenal adenoma.)

3. Key Features

Essentials of Diagnosis

- Hypertension that may be severe or drug resistant
- Hypokalemia (in a minority of patients) may cause polyuria, polydipsia, and muscle weakness
- Elevated plasma and urine aldosterone levels and low plasma renin level

General Considerations

- Excessive aldosterone production
  - Increases sodium retention and suppresses plasma renin
  - Increases renal potassium excretion that can lead to hypokalemia
- Should be suspected with early onset (before age 50 years) hypertension and/or stroke
- Cardiovascular events are more prevalent in patients with hyperaldosteronism (35%) than in those with essential hypertension (11%)
- Hyperaldosteronism may be caused by
  - An aldosterone-producing adrenal adenoma (Conn syndrome), 40% of which have been found to have somatic mutations in a gene involved with the potassium channel
  - Unilateral or bilateral adrenal hyperplasia
- Bilateral hyperaldosteronism may be corticosteroid suppressible due to an autosomal-dominant genetic defect allowing ACTH stimulation of aldosterone production
- Hyperaldosteronism may rarely be due to a malignant ovarian tumor
- The Endocrine Society's Clinical Practice Guidelines recommend screening in patients with any of the following
  - Blood pressure over 160/100 mm Hg
  - Drug-resistant hypertension
  - Early-onset hypertension
  - Hypertension with spontaneous or diuretic-induced hypokalemia
  - Hypertension with adrenal incidentaloma
  - Hypertension with a family history of early-onset hypertension or cerebrovascular accident before age 40 years
  - Hypertension with a first-degree relative with primary hyperaldosteronism

Demographics

- Accounts for 5% to 10% of all cases of hypertension and for 20% of cases of resistant hypertension
- Patients of all ages may be affected, but the peak incidence is between 30 and 60 years

4. Symptoms and Signs

- Hypertension is typically moderate but may be severe
- Some patients have only diastolic hypertension, without other symptoms and signs
- Edema (rare)
- Muscular weakness (at times with paralysis simulating periodic paralysis), paresthesias with frank tetany, headache, polyuria, and polydipsia may be seen in patients with hypokalemia

5. Differential Diagnosis

- Essential hypertension
- Hypokalemic thyrotoxic periodic paralysis
- Renal vascular hypertension (hypertension and hypokalemia, but plasma renin activity is high)
- Hypokalemia from another cause, eg, diuretic use
- Secondary hyperaldosteronism (dehydration, heart failure)
- Congenital adrenal hyperplasia: 11β-hydroxylase deficiency, 17α-hydroxylase deficiency
- Cushing syndrome
- Excessive real licorice ingestion
- Syndrome of cortisol resistance

6. Laboratory, Imaging, and Procedural Findings

Laboratory Tests

- Obtain a plasma potassium level in all hypertensive individuals
- Hypokalemia and elevation of serum bicarbonate (HCO_3^-) concentration may suggest hyperaldosteronism
- Consider evaluation for hyperaldosteronism those normokalemic hypertensive patients who have
  — Treatment-resistant hypertension (despite three drugs)
  — Severe hypertension: > 160 mm Hg systolic or > 100 mm Hg diastolic
  — Early-onset hypertension
  — Low-renin hypertension
  — Hypertension with an adrenal mass
  — Hypertension with a family history of early-onset hypertension or cerebrovascular accident before age 40 years
  — First-degree relatives with aldosteronism
- Initial screening includes aldosterone and plasma renin activity (PRA) to determine an aldosterone-to-renin ratio
- Testing protocol
  — For 3 to 6 weeks prior to testing, patients should consume a diet high in NaCl (> 6 g/d) and hold certain medications: all diuretics, ACEIs, ARBs (stimulate PRA); β-blockers, clonidine, NSAIDs (suppress PRA)
  — Antihypertensives that do not impact the test include amlodipine, verapamil, hydralazine, and doxazosin
  — The patient should be out of bed for at least 2 hours and seated for 15 to 60 minutes before the blood draw, which should be obtained between 8 AM and 10 AM
  — Renin is measured as either PRA or direct renin concentration
- Serum aldosterone should be measured with a tandem mass spectrometry assay
- Serum aldosterone (ng/dL)-to-PRA (ng/mL/hr) ratios < 24 exclude primary hyperaldosteronism, whereas ratios between 24 and 67 are suspicious and ratios > 67 are very suggestive of the diagnosis
- A high aldosterone-to-renin ratio indicates primary hyperaldosteronism; elevated aldosterone and PRA values without an elevated ratio indicate secondary hyperaldosteronism

- When the aldosterone:renin ratio is high, a 24-hour urine collection in an acidified container is assayed for aldosterone, free cortisol, and creatinine

Imaging Studies
- Thin-section computed tomography scan
  - Used to screen for a rare adrenal carcinoma
  - In the absence of a large adrenal carcinoma, scanning cannot reliably distinguish unilateral from bilateral sources of aldosterone excess

Diagnostic Procedures
- Adrenal vein sampling
  - Most accurate way to determine whether primary hyperaldosteronism is due to unilateral aldosterone excess
  - Indicated only to direct the surgeon to the correct adrenal gland and should be performed only if surgery is contemplated
  - Useful for patients who are not hypokalemic, over age 40 years, or who have an adrenal adenoma < 1 cm diameter

7. Treatments

Medications
- Spironolactone or eplerenone
  - Long-term therapy is an option for Conn syndrome
  - Used to treat bilateral adrenal hyperplasia
    - Spironolactone
      - Has antiandrogen activity and frequently causes breast tenderness, gynecomastia, or reduced libido
      - Initial dose: 12.5 to 25 mg once daily orally
      - Dose may be titrated upward to 200 mg daily
      - Contraindicated in pregnant women
    - Eplerenone
      - Does not have antiandrogen effects
      - Must be given twice daily in oral doses of 25 to 50 mg due to short half-life
- Amiloride (10 to 15 mg orally daily) is effective and preferred for resistant hypertension caused by hyperaldosteronism during pregnancy
  - Suppression with low-dose dexamethasone for glucocorticoid-remediable hyperaldosteronism (which is very rare)

Surgery
- Laparoscopic adrenalectomy for Conn syndrome (unilateral aldosterone-secreting adrenal adenoma)

8. Outcomes

Complications
- The incidence of cardiovascular complications from hypertension is higher in primary hyperaldosteronism than in idiopathic hypertension
- Following unilateral adrenalectomy for Conn syndrome, suppression of the contralateral adrenal may result in temporary postoperative hypohyperaldosteronism, characterized by hyperkalemia and hypotension

Prognosis
- Hypertension remits after surgery in about two-thirds of cases but persists or returns despite surgery in one-third
- Prognosis much improved by early diagnosis and treatment
- Only 2% of aldosterone-secreting adrenal tumors are malignant

SUGGESTED REFERENCES

Chao CT et al. Diagnosis and management of primary aldosteronism: an updated review. *Ann Med.* 2013 Jun;45(4):375–383. [PMID: 23701121]

Fourkiotis V et al; Mephisto Study Group. Effectiveness of eplerenone or spironolactone treatment in preserving renal function in primary aldosteronism. *Eur J Endocrinol.* 2012 Dec 10;168(1):75–81. [PMID: 23033260]

Harvey AM. Hyperaldosteronism: diagnosis, lateralization, and treatment. *Surg Clin North Am.* 2012 Jun;94(3):643–656. [PMID: 24857581]

Jansen PM et al. Test characteristics of the aldosterone-to-renin ratio as a screening test for primary aldosteronism. *J Hypertens.* 2014 Jan;32(1):115–126. [PMID: 24018605]

Krysiak R et al. Primary aldosteronism in pregnancy. *Acta Clin Belg.* 2012 Mar–Apr;67(2):130–134. [PMID: 22712170]

Monticone S et al. Primary aldosteronism: who should be screened? *Horm Metab Res.* 2012 Mar;44(3):163–169. [PMID: 22120135]

Rossi GP et al. Clinical management of primary aldosteronism: 2013 Practical Recommendations of the Italian Society of Hypertension (SIIA). *High Blood Press Cardiovasc Prev.* 2014 Mar;21(1):71–75. [PMID: 24464387]

Salvà M et al. Primary aldosteronism: the role of confirmatory tests. *Horm Metab Res.* 2012 Mar;44(3):177–180. [PMID: 22395800]

Steichen O et al. Outcomes of adrenalectomy in patients with unilateral primary aldosteronism: a review. *Horm Metab Res.* 2012 Mar;44(3):221–227. [PMID: 22395801]

Hypercalcemia

70

A 71-year-old woman with lung cancer presents to her primary care clinician with complaints of constipation, nausea, and increased urination. She also has new depression and generalized weakness. Her only medication is calcium carbonate, which she takes for prevention of osteoporosis. On cardiac examination, she has frequent ectopy. Her serum calcium level is elevated at 13.5 mg/dL, her serum parathyroid hormone (PTH) level is low, and her serum PTH-related protein (PTH-rP) level is elevated.

LEARNING OBJECTIVES

▶ Learn the clinical manifestations and objective findings of hypercalcemia
▶ Understand the diseases and medications that predispose to hypercalcemia
▶ Know the differential diagnosis and etiology of hypercalcemia
▶ Understand how to use laboratory testing to differentiate the cause of hypercalcemia
▶ Learn the long- and short-term treatments for hypercalcemia

QUESTIONS

1. What are the salient features of this patient's problem?

2. How do you think through her problem?

3. What are the key features, including essentials of diagnosis and general considerations, of hypercalcemia?

4. What are the symptoms and signs of hypercalcemia?

5. What is the differential diagnosis of hypercalcemia?

6. What are laboratory, imaging, and procedural findings in hypercalcemia?

7. What are the treatments for hypercalcemia?

8. What are the outcomes, including follow-up, complications, prognosis, and prevention, of hypercalcemia?

9. When should patients with hypercalcemia be referred to a specialist or admitted to the hospital?

ANSWERS

1. Salient Features

Constipation, nausea, polyuria, weakness, depression, ectopy; known malignancy; elevated serum calcium; elevated serum PTH-rP and low serum PTH levels

2. How to Think Through

Rapid diagnosis of hypercalcemia requires recognition of a constellation of symptoms. What are the broad categories of symptoms caused by hypercalcemia? (Gastrointestinal [GI], eg, constipation, nausea; neuropsychiatric, eg, fatigue, weakness, and altered mental status; renal, eg, nephrolithiasis and polyuria; and cardiac, eg, shortened QT interval and ectopy.)

The cause of hypercalcemia is determined by a differential diagnosis with several key branch points; it is helpful to recall that most cases are caused by primary hyperparathyroidism or malignancy. The PTH was likely the first laboratory result in this case, with her low value ruling out hyperparathyroidism. From there, what causes were likely next considered? (Malignancy, granulomatous disease, hypervitaminosis D, milk-alkali syndrome, thyrotoxicosis.) Malignancy, the most common cause of hypercalcemia with a suppressed PTH level, is a concern here given the degree of serum calcium elevation. The elevated PTH-rP confirms this suspicion. What three cancer types most frequently cause hypercalcemia? (Breast and lung carcinoma, and multiple myeloma.)

How should she be managed in the short term? (She should be admitted to the hospital for expedited diagnostic workup and therapy to lower her serum calcium, including aggressive intravenous saline hydration and, once well hydrated, treatment with a bisphosphonate.)

3. Key Features

Essentials of Diagnosis

- Serum calcium level > 10.5 mg/dL (> 2.6 mmol/L)
- Serum ionized calcium > 5.3 mg/dL (> 1.32 mmol/L)
- Primary hyperparathyroidism and malignancy-associated hypercalcemia are the most common causes
- Hypercalciuria usually precedes hypercalcemia
- Most often, asymptomatic, mild hypercalcemia (≥ 10.5 mg/dL [or 2.6 mmol/L]) is due to primary hyperparathyroidism, whereas the symptomatic, severe hypercalcemia (≥ 14 mg/dL [or 3.5 mmol/L]) is due to hypercalcemia of malignancy

General Considerations

- Primary hyperparathyroidism and malignancy account for 90% of cases
- Chronic hypercalcemia (over 6 months) or some other manifestations such as nephrolithiasis suggest a benign cause
- Tumor production of PTH-rP is the most common paraneoplastic endocrine syndrome, accounting for most cases of hypercalcemia in inpatients
- Granulomatous diseases, such as sarcoidosis and tuberculosis, cause hypercalcemia from production of active vitamin D_3 (1,25 dihydroxyvitamin D_3) by the granulomas
- Milk-alkali syndrome has had a resurgence related to calcium ingestion for prevention of osteoporosis
- Hypercalcemia can cause nephrogenic diabetes insipidus and volume depletion, which further worsen hypercalcemia

4. Symptoms and Signs

- May affect GI, kidney, neurologic, and cardiac function
- Mild hypercalcemia is often asymptomatic
- Symptoms usually occur if the serum calcium is > 12 mg/dL (or > 3 mmol/L) and tend to be more severe if hypercalcemia develops acutely
- Constipation
- Nephrolithiasis with hematuria and renal colic; polyuria

- Polyuria from hypercalciuria-induced nephrogenic diabetes insipidus can result in volume depletion and acute kidney injury
- Polyuria is absent in hypocalciuric hypercalcemia
- GI symptoms include
  — Nausea
  — Vomiting
  — Anorexia
  — Peptic ulcer disease
- Neurologic manifestations may range from mild drowsiness to weakness, depression, lethargy, stupor, and coma in severe cases
- Ventricular ectopy and idioventricular rhythm occur and can be accentuated by digitalis

5. Differential Diagnosis

Etiology of Hypercalcemia

- Endocrine disorders
  — Primary and secondary hyperparathyroidism
  — Acromegaly
  — Adrenal insufficiency
  — Pheochromocytoma
  — Thyrotoxicosis
- Neoplastic diseases
  — Tumor production of PTH-rP (ovary, kidney, lung)
  — Multiple myeloma (osteoclast-activating factor)
  — Lymphoma
- Miscellaneous causes
  — Thiazide diuretics
  — Granulomatous diseases
  — Paget disease
  — Hypophosphatasia
  — Immobilization
  — Increased calcium intake or absorption: milk-alkali syndrome, vitamin D or A excess
  — Familial hypocalciuric hypercalcemia
  — Complications of kidney transplantation
  — Lithium intake

6. Laboratory, Imaging, and Procedural Findings

Laboratory Tests

- Serum calcium level > 10.5 mg/dL (> 2.6 mmol/L)
- Serum ionized calcium > 5.3 mg/dL (> 1.32 mmol/L)
- Severe hypercalcemia (≥ 15 mg/dL [or > 3.75 mmol/L]) generally occurs in malignancy
- A high serum chloride concentration and a low serum phosphate concentration (ratio > 33:1 [or > 102 if SI units are utilized]) suggest primary hyperparathyroidism because PTH decreases proximal tubular phosphate reabsorption
- A low serum chloride concentration with a high serum bicarbonate concentration, along with blood urea nitrogen and serum creatinine elevations, suggests milk-alkali syndrome
- Urinary calcium excretion
  — > 300 mg (7.5 mmol) per day suggests hypercalciuria
  — < 100 mg (2.5 mmol) per day suggests hypocalciuria
- Hypercalciuria from malignancy or from vitamin D therapy frequently results in hypercalcemia when volume depletion occurs
- Measurements of PTH and PTH-rP levels help distinguish between hyperparathyroidism (elevated PTH) and malignancy-associated hypercalcemia (suppressed PTH and elevated PTH-rP) (see *Hyperparathyroidism*)
- Serum phosphate may or may not be low, depending on the cause

Imaging Studies
• Chest radiograph: to exclude malignancy or granulomatous disease

Diagnostic Procedure
• Electrocardiogram: shortened QT interval

7. Treatments

Medications

Emergency Treatment
• Establish euvolemia to induce renal excretion of Na^+, which is accompanied by excretion of Ca^{2+}
• In dehydrated patients with normal cardiac and renal function, infuse 0.45% saline or 0.9% saline rapidly (250–500 mL/h)
• Furosemide intravenously is often administered but its efficacy and safety were questioned in one meta-analysis
• Thiazides can actually worsen hypercalcemia (as can furosemide if inadequate saline is given)
• In the treatment of hypercalcemia of malignancy
  — Bisphosphonates are the mainstay, although they may require up to 48 to 72 hours before reaching full therapeutic effect
  — Calcitonin may be helpful to treat hypercalcemia before the onset of action of bisphosphonates
  — Denosumab is indicated for hypercalcemia from solid tumor-associated bone metastases

Therapeutic Procedures
• In emergency cases, dialysis with low or no calcium dialysate may be needed

8. Outcomes

Follow-Up
• Monitor serum calcium at least every 6 months during medical therapy of hyperparathyroidism

Complications
• Pathologic fractures are more common in individuals with hyperthyroidism than the general population
• Renal calculi
• Chronic kidney disease
• Peptic ulcer disease
• Pancreatitis
• Precipitation of calcium throughout the soft tissues
• Gestational hypercalcemia produces neonatal hypocalcemia

Prognosis
• Depends on the underlying disease
• Poor prognosis in malignancy

Prevention
• Prevent dehydration that can further aggravate hypercalcemia

9. When to Refer and When to Admit

When to Refer
• Patients may require referral to an oncologist or endocrinologist depending on the underlying cause of hypercalcemia
• Patients with granulomatous diseases (eg, tuberculosis and other chronic infections, granulomatosis with polyangiitis [formerly Wegener granulomatosis], sarcoidosis) may require consultation with infectious disease specialist, rheumatologist, or pulmonologist

When to Admit

• Patients with symptomatic or severe hypercalcemia require immediate treatment
• Unexplained hypercalcemia with associated conditions, such as acute kidney injury or suspected malignancy, may also require urgent treatment and expedited evaluation

SUGGESTED REFERENCES

Crowley R et al. How to approach hypercalcaemia. *Clin Med*. 2013 Jun;13(3):287–290. [PMID: 23760705]

Hu MI et al. Denosumab for treatment of hypercalcemia of malignancy. *J Clin Endocrinol Metab*. 2014 Sep;99(9):3144–3152. [PMID: 24915117]

Marcocci C et al. Clinical practice. Primary hyperparathyroidism. *N Engl J Med*. 2011 Dec 22;365(25):2389–2397. [PMID: 22187986]

Rosner MH et al. Electrolyte disorders associated with cancer. *Adv Chronic Kidney Dis*. 2014 Jan;21(1):7–17. [PMID: 24359982]

71 Primary Hyperparathyroidism

A 56-year-old woman presents to her primary care clinician complaining of progressive fatigue, weakness, and diffuse bony pain. She says that her symptoms have been getting worse over the last 2 months. Her medical history is notable for well-controlled hypertension and recurrent renal stones. Physical examination is unremarkable. A serum calcium level is elevated.

LEARNING OBJECTIVES

▶ Learn the clinical manifestations and objective findings of mild and severe hyperparathyroidism and resulting hypercalcemia

▶ Understand the primary, secondary, tertiary, and genetic causes of hyperparathyroidism

▶ Know the differential diagnosis of hyperparathyroidism

▶ Learn the treatments for hyperparathyroidism and its complications

▶ Know which patients to refer for surgery

QUESTIONS

1. What are the salient features of this patient's problem?

2. How do you think through her problem?

3. What are the key features, including essentials of diagnosis, general considerations, and demographics, of hyperparathyroidism?

4. What are the symptoms and signs of hyperparathyroidism?

5. What is the differential diagnosis of hyperparathyroidism?

6. What are laboratory and imaging findings in hyperparathyroidism?

7. What are the treatments for hyperparathyroidism?

8. What are the outcomes, including follow-up, complications, and prognosis, of hyperparathyroidism?

9. When should patients with hyperparathyroidism be referred to a specialist or admitted to the hospital?

ANSWERS

1. Salient Features

Female sex; fatigue; weakness; bone pain; renal stones; elevated serum calcium

2. How to Think Through

The diagnosis of hypercalcemia requires recognition of a constellation of common symptoms. In addition to her fatigue, weakness, diffuse bony pain, and nephrolithiasis, what other symptoms should be elicited? (Other neuromuscular or psychiatric symptoms including depression; other renal symptoms including polyuria; gastrointestinal symptoms including anorexia.) Because the differential diagnosis of hypercalcemia is complex, it is useful to remember that two causes account for 90% of cases. What are these two causes? (Primary hyperparathyroidism and malignancy.)

How should an elevated serum calcium level be confirmed? (By repeating the serum calcium level after an overnight fast along with a serum albumin level and correcting for a low albumin, if present.) Often a serum phosphate level is available with the initial calcium value; how can this guide the differential diagnosis? (Primary hyperparathyroidism and malignancy with an elevated parathyroid hormone-related protein [PTH-rP] both increase renal excretion of phosphate, leading to a low serum phosphate. Other causes of hypercalcemia generally lead to an elevated serum phosphate.)

If the serum PTH level is found to be elevated in this case, what is the likelihood of malignant hypercalcemia? (Very low. Cancer leads to hypercalcemia by secretion of PTH-rP or by bony metastasis; the serum PTH level is suppressed in almost all such cases. A PTH-secreting tumor is the rare exception.) What is the most likely diagnosis here, and how should this be confirmed? (Primary hyperparathyroidism is most likely, confirmed by an elevated serum PTH. A 24-hour urinary calcium collection is also needed to exclude familial hypocalciuric hypercalcemia.) How should she be treated? (Parathyroidectomy, since she is symptomatic.)

3. Key Features

Essentials of Diagnosis

- Hypercalcemia is frequently detected incidentally by screening
- Renal stones, polyuria, hypertension, constipation, mental changes
- Bone pain
- Urine calcium is elevated; urine phosphate is high with low or normal serum phosphate; serum alkaline phosphatase is normal or elevated
- Elevated or high-normal serum PTH level

General Considerations

- Primary hyperparathyroidism
  — PTH hypersecretion is usually caused by a parathyroid adenoma, less commonly, by hyperplasia or carcinoma (< 1%; more common in familial hyperparathyroidism or multiple endocrine neoplasia [MEN])
  — If age < 30 years, there is a higher incidence of multiglandular disease (36%) and parathyroid carcinoma (5%) responsible for hyperparathyroidism
- Secondary or tertiary hyperparathyroidism
  — Chronic kidney disease (CKD): hyperphosphatemia and diminished renal vitamin D production decrease serum ionized serum calcium, thus stimulating the parathyroids
  — Renal osteodystrophy: bone disease of secondary hyperparathyroidism and CKD
- MEN
  — Hyperparathyroidism is familial in about 10% of cases; parathyroid hyperplasia may arise in MEN types 1, 2, and 4
  — In MEN 1, multiglandular hyperparathyroidism is usually the initial manifestation and ultimately occurs in over 90% of affected individuals
  — Hyperparathyroidism in MEN 2 is less frequent than in MEN 1 and is usually milder
  — MEN 4 patients develop adenomas of the parathyroid and pituitary glands, neuroendocrine tumors of the pancreas, as well as adrenal tumors, renal tumors, testicular cancer, and neuroendocrine cervical carcinoma
- Hyperparathyroidism–jaw tumor syndrome is autosomal dominant and associated with recurrent parathyroid adenomas (5% malignant), benign jaw tumors, and renal cysts

Demographics

- Hyperparathyroidism is the most common cause of hypercalcemia, with a prevalence of 1 to 4 cases per 1000 persons
- It occurs at all ages but most commonly in the seventh decade and in women (74%)
- Before age 45, the prevalence is similar in men and women
- It is more prevalent in blacks, followed by whites, then other races

4. Symptoms and Signs

- Frequently asymptomatic
- Symptoms include problems with "bones, stones, abdominal groans, psychic moans, fatigue overtones"
- Bone pain and arthralgias are common
- Severe, chronic hyperparathyroidism can cause diffuse demineralization, pathologic fractures, and cystic bone lesions throughout the skeleton, a condition known as osteitis fibrosa cystica
- Postmenopausal women are prone to asymptomatic vertebral fractures
- Mild hypercalcemia
  — May be asymptomatic
  — Some patients can have significant symptoms, particularly depression, constipation, and bone and joint pain
- Hypercalcemia in patients with hyperparathyroidism usually causes a variety of manifestations whose severity is not entirely predictable by the level of serum calcium or PTH in patients with hyperparathyroidism
  — Paresthesias, muscular weakness, and diminished deep tendon reflexes
  — Malaise, fatigue, intellectual weariness, depression, increased sleep requirement, progressing to cognitive impairment, disorientation, psychosis, or stupor
  — Hypertension; ECG findings of prolonged P-R interval, shortened Q-T interval, sensitivity to arrhythmic effects of digitalis, bradyarrhythmias, heart block, asystole
  — Polyuria and polydipsia, caused by hypercalcemia-induced nephrogenic diabetes insipidus; nephrocalcinosis and renal failure can occur
  — Anorexia, nausea, vomiting, abdominal pain, weight loss, constipation, and obstipation; pancreatitis (in 3%)
  — Pruritus may be present
  — Calcium may precipitate in the corneas ("band keratopathy"); may also precipitate in extravascular tissues as well as in small arteries, causing small vessel thrombosis and skin necrosis (calciphylaxis)

5. Differential Diagnosis

- Hypercalcemia of malignancy (most frequently with breast, lung, pancreatic, uterine, and renal cell carcinomas, paraganglioma, and multiple myeloma)
- Hypercalcemia from other conditions
  — Vitamin D intoxication
  — Granulomatous diseases (sarcoidosis, tuberculosis)
  — Immobilization
  — Hyperthyroidism
  — High-dose corticosteroid therapy in patients taking thiazide diuretics
  — Milk-alkali syndrome
- Vitamin D deficiency can cause high serum PTH with normal serum calcium

6. Laboratory and Imaging Findings

Laboratory Tests

- In hyperparathyroidism, serum adjusted total calcium > 10.5 mg/dL
- Confirm with serum calcium drawn after overnight fast along with a serum protein, albumin, and triglyceride while ensuring that the patient is well-hydrated

- The serum adjusted total calcium = measured serum calcium in mg/dL + [0.8 × (4.0 − patient's serum albumin in g/dL)]
- Elevated or high-normal PTH confirms the diagnosis. Immunoradiometric assay (IRMA) for PTH is most specific and sensitive
- Serum phosphate is often low (< 2.5 mg/dL) in primary hyperparathyroidism
- Serum phosphate is often high in secondary hyperparathyroidism (CKD)
- Urine calcium excretion is high or normal (average 250 mg/g creatinine), but low for the degree of hypercalcemia
- Urine phosphate is high despite low to low normal serum phosphate
- Serum alkaline phosphatase is elevated only if bone disease present
- Plasma chloride and uric acid may be elevated
- Exclude familial benign hypocalciuric hypercalcemia (FHH) with 24-hour urine for calcium and creatinine. Discontinue thiazide diuretics prior to this test. In FHH, urine calcium excretion is low.

Imaging Studies
- Ultrasound of the neck
  — Should be performed with a high-resolution transducer (5–15 MHz) and should scan the neck from the mandible to the superior mediastinum in an effort to locate ectopic parathyroid adenomas
  — Has a sensitivity of 79% for single adenomas but only 35% for multiglandular disease
- Sestamibi scintigraphy can help locate parathyroid adenomas preoperatively
- CT and MRI are not as sensitive as ultrasound or sestamibi imaging
  — However, four-dimensional CT has been developed and is useful for preoperative imaging in patients who have had prior neck surgery and in those with ectopic glands
  — MRI may also be useful for repeat neck operations and when ectopic parathyroid glands are suspected; it also has the advantage of delivering no radiation and showing better soft tissue contrast than CT
- Noncontrast-enhanced CT scanning of the kidneys recommended for all patients to determine whether calcium-containing stones are present
- Bone radiographs
  — Usually normal and not required
  — However, may show demineralization, subperiosteal bone resorption, loss of lamina dura of the teeth, cysts throughout skeleton, mottling of skull, or pathologic fractures
  — Articular cartilage calcification (chondrocalcinosis) is sometimes found
- In renal osteodystrophy, bone radiographs may show
  — Ectopic calcifications around joints or soft tissue
  — Osteopenia
  — Osteitis fibrosa
  — Osteosclerosis
- Bone densitometry of wrist, hip, and spine may reveal low bone mineral density

7. Treatments
Medications
- Bisphosphonates
  — Pamidronate, 30 to 90 mg (in 0.9% saline) intravenously (IV) over 2 to 4 hours
  — Zoledronic acid 2 to 4 mg IV over 15 to 20 minutes is quite effective but also very expensive
  — Oral bisphosphonates, such as alendronate, are not effective for treating the hypercalcemia or hypercalciuria of hyperparathyroidism
  — However, oral alendronate has been shown to improve bone mineral density in the lumbar spine and hip (not distal radius) and may be used for asymptomatic patients with hyperparathyroidism who have a low bone mineral density

- Cinacalcet hydrochloride
  — Given to patients with severe hypercalcemia due to parathyroid carcinoma
    ○ Initial doses is 30 mg twice daily orally
    ○ Dose is increased progressively to 60 mg twice daily, then 90 mg twice daily, then to a maximum of 90 mg every 6 to 8 hours
  — Usually well-tolerated but may cause nausea and vomiting, which are usually transient
- Vitamin D replacement, 800 to 2000 units daily or more to achieve serum 25-OH vitamin D levels ≥ 30 ng/mL for patients with vitamin D deficiency
- Calcitriol
  — Used in secondary and tertiary hyperparathyroidism associated with azotemia
  — Given orally or IV after dialysis, suppresses parathyroid hyperplasia of kidney disease
  — For patients with near-normal serum calcium levels, it is given orally in starting at doses of 0.25 µg on alternate days or daily
- Doxercalciferol
  — Used in secondary or tertiary hyperparathyroidism associated with azotemia
  — Administer IV three times weekly during hemodialysis to patients with secondary hyperparathyroidism due to CKD
    ○ Starting dose: 4 µg three times weekly to maximum dose of 18 µg three times weekly
    ○ Alternatively, administered orally three times weekly at dialysis, starting with 10 µg at each dialysis to a maximum of 60 µg/wk
- Paricalcitol
  — Used in secondary or tertiary hyperparathyroidism associated with azotemia
  — Administer IV during dialysis three times weekly in starting doses of 0.04 to 0.1 µg/kg body weight to a maximum dose of 0.24 µg/kg three times weekly
- Propranolol may prevent adverse cardiac effects of hypercalcemia

Surgery
- Parathyroidectomy is indicated for patients with symptomatic hyperparathyroidism, kidney stones, or bone disease
- Consider parathyroidectomy for asymptomatic patients if
  — Serum calcium > 1 mg/dL (0.25 mmol/L) above normal and urine calcium excretion > 50 mg/24 h off thiazide diuretics
  — Urine calcium > 400 mg/24 h
  — Creatinine clearance < 60 mL/min
  — Cortical bone (wrist, hip) density > 2 SD below normal or previous fragility bone fracture
  — Age < 50 to 60 years
  — Difficulty ensuring medical follow-up
  — Pregnancy (second trimester)
- Minimally invasive parathyroidectomy surgery usually suffices if an adenoma is identified preoperatively
- Subtotal parathyroidectomy (3½ glands removed) is done for patients with resistant parathyroid hyperplasia

Therapeutic Procedures
- Patients with mild, asymptomatic hyperparathyroidism are advised to
  — Keep active; avoid immobilization
  — Drink adequate fluids
  — Avoid thiazides, large doses of vitamin A, calcium-containing antacids, or calcium supplements

8. Outcomes
Follow-Up
- In mild, asymptomatic hyperparathyroidism, check
  — X-ray, ultrasound, or CT scan to identify any nephrolithiasis or nephrocalcinosis
  — Serum calcium and albumin twice yearly

— Renal function and urine calcium once yearly
— Bone density (distal radius) every 2 years
• Postoperatively
  — Keep patients hospitalized overnight
  — Monitor serum calcium and PTH
  — Oral calcium and calcitriol 0.25 mg/d for 2 weeks helps prevent tetany
  — Treat symptomatic hypocalcemia with oral calcium carbonate and calcitriol 0.25 to 1.0 μg once daily orally
  — Secondary hyperparathyroidism occurs in ~12% and is treated with calcium and vitamin D, usually for 3 to 6 months
  — Hyperthyroidism immediately following parathyroid surgery may require short-term propranolol

Complications
• Forearm and hip fractures
• Urinary tract infection due to obstruction by stones
• Confusion, acute kidney injury, and soft tissue calcinosis from rapidly rising serum calcium
• Renal osteodystrophy from hyperphosphatemia
• Peptic ulcer disease
• Pancreatitis
• Pseudogout before or after surgery
• Disseminated calcification in skin, soft tissues, and arteries (calciphylaxis) can result in gangrene, arrhythmias, and respiratory failure
• Nephrolithiasis, hyperemesis, pancreatitis, muscle weakness, cognitive changes, and hypercalcemic crisis seen in some pregnant women
• About 80% of fetuses experience complications of maternal hyperparathyroidism, including
  — Fetal demise
  — Preterm delivery
  — Low birth weight
  — Postpartum neonatal tetany
  — Permanent hypoparathyroidism

Prognosis
• Asymptomatic mild hypercalcemia
  — Remains stable with follow-up in two-thirds of patients
  — However, worsening hypercalcemia, hypercalciuria and reductions in cortical bone mineral density may develop in one-third of patients
  — Must be monitored and treated with oral hydration and mobilization
• Resection of sporadic parathyroid adenoma generally results in cure
• Despite severe cyst formation or fracture, bones heal if parathyroid adenoma is removed
• Occurrence of pancreatitis increases mortality rate
• Significant renal damage may progress even after adenoma removal
• Parathyroid carcinoma
  — Associated with a 5-year survival of about 80% if surgical margins are clear and no detectable metastases postoperatively. Conversely, positive surgical margins or metastases predict a very poor 5-year survival
  — Tends to invade local structures and may metastasize
  — Repeat surgical resections and medical therapy can prolong life
  — Metastases are relatively radiation-resistant
  — Factors associated with a worsened mortality rate include
    ◦ Lymph node or distant metastases
    ◦ High number of recurrences
    ◦ Higher serum calcium levels at recurrence

9. When to Refer and When to Admit

When to Refer

- Refer to parathyroid surgeon for parathyroidectomy

When to Admit

- Patients with severe hypercalcemia for IV hydration

SUGGESTED REFERENCES

Bilezikian JP et al. Guidelines for the management of asymptomatic primary hyperparathyroidism: summary statement from the Fourth International Workshop. *J Clin Endocrinol Metab*. 2014 Oct;99(10):3561–3569. [PMID: 25162665]

Diaz-Soto G et al. Primary hyperparathyroidism in pregnancy. *Endocrine*. 2013 Dec;44(3):591–597. [PMID: 23670708]

Duntas LH et al. Cinacalcet as alternative treatment of primary hyperparathyroidism: achievements and prospects. *Endocrine*. 2011 Jun;39(3):199–204. [PMID: 21442382]

Kuntsman JW et al. Parathyroid localization and implications for clinical management. *J Clin Endocrinol Metab*. 2013 Mar;98(3):902–912. [PMID: 23345096]

Marcocci C et al. Medical management of primary hyperparathyroidism: proceedings of the Fourth International Workshop on the management of asymptomatic primary hyperparathyroidism. *J Clin Endocrinol Metab*. 2014 Oct;99(10):3607–3618. [PMID: 25162668]

McVeigh T et al. Changing practices in the surgical management of hyperparathyroidism. *Surgeon*. 2012 Dec;10(6):314–320. [PMID: 22105046]

Pepe J et al. Sporadic and hereditary primary hyperparathyroidism. *J Endocrinol Invest*. 2011 Jul; 34(7 suppl):40–44. [PMID: 21985979]

Taieb D et al. Parathyroid scintigraphy: when, how, and why? A concise systematic review. *Clin Nucl Med*. 2012 Jun;37(6):568–574. [PMID: 22614188]

Vestergaard P et al. Medical treatment of primary, secondary, and tertiary hyperparathyroidism. *Curr Drug Saf*. 2011 Apr;6(2):108–113. [PMID: 21524244]

Wei CH et al. Parathyroid carcinoma: update and guidelines for management. *Curr Treat Options Oncol*. 2012 Mar;13(1):11–23. [PMID: 22327883]

Hyperthyroidism

72

A 25-year-old African American woman presents with a complaint of rapid weight loss despite a voracious appetite. Physical examination reveals tachycardia (pulse rate 110 bpm at rest), fine moist skin, symmetrically enlarged thyroid, mild bilateral quadriceps muscle weakness, and fine tremor.

LEARNING OBJECTIVES

► Learn the clinical manifestations and objective findings of hyperthyroidism

► Understand the factors and medications that predispose to hyperthyroidism

► Learn how to distinguish the causes of hyperthyroidism

► Know the differential diagnosis of hyperthyroidism

► Learn the treatments for each cause of hyperthyroidism

QUESTIONS

1. What are the salient features of this patient's problem?

2. How do you think through her problem?

3. What are the key features, including essentials of diagnosis and general considerations, of hyperthyroidism?

4. What are the symptoms and signs of hyperthyroidism?

5. What is the differential diagnosis of hyperthyroidism?

6. What are laboratory and imaging findings in hyperthyroidism?

7. What are the treatments for hyperthyroidism?

8. What are the outcomes, including follow-up, complications, and prognosis, of hyperthyroidism?

9. When should patients with hyperthyroidism be admitted to the hospital?

ANSWERS

1. Salient Features

Weight loss with increased appetite; tachycardia; moist skin; enlarged thyroid; muscle weakness; tremor

2. How to Think Through

Weight loss, weakness, and tachycardia indicate a systemic process. To avoid anchoring prematurely to thyroid disease as an explanation, what are the other major disease categories that could cause these findings? (Infection, malignancy, connective tissue diseases, vasculitis, medication toxicity.) What other symptoms of hyperthyroidism could you elicit to help confirm your suspicion? (Heat intolerance, restlessness, diarrhea, sleep disturbance, irregular menses.) What additional physical examination signs should be sought when considering hyperthyroidism? (Lid lag, exophthalmos, hyperdefecation, abnormally rapid relaxation phase to deep tendon reflexes, pretibial myxedema.) In this case, examination of the thyroid gland shows symmetrical thyroid enlargement. What are the causes of a symmetrically enlarged gland? (Graves disease, viral thyroiditis, early autoimmune thyroid disease ["hashitoxicosis"], thyroid-stimulating hormone [TSH]-producing pituitary adenoma.) What common causes of hyperthyroidism might present with an asymmetrical examination? (Toxic adenoma, toxic multinodular goiter.)

How should her thyroid function be evaluated? (A serum TSH alone is the most sensitive initial test.) If the TSH is suppressed, what would be the next diagnostic steps? (Serum T3, T4, thyroid-stimulating immunoglobulins [TSIs]; thyroid ultrasound, and possibly a radioactive iodine scan; ophthalmology evaluation.) If the TSH in this patient is found to be suppressed, how should she be treated while awaiting the subsequent studies? (The nonspecific β-blocker propranolol is used to control tachycardia and to improve anxiety.)

What are the complications of untreated hyperthyroidism? (Heart failure, osteoporosis, risk of thyroid storm.) What are the features of thyroid storm? (Fever, delirium, vomiting, diarrhea, tachycardia, heart failure.)

3. Key Features

Essentials of Diagnosis

- Sweating, weight loss or gain, anxiety, palpitations, loose stools, heat intolerance, irritability, fatigue, weakness, menstrual irregularity
- Tachycardia; warm, moist skin; stare; tremor; and, in Graves disease, goiter (often with bruit) and ophthalmopathy
- Suppressed TSH in primary hyperthyroidism; increased T_4, free thyroxine (FT_4), T_3, free triiodothyronine (FT_3)

General Considerations

- Causes
  - Graves disease (most common)
  - Autonomous toxic adenomas, single or multiple
  - Jod–Basedow disease, or iodine-induced hyperthyroidism, may occur with multinodular goiters after significant iodine intake, radiographic contrast, or drugs, eg, amiodarone
  - Subacute de Quervain thyroiditis: hyperthyroidism followed by hypothyroidism
  - Hashimoto thyroiditis may cause transient hyperthyroidism during initial phase and may occur postpartum
  - Lymphocytic ("silent") thyroiditis
    ◦ Also known as subacute lymphocytic thyroiditis or "hashitoxicosis"
    ◦ Can occur spontaneously or be triggered by certain medications, such as axitinib, sorafenib, sunitinib, alemtuzumab
  - Amiodarone-induced hyperthyroidism: can occur quite suddenly at any time during treatment and may even develop several months after it has been discontinued
  - High serum human chorionic gonadotropin levels in first 4 months of pregnancy, molar pregnancy, choriocarcinoma, and testicular malignancies may cause hyperthyroidism
  - Thyrotoxicosis factitia: excessive exogenous thyroid hormone

4. Symptoms and Signs

- Heat intolerance, sweating
- Pruritus
- Frequent bowel movements (hyperdefecation)
- Weight loss (or gain)
- Menstrual irregularities
- Nervousness, fine resting tremor
- Fatigue, weakness
- Muscle cramps, hyperreflexia
- Thyroid
  — Goiter (often with a bruit) in Graves disease
  — Moderately enlarged, tender thyroid in subacute thyroiditis
- Eye
  — Upper eyelid retraction
  — Stare and lid lag with downward gaze
  — Ophthalmopathy (chemosis, conjunctivitis, and mild proptosis) in 20% to 40% of patients with Graves disease
  — Diplopia may be due to coexistent myasthenia gravis
- Skin
  — Moist warm skin
  — Fine hair
  — Onycholysis
  — Dermopathy (myxedema) in 3% of patients with Graves disease
- Heart
  — Palpitations or angina pectoris
  — Arrhythmias
    › Sinus tachycardia
    › Premature atrial contractions
    › Atrial fibrillation or atrial tachycardia (can precipitate heart failure)
  — Thyrotoxic cardiomyopathy due to thyrotoxicosis
- Thyroid storm
- Hypokalemic periodic paralysis (Asian or Native American men)

5. Differential Diagnosis

- General anxiety, panic disorder, mania
- Other hypermetabolic state, eg, cancer, pheochromocytoma
- Exophthalmos due to other cause, eg, orbital tumor
- Atrial fibrillation from another cause
- Acute psychiatric disorders (may falsely increase serum thyroxine)
- High estrogen states, eg, pregnancy
- Hypopituitarism
- Subclinical hyperthyroidism

6. Laboratory and Imaging Findings

Laboratory Tests

- Serum TSH is suppressed in hyperthyroidism
- Serum T_4, FT_4, T_3, FT_3, thyroid resin uptake, and FT_4 index are all usually increased
- FT_4 is sometimes normal but serum T_3 is still elevated
- Obtain serum FT_3 (rather than T_3) in women who are pregnant or taking oral estrogen
- Hypercalcemia
- Increased alkaline phosphatase
- Anemia
- Decreased granulocytes

- Hypokalemia and hypophosphatemia occur in thyrotoxic periodic paralysis
- Serum autoantibodies found in most patients with Graves disease include
  — Thyroid stimulating immunoglobulin (TSI), also known as TSH receptor antibody (TSHrAb)
  — Antinuclear antibody
  — Thyroperoxidase or thyroglobulin antibodies
- Erythrocyte sedimentation rate is often elevated in subacute thyroiditis
- TSH may be elevated or normal despite thyrotoxicosis in a TSH-secreting pituitary tumor
- In **type I amiodarone–induced thyrotoxicosis,** the presence of proptosis and TSI is diagnostic
- In **type II amiodarone–induced thyrotoxicosis,** serum level of interleukin-6 is usually quite elevated

Imaging Studies
- Thyroid radioactive ^{123}I iodine scan
  — Usually indicated for hyperthyroidism
  — High ^{123}I uptake in Graves disease and toxic nodular goiter
    ○ Scan can detect toxic nodule or multinodular goiter
  — Low ^{123}I uptake characteristic of subacute thyroiditis and amiodarone-induced hyperthyroidism
  — Do not perform thyroid radioactive iodine scans in pregnant women
- Thyroid ultrasound
  — Can be helpful in patients with hyperthyroidism, particularly in patients with palpable thyroid nodules
  — Color flow Doppler sonography helps distinguish type 1 from type 2 amiodarone-induced thyrotoxicosis
- Magnetic resonance imaging (MRI) of the orbits is the method of choice to visualize Graves ophthalmopathy affecting the extraocular muscles
- MRI is required only in severe or unilateral cases or in euthyroid exophthalmos that must be distinguished from orbital pseudotumor, tumors, and other lesions

7. Treatments

Medications (by Disease Entity)
Graves Disease
- Propranolol
  — Extended-release formulation
    ○ 60 mg orally once or twice daily, with dosage increases every 2 to 3 days to a maximum daily dose of 320 mg
  — Long-acting formulation
    ○ Initially given every 12 hours for patients with severe hyperthyroidism, due to accelerated metabolism of the propranolol
    ○ May be given once daily as hyperthyroidism improves
- Thioureas (methimazole or propylthiouracil [PTU])
  — Generally used for
    ○ Young adults
    ○ Those with mild thyrotoxicosis, small goiters, or fear of radioactive ^{131}I iodine treatment
    ○ Preparing patients for surgery and elderly patients for radioactive ^{131}I treatment
    ○ Thioureas reverse hyperthyroidism, but do not shrink the goiter. There is a 95% recurrence rate if the drug is stopped
  — Methimazole
    ○ Initial dose: 30 to 60 mg once daily orally
    ○ Some patients with very mild hyperthyroidism may respond well to smaller initial doses: 10 to 20 mg daily

- May also be administered twice daily to reduce the likelihood of gastrointestinal upset
- Preferred over PTU (which can rarely cause acute hepatitis and even fulminant hepatic necrosis)
- Reduce dosage as manifestations of hyperthyroidism resolve and as FT_4 level falls toward normal
- If used during pregnancy or breast-feeding, the dose should not exceed 20 mg daily
— Propylthiouracil (PTU)
  - Initial dose: 300 to 600 mg daily orally in four divided doses
  - Reduce dose and frequency as symptoms of hyperthyroidism resolve and the FT_4 level approaches normal
  - Drug of choice during breast-feeding
  - Preferred over methimazole for pregnant women in first trimester of pregnancy; dose is kept < 200 mg/d to avoid goitrous hypothyroidism in the infant; the patient may be switched to methimazole in second trimester
  - Rare complications include arthritis, systemic lupus erythematosus, aplastic anemia, thrombocytopenia, and hypoprothrombinemia
  - Acute hepatitis occurs rarely and is treated with prednisone but may progress to liver failure from fulminant hepatic necrosis
- Iodinated contrast agents (iopanoic acid [Telepaque] or ipodate sodium [Bilivist, Gastrografin, Oragrafin])
  — 500 mg twice daily orally for 3 days, then 500 mg once daily orally
  — Begin after thiourea is started

Subacute and Lymphocytic (Hashimoto) Thyroiditis

- Propranolol ER 60–80 mg twice daily and increased every 3 days until the heart rate is < 90 beats/min for symptomatic relief
- Ipodate sodium or iopanoic acid, 500 mg orally daily, promptly corrects elevated T_3 levels and is continued for 15 to 60 days until the serum FT_4 level normalizes
- With subacute thyroiditis, pain can usually be managed with nonsteroidal anti-inflammatory drugs, but opioid analgesics are sometimes required

Amiodarone-induced Thyrotoxicosis

- Propranolol ER, methimazole, iopanoic acid, prednisone

Hypokalemic Thyrotoxic Paralysis

- Oral propranolol, 3 mg/kg, normalizes the serum potassium and phosphate levels and reverses the paralysis within 2 to 3 hours
- Continued propranolol, 60 to 80 mg every 8 hours (or sustained-action propranolol ER daily at equivalent daily dosage), along with a thiourea drug such as methimazole
- Intravenous potassium or phosphate infusions are not usually required

Graves Ophthalmopathy

- For mild cases, selenium 100 μg orally twice daily slows progression of the disease
- For acute, progressive exophthalmos,
  — Methylprednisolone is given intravenously, 500 mg weekly for 6 weeks, then 250 mg weekly for 6 weeks
  — If oral prednisone is chosen for treatment, it must be given promptly in daily doses of 40 to 60 mg/d orally, with dosage reduction over several weeks
  — Higher initial prednisone doses of 80 to 120 mg/d are used when there is optic nerve compression
- For corticosteroid-resistant acute Graves orbitopathy
  — Rituximab may be given by retro-orbital injection, which limits systemic toxicity
  — Recommended dosing: 10 mg by retro-orbital injection into the affected eye weekly for 1 month, followed by a 1-month break, then another series of four weekly injections
- Avoid smoking and thiazolidinediones

Atrial Fibrillation
- Digoxin and β-blockers to control heart rate
- Warfarin
- Cardioversion is unsuccessful until hyperthyroidism is controlled

Thyrotoxic Heart Failure
- Aggressively control hyperthyroidism
- Use digoxin, angiotensin-converting enzyme inhibitors, angiotensin receptor blockers, diuretics

Graves Disease
- Thyroidectomy preferred over radioiodine for
  — Pregnant women whose thyrotoxicosis is not controlled with low-dose thioureas
  — Women desiring pregnancy in very near future
  — Patients with extremely large goiters
  — Those with suspected malignancy
  — Hartley–Dunhill operation
    ○ Procedure of choice
    ○ Total resection of one lobe and a subtotal resection of the other lobe, leaving about 4 g of thyroid tissue

Toxic Solitary Thyroid Nodules
- Partial thyroidectomy for patients aged < 40
- ^{131}I for those aged > 40 years
- Surgery is the definitive treatment for patients with large toxic nodular goiter; pathology reveals unsuspected differentiated thyroid cancer in 18.3% of cases.

Therapeutic Procedures
- Surgery
  — Treat preoperatively with methimazole
  — Six hours later, give ipodate sodium or iopanoic acid (500 mg twice daily orally) to accelerate euthyroidism and reduce thyroid vascularity
  — Iodine (eg, Lugol solution, 2 to 3 gtts daily orally for several days) also reduces vascularity
  — Give propranolol preoperatively until serum T_3 or free T_3 is normal
  — For thyrotoxic patients undergoing surgery, larger doses of propranolol are required perioperatively to reduce possibility of thyroid crisis
- Radioactive ^{131}I therapy
  — Patients usually only take propranolol
  — However, those with coronary disease, aged > 65 years, or severe hyperthyroidism are usually first rendered euthyroid with methimazole
  — Contraindicated in pregnancy
- Discontinue methimazole 4 days before ^{131}I treatment
- Methimazole given after ^{131}I for symptomatic hyperthyroidism until euthyroid

8. Outcome

Follow-Up
- In patients taking thioureas, check WBC periodically to exclude agranulocytosis, particularly in those with sore throat or febrile illness
- Obtain free T_4 levels every 2 to 3 weeks during initial treatment
- Hypothyroidism is common months to years after ^{131}I therapy or subtotal thyroidectomy surgery
- Lifelong clinical follow-up, with TSH and free T_4 measurements, is indicated in all patients

Complications
- Osteoporosis, hypercalcemia
- Temporary decreased libido, diminished sperm motility, gynecomastia

- Cardiac arrhythmias and heart failure
- Thyroid crisis ("storm")
- Ophthalmopathy
- Dermopathy
- Thyrotoxic hypokalemic periodic paralysis
- Osteoporosis, even in chronic subclinical hyperthyroidism

Prognosis

- Posttreatment hypothyroidism common, especially after ^{131}I therapy or subtotal thyroid-ectomy surgery
- Recurrence of hyperthyroidism occurs most commonly after thioureas (~50%)
- Subacute thyroiditis usually subsides spontaneously in weeks to months
- Graves disease usually progresses, but may rarely subside spontaneously or even result in hypothyroidism
- Despite subtotal thyroidectomy of both lobes, recurrence of hyperthyroidism occurs in 9%
- Despite treatment, there is an increased risk of death from cardiovascular disease, stroke, and femur fracture in women
- Mortality rate from thyroid storm is high
- Subclinical hyperthyroidism: good prognosis; most patients do not have accelerated bone loss

9. When to Admit

- Thyroid storm
- Hyperthyroidism-induced atrial fibrillation with severe tachycardia
- Thyroidectomy

SUGGESTED REFERENCES

Bahn RS et al. Hyperthyroidism and other causes of thyrotoxicosis: management guidelines of the American Thyroid Association and American Association of Clinical Endocrinologists. *Thyroid.* 2011 Jun;21(6):593–646. [PMID: 21510801]

Barbesino G et al. Clinical review: clinical utility of TSH receptor antibodies. *J Clin Endocrinol Metab.* 2013 Jun;98(6):2247–2255. [PMID: 23539719]

Bogazzi F et al. Amiodarone and the thyroid: a 2012 update. *J Endocrinol Invest.* 2012 Mar;35(3): 340–348. [PMID: 22433945]

De Groot L et al. Management of thyroid dysfunction during pregnancy and postpartum: an Endocrine Society clinical practice guideline. *J Clin Endocrinol Metab.* 2012 Aug;97(8):2543–2565. [PMID: 22869843]

Falhammar H et al. Thyrotoxic periodic paralysis: clinical and molecular aspects. *Endocrine.* 2013 Apr;43(2):274–284. [PMID: 22918841]

Franklyn JA et al. Thyrotoxicosis. *Lancet.* 2012 Mar 24;379(9821):1155–1166. [PMID: 22394559]

Melcescu E et al. Graves orbitopathy: update on diagnosis and therapy. *South Med J.* 2014 Jan;107(1): 34–43. [PMID: 24389785]

Minakaran N et al. Rituximab for thyroid-associated ophthalmopathy. *Cochrane Database Syst Rev.* 2013 May;5:CD009226. [PMID: 23728689]

Nakamura H et al. Analysis of 754 cases of antithyroid drug-induced agranulocytosis over 30 years in Japan. *J Clin Endocrinol Metab.* 2013 Dec;98(12):4776–4783. [PMID: 24057289]

Seigel SC et al. Thyrotoxicosis. *Med Clin North Am.* 2012 Mar;96(2):175–201. [PMID: 22443970]

Smith JJ et al. Toxic nodular goiter and cancer: a compelling case for thyroidectomy. *Ann Surg Oncol.* 2013 Apr;20(4):1336–1340. [PMID: 23108556]

Sundaresh V et al. Comparative effectiveness of therapies for Graves' hyperthyroidism: a systematic review and network meta-analysis. *J Clin Endocrinol Metab.* 2013 Sep;98(9):3671–3677. [PMID: 23824415]

Wirth CD et al. Subclinical thyroid dysfunction and the risk for fractures: a systematic review and meta-analysis. *Ann Intern Med.* 2014 Aug;161(3):189–199. [PMID: 25089863]

Zhu W et al. A prospective, randomized trial of intravenous glucocorticoids therapy with different protocols for patients with Graves' ophthalmopathy. *J Clin Endocrinol Metab.* 2014 Jun;99(6): 1999–2007. [PMID: 24606088]

73

Hypothyroidism

A 45-year-old woman presents complaining of fatigue, 30 pounds of weight gain despite dieting, constipation, thinning hair, and menorrhagia. On physical examination, the thyroid gland is not palpable; the skin is cool, dry, and rough; the heart sounds are quiet; and the pulse rate is 50 bpm; the deep tendon reflexes show a delayed relaxation phase. The rectal and pelvic examinations are normal, and the stool is guaiac negative. The clinical findings suggest hypothyroidism.

LEARNING OBJECTIVES

▶ Learn the common and uncommon clinical manifestations of hypothyroidism
▶ Understand the difference between primary and secondary hypothyroidism, and the causes for each
▶ Know the differential diagnosis of hypothyroidism
▶ Learn the treatments and monitoring for hypothyroidism and myxedema
▶ Know the medications and supplements that affect the metabolism of L-thyroxine

QUESTIONS

1. What are the salient features of this patient's problem?

2. How do you think through her problem?

3. What are the key features, including essentials of diagnosis and general considerations, of hypothyroidism?

4. What are the symptoms and signs of hypothyroidism?

5. What is the differential diagnosis of hypothyroidism?

6. What are laboratory findings in hypothyroidism?

7. What are the treatments for hypothyroidism?

8. What are the outcomes, including follow-up, complications, and prognosis, of hypothyroidism?

9. When should patients with hypothyroidism be referred to a specialist or admitted to the hospital?

ANSWERS

1. Salient Features

Middle-aged female; weight gain; constipation; menorrhagia; thinning hair; dry skin; bradycardia; delayed relaxation phase of deep tendon reflexes

2. How to Think Through

What major disease categories might present with fatigue and weight gain? (Depression, Cushing syndrome, hypothyroidism.) In addition to the fatigue, constipation, weight gain, alopecia, and menorrhagia, what other symptoms should be sought in this case? (Cold intolerance, mental clouding, muscle weakness or cramping.)

What are common causes of hypothyroidism? (Autoimmune [Hashimoto] thyroiditis is most common; drug toxicity including amiodarone and lithium; iodine deficiency; surgical resection or radioablation of the thyroid gland.) If the thyroid-stimulating hormone (TSH) value in this case proves to be low normal, what diagnosis should we consider? (Secondary hypothyroidism due to a pituitary process such as a mass effect from a prolactin [PRL]-producing pituitary adenoma.) Is this patient at risk for autoimmune hypothyroidism? (Yes, given her age and sex.)

How should she be evaluated? (A serum TSH alone is the appropriate initial test; an abnormal TSH should be followed by a free T4. Tests for thyroperoxidase and thyroglobulin antibodies are positive in most cases of autoimmune thyroiditis, but are nonspecific and may be positive in the setting of acute illness.)

If this patient's TSH value is elevated, and her free T4 is low, how should thyroid replacement therapy be initiated? (*Start low, go slow.* The primary concern is that coronary artery disease can be "unmasked" if the metabolic rate accelerates too quickly.) What are other risks of overtreatment? (Osteoporosis, atrial fibrillation.)

3. Key Features

Essentials of Diagnosis

- Weakness, cold intolerance, constipation, depression, menorrhagia, hoarseness
- Dry skin, bradycardia, delayed relaxation phase of deep tendon reflexes
- Anemia, hyponatremia, hyperlipidemia
- Free tetraiodothyronine (FT_4) low
- TSH elevated in primary hypothyroidism

General Considerations

- **Primary** hypothyroidism is due to thyroid gland disease
- **Secondary** hypothyroidism is due to lack of pituitary TSH
- **Maternal** hypothyroidism during pregnancy results in cognitive impairment in the child
- Radiation therapy to the head-neck-chest-shoulder region can cause hypothyroidism with or without goiter or thyroid cancer many years later
- TSH may be mildly elevated in some euthyroid individuals, especially elderly women (10% incidence)
- Amiodarone, with its very high iodine content, causes clinical hypothyroidism in 15% to 20% of patients receiving it.
- High iodine intake from other sources may also cause hypothyroidism, especially in those with underlying lymphocytic thyroiditis
- Myxedema is caused by interstitial accumulation of hydrophilic mucopolysaccharides, leading to fluid retention and lymphedema

4. Symptoms and Signs

- **Common manifestations**
  — Weight gain, fatigue, lethargy, depression
  — Weakness, dyspnea on exertion

— Arthralgias or myalgias, muscle cramps
— Cold intolerance
— Constipation
— Dry skin
— Headache
— Paresthesias, carpal tunnel syndrome
— Menorrhagia
— Bradycardia; diastolic hypertension
— Thin, brittle nails
— Thinning of hair
— Peripheral edema, puffy face and eyelids
— Skin pallor or yellowing (carotenemia)
— Delayed relaxation phase of deep tendon reflexes
— Palpably enlarged thyroid (goiter) that arises due to elevated serum TSH levels or underlying thyroid pathology, such as Hashimoto thyroiditis
• **Less common manifestations**
— Diminished appetite and weight loss
— Hoarseness
— Decreased sense of taste and smell and diminished auditory acuity
— Dysphagia or neck discomfort
— Menorrhagia, scant menses, or amenorrhea
— Thinning of the outer halves of the eyebrows
— Thickening of the tongue
— Hard pitting edema
— Effusions into the pleural and peritoneal cavities as well as into joints
— Galactorrhea
— Cardiac enlargement ("myxedema heart") and pericardial effusions
— Psychosis ("myxedema madness")
— Pituitary enlargement

5. Differential Diagnosis

• Causes of **hypothyroidism with goiter**
— Hashimoto thyroiditis
— Subacute (de Quervain thyroiditis) (after initial hyperthyroidism)
— Riedel thyroiditis
— Iodine deficiency
— Genetic thyroid enzyme defects
— Hepatitis C
— Drugs
  ○ Amiodarone, interferon-alfa, interferon-beta, lithium, methimazole, propylthiouracil, sulfonamides
— Food goitrogens in iodide-deficient areas
— Peripheral resistance to thyroid hormone
— Infiltrating diseases
• Causes of **hypothyroidism without goiter**
— Thyroid surgery, irradiation, or radioiodine treatment
— Deficient pituitary TSH
— Severe illness

6. Laboratory Findings

Laboratory Tests
• Serum TSH is increased in primary hypothyroidism but low or normal in secondary hypothyroidism (hypopituitarism)

- Serum FT_4 may be low or low normal
- Other laboratory abnormalities include
  — Hyponatremia
  — Hypoglycemia
  — Anemia (with normal or increased mean corpuscular volume)
- Additional findings frequently include increased serum levels of
  — LDL cholesterol, triglycerides, lipoprotein (a)
  — Liver enzymes
  — Creatine kinase
  — Prolactin
- During pregnancy
  — Serum TSH levels normally drop while serum FT_4 rises during the first trimester; most women with a low serum TSH in the first trimester are clinically euthyroid
  — Serum FT_4 is helpful in evaluating the thyroid status of pregnant women, particularly in the first trimester
  — Check serum TSH frequently (eg, every 4 to 6 weeks) to ensure adequate replacement
  — Postpartum, levothyroxine replacement requirement ordinarily returns to prepregnancy level

Imaging
- Radiologic imaging is usually not necessary
- CT or MRI
  — Chest CT or MRI may show a goiter in the neck or in the mediastinum (retrosternal goiter)
    ◦ An enlarged thymus is frequently seen in the mediastinum in cases of autoimmune thyroiditis
  — On head MRI, the pituitary is often quite enlarged in primary hypothyroidism due to reversible hyperplasia of TSH-secreting cells

7. Treatments

Medications
- Levothyroxine (T_4)
  — Treatment of choice after excluding adrenal insufficiency and angina, which require treatment first
  — Traditionally taken before breakfast; consistent timing of the dose is important
  — Take at least 4 hours before or after binding substances, eg, iron, aluminum hydroxide antacids, calcium supplements, or soy milk; or with bile acid-binding resins (eg, cholestyramine)
  — Starting dose
    ◦ 25 to 75 μg orally every morning if no coronary disease and age < 60 years
    ◦ 100 to 150 μg orally every morning if hypothyroid during pregnancy
    ◦ 25 to 50 μg orally every morning if coronary disease or age > 60
  — Dose titrated up by 25 μg every 1 to 3 weeks until patient is euthyroid, usually at 100 to 250 μg every morning
  — Elevated TSH usually indicates underreplacement
  — Before increasing T_4 dosage, assess for angina, diarrhea, or malabsorption
  — Once a maintenance dose is determined, continue with the same brand owing to slight differences in absorption
  — T_4 requirements increase with oral estrogen therapy
  — Increase T_4 dose 30% as soon as pregnancy is confirmed
  — T_4 dosage requirements can rise, owing to increased hepatic metabolism of thyroxine induced by certain medications
    ◦ Carbamazepine
    ◦ Phenobarbital
    ◦ Primidone

- ○ Phenytoin
- ○ Rifabutin
- ○ Rifampin
- ○ Sunitinib and other tyrosine kinase inhibitors
- — T_4 dosage may need to be titrated downward for patients who start taking teduglutide for short bowel syndrome
- — T_4 dosages must usually be reduced for women who experience decreased estrogen levels after delivery, after bilateral oophorectomy or natural menopause, after cessation of oral estrogen replacement, when switching from oral to transdermal estrogen therapy, or during therapy with GnRH agonists
- — Suppressed TSH may indicate T_4 overreplacement
  - ○ Assess for severe nonthyroidal illness
  - ○ Assess other medications (eg, nonsteroidal anti-inflammatory drugs, opioids, nifedipine, verapamil, and corticosteroids)
- — Hypothyroid patients with ischemic heart disease should begin T_4 *after* coronary artery angioplasty or bypass
- Some otherwise healthy hypothyroid patients taking levothyroxine with a normal serum TSH continue to have hypothyroid-type symptoms
  - — After ruling out concurrent conditions, a serum T3 or free T3 level is often helpful
  - — Low serum T3 levels may reflect inadequate peripheral deiodinase activity to convert inactive T4 to active T3
  - — Consider a clinical trial of a higher dose of levothyroxine that results in a normal serum T3 but a slightly low serum TSH
  - — More controversial is the supplementation of levothyroxine with triiodothyronine (5 to10 µg/d)
  - — Dessicated natural porcine thyroid preparations containing both T4 and T3 (eg, Armour Thyroid, Nature-Throid, NP Thyroid) are discouraged by professional medical societies, but some patients prefer them
- Amiodarone-induced hypothyroidism: treat with just enough T_4 to relieve symptoms
- **Myxedema crisis**
  - — Levothyroxine (T4) sodium, 400 µg intravenous (IV) loading dose, then 50 to 100 µg IV once daily
  - — The lower dose (50 µg) is for patients with coronary artery disease
- **Myxedema coma**
  - — Liothyronine (T_3, Triostat) can be given in doses of 5 to 10 µg IV every 8 hours for the first 48 hours
  - — If hypothermic, warm only with blankets
  - — If hypercapnic, institute mechanical ventilation
  - — Treat infections aggressively
  - — If adrenal insufficiency is suspected, give hydrocortisone, 100 mg IV, then 25 to 50 mg IV every 8 hours

8. Outcomes

Follow-Up

- Continue T_4 for life; reassess dosage requirements periodically by clinical examination and by serum TSH
- Surveillance for atrial arrhythmias and for osteoporosis, especially in patients who require high doses of T_4
- Monitor patients with subclinical hypothyroidism for subtle signs (eg, fatigue, depression, hyperlipidemia)
- Clinical hypothyroidism later develops in ~18%

Complications

- Cardiac complications may occur as a result of preexistent coronary artery disease and heart failure, which may be exacerbated by T_4 therapy

- Increased susceptibility to infection in hypothyroidism
- Megacolon in long-standing hypothyroidism
- Organic psychoses with paranoid delusions ("myxedema madness")
- Adrenal crisis precipitated by thyroid replacement
- Infertility (rare), miscarriage in untreated hypothyroidism
- Sellar enlargement and TSH-secreting tumors in untreated cases

Prognosis
- Excellent prognosis with early treatment, but relapses may occur if treatment is interrupted
- Mortality rate for myxedema coma is high

9. When to Refer and When to Admit

When to Refer
- Difficulty titrating T_4 replacement to normal TSH or clinically euthyroid state
- Any patient with significant coronary disease needing T_4

When to Admit
- Suspected myxedema coma
- Hypercapnia

SUGGESTED REFERENCES

Almandoz JP et al. Hypothyroidism: etiology, diagnosis, and management. *Med Clin North Am.* 2012 Mar;96(2):203–221. [PMID: 22443971]

Biondi B et al. Combination treatment with T4 and T3: toward personalized replacement therapy in hypothyroidism? *J Clin Endocrinol Metab.* 2012 Jul;97(7):2256–2271. [PMID: 22593590]

De Groot L et al. Management of thyroid dysfunction during pregnancy and postpartum: an Endocrine Society clinical practice guideline. *J Clin Endocrinol Metab.* 2012 Aug;97(8):2543–2565. [PMID: 22869843]

Koulouri O et al. Pitfalls in the measurement and interpretation of thyroid function tests. *Best Pract Res Clin Endocrinol Metab.* 2013 Dec;27(6):745–762. [PMID: 24275187]

Samuels MH et al. The effects of levothyroxine replacement or suppressive therapy on health status, mood, and cognition. *J Clin Endocrinol Metab.* 2014 Mar;99(3):843–851. [PMID: 24423358]

Wiersinga WM. Paradigm shifts in thyroid hormone replacement therapies for hypothyroidism. *Nat Rev Endocrinol.* 2014 Mar;10(3):164–174. [PMID: 24419358]

74

Obesity

A 53-year-old woman came to the clinic to get help managing her weight. She has been overweight since childhood and has continued to gain weight throughout her adult life. She has tried numerous diets without lasting success. She initially loses weight, but then regains it after a few months. She is otherwise healthy and is not taking any medications. Other family members are also overweight or obese. She does not do any regular exercise and has a sedentary office job. On examination, she is 5 feet 3 inches tall and 260 pounds, with a body mass index (BMI) of 46.2 (normal < 25).

LEARNING OBJECTIVES

▶ Learn the clinical manifestations and objective findings of obesity
▶ Understand the factors that predispose to obesity
▶ Know the differential diagnosis of obesity
▶ Learn the treatment for obesity

QUESTIONS

1. What are the salient features of this patient's problem?

2. How do you think through her problem?

3. What are the key features, including essentials of diagnosis, general considerations, and demographics, of obesity?

4. What are the symptoms and signs of obesity?

5. What is the differential diagnosis of obesity?

6. What are laboratory and procedural findings in obesity?

7. What are the treatments for obesity?

8. What are the outcomes, including complications and prognosis, of obesity?

9. When should patients with obesity be referred to a specialist or admitted to the hospital?

ANSWERS

1. Salient Features

Long-standing obesity; multiple failed diets; family history of overweight or obesity; sedentary lifestyle; elevated BMI

2. How to Think Through

A BMI of 46 places her into which class of obesity? (Extreme.) In addition to excess caloric intake and inadequate exercise, what are the important causes of obesity to consider in your evaluation of this patient? What are the potential endocrine causes? (Hypothyroidism and Cushing syndrome.) What medications cause weight gain? Psychiatric causes? (Depression.)

What are the major medical complications of obesity and how would you screen for each? (Hypertension, dyslipidemia, diabetes mellitus, coronary artery disease, degenerative joint disease, cholelithiasis.) Does obesity increase her risk of any cancers?

What are the elements of a comprehensive treatment strategy? (Nutrition education, exercise program, and weight loss counseling, including a diet log, exercise log, motivational interviewing, and changes to environmental cues.) Is there a difference between success of low-fat or low-carbohydrate diets over time? (No.)

If she makes limited progress after 6 months of the above, what are possible next steps? (Medically managed very low-calorie diets and gastric bypass surgery.) Are there pharmacologic agents for weight loss? (Yes, but of limited utility. Orlistat is modestly effective but has frequent gastrointestinal [GI] side effects. Catecholaminergic agents have high abuse and dependence potential.)

3. Key Features

Essentials of Diagnosis
- Defined as excess adipose tissue; BMI = weight (in kg)/height (in m^2) > 30
- Upper body obesity (abdomen and flank) is of greater health consequence than lower body obesity (buttocks and thighs)
- Obesity is associated with health consequences, including diabetes mellitus, hypertension, and hyperlipidemia

General Considerations
- Quantitative evaluation involves determination of BMI, calculated by dividing measured body weight in kilograms by height in meters squared
- BMI accurately reflects the presence of excess adipose tissue
  - Normal: BMI = 18.5 to 24.9
  - Overweight: BMI = 25 to 29.9
  - Class I obesity: BMI = 30 to 34.9
  - Class II obesity: BMI = 35 to 39.9
  - Class III (extreme) obesity: BMI > 40
- Increased abdominal circumference (> 102 cm in men and > 88 cm in women) or high waist/hip ratios (> 1.0 in men and > 0.85 in women) confers greater risk of
  - Diabetes mellitus
  - Stroke
  - Coronary artery disease
  - Early death
- Obesity is associated with significant increases in morbidity and mortality
- Surgical and obstetric risks greater

- The relative risk associated with obesity decreases with age, and excess weight is no longer a risk factor in adults aged > 75

Demographics
- 68% of Americans are overweight
- 33.8% of Americans are obese
- Approximately 60% of individuals with obesity in the United States have the "metabolic syndrome" (obesity plus hypertension, hyperlipidemia and insulin resistance [diabetes mellitus])
- As much as 40% to 70% of obesity may be explained by genetic influences

4. Symptoms and Signs
- Assess BMI
- Assess degree and distribution of body fat
- Assess overall nutritional status
- Signs of secondary causes of obesity (hypothyroidism and Cushing syndrome) are found in < 1%

5. Differential Diagnosis
- Increased caloric intake
- Fluid retention: heart failure, cirrhosis, nephrotic syndrome
- Cushing syndrome
- Hypothyroidism
- Diabetes mellitus (type 2)
- Drugs, eg, antipsychotics, antidepressants, corticosteroids
- Insulinoma
- Depression
- Binge eating disorder

6. Laboratory and Procedural Findings

Laboratory Tests
- Endocrinologic evaluation, including serum thyroid-stimulating hormone and dexamethasone suppression test in obese patients with unexplained recent weight gain or clinical features of endocrinopathy, or both
- Assessment for medical consequences such as the "metabolic syndrome," by checking
  — Blood pressure
  — Fasting serum glucose
  — Fasting serum low-density and high-density cholesterol levels
  — Fasting serum triglyceride level

Diagnostic Procedures
- Calculation of BMI
- Measurement of waist circumference

7. Treatments

Medications
- Catecholaminergic or serotonergic medications
  — Amphetamines (high abuse potential)
  — Nonamphetamine schedule IV appetite suppressants (phentermine, diethylpropion, benzphetamine, and phendimetrazine) are approved for short-term use only and have limited utility
  — These medications are sometimes used in patients with BMI > 30 or in patients with BMI > 27 who have obesity-related health risks
  — Average weight loss approximately 3 to 5 kg more than placebo
  — No evidence of long-term benefit

- Orlistat (120 mg orally three times daily with meals)
  — Reduces fat absorption in the GI tract by inhibiting intestinal lipase
  — Side effects include diarrhea, gas, and cramping and perhaps reduced absorption of fat-soluble vitamins
  — A lower dose formulation (Alli 60 mg, 1 capsule orally up to three times daily with each fat-containing meal; maximum of three capsules per day) is available without a prescription
- Lorcaserin
  — Associated with modest weight loss, about 3% of initial weight more than placebo
  — Approximately twice as many patients (38% vs 16%) lose > 5% of initial weight on lorcaserin compared to placebo
  — Post-marketing surveillance is focused on concerns regarding increased breast tumors (in animal studies), increased valvular heart disease in earlier drugs of this class, and psychiatric side effects

- Phentermine plus topiramate
  — Patients on a lower dose lost 5% more weight than placebo
  — With a higher dose, 15% more weight was lost than placebo
  — The combination is associated with increased birth defects and should not be used during pregnancy
  — Clinicians prescribing this combination are required to take an online training module and use only one of three mail order pharmacies
  — Other side effects include mood changes, fatigue, and insomnia
  — Post-marketing surveillance focuses on cardiovascular risk since the medications increases heart rate
- Bupropion plus naltrexone
  — Clinical trials demonstrated a 2% to 4% weight loss compared to placebo after 1 year
  — However, the combination may cause suicidal thoughts and behaviors, other neuropsychiatric effects, seizures, and elevations of blood pressure and heart rate
  — Other side effects include nausea and vomiting, diarrhea and constipation, headache, and dry mouth
  — A cardiovascular outcome trial is in progress to further assess safety
- Liraglutide
  — An injectable incretin (a glucagon-like peptide-1 receptor agonist)
  — Clinical trials demonstrated a 3.7% to 4.5% weight loss compared to placebo at 1 year
  — However, liraglutide may cause thyroid tumors (in animals), pancreatitis, gallbladder disease, renal impairment, suicidal thoughts, and increased heart rate
  — Other side effects include nausea and vomiting, diarrhea and constipation, and hypoglycemia
  — A cardiovascular outcomes trial is being conducted

Surgery
- Consider for patients with BMI > 40, or BMI > 35 if obesity-related comorbidities are present
- Effective surgical procedures (each can be done laparoscopically)
  — Roux-en-Y gastric bypass
  — Vertical banded gastroplasty
  — Gastric banding
  — Sleeve gastrectomy
- Surgical complications are common and include
  — Peritonitis due to anastomotic leak
  — Abdominal wall hernias
  — Staple line disruption
  — Gallstones
  — Neuropathy
  — Marginal ulcers
  — Stomal stenosis

— Wound infections
— Thromboembolic disease
— Nutritional deficiencies
— GI symptoms
- Surgical mortality (30 day) ranges from nil to 1%; 1-year mortality is higher, especially in high-risk and older patients

Therapeutic Procedures
- Multidisciplinary approach
  — Hypocaloric diets
  — Behavior modification
  — Exercise
  — Social support
- Limit foods that provide large amounts of calories without other nutrients, ie, fat, sucrose, and alcohol
- No special advantage to carbohydrate-restricted or high-protein diets, nor to ingestion of foods one at a time
- Plan and keep records of menus and exercise sessions
- Aerobic exercise useful for long-term weight maintenance
- For BMI > 35
  — Consider very low-calorie diets (typically 800 to 1000 kcal/d) for 4 to 6 months
  — Side effects include fatigue, orthostatic hypotension, cold intolerance, and fluid and electrolyte disorders
  — Less-common complications include gout, gallbladder disease, and cardiac arrhythmias

8. Outcomes

Complications
- Hypertension
- Type 2 diabetes mellitus
- Hyperlipidemia
- Coronary artery disease
- Degenerative joint disease
- Psychosocial disability
- Cancers (colon, rectum, prostate, uterus, biliary tract, breast, ovary)
- Thromboembolic disorders
- Digestive tract diseases (gallstones, reflux esophagitis)
- Skin disorders

Prognosis
- Only 20% of patients will lose 20 lb and maintain the loss for > 2 years; only 5% will maintain a 40-lb loss
- With very low-calorie diets, patients lose an average of 2 lb/wk; long-term weight maintenance following meal replacement programs is less predictable and requires concurrent behavior modification and exercise
- Orlistat, 120 mg orally three times daily with each fat-containing meal, for up to 2 years results in 2 to 4 kg greater weight loss than placebo
- Roux-en-Y gastric bypass leads to substantial weight loss—close to 50% of initial body weight

9. When to Refer and When to Admit

When to Refer
- Refer for bariatric surgery for BMI > 40, or BMI > 35 with comorbid conditions

When to Admit
- For bariatric surgery

SUGGESTED REFERENCES

Gloy VL et al. Bariatric surgery versus non-surgical treatment for obesity: a systematic review and meta-analysis of randomised controlled trials. *BMJ*. 2013 Oct 22;347:f5934. [PMID: 24149519]

Gray LJ et al. A systematic review and mixed treatment comparison of pharmacological interventions for the treatment of obesity. *Obes Rev*. 2012 Jun;13(6):483–498. [PMID: 22288431]

Jensen MD et al. 2013 AHA/ACC/TOS guideline for the management of overweight and obesity in adults: a report of the American College of Cardiology/American Heart Association Task Force on Practice Guidelines and The Obesity Society. *Circulation*. 2014 Jun 24;129(25 suppl 2):S102–S138. [PMID: 24222017]

Johansson K et al. Effects of anti-obesity drugs, diet, and exercise on weight-loss maintenance after a very-low-calorie diet or low-calorie diet: a systematic review and meta-analysis of randomized controlled trials. *Am J Clin Nutr*. 2014 Jan;99(1):14–23. [PMID: 24172297]

Johnston BC et al. Comparison of weight loss among named diet programs in overweight and obese adults: a meta-analysis. *JAMA*. 2014 Sep 3;312(9):923–933. [PMID: 25182101]

Kushner RF et al. Assessment and lifestyle management of patients with obesity: clinical recommendations from systematic reviews. *JAMA*. 2014 Sep 3;312(9):943–952. Erratum in: *JAMA*. 2014 Oct 15;312(15):1593. [PMID: 25182103]

Ogden CL et al. Prevalence of obesity in the United States. *JAMA*. 2014 Jul;312(2):189–190. [PMID: 25005661]

Tsai AG et al. In the clinic: obesity. *Ann Intern Med*. 2013 Sep 3;159(5):ITC3-1–15. [PMID: 24026335]

Unick JL et al; Look AHEAD Research Group. The long-term effectiveness of a lifestyle intervention in severely obese individuals. *Am J Med*. 2013 Mar;126(3):236–242. [PMID: 23410564]

Yanovski SZ et al. Long-term drug treatment for obesity: a systematic and clinical review. *JAMA*. 2014 Jan 1;311(1):74–86. [PMID: 24231879]

75 Osteoporosis

A 72-year-old woman presents to the emergency room after falling in her home. She slipped on spilled water in her kitchen. She was unable to get up after her fall and was found on the floor in her kitchen by her son, who stopped by after work. She complains of severe right hip pain. Her medical history includes giant cell arteritis, for which she has taken daily prednisone for > 1 year. On examination, she has bruising over her right hip. Range of motion in her right hip is markedly decreased, with pain on both internal and external rotation. X-ray film reveals a hip fracture and probable low bone mass.

LEARNING OBJECTIVES

▶ Learn the common presentations and objective findings of osteoporosis
▶ Understand the patient characteristics, diseases, and medications that predispose to osteoporosis
▶ Know how to screen for osteoporosis and to rule out causes of bone loss
▶ Learn the treatments of osteoporosis, including medications for patients intolerant of oral bisphosphonates

QUESTIONS

1. What are the salient features of this patient's problem?
2. How do you think through her problem?
3. What are the key features, including essentials of diagnosis, general considerations, and demographics, of osteoporosis?
4. What are the symptoms and signs of osteoporosis?
5. What is the differential diagnosis of osteoporosis?
6. What are laboratory and imaging findings in osteoporosis?
7. What are the treatments for osteoporosis?
8. What are the outcomes, including follow-up, complications, and prognosis, of osteoporosis?

ANSWERS

1. Salient Features

Elderly; female sex; sex; long-term glucocorticoid use; fall with fracture of hip; radiograph shows low bone mass

2. How to Think Through

Osteoporosis is a common, underdiagnosed problem. In the absence of screening for osteoporosis, the loss of bone density goes untreated and, as in this case, can lead to fracture. Fractures, in turn, precipitate significant morbidity in the elderly. This patient is an older woman with a history of chronic corticosteroid use. What are the other major risk factors for osteoporosis that should be explored in her history? (Tobacco use, hyperthyroidism, inflammatory bowel and celiac disease, and premenopausal estrogen deficiency [eg, eating disorders, hypopituitarism, and premature ovarian failure].)

What is the screening test for osteoporosis? (Dual-energy x-ray absorptiometry—DEXA.) Can osteoporosis be diagnosed without DEXA testing? (Yes. An older woman, such as the patient in this case, with a "fragility" or "low-trauma" fracture, can be considered to have the osteoporosis and should be so treated.)

How should this patient be treated? (Bisphosphonates are the mainstay. Selective estrogen receptor modulators and parathyroid hormone [PTH] are considered in severe cases or with bisphosphonate intolerance.) When the decision to treat is unclear, consider the many other risk factors for fracture. These include age, prior fracture, family history of fracture, low body mass index, and alcoholism. Clinical formulas such as the FRAX algorithm incorporate these factors, along with the DEXA result, to determine risk of major osteoporotic fracture.

3. Key Features

Essentials of Diagnosis

- Propensity to fracture of spine, hip, pelvis, and wrist from demineralization
- Serum PTH, calcium, phosphorus, and alkaline phosphatase are all usually normal
- Serum 25-hydroxyvitamin D level is often low as a comorbid condition

General Considerations

- Osteoporosis causes approximately 2 million fractures annually in the United States, mainly of the spine and hip
- Morbidity and indirect mortality rates are very high
- Bone densitometry screening is recommended for all postmenopausal women, men over age 70 years, and younger patients who have pathologic fractures or radiographic evidence of diminished bone density
- Rate of bone formation is often normal, but rate of bone resorption is increased
- Most common causes
  — Aging
  — High-dose corticosteroid administration
  — Alcoholism
  — Smoking
  — Sex hormone deficiency, particularly menopause in women
  — See Table 75-1
- Osteogenesis imperfecta
  — Caused by a major mutation in the gene encoding for type I collagen, the major collagen constituent of bone
  — Causes severe osteoporosis

Table 75–1. Causes of osteoporosis.

Hormone deficiency	**Genetic disorders**
Estrogen (women)	Aromatase deficiency
Androgen (men)	Collagen disorders
Hormone excess	Ehlers–Danlos syndrome
Cushing syndrome or corticosteroid administration	Homocystinuria
Thyrotoxicosis	Hypophosphatasia
Hyperparathyroidism	Idiopathic juvenile and adult osteoporosis
Alcoholism	Marfan syndrome
Immobilization and microgravity	Osteogenesis imperfecta
Inflammatory bowel disease	**Miscellaneous**
Malignancy, especially multiple myeloma	Anorexia nervosa
Tobacco	Celiac disease
Medications (chronic)	Copper deficiency
Aromatase inhibitors	Diabetes mellitus (uncontrolled)
Heparin	Hyponatremia (chronic)
Pioglitazone	Liver disease (chronic)
Selective serotonin	Mastocytosis (systemic)
reuptake inhibitors	Protein-calorie malnutrition
Vitamin A excess	Rheumatoid arthritis
Vitamin D excess	Vitamin C deficiency

Demographics

- Clinically evident in middle life and beyond
- Women are more frequently affected than men

4. Symptoms and Signs

- Usually asymptomatic until fractures occur
- May present as back pain of varying degrees of severity or as spontaneous fracture or collapse of a vertebra
- Loss of height common secondary to vertebral fractures
- Fractures of femoral neck and distal radius also common
- Once osteoporosis is identified, careful history and physical examination are required to determine its cause

5. Differential Diagnosis

- Rickets (eg, from vitamin D deficiency in childhood)
- Osteomalacia (inadequate mineralization of existing bone matrix [osteoid])
- Multiple myeloma
- Metastatic cancer
- Paget disease of bone
- Renal osteodystrophy

6. Laboratory and Imaging Findings

Laboratory Tests

- Serum calcium, phosphate, and PTH normal
- Alkaline phosphatase usually normal but may be slightly elevated, especially following fracture
- Vitamin D deficiency is very common
- Testing for thyrotoxicosis and hypogonadism may be required
- Screen for celiac disease (gluten enteropathy) with serum immunoglobulin A (IgA) anti-tissue transglutaminase

Imaging Studies

- Radiographs of spine and pelvis may show demineralization; in skull and extremities, demineralization is less marked

- Radiographs of spine may show compression of vertebrae
- DEXA is quite accurate and delivers negligible radiation
  — Generally measured at two or three sites, including total lumbar spine and total hip
  — DXA of the nondominant distal radius can be done for patients with hyperparathyroidism, men receiving androgen deprivation therapy, and for conditions causing DXA artifacts (eg, hip arthroplasties, or spinal orthopedic hardware, severe spinal arthritis, or lumbar vertebral compression fractures)
- Osteoporosis: bone densitometry T score ≤ –2.5; osteopenia: T score ≤ –1.0 to –2.5
- Quantitative computed tomography delivers more radiation but is highly accurate

7. Treatments

Medications

- Calcium and vitamin D to prevent or treat osteoporosis
  — Calcium: the daily recommendation of 1200 mg for postmenopausal women and men older than age 70 years is achieved with most healthy diets, though supplementation is recommended if dairy products, dark leafy greens, sardines, tofu, or fortified foods are not included
  — Calcium citrate causes less gastrointestinal intolerance and does not require acid for absorption (recommended with concurrent acid suppression treatment)
  — Vitamin D (600 to 800 U/d) is difficult to obtain with diet and sun exposure alone; supplement with daily vitamin D3 (cholecalciferol) (800 to 2000 IU or in doses titrated to achieve serum levels of 25-hydroxyvitamin D between 30 and 60 ng/mL) for both prevention and treatment
- Bisphosphonates
  — Increase bone density, reduce fracture risk
  — Reduce corticosteroid-induced osteoporosis
  — Take in morning with ≥ 8 oz water, 30 to 60 minutes before any other food or liquid
  — Must remain upright for 30 minutes after taking to reduce risk of pill-induced esophagitis
  — Doses:
    ◦ Alendronate, 70 mg orally every week
    ◦ Risedronate, 35 mg orally every week
    ◦ Ibandronate sodium, 150 mg orally once monthly
    ◦ Zoledronic acid, 5 mg, can be administered intravenously every 12 months if patient cannot tolerate oral bisphosphonates
  — All patients taking bisphosphonates should receive oral calcium with evening meal and vitamin D
- Consider estrogen or raloxifene for women with hypogonadism
  — Raloxifene, 60 mg once daily orally, decreases risk of vertebral, but not nonvertebral, fractures
- Teriparatide
  — Stimulates production of new collagenous bone matrix that must be mineralized
  — Patients must have sufficient intake of vitamin D and calcium
  — Administer 20 µg/d subcutaneously for 2 years, then discontinue and substitute a bisphosphonate
  — May also be used to promote healing of atypical femoral chalkstick fractures associated with bisphosphonate therapy
  — Avoid in patients with
    ◦ Increased risk of osteosarcoma
    ◦ Hypercalcemia
  — Use with caution in patients taking corticosteroids or thiazide diuretics along with oral calcium supplementation therapy because hypercalcemia may develop
- Denosumab
  — Dose: 60 mg subcutaneously every 6 months
  — Its efficacy is comparable to bisphosphonates

— However, its long-term safety remain unknown, so it is reserved for patients with severe osteoporosis who have not tolerated or not responded to bisphosphonates
- Nasal calcitonin-salmon (Miacalcin) can be given if the patient is unable to tolerate bisphosphonates; usual dose is one puff (0.09 mL, 200 international units) once daily, alternating nostrils

Therapeutic Procedures
- Diet adequate in protein, total calories, calcium, and vitamin D
- Discontinue or reduce doses of corticosteroids, if possible
- Smoking cessation
- Avoidance of excessive alcohol intake
- High-impact physical activity (eg, jogging), stair climbing, and weight training increase bone density
- Fall-avoidance measures (eg, handrails and lighting)
- Minimization of medications that cause orthostasis, dizziness, or confusion

8. Outcomes

Follow-Up
- DEXA bone densitometry every 2 to 3 years
- Monitor patients taking corticosteroids or thiazides or who have kidney disease for development of hypercalcemia when given calcium supplements
- Reduce bisphosphonate dosage in chronic kidney disease, and monitor serum phosphate

Complications
- Fractures common, especially femur, vertebrae, and distal radius
- Calcium supplements (with and without coadministered vitamin D) are associated with a modest increased risk of myocardial infarction in some reports, though not in the Women's Health Initiative
- Bisphosphonates
  — Oral can cause esophagitis, gastritis, and abdominal pain
  — Oral and intravenous can cause fatigue, bone, joint, muscle pain, or osteonecrosis of the jaw
    ∘ Bone, joint, muscle pains can be migratory or diffuse, mild to incapacitating
    ∘ Onset of pain occurs 1 day to 1 year after therapy is initiated, with a mean of 14 days
    ∘ Pain can be transient, lasting several days and resolving spontaneously, but typically recurs with subsequent doses
    ∘ Most experience gradual pain relief when medication is stopped
    ∘ Osteonecrosis of the jaw is a rare (1:100,000) complication of bisphosphonate therapy for osteoporosis. A painful, necrotic, nonhealing lesion of the jaw occurs, particularly after tooth extraction.
- Raloxifene
  — Increases the risk for thromboembolism
  — Aggravates hot flashes
  — Nausea
  — Weight gain
  — Depression
  — Insomnia
  — Leg cramps
  — Rash
- Teriparatide
  — Orthostatic hypotension
  — Asthenia
  — Nausea
  — Leg cramps

— Hypercalcemia (if taken along with corticosteroids, thiazide diuretics, and calcium supplementation)

— Must not be given to patients with Paget disease or a history of osteosarcoma or chondrosarcoma

• Nasal calcitonin-salmon can cause

— Bronchospasm and allergic reactions

— Rhinitis

— Epistaxis

— Back pain

— Arthralgias

• Estrogen replacement

— Increases risk of thromboembolism and myocardial infarction, breast and endometrial cancer

— Cholestatic jaundice, hypertriglyceridemia, pancreatitis

— Enlargement of uterine fibroids, migraines, edema

Prognosis

• Bisphosphonates and raloxifene

— Can reverse progressive osteopenia and osteoporosis

— Can decrease fracture risk

• Give calcium supplements with meals to reduce risk of calcium oxalate nephrolithiasis

• Bone pain reduction may be noted within 2 to 4 weeks on nasal calcitonin

SUGGESTED REFERENCES

Ensrud KE et al; Osteoporotic Fractures in Men Study Group. Implications of expanding indications for drug treatment to prevent fracture in older men in United States: cross sectional and longitudinal analysis of prospective cohort study. *BMJ*. 2014 Jul 3;349:g4120. [PMID: 24994809]

Khosla S et al. Benefits and risks of bisphosphonate therapy for osteoporosis. *J Clin Endocrinol Metab*. 2012 Jul;97(7):2272–2282. [PMID: 22523337]

Knopp-Sihota JA et al. Calcitonin for treating acute and chronic pain of recent and remote osteoporotic vertebral compression fractures: a systematic review and meta-analysis. *Osteoporos Int*. 2012 Jan;23(1):17–38. [PMID: 21660557]

Leder BZ et al. Two years of denosumab and teriparatide administration in postmenopausal women with osteoporosis (The DATA Extension Study): a randomized controlled trial. *J Clin Endocrinol Metab*. 2014 May;99(5):1694–1700. [PMID: 24517156]

Lekamwasam S et al; Joint IOF-ECTS GIO Guidelines Working Group. A framework for the development of guidelines for the management of glucocorticoid-induced osteoporosis. *Osteoporos Int*. 2012 Sep;23(9):2257–2276. [PMID: 22434203]

Moyer VA et al. Vitamin D and calcium supplementation to prevent fractures in adults: U.S. Preventive Services Task Force recommendation statement. *Ann Intern Med*. 2013 May 7;158(9):691–696. [PMID: 23440163]

Murad MH et al. Clinical review. Comparative effectiveness of drug treatments to prevent fragility fractures: a systematic review and network meta-analysis. *J Clin Endocrinol Metab*. 2012 Jun;97(6):1871–1880. [PMID: 22466336]

Salam SN et al. Fragility fractures and osteoporosis in CKD: pathophysiology and diagnostic methods. *Am J Kidney Dis*. 2014 Jun;63(6):1049–1059. [PMID: 24631043]

Scott LJ. Denosumab: a review of its use in postmenopausal women with osteoporosis. *Drugs Aging*. 2014 Jul;31(7):555–576. [PMID: 24935243]

Sugerman DT. JAMA patient page. Osteoporosis. *JAMA*. 2014 Jan 1;311(1):104. [PMID: 24381978]

Sun LM et al. Calcitonin nasal spray and increased cancer risk: a population-based nested case-control study. *J Clin Endocrinol Metab*. 2014 Nov;99(11):4259–4264. [PMID: 25144633]

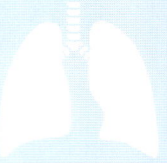

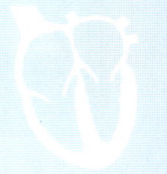

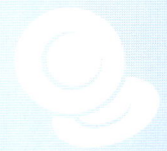

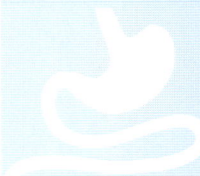

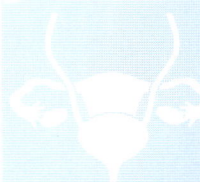

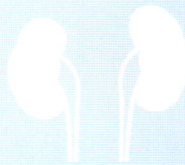

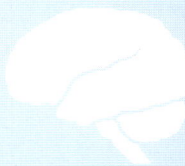

Infectious Disorders

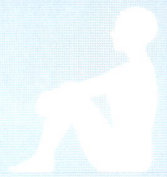

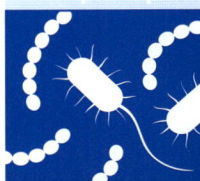

76

Fever

A 28-year-old woman presents to her primary care clinician because of intermittent fevers for the past 3 days, reaching 39°C. She reports sore throat, myalgias, and stomach upset. She had unprotected sex with a new partner 2 weeks prior. On physical examination, there is diffuse, nontender lymphadenopathy in the axillary, cervical, and occipital regions, and an erythematous throat without tonsillar exudates. HIV enzyme-linked immunosorbent assay (ELISA) test result is negative, but HIV viral load shows 150,000 copies/mL.

LEARNING OBJECTIVES

▶ Learn the clinical manifestations and objective findings that can suggest an etiology for the fever

▶ Understand the patient factors that predispose to the different causes of fever

▶ Know the infectious and noninfectious causes of fever

▶ Learn how to diagnose the etiology of fever

▶ Know which patients with fever to treat empirically with antibiotic therapy

QUESTIONS

1. What are the salient features of this patient's problem?

2. How do you think through her problem?

3. What are the key features, including essentials of diagnosis and general considerations, of fever?

4. What are the symptoms and signs of fever?

5. What is the differential diagnosis of fever?

6. What are laboratory, imaging, and procedural findings in fever?

7. What are the treatments for fever?

8. What is the outcome, including prognosis, of fever?

9. When should patients with fever be referred to a specialist or admitted to the hospital?

ANSWERS

1. Salient Features

Young woman; fever accompanied by systemic symptoms; myalgias; sore throat without tonsillar exudates; unprotected sex; lymphadenopathy; negative HIV ELISA with positive viral load indicating acute HIV infection

2. How to Think Through

While most acute febrile illnesses are self-limiting, many serious illnesses can present with fever. A broad framework is essential for clinical reasoning. What broad categories of disease could account for the initial presentation of the patient in this case—fever, plus pharyngitis, myalgias, gastrointestinal symptoms, and lymphadenopathy? (Infection, such as infectious mononucleosis, cytomegalovirus, streptococcal pharyngitis, or acute HIV infections; malignancy, such as lymphoma; inflammatory disease, such as lupus or sarcoidosis.)

Most patients with acute fever can be managed with supportive care, but only after assessment of risk factors and "red flag" symptoms. What exposures and social risk factors should be assessed? (High-risk sexual activity, as in this case; injection drug use; substance use; medications; travel; occupational exposures; contact with ill persons.)

Physical examination is important for localizing the source of fever, and for refining the differential diagnosis. What examination elements should be included? (Mental status, neck range of motion, cardiac, lung, abdominal, skin, and joint examinations.) At this patient's initial presentation, what diagnostic testing would have been appropriate, in addition to the HIV antibody test? (Complete blood count [CBC], rapid strep test, heterophile test. Blood cultures and liver tests should also be considered in febrile patients.)

Here, the diagnosis is acute HIV infection. Both medical and social resources need to be marshaled. What initial testing is needed to begin planning her care? (CBC, CD4 T-cell lymphocyte count, HIV genotype, serum creatinine, liver tests, hepatitis B serologies, hepatitis C antibody, toxoplasmosis IgG, G6PD level, and tuberculin skin test.)

3. Key Features

Essentials of Diagnosis

- In patients with fever, inquire about
  — Age
  — Localizing symptoms
  — Weight loss
  — Joint pain
  — Injection substance use
  — Immunosuppression or neutropenia
  — History of cancer
  — Medications
  — Travel history
  — Sexual contacts history

General Considerations

- Fever is a regulated rise to a new "set point" of body temperature mediated by pyrogenic cytokines acting on the hypothalamus
- The fever pattern is of marginal value, except for the relapsing fever of malaria, borreliosis, and lymphoma (especially Hodgkin disease)
- Most febrile illnesses are
  — Caused by common infections
  — Short-lived
  — Relatively easy to diagnose

- The term FUO ("fever of undetermined origin") refers to cases of unexplained fever exceeding 38.3°C on several occasions for at least 3 weeks in patients without neutropenia or immunosuppression
- In HIV-infected individuals, prolonged unexplained fever is usually due to infections
  — Disseminated *Mycobacterium avium-intracellulare*
  — *Pneumocystis jiroveci*
  — Cytomegalovirus
  — Disseminated histoplasmosis
- Lymphoma is another common cause of prolonged FUO in HIV-infected persons
- In the returned traveler, consider
  — Malaria
  — Dysentery
  — Hepatitis
  — Dengue fever

4. Symptoms and Signs

- Fever is defined as an elevated body temperature above 38.3°C
- The average normal oral body temperature taken in midmorning 36.7°C (range 36.0°C–37.4°C)
- The normal rectal or vaginal temperature is 0.5°C higher; the axillary temperature is 0.5°C lower
- Rectal is more reliable than oral temperature, particularly in patients who breathe through their mouth or in tachypneic states
- The normal diurnal temperature variation is 0.5°C to 1.0°C—lowest in the early morning and highest in the evening
- There is a slight sustained temperature rise following ovulation, during the menstrual cycle, and in the first trimester of pregnancy

5. Differential Diagnosis

Common Causes

- Infections
  — Bacterial (including tuberculosis)
  — Viral
  — Rickettsial
  — Fungal
  — Parasitic
- Autoimmune diseases
- CNS diseases
  — Head trauma
  — Mass lesions
- Malignant disease
  — Renal cell carcinoma
  — Primary or metastatic liver cancer
  — Leukemia
  — Lymphoma
- Cardiovascular diseases
  — Myocardial infarction
  — Thrombophlebitis
  — Pulmonary embolism
- Gastrointestinal diseases
  — Inflammatory bowel disease
  — Alcoholic hepatitis
  — Granulomatous hepatitis

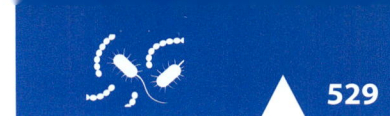

- Miscellaneous diseases
  — Drug fever
  — Sarcoidosis
  — Familial Mediterranean fever
  — Tissue injury
  — Hematoma
  — Factitious fever

Hyperthermia

- Peripheral thermoregulatory disorders
  — Heat stroke
  — Malignant hyperthermia of anesthesia
  — Malignant neuroleptic syndrome

6. Laboratory, Imaging, and Procedural Findings

Laboratory Tests

- Obtain
  — CBC with differential
  — Erythrocyte sedimentation rate (ESR) or C-reactive protein level
  — Urinalysis
  — Liver tests (alkaline phosphatase, alanine aminotransferase, γ-glutamyl transpeptidase, total bilirubin)
  — Blood and urine cultures

Imaging Studies

- Obtain chest radiograph
- Consider
  — Abdominal ultrasound and CT scan
  — Radionuclide-labeled leukocyte, gallium-67, and radiolabeled human immunoglobulin tests

Diagnostic Procedures

- Consider temporal artery biopsy in febrile patients aged 65 years and older with elevated ESR

7. Treatments

Medications

- Antipyretic therapy with aspirin or acetaminophen, 325 to 650 mg every 4 hours orally
- After obtaining blood and urine cultures, empiric broad-spectrum antibiotic therapy is indicated in patients who are
  — Clinically unstable
  — Hemodynamic unstable
  — Neutropenic (neutrophils < 500/μL)
  — Asplenic (from surgery or sickle-cell disease)
  — Immunosuppressed (including persons taking systemic corticosteroids, azathioprine, cyclosporine, or other immunosuppressive medications, and those who are HIV infected)
  — Likely to have a clinically significant infection
- Outpatient parenteral antimicrobial therapy can be given to patients with fever and neutropenia after chemotherapy
  — In low-risk patients, single agents can be used
    ◦ Cefepime
    ◦ Piperacillin/tazobactam
    ◦ Imipenem
    ◦ Meropenem
    ◦ Doripenem

— In high-risk patients, a combination of agents such as an aminoglycoside plus one of the following agents:
  ◦ Piperacillin/tazobactam
  ◦ Cefepime (or ceftazidime)
  ◦ Imipenem
  ◦ Meropenem (or doripenem)
— Alternatively, in high-risk patients, a combination of agents such as vancomycin plus one of the following agents:
  ◦ Piperacillin/tazobactam
  ◦ Cefepime (or ceftazidime)
  ◦ Imipenem
  ◦ Meropenem
  ◦ Aztreonam plus an aminoglycoside
  ◦ Ciprofloxacin plus an aminoglycoside
— Carefully selected outpatients determined to be at low risk by a validated risk index (MASCC score or Talcott rules) can be treated with
  ◦ Oral fluoroquinolone plus amoxicillin/clavulanate
    or, if penicillin allergic
  ◦ Oral fluoroquinolone plus clindamycin,
    Exception: Patients receiving fluoroquinolone prophylaxis before fever developed
• If a fungal infection is suspected, add fluconazole or amphotericin B

Therapeutic Procedures
• Most fever is well tolerated
• When temperature is < 40°C, symptomatic treatment
• When temperature is > 41°C, emergent management of hyperthermia is indicated
— Alcohol sponges
— Cold sponges
— Ice bags
— Ice-water enemas
— Ice baths

8. Outcome

Prognosis
• After extensive evaluation
— 25% of patients with FUO have chronic or indolent infection
— 25% have autoimmune disease
— 10% have malignancy
— The remainder have other miscellaneous disorders or no definitive diagnosis
• Long-term follow-up of patients with initially undiagnosed FUO demonstrates that
— 50% become symptom-free during evaluation
— 20% reach a definitive diagnosis (usually within 2 months)
— 30% have persistent or recurring fever for months or years

9. When to Refer and When to Admit

When to Refer
• Once the diagnosis of FUO is made, referral to infectious disease specialist or rheumatologist may be appropriate to guide specific additional tests

When to Admit
• Neuroleptic malignant syndrome; serotonin syndrome; malignant hyperthermia of anesthesia
• Heat stroke
• For measures to control temperature when it is above 41°C or when fever is associated with seizure or other mental status changes

SUGGESTED REFERENCES

Affronti M et al. Low-grade fever: how to distinguish organic from non-organic forms. *Int J Clin Pract*. 2010 Feb;64(3):316–321. [PMID: 20456171]

Hocker SE et al. Indicators of central fever in the neurologic intensive care unit. *JAMA Neurol*. 2013 Dec;70(12):1499–1504. [PMID: 24100963]

Kim YJ et al. Diagnostic value of 18F-FDG PET/CT in patients with fever of unknown origin. *Intern Med J*. 2012 Jul;42(7):834–837. [PMID: 22805689]

Siikamäki HM et al. Fever in travelers returning from malaria-endemic areas: don't look for malaria only. *J Travel Med*. 2011 Jul–Aug;18(4):239-244. [PMID: 21722234]

Worth LJ et al; Australian Consensus Guidelines 2011 Steering Committee. Use of risk stratification to guide ambulatory management of neutropenic fever. *Intern Med J*. 2011 Jan;41(1b):82–89. [PMID: 21272172]

77

HIV-AIDS

A 31-year-old male injection drug user presents to the emergency department with a chief complaint of shortness of breath. He describes a 1-month history of intermittent fevers and night sweats associated with a nonproductive cough. He has become progressively more short of breath, initially only with exertion, but now he feels dyspneic at rest. He appears to be in moderate respiratory distress. His vital signs are abnormal, with fever to 39°C, heart rate of 112 bpm, respiratory rate of 20/min, and oxygen saturation of 88% on room air. Physical examination is otherwise unremarkable. Notably, the lung examination is normal. Chest x-ray film reveals a diffuse interstitial infiltrate in a "bat's wing" or "butterfly" pattern.

LEARNING OBJECTIVES

► Learn the clinical manifestations and objective findings of HIV
► Understand the factors that predispose to HIV
► Know the differential diagnosis of HIV
► Learn the treatment for HIV
► Know how to prevent HIV and related complications

QUESTIONS

1. What are the salient features of this patient's problem?

2. How do you think through his problem?

3. What are the key features, including essentials of diagnosis, general considerations, and demographics, of HIV?

4. What are the symptoms and signs of HIV?

5. What is the differential diagnosis of HIV?

6. What are laboratory and procedural findings in HIV?

7. What are the treatments for HIV?

8. What are the outcomes, including follow-up, prognosis, and prevention, of HIV?

9. When should patients with HIV be referred to a specialist or admitted to the hospital?

ANSWERS

1. Salient Features

Injection drug use; 1-month duration of intermittent fevers and night sweats; pneumonia symptoms (slowly progressive dyspnea, fever, tachycardia, hypoxia) and abnormal chest radiograph suggesting a possible opportunistic infection

2. How to Think Through

What are the broad categories in the differential diagnosis for this presentation—1 month of fevers, night sweats, cough, dyspnea, and hypoxia? Among infections, what are possible causes? Could this be a typical bacterial pneumonia? (Unlikely, given the duration.) How about TB or a fungal infection (eg, coccidioidomycosis)? What elements of the case strongly suggest pneumocystis? (The x-ray pattern, hypoxia despite normal lung sounds.) At what CD4+ T-cell count does pneumocystis become more likely? (< 200 cells/μL). How is the diagnosis of pneumocystis definitively made? (Sputum induction or bronchoscopy.)

When unusual infections enter the differential, one MUST think of HIV—even in the absence of known risk factors. Which test is used to diagnose HIV and which to confirm the diagnosis? (HIV antibody by ELISA, confirmed by Western blot) When, after exposure, is HIV antibody detectable? (95% of persons develop antibodies within 6 weeks after infection) At what CD4+ T-cell count is the diagnosis of AIDS made? (< 200/μL). If this patient's CD4 count is 50 cells/μL, what other infectious and noninfectious complications might he develop? (See below and generate a list for each of the following organ systems: ocular, oral, pulmonary, gastrointestinal, hepatic and biliary, central and peripheral nervous system, endocrine, cutaneous, malignancies.)

3. Key Features

Essentials of Diagnosis
- Risk factors include
  - Sexual contact with an infected person
  - Parenteral exposure to infected blood by transfusion or needle sharing
  - Perinatal exposure
- Prominent systemic complaints such as sweats, diarrhea, weight loss, and wasting
- Opportunistic infections
  - Due to diminished cellular immunity
  - Often life-threatening
- Aggressive cancers, particularly Kaposi sarcoma, and extranodal lymphoma
- Neurologic manifestations
  - Dementia
  - Aseptic meningitis
  - Neuropathy

General Considerations
- Etiology: HIV-1, a retrovirus
- Definition: Centers for Disease Control and Prevention AIDS case definition (Table 77-1)

Demographics
- An estimated 1,201,100 Americans aged 13 years or older are infected with HIV
- There are about 50, 000 new infections each year
- An estimated 494,602 persons in the United States are living with AIDS
  - Of those, 76% are men, of whom 64% were exposed through male-to-male sexual contact, 15% were exposed through injection drug use, 11% were exposed through heterosexual contact, and 8% were exposed through male-to-male sexual contact and injection drug use

Table 77-1. CDC AIDS case definition for surveillance of adults and adolescents.

Definitive AIDS Diagnoses (With or Without Laboratory Evidence of HIV Infection)

1. Candidiasis of the esophagus, trachea, bronchi, or lungs
2. Cryptococcosis, extrapulmonary
3. Cryptosporidiosis with diarrhea persisting > 1 mo
4. Cytomegalovirus disease of an organ other than liver, spleen, or lymph nodes
5. Herpes simplex virus infection causing a mucocutaneous ulcer that persists longer than 1 mo; or bronchitis, pneumonitis, or esophagitis of any duration
6. Kaposi sarcoma in a patient < 60 y of age
7. Lymphoma of the brain (primary) in a patient < 60 y of age
8. *Mycobacterium avium* complex or *M kansasii* disease, disseminated (at a site other than or in addition to lungs, skin, or cervical or hilar lymph nodes)
9. *Pneumocystis jiroveci* pneumonia
10. Progressive multifocal leukoencephalopathy
11. Toxoplasmosis of the brain

Definitive AIDS Diagnoses (With Laboratory Evidence of HIV Infection)

1. Coccidioidomycosis, disseminated (at a site other than or in addition to lungs or cervical or hilar lymph nodes)
2. HIV encephalopathy
3. Histoplasmosis, disseminated (at a site other than or in addition to lungs or cervical or hilar lymph nodes)
4. Isosporiasis with diarrhea persisting > 1 mo
5. Kaposi sarcoma at any age
6. Lymphoma of the brain (primary) at any age
7. Other non-Hodgkin lymphoma of B cell or unknown immunologic phenotype
8. Any mycobacterial disease caused by mycobacteria other than *Mycobacterium tuberculosis*, disseminated (at a site other than or in addition to lungs, skin, or cervical or hilar lymph nodes)
9. Disease caused by extrapulmonary *M tuberculosis*
10. *Salmonella* (nontyphoid) septicemia, recurrent
11. HIV wasting syndrome
12. CD4 lymphocyte count below 200 cells/μL or a CD4 lymphocyte percentage < 14%
13. Pulmonary tuberculosis
14. Recurrent pneumonia
15. Invasive cervical cancer

Presumptive AIDS Diagnoses (With Laboratory Evidence of HIV Infection)

1. Candidiasis of esophagus: (a) recent onset of retrosternal pain on swallowing; and (b) oral candidiasis
2. Cytomegalovirus retinitis. A characteristic appearance on serial ophthalmoscopic examinations
3. Mycobacteriosis. Specimen from stool or normally sterile body fluids or tissue from a site other than lungs, skin, or cervical or hilar lymph nodes, showing acid-fast bacilli of a species not identified by culture
4. Kaposi sarcoma. Erythematous or violaceous plaque-like lesion on skin or mucous membrane
5. *Pneumocystis jiroveci* pneumonia: (a) a history of dyspnea on exertion or nonproductive cough of recent onset (within the past 3 mo); and (b) chest x-ray evidence of diffuse bilateral interstitial infiltrates or gallium scan evidence of diffuse bilateral pulmonary disease; and (c) arterial blood gas analysis showing an arterial oxygen partial pressure of < 70 mm Hg or a low respiratory diffusing capacity of < 80% of predicted values or an increase in the alveolar-arterial oxygen tension gradient; and (d) no evidence of a bacterial pneumonia
6. Toxoplasmosis of the brain: (a) recent onset of a focal neurologic abnormality consistent with intracranial disease or a reduced level of consciousness; and (b) brain imaging evidence of a lesion having a mass effect or the radiographic appearance of which is enhanced by injection of contrast medium; and (c) serum antibody to toxoplasmosis or successful response to therapy for toxoplasmosis
7. Recurrent pneumonia: (a) more than one episode in a 1-y period; and (b) acute pneumonia (new symptoms, signs, or radiologic evidence not present earlier) diagnosed on clinical or radiologic grounds by the patient's clinician
8. Pulmonary tuberculosis: (a) apical or miliary infiltrates and (b) radiographic and clinical response to antituberculous therapy

— Women account for 24% of living persons with HIV infection, of whom 69% were infected through heterosexual contact, and 28% were exposed through injection drug use

4. Symptoms and Signs

- HIV-related infections and neoplasms affect virtually every organ
- Many HIV-infected persons remain asymptomatic for years even without antiretroviral therapy: mean of ~10 years between infection with HIV and development of AIDS
- Symptoms protean and nonspecific
- Fever, night sweats, and weight loss
- Shortness of breath, cough, and fever from pneumonia
- Anorexia, nausea and vomiting, and increased metabolic rate contribute to weight loss
- Diarrhea from bacterial, viral, or parasitic infections
- Physical examination may be normal
- Conditions highly suggestive of HIV infection
  - Hairy leukoplakia of the tongue
  - Disseminated Kaposi sarcoma
  - Cutaneous bacillary angiomatosis
  - Generalized lymphadenopathy early in infection
- Ocular
  - Cytomegalovirus (CMV)
  - Herpesvirus
  - Toxoplasmosis retinitis
- Oral
  - Candidiasis, pseudomembranous (removable white plaques) and erythematous (red friable plaques)
  - Hairy leukoplakia
  - Angular cheilitis
  - Gingivitis or periodontitis
  - Aphthous ulcers
  - Kaposi sarcoma (usually on the hard palate)
  - Warts
- Sinuses: chronic sinusitis
- Lungs
  - Bacterial (eg, *Streptococcus pneumoniae, Haemophilus influenzae*)
  - Mycobacterial (eg, *M tuberculosis, M avium* complex [MAC])
  - Fungal (eg, *P jiroveci*)
  - Viral pneumonias
  - Noninfectious
    - Kaposi sarcoma
    - Non-Hodgkin lymphoma
    - Interstitial pneumonitis
- Gastrointestinal
  - Esophagitis (*Candida*, herpes simplex, CMV)
  - Gastropathy
  - Malabsorption
- Enterocolitis
  - Bacteria (*Campylobacter, Salmonella, Shigella*)
  - Viruses (CMV, adenovirus, HIV)
  - Protozoans (*Cryptosporidium, Entamoeba histolytica, Giardia, Isospora, Microsporidia*)
- Hepatic
  - Liver infections (mycobacterial, CMV, hepatitis B and C viruses) and neoplasms (lymphoma)
  - Medication-related hepatitis

- Biliary
  - Cholecystitis
  - Sclerosing cholangitis
  - Papillary stenosis (CMV, *Cryptosporidium*, and *Microsporidia*)
- Central nervous system (CNS)
  - Intracerebral space-occupying lesions
    - Toxoplasmosis
    - Bacterial and *Nocardia* abscesses
    - Cryptococcomas
    - Tuberculomas
  - HIV encephalopathy
  - Meningitis
  - CNS (non-Hodgkin) lymphoma
  - Progressive multifocal leukoencephalopathy (PML)
- Spinal cord: HIV myelopathy
- Peripheral nervous system
  - Inflammatory polyneuropathies, sensory neuropathies, and mononeuropathies
  - CMV polyradiculopathy
  - Transverse myelitis (herpes zoster or CMV)
- Endocrinologic
  - Adrenal insufficiency from infection (eg, CMV and MAC), infiltration (Kaposi sarcoma), hemorrhage, and presumed autoimmune injury
  - Isolated mineralocorticoid defect
  - Thyroid function test abnormalities (high T_3, T_4, and thyroxine-binding globulin, and low reverse-T_3)
- Gynecologic
  - Vaginal candidiasis
  - Cervical dysplasia and carcinoma
  - Pelvic inflammatory disease
- Malignancies
  - Kaposi sarcoma
  - Non-Hodgkin and Hodgkin lymphoma
  - Primary CNS lymphoma
  - Cervical dysplasia and invasive cervical carcinoma
  - Anal dysplasia and squamous cell carcinoma
- Skin
  - Viral
    - Herpes simplex
    - Herpes zoster
    - Molluscum contagiosum
  - Bacterial
    - *Staphylococcus* folliculitis, furuncles, bullous impetigo, dissemination with sepsis
    - Bacillary angiomatosis caused by *Bartonella henselae* and *B quintana*
  - Fungal
    - *Candida*
    - Dermatophytes
    - *Malassezia furfur/Pityrosporum ovale* seborrheic dermatitis
  - Neoplastic (Kaposi sarcoma)
  - Nonspecific (psoriasis, severe pruritus, and xerosis) dermatitides
- Musculoskeletal
  - Myopathy
  - Arthritis of single or multiple joints, with or without effusions
  - Reactive arthritis (Reiter syndrome)

— Psoriatic arthritis
— Sicca syndrome
— Systemic lupus erythematosus

5. Differential Diagnosis

• Depends on mode of presentation

Constitutional symptoms

— Cancer
— Tuberculosis
— Endocarditis
— Endocrinologic diseases (eg, hyperthyroidism)
• Pulmonary processes
— Acute and chronic lung infections
— Other causes of diffuse interstitial pulmonary infiltrates
• Neurologic disease
— Causes of mental status changes
— Causes of neuropathy
• Diarrhea
— Infectious enterocolitis
— Antibiotic-associated colitis
— Inflammatory bowel disease
— Malabsorption syndromes

6. Laboratory and Procedural Findings

Laboratory Tests

• See Table 77-2
• HIV antibody by ELISA, confirmed by Western blot (sensitivity > 99.9%, specificity ~100%)
• About 95% of persons develop antibodies within 6 weeks after infection
• Absolute CD4 lymphocyte count: as counts decrease, risk of serious opportunistic infection increases

Table 77-2. Laboratory findings with HIV infection.

Test	Significance
HIV enzyme-linked immunosorbent assay (ELISA)	Screening test for HIV infection. Of ELISA tests, 50% are positive within 22 d after HIV transmission; 95% are positive within 6 wk after transmission. Sensitivity > 99.9%; to avoid false-positive results, repeatedly reactive results must be confirmed with Western blot
Western blot	Confirmatory test for HIV. Specificity when combined with ELISA > 99.99%. Indeterminate results with early HIV infection, HIV-2 infection, autoimmune disease, pregnancy, and recent tetanus toxoid administration
HIV rapid antibody test	Screening test for HIV. Produces results in 10 to 20 min. Can be performed by personnel with limited training. Positive results must be confirmed with standard HIV test (ELISA and Western blot)
Complete blood count	Anemia, neutropenia, and thrombocytopenia common with advanced HIV infection
Absolute CD4 lymphocyte count	Most widely used predictor of HIV progression. Risk of progression to an AIDS opportunistic infection or malignancy is high with CD4 < 200 cells/μL in the absence of treatment
CD4 lymphocyte percentage	Percentage may be more reliable than the CD4 count. Risk of progression to an AIDS opportunistic infection or malignancy is high with percentage < 14% in the absence of treatment
HIV viral load tests	These tests measure the amount of actively replicating HIV virus. Correlate with disease progression and response to antiretroviral drugs. Best tests available for diagnosis of acute HIV infection (prior to seroconversion); however, caution is warranted when the test result shows low-level viremia (ie, < 500 copies/mL) as this may represent a false-positive test

Diagnostic Procedures

- For *P jiroveci* pneumonia
  — Arterial blood gases
  — Serum lactate dehydrogenase
  — Chest radiograph
  — Wright–Giemsa stain of induced sputum
  — Bronchoalveolar lavage
  — Diffusing capacity of carbon monoxide (DLco)
  — High-resolution CT scan
- For CNS toxoplasmosis
  — Head CT scan
  — Stereotactic brain biopsy
- For cryptococcal meningitis
  — Cerebrospinal fluid (CSF) culture
  — CSF, serum cryptococcal antigen (CRAG)
- For HIV meningitis: CSF cell count
- For HIV myelopathy
  — Lumbar puncture
  — Head MRI or CT scan
- For AIDS dementia complex, depression: neuropsychiatric testing
- For myopathy
  — Serum creatine kinase
  — Muscle biopsy
- For hepatic dysfunction
  — Percutaneous liver biopsy
  — Blood culture
  — Biopsy of a more accessible site
- For enterocolitis
- Stool culture and multiple ova and parasite examinations
- Colonoscopy and biopsy

7. Treatments

Medications

- Fever: antipyretics
- Anorexia: megestrol acetate, 80 mg four times daily orally or dronabinol, 2.5 to 5.0 mg three times daily
- Weight loss
  — Food supplementation with high-calorie drinks
  — Growth hormone, 0.1 mg/kg/d subcutaneously for 12 weeks, or anabolic steroids—oxandrolone, 15 to 20 mg orally in 2 to 4 divided doses
  — Testosterone enanthate or cypionate, 100 to 200 mg intramuscularly every 2 to 4 weeks, or testosterone patches or gel
- Nausea
  — Prochlorperazine, 10 mg three times daily orally before every meal
  — Metoclopramide, 10 mg three times daily orally before every meal
  — Ondansetron, 8 mg three times daily orally before every meal
  — Dronabinol, 5 mg three times daily, or medical cannabis
  — Empiric oral antifungal agent
- It is now recommended that antiretroviral treatment be started in all HIV-infected persons regardless of CD4 count due to the recognition that HIV damages the immune system from the beginning of infection even when the damage is not easily measured by conventional tests
- Resistance testing is recommended for all patients prior to initiating ART
- Presence of an acute opportunistic infection does not preclude the initiation of ART (Table 77-3)

Table 77–3. Antiretroviral therapy.

Medication	Dose	Common Side Effects	Special Monitoring[a]
Nucleoside reverse transcriptase inhibitors			
Abacavir (Ziagen)	300 mg orally twice daily	Rash, fever—if occur, rechallenge may be fatal	No special monitoring
Didanosine (ddI) (Videx)	400 mg orally daily (enteric-coated capsule) for persons ≥ 60 kg	Peripheral neuropathy, pancreatitis, dry mouth, hepatitis	Bimonthly neurologic questionnaire for neuropathy, K$^+$, amylase, bilirubin, triglycerides
Emtricitabine (Emtriva)	200 mg orally once daily	Skin discoloration palms/soles (mild)	No special monitoring
Lamivudine (3TC) (Epivir)	150 mg orally twice daily or 300 mg daily	Rash, peripheral neuropathy	No special monitoring
Stavudine (d4T) (Zerit)	40 mg orally twice daily for persons ≥ 60 kg	Peripheral neuropathy, hepatitis, pancreatitis	Monthly neurologic questionnaire for neuropathy, amylase
Zidovudine (AZT) (Retrovir)	600 mg orally daily in two divided doses	Anemia, neutropenia, nausea, malaise, headache, insomnia, myopathy	No special monitoring
Nucleotide reverse transcriptase inhibitors			
Tenofovir (Viread)	300 mg orally once daily	Gastrointestinal distress	Creatinine every 3–4 mo, urine analysis every 6–12 mo
Nonnucleoside reverse transcriptase inhibitors (NNRTIs)			
Delavirdine (Rescriptor)	400 mg orally three times daily	Rash	No special monitoring
Efavirenz (Sustiva)	600 mg orally daily	Neurologic disturbances, rash	No special monitoring
Etravirine (Intelence)	200 mg orally twice daily	Rash, peripheral neuropathy	No special monitoring
Nevirapine (Viramune)	200 mg orally daily for 2 wk, then 200 mg orally twice daily	Rash	No special monitoring
Rilpivirine (Edurant)	25 mg daily	Depression, rash	No special monitoring
Protease inhibitors (PIs)			
Fosamprenavir (Lexiva)	**For PI-experienced patients:** 700 mg orally twice daily and 100 mg of ritonavir orally twice daily. **For PI-naïve patients:** above or 1400 mg orally twice daily or 1400 mg orally once daily and 200 mg of ritonavir orally once daily	Gastrointestinal, rash	No special monitoring
Indinavir (Crixivan)	800 mg orally three times daily	Renal calculi	Bilirubin level every 3–4 mo
Lopinavir/ritonavir (Kaletra)	400 mg/100 mg orally twice daily	Diarrhea	No special monitoring
Nelfinavir (Viracept)	750 mg orally three times daily or 1250 mg twice daily	Diarrhea	No special monitoring
Ritonavir (Norvir)	600 mg orally twice daily or in lower doses (eg, 100 mg orally once or twice daily) for boosting other PIs	Gastrointestinal distress, peripheral paresthesias	No special monitoring
Saquinavir hard gel (Invirase)	1000 mg orally twice daily with 100 mg ritonavir orally twice daily	Gastrointestinal distress	No special monitoring
Atazanavir (Reyataz)	400 mg orally once daily or 300 mg atazanavir with 100 mg ritonavir daily.	Hyperbilirubinemia	Bilirubin level every 3–4 mo
Darunavir/ritonavir (Prezista/Norvir)	**For PI-experienced patients:** 600 mg of darunavir and 100 mg of ritonavir orally twice daily. **For PI-naïve patients:** 800 mg of darunavir and 100 mg of ritonavir orally daily.	Rash	No special monitoring
Tipranavir/ritonavir (Aptivus/Norvir)	500 mg of tipranavir and 200 mg of ritonavir orally twice daily	Gastrointestinal, rash	No special monitoring

(continued)

Table 77–3. Antiretroviral therapy. (continued)

Medication	Dose	Common Side Effects	Special Monitoring[a]
Entry inhibitors			
Enfuvirtide (Fuzeon)	90 mg subcutaneously twice daily	Injection site pain and allergic reaction	No special monitoring
Maraviroc (Selzentry)	150–300 mg orally daily	Cough, fever, rash	No special monitoring
Integrase inhibitors			
Raltegravir (Isentress)	400 mg orally twice daily	Diarrhea, nausea, headache	No special monitoring
Elvitegravir (available only in a fixed medication combination with cobicistat, tenofovir, emtricitabine, Stribild)	Elvitegravir 150 mg+ Cobicistat 150 mg+ Tenofovir 300 mg+ Emtricitabine 200 mg (One tablet daily)	Serum elevation of creatinine, diarrhea, rash	Creatinine every 3–4 mo; urine analysis at initiation and first follow-up.
Dolutegravir (Tivicay)	Treatment-naïve or integrase-naïve patients: 50 mg daily. When administered with efavirenz, forsamprenavir/ritonavir, tipranavir/ritonavir, or rifampin: 50 mg twice daily. When administered to integrase-experienced patients with suspected integrase resistance: 50 mg twice daily.	Hypersensitivity, rash	No special monitoring

[a]Standard monitoring is complete blood count (CBC) and differential, serum aminotransferases every 3–4 mo, and cholesterol (total, LDL, HDL), and triglycerides 6 mo after starting ART and annually among those over age 40 y.

Average wholesale price (AWP, for AB-rated generic when available) for quantity listed. Source: *Red Book Online, 2013, Truven Health Analytics, Inc.* AWP may not accurately represent the actual pharmacy cost because wide contractual variations exist among institutions.

- Antiretrovirals should never be used alone as a single agent, and at least three active agents should be used at all times
- Most clinicians use fixed-dose combinations (see Tables 77–4 and 77-5) which can be given once a day.
- The primary goal of therapy should be complete suppression of viral replication as measured by the serum viral load
- See Figure 77-1 for an approach to initial and subsequent antiretroviral therapy.
- See Table 77-6 for treatment of common opportunistic infections and malignancies

Table 77–4. Fixed dose antiretroviral combinations.

Name	Components	Dosing and Special Considerations	Cost Per Month
Truvada	Tenofovir 300 mg Emtricitabine 200 mg	One pill daily with an NNRTI, protease inhibitor, integrase inhibitor, or maraviroc (entry inhibitor). Most commonly used nucleoside/nucleotide reverse transcriptase inhibitor backbone	$1539.90
Epzicom	Abacavir 600 mg Lamivudine 300 mg	One pill daily with a NNRTI, protease inhibitor, integrase inhibitor, or maraviroc (entry inhibitor)	$1324.93
Trizivir	Abacavir 300 mg Lamivudine 150 mg Zidovudine 300 mg	One tablet twice daily with a NNRTI, protease inhibitor, integrase inhibitor, or maraviroc (entry inhibitor). Although it contains three medications it does not constitute a complete treatment	$1931.64
Atripla	Tenofovir 300 mg Emtricitabine 200 mg Efavirenz 600 mg	One pill daily constitutes a complete regimen	$2402.04
Stribild	Tenofovir 300 mg Emtricitabine 200 mg Elvitegravir 150 mg Cobicistat 150 mg	One pill daily constitutes a complete regimen. Although it contains four medications, one component (Cobicistat) is a medication booster only	$2948.70
Complera	Tenofovir 300 mg Emtricitabine 200 mg Rilpivirine 25 mg	One pill daily constitutes complete regimen. Only for patients with HIV viral load < 100,000/mL	$2463.37

Table 77-5. Recommended initial antiretroviral regimens.[a]

Regimen	Advantages	Disadvantages
Atripla (tenofovir/ emtricitabine/efavirenz)	Single tablet once-a-day regimen Longest term clinical experience Highly effective across broad range of initial CD4 counts and viral loads	Avoid in patients with transmitted K103N Neuropsychiatric symptoms common and can be persistent
Epzicom (abacavir/lamivudine) + efavirenz (600 mg daily)[b]	Can be used instead of Atripla in patients who should be spared tenofovir because of decreased creatinine clearance or use of other nephrotoxic drugs.	Less effective than Atripla for patients with viral load greater than 100,000/µL Avoid in patients with transmitted K103N. Neuropsychiatric symptoms common and can be persistent. Abacavir should only be used in HLA-B*5701 – negative patients.
Complera (tenofovir/ emtricitabine/rilpivirine)	Single tablet once-a-day regimen Noninferior to Atripla in patients with baseline viral load less than 100,000/µL Limited metabolic side effects	Requires taking with a meal Cannot be used with proton-pump inhibitors Do not use in patients with viral loads greater than 100,000/µL
Atazanavir (300 mg daily) with ritonavir (100 mg daily) boosting + Truvada (emtricitabine/tenofovir)	Once-a-day regimen Limited risk of resistance with poor adherence Resistance to atazanavir generally does not confer resistance to other PI	Not available as a single tablet Increases in bilirubin (nonpathologic) Increased risk of cholelithiasis, nephrolithiasis, and chronic kidney injury. Has metabolic side effects. Should be taken with food and H2-blockers and proton pumps should be avoided.
Atazanavir (300 mg daily) with ritonavir (100 mg daily) boosting + Epzicom (abacavir/lamivudine)	Limited risk of resistance with poor adherence Resistance to atazanavir generally does not confer resistance to other PI	Not available as a single table Increases in bilirubin (nonpathologic) Increase in cholelithiasis, nephrolithiasis, and chronic kidney injury. Has metabolic side effects Abacavir should only be used in HLA-B*5701- negative patients
Darunavir (800 mg daily) with ritonavir (100 mg daily) boosting + Truvada (emtricitabine/tenofovir)	Potent boosted PI Can be given once daily Limited risk of resistance with poor adherence	Not available as a single tablet May cause rash in patients with sulfa allergy Ritonavir boosting required Has metabolic side effects
Raltegravir (400 mg twice daily) + Truvada (emtricitabine/ tenofovir)	Metabolically neutral Superior to Atripla over 5-y of follow-up	Requires twice a day dosing No single tablet available
Stribild (emtricitabine/ tenofovir/elvitegravir with cobicistat boosting)	Single tablet once-a-day regimen Excellent response across broad range of CD4 and viral loads	Cobicistat boosting causes similar drug–drug interactions as ritonavir; increases in serum creatinine (nonpathologic); requires estimated glomerular filtration rate equal to or greater than 70 mL/min
Dolutegravir (50 mg daily)+ Epzicom (abacavir/ lamivudine)	A single once-a-day tablet will soon be available Has activity in some patients with integrase resistance Superior to Atripla; Dolutegravir plus either Epzicom or Truvada was superior to darunavir/ritonavir plus either Epzicom or Truvada	Abacavir should be used only in HLA-B*5701- negative persons. When used in patients with integrase resistance or combined with certain other medications, requires twice a day dosing. Avoid antacids and other medications with divalent cations (Ca^{2+},Mg++, Al++, Fe++)
Dolutegravir (50 mg daily)+ emtricitabine/ tenofovir	Has activity in some patients with integrase resistance. Once-a-day regimen	No single tablet available. When used in patients with integrase resistance or combined with certain other medications, requires twice a day dosing Avoid antacids and other medications with divalent cations (Ca^{2+},Mg++, Al++, Fe++)

[a]These 10 regimens have been recommended by the USA Panel of the International Antiviral Society.

[b]Usual medication doses are supplied when not part of a fixed dose preparation

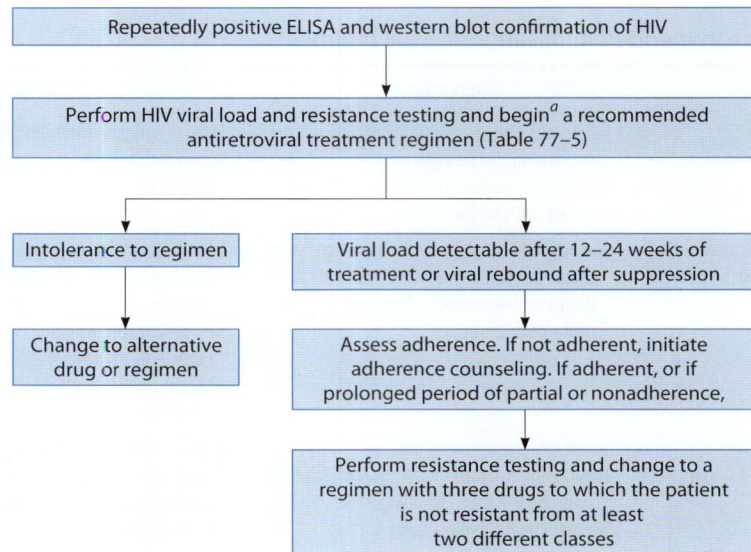

Figure 77–1. Approach to initial and subsequent antiretroviral therapy.

Table 77–6. Treatment of AIDS-related opportunistic infections and malignancies.[a]

Infection or Malignancy	Treatment	Complications
Pneumocystis jirovecii infection[b]	Trimethoprim-sulfamethoxazole, 15 mg/kg/d (based on trimethoprim component) orally or intravenously for 14–21 d	Nausea, neutropenia, anemia, hepatitis, rash, Stevens–Johnson syndrome
	Pentamidine, 3–4 mg/kg/d intravenously for 14–21 d	Hypotension, hypoglycemia, anemia, neutropenia, pancreatitis, hepatitis
	Trimethoprim, 15 mg/kg/d orally, with dapsone, 100 mg/d orally, for 14–21 d[3]	Nausea, rash, hemolytic anemia in G6PD[c]-deficient patients Methemoglobinemia (weekly levels should be < 10% of total hemoglobin)
	Primaquine, 15–30 mg/d orally, and clindamycin, 600 mg every 8 h orally, for 14–21 d	Hemolytic anemia in G6PD-deficient patients Methemoglobinemia, neutropenia, colitis
	Atovaquone, 750 mg orally three times daily for 14–21 d	Rash, elevated aminotransferases, anemia, neutropenia
	Trimetrexate, 45 mg/m² intravenously for 21 d (given with leucovorin calcium) if intolerant of all other regimens	Leukopenia, rash, mucositis
Mycobacterium avium complex infection	Clarithromycin, 500 mg orally twice daily with ethambutol, 15 mg/kg/d orally (maximum, 1 g). May also add:	Clarithromycin: hepatitis, nausea, diarrhea; ethambutol: hepatitis, optic neuritis
	Rifabutin, 300 mg orally daily	Rash, hepatitis, uveitis
Toxoplasmosis	Pyrimethamine, 100–200 mg orally as loading dose, followed by 50–75 mg/d, combined with sulfadiazine, 4–6 g orally daily in four divided doses, and folinic acid, 10 mg orally daily for 4–8 wk; then pyrimethamine, 25–50 mg/d, with clindamycin, 2–2.7 g/d in three or four divided doses, and folinic acid, 5 mg/d, until clinical and radiographic resolution is achieved	Leukopenia, rash
Lymphoma	Combination chemotherapy (eg, modified CHOP, M-BACOD, with or without G-CSF or GM-CSF). Central nervous system disease: radiation treatment with dexamethasone for edema	Nausea, vomiting, anemia, leukopenia, cardiac toxicity (with doxorubicin)
Cryptococcal meningitis	Amphotericin B, 0.6 mg/kg/d intravenously, with or without flucytosine, 100 mg/kg/d orally in four divided doses for 2 wk, followed by:	Fever, anemia, hypokalemia, azotemia
	Fluconazole, 400 mg orally daily for 6 wk, then 200 mg orally daily	Hepatitis

(continued)

Table 77–6. Treatment of AIDS-related opportunistic infections and malignancies.[a] (continued)

Infection or Malignancy	Treatment	Complications
Cytomegalovirus infection	Valganciclovir, 900 mg orally twice a day for 21 d with food (induction), followed by 900 mg daily with food (maintenance)	Neutropenia, anemia, thrombocytopenia
	Ganciclovir, 10 mg/kg/d intravenously in two divided doses for 10 d, followed by 6 mg/kg 5 d a week indefinitely. (Decrease dose for kidney disease.) May use ganciclovir as maintenance therapy (1 g orally with fatty foods three times a day)	Neutropenia (especially when used concurrently with zidovudine), anemia, thrombocytopenia
	Foscarnet, 60 mg/kg intravenously every 8 h for 10–14 d (induction), followed by 90 mg/kg once daily. (Adjust for changes in kidney function)	Nausea, hypokalemia, hypocalcemia, hyperphosphatemia, azotemia
Esophageal candidiasis or recurrent vaginal candidiasis	Fluconazole, 100–200 mg orally daily for 10–14 d	Hepatitis, development of imidazole resistance
Herpes simplex infection	Acyclovir, 400 mg orally three times daily until healed; or acyclovir, 5 mg/kg intravenously every 8 h for severe cases	Resistant herpes simplex with long-term therapy
	Famciclovir, 500 mg orally twice daily until healed	Nausea
	Valacyclovir, 500 mg orally twice daily until healed	Nausea
	Foscarnet, 40 mg/kg intravenously every 8 h, for acyclovir-resistant cases. (Adjust for changes in kidney function)	Nausea, hypokalemia, hypocalcemia, hyperphosphatemia, azotemia
Herpes zoster	Acyclovir, 800 mg orally four or five times daily for 7 d. Intravenous therapy at 10 mg/kg every 8 h for ocular involvement, disseminated disease	Resistant herpes simplex with long-term therapy
	Famciclovir, 500 mg orally three times daily for 7 d	Nausea
	Valacyclovir, 500 mg orally three times daily for 7 d	Nausea
	Foscarnet, 40 mg/kg intravenously every 8 h for acyclovir-resistant cases. (Adjust for changes in kidney function)	Nausea, hypokalemia, hypocalcemia, hyperphosphatemia, azotemia
Kaposi sarcoma		
Limited cutaneous disease	Observation, intralesional vinblastine	Inflammation, pain at site of injection
Extensive or aggressive cutaneous disease	Systemic chemotherapy (eg, liposomal doxorubicin). Interferon-alfa (for patients with CD4 > 200 cells/μL and no constitutional symptoms). Radiation (amelioration of edema)	Bone marrow suppression, peripheral neuritis, flu-like syndrome
Visceral disease (eg, pulmonary)	Combination chemotherapy (eg, daunorubicin, bleomycin, vinblastine)	Bone marrow suppression, cardiac toxicity, fever

[a]For treatment of *M tuberculosis* infection, see Chapter 9.

[b]For moderate-to-severe *P jirovecii* infection (oxygen saturation < 90%), corticosteroids should be given with specific treatment. The dose of prednisone is 40 mg orally twice daily for 5 d, then 40 mg daily for 5 d, and then 20 mg daily until therapy is complete.

[c]When considering use of dapsone, check glucose-6-phosphate dehydrogenase (G6PD) level in black patients and those of Mediterranean origin.

CHOP, cyclophosphamide, doxorubicin (hydroxydaunomycin), vincristine (Oncovin), and prednisone; G-CSF, granulocyte-colony stimulating factor (filgrastim); GM-CSF, granulocyte-macrophage colony-stimulating factor (sargramostim); modified M-BACOD, methotrexate, bleomycin, doxorubicin (Adriamycin), cyclophosphamide, vincristine (Oncovin), and dexamethasone.

8. Outcomes

Follow-Up
- CD4 cell count and HIV viral load 1 to 2 months after initiation or change in ART, then every 3 to 6 months in stable patients
- Health care maintenance (see Table 77-7)

Prognosis
- The efficacy of antiretroviral treatments—especially protease inhibitors and nonnucleoside reverse transcriptase inhibitors—has improved prognosis
- The life expectancy of HIV-infected persons approaches that of the uninfected if treatment is initiated early in the course of the disease

Table 77-7. Health care maintenance of HIV-infected individuals.

For all HIV-infected individuals:
CD4 counts every 3–6 mo (Can decrease to every 12 mo if viral load suppressed on ART for 2 y and CD4 count > 300 cells)
Viral load tests every 3–6 mo and 1 mo following a change in therapy
Genotypic resistance testing at baseline and if viral load not fully suppressed and patient taking ART.
Complete blood count, chemistry profile, fasting glucose or hemoglobin A1C, liver function tests, creatinine, BUN, urinalysis at baseline.
Cholesterol and triglycerides at baseline, 6–12 mo after starting antiretroviral therapy, and annually for everyone over 40 y of age
PPD annually
INH for those with positive PPD and normal chest radiograph
RPR or VDRL
Toxoplasma IgG serology at baseline
Hepatitis serologies: hepatitis A antibody, hepatitis B surface antigen, hepatitis B surface antibody, hepatitis B core antibody, hepatitis C antibody
Pneumococcal vaccine
Inactivated influenza vaccine annually in season
Hepatitis A vaccine for those without immunity to hepatitis A
Hepatitis B vaccine for those who are hepatitis B surface antigen and antibody negative. (Use 40 μg formulation at 0, 1, and 6 mo; repeat if no immunity 1 mo after three-shot series)
Combined tetanus, diphtheria, pertussis vaccine
Human papillomavirus vaccine for HIV-infected women age 26 y or less
Haemophilus influenzae type b vaccination
Bone mineral density monitoring for women and men over 50 y of age
Papanicolaou smears every 6 mo for women
Consider anal swabs for cytologic evaluation
For HIV-infected individuals with CD4 < 200 cells/μL:
Pneumocystis jiroveci prophylaxis (see Table 77-6)
For HIV-infected Individuals with CD4 < 75 cells/μL:
M avium complex prophylaxis (see Table 77-4)
For HIV-infected individuals with CD4 < 50 cells/μL:
Consider CMV prophylaxis

CMV, cytomegalovirus; IgG, immunoglobulin G; INH, isoniazid; PPD, purified protein derivative; RPR, rapid plasma reagin; VDRL, Venereal Disease Research Laboratories

Prevention

Primary Prevention

- Precautions regarding sexual practices and injection drug use (safer sex, latex condoms, and clean needle use)
- Perinatal HIV prophylaxis
- Screening of blood products
- Infection control practices in the health care setting
- Besides preventing progression of HIV disease, effective antiretroviral therapy likely decreases the risk of HIV transmission between sexual partners
- Postexposure prophylaxis for sexual and drug use exposures to HIV

Secondary Prevention

- For MAC infection when CD4 counts < 75 to 100 cells/μL: azithromycin (1200 mg orally every week), or clarithromycin (500 mg twice daily orally)
- For M *tuberculosis* infection when positive PPD reactions > 5 mm of induration: isoniazid, 300 mg once daily orally plus pyridoxine, 50 mg once daily orally for 9 to 12 months
- For toxoplasmosis when positive IgG toxoplasma serology when CD4 counts < 100 cells/μL: trimethoprim–sulfamethoxazole (1 double-strength tablet once daily

Table 77–8. *Pneumocystis jirovecii* prophylaxis in order of preference.

Medication	Dose	Side Effects	Limitations
Trimethoprim-sulfamethoxazole	One double-strength tablet three times a week to one tablet daily	Rash, neutropenia, hepatitis, Stevens–Johnson syndrome	Hypersensitivity reaction is common but, if mild, it may be possible to treat through
Dapsone	50–100 mg orally daily or 100 mg two or three times per week	Anemia, nausea, methemoglobinemia, hemolytic anemia	Less effective than above. Glucose-6-phosphate dehydrogenase (G6PD) level should be checked prior to therapy. Check methemoglobin level after 1 month of treatment
Atovaquone	1500 mg orally daily with a meal	Rash, diarrhea, nausea	Less effective than suspension trimethoprim-sulfamethoxazole; equal efficacy to dapsone, but more expensive
Aerosolized pentamidine	300 mg monthly	Bronchospasm (pretreat with bronchodilators); rare reports of pancreatitis	Apical *P jirovecii* pneumonia, extrapulmonary *P jirovecii* infections, pneumothorax

orally), or pyrimethamine, 50 mg orally every week plus dapsone, 50 mg once daily orally plus leucovorin 25 mg every week orally

- For *P jiroveci* pneumonia when CD4 counts < 200 cells/µL, a CD4 lymphocyte percentage < 14%, or weight loss or oral candidiasis: trimethoprim–sulfamethoxazole, dapsone, or atovaquone (see Table 77-6)

9. When to Refer and When to Admit

When to Refer

- For advice regarding change of antiretroviral therapy, including interpretation of resistance tests
- For management of complicated opportunistic infections

When to Admit

- For new unexplained fever if bacterial infection requiring intravenous antibiotics is suspected
- For acute organ system dysfunction or acute change in mental status

SUGGESTED REFERENCES

AIDSinfo. Guidelines for the prevention and treatment of opportunistic infections in HIV-infected adults and adolescents. 2014 Oct 28. http://aidsinfo.nih.gov/contentfiles/lvguidelines/adult_oi.pdf

Baeten JM et al; Partners PrEP Study Team. Antiretroviral prophylaxis for HIV prevention in heterosexual men and women. *N Engl J Med*. 2012 Aug 2;367(5):399–410. [PMID: 22784037]

Eron JJ et al; BENCHMRK Study Teams. Efficacy and safety of raltegravir for treatment of HIV for 5 years in the BENCHMRK studies: final results of two randomised, placebo-controlled trials. *Lancet Infect Dis*. 2013 Jul;13(7):587–596. [PMID: 23664333]

Günthard HF et al. Antiretroviral treatment of adult HIV infection: 2014 recommendations of the International Antiviral Society-USA Panel. *JAMA*. 2014 Jul 23–30;312(4):410–425. [PMID: 25038359]

Marrazzo JM et al. HIV prevention in clinical care settings: 2014 recommendations of the International Antiviral Society-USA Panel. *JAMA*. 2014 Jul 23–30;312(4):390–409. Erratum in: *JAMA*. 2014 Aug 13;312(6):652. [PMID: 25038358]

New York State Department of Health AIDS Institute. HIV prophylaxis following non-occupational exposure. October 2014 update. http://www.hivguidelines.org/wp-content/uploads/2014/12/hiv-prophylaxis-following-non-occupational-exposure.pdf

Patel DA et al. 48-week efficacy and safety of dolutegravir relative to commonly used third agents in treatment-naive HIV-1-infected patients: a systematic review and network meta-analysis. *PLoS One*. 2014 Sep 4;9(9):e105653. [PMID: 25188312]

Raffi F et al; extended SPRING-2 Study Group. Once-daily dolutegravir versus twice-daily raltegravir in antiretroviral-naive adults with HIV-1 infection (SPRING-2 study): 96 week results from a randomised, double-blind, non-inferiority trial. *Lancet Infect Dis*. 2013 Nov;13(11):927–935. [PMID: 24074642]

Saunders KO. The design and evaluation of HIV-1 vaccines. *AIDS*. 2012 Jun 19;26(10):1293–1302. [PMID: 22706011]

U.S. Department of Health and Human Services. Guidelines for the use of antiretroviral agents in HIV-1-infected adults and adolescents. http://aidsinfo.nih.gov/guidelines/html/1/adult-and-adolescent-arv-guidelines/11/what-to-start

U.S. Food and Drug Administration. FDA Drug Safety Communication: interactions between certain HIV or hepatitis C drugs and cholesterol-lowering statin drugs can increase the risk of muscle injury. http://www.fda.gov/Drugs/DrugSafety/ucm293877.htm

U.S. Preventive Services Task Force. Screening for HIV: U.S. Preventive Services Task Force Recommendation Statement. April 2013. http://www.uspreventiveservicestaskforce.org/uspstf13/hiv/hivfinalrs.htm

U.S. Public Health Service. Preexposure prophylaxis for the prevention of HIV infection in the United States—2014: a clinical practice guideline. http://www.cdc.gov/hiv/pdf/PrEPguidelines2014.pdf

Walmsley SL et al; SINGLE Investigators. Dolutegravir plus abacavir-lamivudine for the treatment of HIV-1 infection. *N Engl J Med*. 2013 Nov 7;369(19):1807–1818. [PMID: 24195548]

Health Care-Associated Infections

78

A 71-year-old man is admitted to the intensive care unit for pneumonia, sepsis, and ARDS. He is treated with intravenous ceftriaxone. An initial improvement occurs in his sepsis symptoms and lung function, but on hospital day 6, he becomes febrile to 39°C, tachycardic, and hypotensive. His femoral central venous catheter is found to be erythematous and draining purulent material. The catheter is removed and intravenous vancomycin is administered with resolution of his fever, tachycardia, and hypotension. Blood cultures drawn from the central venous catheter grow methicillin-resistant *Staphylococcus aureus* (MRSA).

LEARNING OBJECTIVES

▶ Learn the clinical manifestations and objective findings of health care-associated infections

▶ Understand the factors that predispose to hospital-associated infections and how they differ from community-acquired infections

▶ Know the differential diagnosis of health care-associated infections

▶ Learn how to treat common health care-associated infections and when to replace venous and urinary catheters

▶ Know the strategies to prevent health care-associated infections

QUESTIONS

1. What are the salient features of this patient's problem?

2. How do you think through his problem?

3. What are the key features, including essentials of diagnosis, general considerations, and demographics, of health care-associated infections?

4. What are the symptoms and signs of health care-associated infections?

5. What is the differential diagnosis of health care-associated infections?

6. What are laboratory and imaging findings in health care-associated infections?

7. What are the treatments for health care-associated infections?

8. What are the outcomes, including follow-up and prevention, of health care-associated infections?

9. When should patients with health care-associated infections be referred to a specialist?

ANSWERS

1. Salient Features

Recurrent symptoms of sepsis while hospitalized despite initial improvement; central venous catheter with erythema and drainage; blood cultures growing MRSA; resolution with vancomycin

2. How to Think Through

What major causes of new fever, tachycardia, and hypotension should be considered in this case besides the purulent central line? (Medication toxicity, pulmonary embolism, and infection.) Within the category of infection, treatment of the pneumonia may be inadequate due to insufficient antibiotic coverage, dosing, or penetration of the infected tissue. An example of the latter would be development of empyema. The patient may have also developed a new, health care-associated infection. Health care-associated infection possibilities include ventilator-associated pneumonia, infection spread by contact such as *Clostridium difficile*, Foley catheter-associated urinary tract infection, intravenous catheter-associated bloodstream infection, and infection from inadequately sterilized diagnostic equipment (eg, duodenoscopes used in cholangiopancreatography). In this case, a femoral central venous catheter is the leading possibility. Line placement at a femoral site has a higher infection risk than one at a subclavian or internal jugular site.

How can "differential time to positivity" of blood cultures help make the diagnosis of line infection? (A blood culture specimen from a central line that becomes positive at least 120 minutes prior to a blood culture simultaneously drawn from a peripheral vein, indicates a higher organism burden within the catheter.) Removal of a central line is not a trivial consideration—venous access may be difficult to obtain and it may be essential for treatment. When should a central line be removed? (If there is purulence at the exit site; if the organism is *S aureus,* a gram-negative rod, or a *Candida* species; if there is persistent bacteremia; if septic thrombophlebitis, endocarditis, or metastatic abscesses occur.)

3. Key Features

Essentials of Diagnosis

- Health care-associated infections are acquired during the course of receiving health care treatment for other conditions
- Health care-associated infections are defined as those not present (or incubating) at the time of hospital admission and developing at least 48 hours or more after admission
- Most health care-associated infections are preventable
- Hand washing is the most effective means of preventing health care-associated infections and should be done routinely even when gloves are worn

General Considerations

- Although most fevers are due to infections, about 25% of patients will have fever of non-infectious origin
- Many infections are a direct result of the use of invasive devices for diagnosis, monitoring or therapy such as
  — Intravenous catheters
  — Foley catheters
  — Catheters placed by interventional radiology for drainage
  — Orotracheal tubes for ventilatory support
  — Duodenoscopes used in cholangiopancreatography
- Early removal of such devices reduces infection
- Proper sterilization of equipment used repeatedly with different patients is key
- Patients in whom health care-associated infections develop

— Are often critically ill

— Have been hospitalized for extended periods

— Have received several courses of broad-spectrum antibiotic therapy

• As a result, the causative organisms are often multidrug resistant and different from those in community-acquired infections

— *S aureus* and *Staphylococcus epidermidis* (a frequent cause of prosthetic device infection) may be resistant to nafcillin and cephalosporins and require vancomycin for therapy

— *Enterococcus faecium* resistant to ampicillin and vancomycin

— Gram-negative infections caused by *Pseudomonas, Citrobacter, Acinetobacter, Stenotrophomonas,* and *Enterobacter,* including carbapenem-resistant *Enterobacteriaceae* (CRE) may be resistant to most (or, with CRE, all) currently available antibacterials

Demographics

• In the United States, approximately 5% of patients who enter the hospital free of infection acquire a health care-associated infection resulting in

— Prolongation of the hospital stay

— Increase in cost of care

— Significant morbidity

— Even death (5% mortality rate)

4. Symptoms and Signs

• Those of the underlying disease

• All infections: fever, tachycardia, tachypnea, hypotension, systemic inflammatory response syndrome (SIRS), sepsis, and septic shock.

• Ventilator-associated pneumonia: increasing ventilator requirements, focal lung consolidation

• Central venous catheter infections: erythema, warmth, drainage at catheter site

• *C difficile* infection: diarrhea

5. Differential Diagnosis

• Noninfectious

— Drug fever

— Nonspecific postoperative fevers (tissue damage or necrosis)

— Hematoma

— Pancreatitis

— Pulmonary embolism

— Myocardial infarction

— Ischemic bowel

• Urinary tract infections

• Pneumonia

• Bacteremia, eg, indwelling catheter, wound, abscess, pneumonia, genitourinary or gastro-intestinal tract

• Wound infection, eg, pressure ulcer, *C difficile* colitis

6. Laboratory and Imaging Findings

Laboratory Tests

• Blood cultures are universally recommended

• A properly prepared sputum Gram stain and semiquantitative sputum cultures may be useful in selected patients where there is a high pretest probability of pneumonia

• Unreliable or uninterpretable specimens are often obtained for culture that result in unnecessary use of antibiotics

— The best example of this occurrence is in the diagnosis of line-related or bloodstream infection in the febrile patient

— Blood cultures from unidentified sites, a single blood culture from any site, or a blood culture through an existing line will often be positive for *S epidermidis* and this will result in unnecessary therapy with vancomycin

• Unless two separate venipuncture cultures are obtained—*not* through catheters—interpretation of results is impossible and unnecessary therapy is given

• A positive wound culture without signs of inflammation or infection, a positive sputum culture without pulmonary infiltrates on chest radiograph, or a positive urine culture in a catheterized patient without symptoms or signs of pyelonephritis are all likely to represent colonization, not infection

Imaging Studies

• Chest radiographs are frequently obtained

7. Treatments

Medications

• Empiric therapy with vancomycin, 15 mg/kg intravenously twice daily, should be given if there is normal kidney function

• Empiric gram-negative coverage may be considered in patients who are immunocompromised or who are critically ill (Tables 78-1 and 80-1)

• Antibiotic lock therapy

— Involves the instillation of supratherapeutic concentrations of antibiotics with heparin in the lumen of catheters

— Purpose is to achieve adequate concentrations of antibiotics to kill microbes in the biofilm

— Can be used for catheter-related bloodstream infections caused by coagulase-negative staphylococci or enterococci and when the catheter is being retained in a salvage situation

Therapeutic Procedures

• Remove catheters if

— There is purulence at the exit site

— The organism is *S aureus,* a gram-negative rod, or *Candida* species

— There is persistent bacteremia (> 48 hours while receiving antibiotics)

— Complications, such as septic thrombophlebitis, endocarditis, or other metastatic disease exist

• Central venous catheters may be exchanged over a guidewire provided there is no erythema or purulence at the exit site and the patient does not appear to be septic

8. Outcomes

Follow-Up

• Monitoring of high-risk areas by hospital epidemiologists detects increases in infection rates early

Prevention

• Universal precautions against potential blood-borne transmissible disease

• Hepatitis A, hepatitis B, and varicella vaccines should be considered in the appropriate setting

• Peripheral intravenous lines should be replaced every 3 days

• Arterial lines and lines in the central venous circulation (including those placed peripherally) can be left in indefinitely and are changed or removed when

— They are clinically suspected of being infected

— They are nonfunctional

— They are no longer needed

Table 78-1. Examples of initial antimicrobial therapy for acutely ill, hospitalized adults pending identification of causative organism.

Suspected Clinical Diagnosis	Likely Etiologic Diagnosis	Drugs of Choice
Meningitis, bacterial, community-acquired	*Streptococcus pneumoniae* (pneumococcus),[a] *Neisseria meningitidis* (meningococcus)	Cefotaxime,[b] 2–3 g intravenously every 6 h **or** ceftriaxone, 2 g intravenously every 12 h; **plus** vancomycin, 15 mg/kg intravenously every 8 h
Meningitis, bacterial, age > 50, community-acquired	Pneumococcus, meningococcus, *Listeria monocytogenes*,[c] gram-negative bacilli, Group B streptococcus	Ampicillin, 2 g intravenously every 4 h, **plus** cefotaxime, 2–3 g intravenously every 6 h **or** ceftriaxone, 2 g intravenously every 12 h, **plus** vancomycin, 15 mg/kg intravenously every 8 h
Meningitis, postoperative (or posttraumatic)	*S aureus*, gram-negative bacilli, coagulase negative staphylococci, diphtheroids (eg, *Propionibacterium acnes*) (uncommon) (pneumococcus, in posttraumatic)	Vancomycin,[d] 15 mg/kg intravenously every 8 h, **plus** cefepime, 3 g intravenously every 8 h
Brain abscess	Mixed anaerobes, pneumococci, streptococci	Penicillin G, 4 million units intravenously every 4 h, **plus** metronidazole, 500 mg orally every 8 h; **or** cefotaxime, 2–3 g intravenously every 6 h **or** ceftriaxone, 2 g intravenously every 12 h **plus** metronidazole, **500** mg orally every 8 h
Pneumonia, acute, community-acquired, non-ICU hospital admission	Pneumococci, *M pneumoniae*, *Legionella*, *C pneumoniae*	Cefotaxime, 2 g intravenously every 8 h (**or** ceftriaxone, 1 g intravenously every 24 h or ampicillin 2 g intravenously every 6 h) **plus** azithromycin 500 mg intravenously every 24 h; **or** a fluoroquinolone[e] alone
Pneumonia, postoperative or nosocomial	*S aureus*, mixed anaerobes, gram-negative bacilli	Cefepime, 1 g intravenously every 8 h; **or** ceftazidime, 2 g intravenously every 8 h; **or** piperacillin-tazobactam, 4.5 g intravenously every 6 h; **or** imipenem, 500 mg intravenously every 6 h; **or** meropenem, 1 g intravenously every 8 h **plus** tobramycin, 5 mg/kg intravenously every 24 h; **or** ciprofloxacin, 400 mg intravenously every 12 h; **or** levofloxacin, 500 mg intravenously every 24 h plus vancomycin, 15 mg/kg intravenously every 12 h
Endocarditis, acute (including injection drug user)	*S aureus*, *E faecalis*, gram-negative aerobic bacteria, viridans streptococci	Vancomycin, 15 mg/kg intravenously every 12 h, **plus** gentamicin, 1 mg/kg every 8 h
Septic thrombophlebitis (eg, IV tubing, IV shunts)	*S aureus*, gram-negative aerobic bacteria	Vancomycin, 15 mg/kg intravenously every 12 h, plus ceftriaxone, 1 g intravenously every 24 h
Osteomyelitis	*S aureus*	Nafcillin, 2 g intravenously every 4 h; **or** cefazolin, 2 g intravenously every 8 h
Septic arthritis	*S aureus*, *N gonorrhoeae*	Ceftriaxone, 1–2 g intravenously every 24 h
Pyelonephritis with flank pain and fever (recurrent urinary tract infection)	*E coli*, *Klebsiella*, *Enterobacter*, *Pseudomonas*	Ceftriaxone, 1 g intravenously every 24 h; **or** ciprofloxacin, 400 mg intravenously every 12 h (500 mg orally); **or** levofloxacin, 500 mg once daily (intravenously/orally)
Fever in neutropenic patient receiving cancer chemotherapy	*S aureus*, *Pseudomonas*, *Klebsiella*, *E coli*	Ceftazidime, 2 g intravenously every 8 h; **or** cefepime, 2 g intravenously every 8 h

[a]Some strains may be resistant to penicillin.

[b]Most studies on meningitis have been with cefotaxime or ceftriaxone (see text).

[c]TMP-SMZ can be used to treat *Listeria monocytogenes* in patients allergic to penicillin in a dosage of 15–20 mg/kg/d of TMP in three or four divided doses.

[d]In postsurgical or posttraumatic patients receiving dexamethasone, some experts add rifampin to empiric vancomycin.

[e]Levofloxacin 750 mg/d, moxifloxacin 400 mg/d.

- Silver alloy–impregnated Foley catheters reduce the incidence of catheter-associated bacteriuria, and antibiotic-impregnated (minocycline plus rifampin or chlorhexidine plus silver sulfadiazine) venous catheters reduce line infections and bacteremia
- Whether the increased cost of these devices justifies their routine use should be determined by individual institutions based on local infection rates
- Preoperative skin preparation with chlorhexidine and alcohol (but not povidone-iodine) has been shown to reduce the incidence of infection following surgery
- Attentive nursing care (positioning to prevent pressure ulcers, wound care, elevating the head during tube feedings to prevent aspiration) is critical

9. When to Refer

- Any patient with multidrug-resistant infection
- Any patient with fungemia or persistent bacteremia

- Patients with multisite infections
- Patients with impaired or fluctuating kidney function for assistance with dosing of antimicrobials
- Patients with refractory or recurrent *C difficile* colitis

SUGGESTED REFERENCES

Baron EJ et al. A guide to utilization of the microbiology laboratory for diagnosis of infectious diseases: 2013 recommendations by the Infectious Diseases Society of America (IDSA) and the American Society for Microbiology (ASM)(a). *Clin Infect Dis.* 2013 Aug;57(4):e22–e121. [PMID: 23845951]

Cannon CM et al. The GENESIS Project (GENeralized Early Sepsis Intervention Strategies): a multi-center quality improvement collaborative. *J Intensive Care Med.* 2013 Nov–Dec;28(6):355–368. [PMID: 22902347]

Centers for Disease Control and Prevention (CDC). CDC Statement: Los Angeles County/UCLA investigation of CRE transmission and duodenoscopes. 2015 Feb 20. http://www.cdc.gov/hai/outbreaks/cdcstatement-LA-CRE.html

Centers for Disease Control and Prevention (CDC). Healthcare-associated Infections (HAIs): Carbapenem-resistant *Enterobacteriaceae* (CRE) infection. 2015 Feb 23. http://www.cdc.gov/hai/organisms/cre/cre-clinicians.html

Epstein L et al. New Delhi metallo-β-lactamase-producing carbapenem-resistant *Escherichia coli* associated with exposure to duodenoscopes. *JAMA.* 2014 Oct 8;312(14):1447-1455. [PMID: 25291580]

Ferrer R et al. Empiric antibiotic treatment reduces mortality in severe sepsis and septic shock from the first hour: results from a guideline-based performance improvement program. *Crit Care Med.* 2014 Aug;42(8):1749–1755. [PMID: 24717459]

Harris AD et al. Universal glove and gown use and acquisition of antibiotic-resistant bacteria in the ICU: a randomized trial. *JAMA.* 2013 Oct 16;310(15):1571–1580. [PMID: 24097234]

Huang SS et al; CDC Prevention Epicenters Program; AHRQ DECIDE Network and Healthcare-Associated Infections Program. Targeted versus universal decolonization to prevent ICU infection. *N Engl J Med.* 2013 Jun 13;368(24):2255–2265. Erratum in: *N Engl J Med.* 2013 Aug 8;369(6):587. [PMID: 23718152]

Lo E et al. Strategies to prevent catheter-associated urinary tract infections in acute care hospitals: 2014 update. *Infect Control Hosp Epidemiol.* 2014 Sep;35(suppl 2):S32–S47. [PMID: 25376068]

Oostdijk EA et al. Effects of decontamination of the oropharynx and intestinal tract on antibiotic resistance in ICUs: a randomized clinical trial. *JAMA.* 2014 Oct 8;312(14):1429–1437. [PMID: 25271544]

Sinuff T et al; Canadian Critical Care Trials Group. Implementation of clinical practice guidelines for ventilator-associated pneumonia: a multicenter prospective study. *Crit Care Med.* 2013 Jan;41(1):15–23. [PMID: 23222254]

Infective Endocarditis

A 55-year-old man who recently emigrated from China presents to the emergency department with fever. He states that he has had recurring fevers over the past 3 weeks, associated with chills, night sweats, and malaise. Today he developed new painful lesions on the pads of his fingers, prompting him to come to the emergency department. His medical history is remarkable for "being very sick as a child after a sore throat." He has recently had several teeth extracted for severe dental caries. He is taking no medications. On physical examination, he is febrile with temperature 38.5°C, blood pressure 120/80 mm Hg, heart rate 108 bpm, respiratory rate 16/min, and oxygen saturation of 97% on room air. Skin examination is remarkable for painful nodules on the pads of several fingers and toes. He has multiple splinter hemorrhages in the nail beds and painless hemorrhagic macules on the palms of the hands. Ophthalmoscopic examination is remarkable for retinal hemorrhages. Chest examination is clear to auscultation and percussion. Cardiac examination is notable for a grade 3/6 holosystolic murmur heard loudest at the left lower sternal border, with radiation to the axilla.

LEARNING OBJECTIVES

▶ Learn the clinical manifestations and objective findings of infective endocarditis (IE), differentiating autoimmune and embolic phenomena

▶ Understand the factors that predispose to developing IE

▶ Learn the differences between acute and subacute presentations of IE

▶ Know the differential diagnosis of IE

▶ Learn the medical treatments for IE based on causative organism and antibiotic susceptibilities

▶ Know the indications for surgical intervention in IE

QUESTIONS

1. What are the salient features of this patient's problem?

2. How do you think through his problem?

3. What are the key features, including essentials of diagnosis, general considerations, and demographics, of IE?

4. What are the symptoms and signs of IE?

5. What is the differential diagnosis of IE?

6. What are laboratory, imaging, and procedural findings in IE?

7. What are the treatments for IE?

8. What are the outcomes, including follow-up, complications, prognosis, and prevention, of IE?

9. When should patients with IE be referred to a specialist or admitted to the hospital?

ANSWERS

1. Salient Features

Constitutional symptoms (fever, chills, night sweats, malaise); likely history of prior rheumatic heart disease; poor dentition; fever and tachycardia; painful Osler nodes; splinter hemorrhages, painless Janeway lesions; Roth spots on ophthalmoscopy; cardiac murmur

2. How to Think Through

Mortality from IE is high (with rates dependent on the affected valve and the organism). Often, only nonspecific symptoms and signs are apparent at presentation, but delay in diagnosis can be catastrophic. On presentation, this patient had the cardinal constitutional symptoms of fever, chills, night sweats, and malaise. Therefore, IE needs to be considered and a directed history and physical examination performed. What historical risk factors raise the likelihood of IE? (History of rheumatic fever, prosthetic valves, and injection drug use.) The physical findings of IE are crucial in establishing the diagnosis with this otherwise nonspecific presentation. What are the signs associated with IE? (Fever, murmur, embolic lesions, and peripheral stigmata.) IE can lead to embolic lesions in nonvisible locations as well, and detection of these can assist with the diagnosis. What should you look for in your initial evaluation? (Altered mental status, inflammatory arthritis, hematuria, embolic infarctions on chest or abdominal imaging.)

What are the key tests for diagnosis and treatment? (Blood cultures and echocardiography.) How many major Duke criteria for IE does this patient have? (1.) How many minor? (3.) What are the most common organisms in IE? (Viridans strains of streptococci, *Staphylococcus aureus*, enterococci, coagulase-negative staphylococci.) Which organisms tend to present with a more subacute course? (Viridans streptococci, enterococci, and other gram-positive and gram-negative bacilli, yeasts, and fungi.)

3. Key Features

Essentials of Diagnosis

- Risk factors: preexisting organic heart lesion, prosthetic valve, injection drug use
- Fever
- New or changing heart murmur
- Evidence of systemic emboli
- Positive blood cultures
- Evidence of vegetations on echocardiography

General Considerations

- Important factors that determine the clinical presentation
  — Nature of the infecting organism
  — Valve that is infected
  — Route of infection
- Acute presentation
  — Caused by more virulent organisms, particularly *Staphylococcus aureus*
  — Rapidly progressive and destructive infection
  — Acute febrile illnesses

— Early embolization
— Acute valvular regurgitation
— Myocardial abscess
• Subacute presentation
— Caused by viridans strains of streptococci, enterococci, and other gram-positive and gram-negative bacilli, yeasts, and fungi
— Systemic and peripheral manifestations may predominate
• Patients may have underlying cardiac disease, but its prevalence as a risk factor is decreasing
• The initiating event is infection of the valve by bacteria during a transient or persistent bacteremia

Native Valve Endocarditis
• Most commonly due to
— *S aureus* (~40%)
— Viridans streptococci (~30%)
— Enterococci (5%–10%)
• Gram-negative organisms and fungi account for a small percentage
• Injection drug users
— *S aureus* in at least 60% of cases and 80% to 90% of tricuspid valve infections
— Enterococci and streptococci comprise the balance in about equal proportions

Prosthetic Valve Endocarditis
• Early infections (within 2 months of valve implantation) are commonly caused by
— Staphylococci—both coagulase-positive and coagulase-negative
— Gram-negative organisms and fungi
• Late prosthetic valve endocarditis
— Resembles native valve endocarditis
— Most cases caused by streptococci, though coagulase-negative staphylococci cause a significant proportion of cases

Demographics
• Endocarditis occurs in individuals with
— Injection drug use
— Underlying valvular disease (eg, congenital or rheumatic heart disease)
— Prosthetic valve replacement

4. Symptoms and Signs
• Most present with a febrile illness that has lasted several days to 2 weeks
• Heart murmurs
— In most cases, preexisting heart murmurs are stable
— A new or changing murmur is significant diagnostically, but is the exception rather than the rule
• Characteristic peripheral lesions occur in up to 20% to 25% of patients
— Petechiae (on the palate or conjunctiva or beneath the fingernails)
— Subungual ("splinter") hemorrhages
— Osler nodes (painful, violaceous raised lesions of the fingers, toes, or feet)
— Janeway lesions (painless erythematous lesions of the palms or soles)
• Roth spots (exudative, hemorrhagic lesions of the retinas)

5. Differential Diagnosis
• Valvular abnormality without endocarditis
— Rheumatic heart disease
— Mitral valve prolapse
— Bicuspid or calcific aortic valve

- Flow murmur (anemia, pregnancy, hyperthyroidism, and sepsis)
- Atrial myxoma
- Noninfective endocarditis, eg, systemic lupus erythematosus (Libman–Saks endocarditis), marantic endocarditis (nonbacterial thrombotic endocarditis)
- Acute rheumatic fever
- Vasculitis
- Hematuria from other causes, such as
  — Glomerulonephritis
  — Renal cell carcinoma

6. Laboratory, Imaging, and Procedural Findings

Laboratory Tests

- Blood culture
  — Most important diagnostic tool
  — To maximize the yield, obtain three sets of blood cultures from different sites at least 1 hour apart before starting antibiotics
- In acute endocarditis, leukocytosis is common
- In subacute cases, anemia of chronic disease and a normal white blood cell count are the rule
- Hematuria and proteinuria as well as renal dysfunction may result from emboli or immunologically mediated glomerulonephritis
- Duke criteria for the diagnosis of infective endocarditis
  — Major criteria
    ◦ Two positive blood cultures for a typical microorganism of IE
    ◦ Positive echocardiogram (vegetation, myocardial abscess, or new partial dehiscence of a prosthetic valve)
    ◦ New regurgitant murmur
  — Minor criteria
    ◦ Presence of a predisposing condition
    ◦ Fever > 38°C
    ◦ Embolic disease
    ◦ Immunologic phenomena (Osler nodes, Janeway lesions, Roth spots, glomerulonephritis, and rheumatoid factor)
    ◦ Positive blood cultures with an organism not meeting the major criteria or serologic evidence of active infection with an organism that causes endocarditis
  — A definite diagnosis of endocarditis is made with 80% accuracy if two major criteria, or one major criterion and three minor criteria, or five minor criteria are fulfilled
  — Possible endocarditis is defined as the presence of one major and one minor criterion, or three minor criteria
  — If these criteria thresholds are not met and either an alternative explanation for illness is identified or the patient's febrile illness has resolved within 4 days, endocarditis is highly unlikely

Imaging Studies

- Chest radiograph may show findings indicating an underlying cardiac abnormality and, in right-sided endocarditis, pulmonary infiltrates
- Echocardiography
  — Transthoracic echocardiography has only a 55% to 65% sensitivity; therefore, it cannot rule out endocarditis but may confirm a clinical suspicion
  — Transesophageal echocardiography has a 90% sensitivity in detecting vegetations and is particularly useful for identifying myocardial valve ring abscesses, and pulmonary valve and prosthetic valve endocarditis

Diagnostic Procedures

- The ECG is nondiagnostic. Changing conduction abnormalities suggest myocardial abscess formation

7. Treatments

Medications

- For penicillin-susceptible viridans streptococcal endocarditis (ie, MIC ≤ 0.1 µg/mL)
  - Penicillin G, 2 to 3 million units intravenously (IV) every 4 hours for 4 weeks
  - Duration of therapy can be shortened to 2 weeks if gentamicin, 1 mg/kg intravenously every 8 hours, is used with penicillin (do not use 2-week regimen if symptoms are present for at least 3 months or there are complications such as myocardial abscess or extracardiac infection)
  - Ceftriaxone, 2 g once daily IV or intramuscularly for 4 weeks, is also effective therapy and is a convenient regimen for home therapy
  - For the penicillin-allergic patient, vancomycin, 15 mg/kg IV every 12 hours for 4 weeks, is given
- For penicillin-resistant viridans streptococci (ie, MIC > 0.1 µg/mL but ≤ 0.5 µg/mL)
  - Treat for 4 weeks
  - Penicillin G, 3 million units intravenously every 4 hours, is combined with gentamicin, 1 mg/kg intravenously every 8 hours for the first 2 weeks
  - In the patient with IgE-mediated allergy to penicillin, vancomycin alone, 15 mg/kg IV every 12 hours for 4 weeks, should be administered
- *Streptococcus pneumoniae* sensitive to penicillin (MIC < 0.1 µg/mL) can be treated with penicillin alone, 2 to 3 million units IV every 4 hours for 4 to 6 weeks
  - Vancomycin should be effective for endocarditis caused by strains resistant to penicillin
- Group A streptococcal infection can be treated with penicillin, ceftriaxone, or vancomycin for 4 to 6 weeks
- Groups B, C, and G streptococci
  - Tend to be more resistant to penicillin than group A streptococci
  - Some experts recommend adding gentamicin, 1 mg/kg IV every 8 hours, to penicillin for the first 2 weeks of a 4- to 6-week course
- For enterococcal endocarditis
  - Penicillin alone is inadequate; either streptomycin or gentamicin must be included
  - Gentamicin is the aminoglycoside of choice, because streptomycin resistance is more common
  - Ampicillin, 2 g IV every 4 hours, or penicillin G, 3 to 4 million units IV every 4 hours (or, in the penicillin-allergic patient, vancomycin, 15 mg/kg intravenously every 12 hours), plus gentamicin, 1 mg/kg IV every 8 hours, are recommended for 4 to 6 weeks
  - Ampicillin, 2 g IV every 4 hours, plus ceftriaxone, 2 g intravenously every 12 hours, for 4–6 weeks may be as effective and less toxic than the combination of ampicillin and an aminoglycoside
- For methicillin-susceptible *S aureus (MSSA)*
  - Nafcillin or oxacillin, 1.5 to 2 g IV every 4 hours for 6 weeks, is the preferred therapy
  - Uncomplicated tricuspid valve endocarditis probably can be treated for 2 weeks with nafcillin or oxacillin alone
  - For penicillin-allergic patients, cefazolin, 2 g IV every 8 hours, or vancomycin, 30 mg/kg IV divided in 2 or 3 doses, may be used
- For methicillin-resistant *S aureus* (MRSA), vancomycin remains the preferred agent
- For prosthetic valve infection, a combination of vancomycin, 30 mg/kg/d IV divided in 2 or 3 doses for 6 weeks, rifampin, 300 mg every 8 hours for 6 weeks, and gentamicin, 1 mg/kg IV every 8 hours for the first 2 weeks, is recommended
- For endocarditis caused by HACEK organisms
  - Ceftriaxone (or some other third-generation cephalosporin), 2 g IV once daily for 4 weeks is the treatment of choice
  - Prosthetic valve endocarditis should be treated for 6 weeks
  - In the penicillin-allergic patient, experience is limited, but trimethoprim–sulfamethoxazole, quinolones, and aztreonam should be considered

Surgery

- Valve replacement surgery is indicated for
  - Regurgitation resulting in acute heart failure that does not resolve promptly after institution of medical therapy (even if active infection is present), especially if the aortic valve is involved
  - Infections that do not respond to appropriate antimicrobial therapy after 7 to 10 days (ie, persistent fevers, positive blood cultures despite therapy)
- Valve replacement is nearly always necessary for fungal endocarditis
- Valve replacement is more often necessary with
  - Gram-negative bacilli
  - Infection involving the sinus of Valsalva
  - Infection producing septal abscesses
  - Recurrent infection with the same organism, especially with prosthetic valves
  - Continuing embolization when the infection is otherwise responding

Therapeutic Procedures

- Colonoscopy should be performed to exclude colon cancer in patients with endocarditis caused by *S bovis*

8. Outcomes

Follow-Up

- Defervescence occurs in 3 to 4 days on average if infection is caused by
  - Viridans streptococci
  - Enterococci
  - Coagulase-negative staphylococci
- Patients may remain febrile for a week or more if infection is caused by
  - *S aureus*
  - *Pseudomonas aeruginosa*

Complications

- Destruction of infected heart valves
- Myocardial abscesses leading to conduction disturbances
- Systemic embolization
- Metastatic infections
- Mycotic aneurysms
- Right-sided endocarditis, which usually involves the tricuspid valve, often leads to septic pulmonary emboli, causing pulmonary infarction and lung abscesses

Prognosis

- Higher morbidity and mortality is associated with nonstreptococcal organisms, and with aortic or prosthetic valvular infection

Prevention

- Prophylactic antibiotics are given to patients with predisposing congenital, prosthetic or valvular anomalies (Table 79-1) who are to have any of a number of procedures (Table 79-2)
- Current recommendations for endocarditis prophylaxis are given in Table 79-3

9. When to Refer and When to Admit

When to Refer

- Infectious diseases consultation recommended
- Patients with signs of heart failure should be referred for surgical evaluation

When to Admit

- Patients with evidence of heart failure
- Patients with a nonstreptococcal etiology
- For initiation of antimicrobial therapy in suspected, definite, or possible cases

Table 79-1. Cardiac conditions with high risk of adverse outcomes from endocarditis for which prophylaxis with dental procedures is recommended.[a,b]

Prosthetic cardiac valve
Previous infective endocarditis
Congenital heart disease (CHD)[c]
Unrepaired cyanotic CHD, including palliative shunts and conduits
Completely repaired congenital heart defect with prosthetic material or device, whether placed by surgery or by catheter intervention, during the first 6 mo after the procedure[d]
Repaired CHD with residual defects at the site or adjacent to the site of a prosthetic patch or prosthetic device
Cardiac transplantation recipients in whom cardiac valvulopathy develops

[a]Reproduced, with permission, from the American Heart Association. *Circulation*. 2007;116(15):1736–1754.

[b]See Table 79-3 for prophylactic regimens.

[c]Except for the conditions listed above, antibiotic prophylaxis is no longer recommended for other forms of CHD.

[d]Prophylaxis is recommended because endothelialization of prosthetic material occurs within 6 mo after procedure.

Table 79-2. Recommendations for administration of bacterial endocarditis prophylaxis for patients according to type of procedure.[a]

Prophylaxis Recommended	Prophylaxis Not Recommended
Dental procedures	**Dental procedures**
All dental procedures that involve manipulation of gingival tissue or the periapical region of the teeth or perforation of the oral mucosa	Routine anesthetic injections through noninfected tissue, taking dental radiographs, placement of removable prosthodontic or orthodontic appliances, adjustment of orthodontic appliances, placement of orthodontic brackets, shedding of deciduous teeth, and bleeding from trauma to the lips or oral mucosa
Respiratory tract procedures	
Only respiratory tract procedures that involve incision of the respiratory mucosa	
Procedures on infected skin, skin structure, or musculoskeletal tissue	**Gastrointestinal tract procedures**
	Genitourinary tract procedures

[a]Reproduced, with permission, from the American Heart Association. *Circulation*. 2007;116(15):1736–1754.

Table 79-3. American Heart Association recommendations for endocarditis prophylaxis for dental procedures for patients with cardiac conditions.[a–c]

Oral	Amoxicillin	2 g 1 h before procedure
Penicillin allergy	Clindamycin	600 mg 1 h before procedure
	or	
	Cephalexin	2 g 1 h before procedure (contraindicated if there is history of a β-lactam immediate hypersensitivity reaction)
	or	
	Azithromycin or clarithromycin	500 mg 1 h before procedure
Parenteral	Ampicillin	2 g intramuscularly or intravenously 30 min before procedure
Penicillin allergy	Clindamycin	600 mg intravenously 1 h before procedure
	or	
	Cefazolin	1 g intramuscularly or intravenously 30 min before procedure (contraindicated if there is history of a β-lactam immediate hypersensitivity reaction)

[a]Data from the American Heart Association. *Circulation*. 2007;116(15):1736–1754.

[b]For patients undergoing respiratory tract procedures involving incision of respiratory tract mucosa to treat an established infection or a procedure on infected skin, skin structure, or musculoskeletal tissue known or suspected to be caused by *S aureus*, the regimen should contain an anti-staphylococcal penicillin or cephalosporin. Vancomycin can be used to treat patients unable to tolerate a β-lactam or if the infection is known or suspected to be caused by a methicillin-resistant strain of *S aureus*.

[c]See Table 79-1 for list of cardiac conditions.

SUGGESTED REFERENCES

Chirouze C et al. Infective endocarditis epidemiology and consequences of prophylaxis guidelines modifications: the dialectical evolution. *Curr Infect Dis Rep.* 2014 Nov;16(11):440. [PMID: 25233804]

Chu VH et al; International Collaboration on Endocarditis (ICE) Investigators*. Association between surgical indications, operative risk, and clinical outcome in infective endocarditis: a prospective study from the international collaboration on endocarditis. *Circulation.* 2015 Jan 13;131(2):131–140. [PMID: 25480814]

Dayer MJ et al. Incidence of infective endocarditis in England, 2000–13: a secular trend, interrupted time-series analysis. *Lancet.* 2015 Mar 28;385(9974):1219–1228. [PMID: 25467569]

Desimone DC et al; Mayo Cardiovascular Infections Study Group. Incidence of infective endocarditis caused by viridans group streptococci before and after publication of the 2007 American Heart Association's endocarditis prevention guidelines. *Circulation.* 2012 Jul 3;126(1):60–64. [PMID: 22689929]

Duval X et al; AEPEI Study Group. Temporal trends in infective endocarditis in the context of prophylaxis guideline modifications: three successive population-based surveys. *J Am Coll Cardiol.* 2012 May 29;59(22):1968–1976. [PMID: 22624837]

Krzyściak W et al. The pathogenicity of the Streptococcus genus. *Eur J Clin Microbiol Infect Dis.* 2013 Nov;32(11):1361–1376. [PMID: 24141975]

Ohlsson A et al. Intrapartum antibiotics for known maternal Group B streptococcal colonization. *Cochrane Database Syst Rev.* 2013 Jan 31;1:CD007467. [PMID: 23440815]

Thuny F et al. Infective endocarditis: prevention, diagnosis, and management. *Can J Cardiol.* 2014 Sep;30(9):1046-1057. [PMID: 25151287]

Sepsis

80

A 65-year-old woman is admitted to the hospital with community-acquired pneumonia. She is treated with intravenous antibiotics and is given oxygen by nasal cannula. A Foley catheter is placed in her bladder. On the third hospital day she is switched to oral antibiotics in anticipation of discharge. On the evening of hospital day 3, she develops fever and tachycardia. Blood and urine cultures are obtained. The following morning, she is lethargic and difficult to arouse. Her temperature is 35°C, blood pressure 85/40 mm Hg, heart rate 110 bpm, and respiratory rate 25/min. Lung examination is unchanged from admission, with rales in the left base. Cardiac examination is notable for a rapid but regular rhythm, without murmurs, gallops, or rubs. Abdominal examination is normal. Extremities are warm. Neurologic examination is nonfocal. The patient is transferred to the ICU for management of presumed sepsis and given intravenous fluids and broad spectrum antibiotics. Blood and urine cultures are positive for gram-negative rods.

LEARNING OBJECTIVES

▶ Learn the clinical manifestations and objective findings that are diagnostic of systemic inflammatory response syndrome (SIRS), sepsis, and septic shock

▶ Understand the factors that predispose to higher mortality in sepsis and the common infectious sources for gram-negative organisms

▶ Know the differential diagnosis of sepsis

▶ Learn the empiric treatment for sepsis

▶ Know the possible complications of sepsis

QUESTIONS

1. What are the salient features of this patient's problem?

2. How do you think through her problem?

3. What are the key features, including essentials of diagnosis and general considerations, of sepsis?

4. What are the symptoms and signs of sepsis?

5. What is the differential diagnosis of sepsis?

6. What are laboratory, imaging, and procedural findings in sepsis?

7. What are the treatments for sepsis?

8. What are the outcomes, including complications and prognosis, of sepsis?

9. When should patients with sepsis be admitted to the hospital?

ANSWERS

1. Salient Features

Foley catheter placement; hypothermia, tachycardia, tachypnea; hypotension; warm extremities suggesting decreased systemic vascular resistance (SVR); presumptive treatment with antibiotics and IV fluids; bacteremia; blood and urine cultures are diagnostic

2. How to Think Through

First, consider other causes of shock (hypovolemic, cardiogenic, obstructive, and other distributive) to avoid prematurely settling on septic shock as the cause of her deterioration. What examination finding makes blood loss or cardiogenic shock less likely? (These are states of high SVR, but her skin is warm.) A high suspicion for sepsis is important, since early intervention improves outcomes. Consider how to differentiate SIRS, sepsis, and septic shock. What are the key management components? (Restore perfusion; ensure adequate oxygenation; institute early a goal-directed therapy protocol; identify and treat the infection [use broad-spectrum antibiotics initially, followed by more targeted coverage based on blood cultures].)

Initially, intravascular fluids should be aggressively repleted, but ongoing assessment of volume status becomes a central challenge in sepsis. When a patient remains hypotensive despite fluid resuscitation, vasopressors must be employed. What end-organ effects of poor perfusion can one evaluate and monitor? (Mental status; urine output; lactic acidemia; electrocardiographic evidence of cardiac ischemia or arrhythmia; peripheral perfusion [pulses and capillary refill].) What are the important complications of sepsis? (Disseminated intravascular coagulation [DIC]; renal hypoperfusion; hepatic hypoperfusion; acute respiratory distress syndrome [ARDS].)

3. Key Features

Essentials of Diagnosis

- Fever, tachycardia, and/or increased respiratory rate; elevated white blood cell (WBC) count
- Proven or probable source of infection
- Bacteremia with positive blood cultures
- Elevated lactate or end-organ dysfunction in severe disease
- Hypotension in septic shock

General Considerations

- Sepsis is defined as meeting SIRS criteria with a known source of infection
- SIRS is defined by meeting two or more of the four following criteria: temperature $< 36°C$ or $> 38°C$; heart rate > 90 bpm; respiratory rate > 20/min or $Paco_2 < 32$ mm Hg; WBC count $< 4000/\mu L$ or $> 12,000/\mu L$ or differential with $> 10\%$ immature polymorphonuclear leukocytes ("bands")
- Gram-negative bacteremia usually originates from the genitourinary system, hepatobiliary tract, gastrointestinal tract, and lungs, though may also be from wounds and decubitus ulcers
- Mortality rate is significantly higher in those with underlying serious diseases

4. Symptoms and Signs

- Fevers and chills, often with abrupt onset
- Hyperventilation with respiratory alkalosis

- Altered mental status
- Hypotension and shock are late findings and poor prognostic signs
- Symptoms and signs of infectious source, eg, abdominal or urinary symptoms, pneumonia

5. Differential Diagnosis

- Gram-positive sepsis
- Fungal infection
- Acid-fast bacillus infection
- SIRS due to another cause
  — Trauma
  — Burns
  — Pancreatitis
  — Myocardial or bowel ischemia
  — Adrenal insufficiency
  — Pulmonary embolism
  — Aortic aneurysm rupture
  — Anaphylaxis
  — Cardiac tamponade
  — Toxic ingestion
- Shock from another cause
  — Cardiogenic
  — Neurogenic
  — Hypovolemic
  — Anaphylactic

6. Laboratory, Imaging, and Diagnostic Findings

Laboratory Tests

- Complete blood count (CBC) may show neutropenia or neutrophilia and immature poly-morphonuclear leukocytes ("bands")
- Thrombocytopenia
- Coagulation panel may show coagulation dysfunction with or without disseminated intravascular coagulation (DIC)
- Lactic acid elevation
- Three blood cultures should be obtained before starting antimicrobials, if possible

Imaging Studies

- Chest radiograph to look for pulmonary infection

Diagnostic Procedures

- Urinalysis with culture, which may show positive leukocyte esterase, elevated WBCs, and positive nitrite
- Culture of fluid from abscess, if applicable

7. Treatments

Medications

- Antibiotic therapy should be given as soon as the diagnosis is suspected, as delayed antibiotic therapy leads to increased mortality rates
- Initial antibiotic therapy should cover both gram-positive and gram-negative bacteria
- Table 80-1 lists examples of initial antimicrobial therapy for acutely ill, hospitalized adults pending identification of causative organism
- After initial empiric therapy, narrow antibiotics based on culture and sensitivity data
- Aggressive initial intravenous fluid repletion; vasopressors to maintain blood pressure if not responsive to IV fluid repletion
- Institute goal-directed therapy early using a set protocol for the treatment of septic shock by adjusting the use of fluids, vasopressors, inotropes, and blood transfusions to meet

Table 80-1. Examples of initial antimicrobial therapy for acutely ill, hospitalized adults pending identification of causative organism.

Suspected Clinical Diagnosis	Likely Etiologic Diagnosis	Drugs of Choice
Meningitis, bacterial, community-acquired	Pneumococcus,[a] meningococcus	Cefotaxime,[b] 2–3 g intravenously every 6 h; or ceftriaxone, 2 g intravenously every 12 h plus vancomycin, 15 mg/kg intravenously every 8 h
Meningitis, bacterial, age > 50, community-acquired	Pneumococcus, meningococcus, Listeria monocytogenes,[c] gram-negative bacilli	Ampicillin, 2 g intravenously every 4 h, plus cefotaxime, 2–3 g intravenously every 6 h; or ceftriaxone, 2 g intravenously every 12 h plus vancomycin, 15 mg/kg intravenously every 8 h
Meningitis, postoperative (or posttraumatic)	S aureus, gram-negative bacilli (pneumococcus, in posttraumatic)	Vancomycin, 15 mg/kg intravenously every 8 h, plus cefepime, 3 g intravenously every 8 h
Brain abscess	Mixed anaerobes, pneumococci, streptococci	Penicillin G, 4 million units intravenously every 4 h, plus metronidazole, 500 mg orally every 8 h; or cefotaxime, 2–3 g intravenously every 6 h or ceftriaxone, 2 g intravenously every 12 h plus metronidazole, 500 mg orally every 8 h
Pneumonia, acute, community-acquired, non-ICU hospital admission	Pneumococci, M pneumoniae, Legionella, C pneumoniae	Cefotaxime, 2 g intravenously every 8 h (or ceftriaxone, 1 g intravenously every 24 h or ampicillin 2 g intravenously every 6 h) plus azithromycin 500 mg intravenously every 24 h; or a fluoroquinolone[d] alone
Pneumonia, postoperative or nosocomial	S aureus, mixed anaerobes, gram-negative bacilli	Cefepime, 1 g intravenously every 8 h; or ceftazidime, 2 g intravenously every 8 h; or piperacillin-tazobactam, 4.5 g intravenously every 6 h; or imipenem, 500 mg intravenously every 6 h; or meropenem, 1 g intravenously every 8 h plus tobramycin, 5 mg/kg intravenously every 24 h; or ciprofloxacin, 400 mg intravenously every 12 h; or levofloxacin, 500 mg intravenously every 24 h plus vancomycin, 15 mg/kg intravenously every 12 h
Endocarditis, acute (including injection drug user)	S aureus, E faecalis, gram-negative aerobic bacteria, viridans streptococci	Vancomycin, 15 mg/kg intravenously every 12 h, plus gentamicin, 1 mg/kg every 8 h
Septic thrombophlebitis (eg, IV tubing, IV shunts)	S aureus, gram-negative aerobic bacteria	Vancomycin, 15 mg/kg intravenously every 12 h plus ceftriaxone, 1 g intravenously every 24 h
Osteomyelitis	S aureus	Nafcillin, 2 g intravenously every 4 h; or cefazolin, 2 g intravenously every 8 h
Septic arthritis	S aureus, N gonorrhoeae	Ceftriaxone, 1–2 g intravenously every 24 h
Pyelonephritis with flank pain and fever (recurrent urinary tract infection)	E coli, Klebsiella, Enterobacter, Pseudomonas	Ceftriaxone, 1 g intravenously every 24 h; or ciprofloxacin, 400 mg intravenously every 12 h (500 mg orally); or levofloxacin, 500 mg once daily (intravenously/orally)
Fever in neutropenic patient receiving cancer chemotherapy	S aureus, Pseudomonas, Klebsiella, E coli	Ceftazidime, 2 g intravenously every 8 h; or cefepime, 2 g intravenously every 8 h
Intra-abdominal sepsis (eg, postoperative, peritonitis, cholecystitis)	Gram-negative bacteria, Bacteroides, anaerobic bacteria, streptococci, clostridia	Piperacillin-tazobactam, 4.5 g intravenously every 6 h, or ertapenem, 1 g every 24 h

[a]Some strains may be resistant to penicillin.

[b]Most studies on meningitis have been with cefotaxime or ceftriaxone (see *Bacterial Meningitis*).

[c]TMP-SMZ can be used to treat *Listeria monocytogenes* in patients allergic to penicillin in a dosage of 15–20 mg/kg/d of TMP in three or four divided doses.

[d]Levofloxacin 750 mg/d, moxifloxacin 400 mg/d.

hemodynamic targets (MAP > 65 mm Hg, CVP 8–12 mm Hg, ScvO$_2$ > 70%,) and provides a significant mortality benefit; however, some data exist that the blood transfusion goals may do more harm than good

- Corticosteroids
  - Based on available data, cosyntropin stimulation testing is not recommended in patients with septic shock
  - Stress-dose hydrocortisone may benefit patients with severe septic shock (systolic blood pressure < 90 mm Hg for > 1 hour despite adequate fluid resuscitation and vasopressor administration)
  - However, such corticosteroid administration is unlikely to benefit those with less-severe septic shock

Surgery

- May be required to control source of bacteremia, depending on etiology

Therapeutic Procedures

- Drainage or removal of source of bacteremia, eg, central venous catheter removal, abscess or empyema drainage
- Management of any associated DIC

8. Outcomes

Complications

- DIC
- Acute lung injury/ARDS
- End-organ dysfunction, eg, acute kidney injury

Prognosis

- Mortality is < 5% in patients with no underlying disease; 15% to 20% in patients with cancer (solid tumors), cirrhosis, or aplastic anemia; 40% to 60% in patients with neutropenia or immunocompromised and underlying fatal conditions

9. When to Admit

- All patients who meet sepsis criteria should be admitted to the hospital for management and intravenous antibiotics

SUGGESTED REFERENCES

Caironi P et al; ALBIOS Study Investigators. Albumin replacement in patients with severe sepsis or septic shock. *N Engl J Med*. 2014 Apr 10;370(15):1412–1421. [PMID: 24635772]

Dellinger RP et al; Surviving Sepsis Campaign Guidelines Committee including the Pediatric Subgroup. Surviving Sepsis Campaign: international guidelines for management of severe sepsis and septic shock: 2012. *Crit Care Med*. 2013 Feb;41(2):580–637. [PMID: 23353941]

Havel C et al. Vasopressors for hypotensive shock. *Cochrane Database Syst Rev*. 2011;(5):CD003709. [PMID: 21563137]

Patel GP et al. Efficacy and safety of dopamine versus norepinephrine in the management of septic shock. *Shock*. 2010 Apr;33(4):375–380. [PMID: 19851126]

Patel GP et al. Systemic steroids in severe sepsis and septic shock. *Am J Respir Crit Care Med*. 2012 Jan 15;185(2):133–139. [PMID: 21680949]

Peake SL et al; ARISE Investigators; ANZICS Clinical Trials Group. Goal-directed resuscitation for patients with early septic shock. *N Engl J Med*. 2014 Oct 16;371(16):1496–1506. [PMID: 25272316]

Rivers E et al. Early goal-directed therapy in the treatment of severe sepsis and septic shock. *N Engl J Med*. 2001 Nov;345(19):1368–1377. [PMID: 11794169]

Russell JA et al; VASST Investigators. Vasopressin versus norepinephrine infusion in patients with septic shock. *N Engl J Med*. 2008 Feb 28;358(9):877–887. [PMID: 18305265]

Society of Critical Care Medicine. Surviving sepsis campaign. http://survivingsepsis.org

Yealy DM et al; ProCESS Investigators. A randomized trial of protocol-based care for early septic shock. *N Engl J Med*. 2014 May 1;370(18):1683–1693. [PMID: 24635773]

Index